Metal Ions in Life Sciences

Volume 25

Modern Avenues in Metal-Nucleic Acid Chemistry

Guest Editor
Jens Müller
Westfälische Wilhelms-Universität Münster
Institut für Anorganische und Analytische Chemie
Corrensstr. 28/30
D-48149 Münster
Germany
mueller.j@uni-muenster.de

Bernhard Lippert
Technische Universität Dortmund
Fakultät für Chemie und Chemische Biologie
Otto-Hahn-Str. 6
D-44227 Dortmund
Germany
bernhard.lippert@tu-dortmund.de

Series Editors
Astrid Sigel, Helmut Sigel
Department of Chemistry
Inorganic Chemistry
University of Basel
St. Johanns-Ring 19
CH-4056 Basel
Switzerland
astrid.sigel@unibas.ch,
helmut.sigel@unibas.ch

Eva Freisinger, Roland K. O. Sigel
Department of Chemistry
University of Zürich
Winterthurerstrasse 190
CH-8057 Zürich
Switzerland
freisinger@chem.uzh.ch,
roland.sigel@chem.uzh.ch

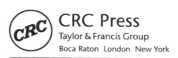

CRC Press is an imprint of the
Taylor & Francis Group, an **informa** business

Cover illustration: The figure represents two metal-assisted DNA-binding modes of peptides directly (top) or indirectly via a co-ligand at the metal species (bottom). Adapted from Chapter 7 by permission of Tim Kench and Ramon Vilar.

First edition published 2023
by CRC Press
6000 Broken Sound Parkway NW, Suite 300, Boca Raton, FL 33487-2742

and by CRC Press
4 Park Square, Milton Park, Abingdon, Oxon, OX14 4RN

CRC Press is an imprint of Taylor & Francis Group, LLC

© 2023 Jens Müller and Bernhard Lippert; individual chapters, the contributors

Reasonable efforts have been made to publish reliable data and information, but the author and publisher cannot assume responsibility for the validity of all materials or the consequences of their use. The authors and publishers have attempted to trace the copyright holders of all material reproduced in this publication and apologize to copyright holders if permission to publish in this form has not been obtained. If any copyright material has not been acknowledged please write and let us know so we may rectify in any future reprint.

Except as permitted under U.S. Copyright Law, no part of this book may be reprinted, reproduced, transmitted, or utilized in any form by any electronic, mechanical, or other means, now known or hereafter invented, including photocopying, microfilming, and recording, or in any information storage or retrieval system, without written permission from the publishers.

For permission to photocopy or use material electronically from this work, access www.copyright.com or contact the Copyright Clearance Center, Inc. (CCC), 222 Rosewood Drive, Danvers, MA 01923, 978-750-8400. For works that are not available on CCC please contact mpkbookspermissions@tandf.co.uk

Trademark notice: Product or corporate names may be trademarks or registered trademarks and are used only for identification and explanation without intent to infringe.

ISBN: 978-1-032-21817-5 (hbk)
ISBN: 978-1-032-21827-4 (pbk)
ISBN: 978-1-003-27020-1 (ebk)

ISSN 1559–0836   e-ISSN 1868-0402

DOI: 10.1201/9781003270201

Typeset in Times New Roman
by codeMantra

About the Editors

Jens Müller holds a Chair of Inorganic Chemistry (2018) at the Department of Chemistry and Pharmacy, Westfälische Wilhelms-Universität Münster, Germany. He obtained his doctoral degree (1999, *summa cum laude*) from the Technische Universität Dortmund, working with Bernhard Lippert. After a postdoctoral stay in the groups of Stephen J. Lippard (MIT) and Gerhard Wagner (Harvard Medical School), he started his independent career at the Technische Universität Dortmund in 2002, funded by the prestigious Emmy Noether Programme. After having received his *Habilitation* in 2008, he became Professor of Inorganic Chemistry at the Westfälische Wilhelms-Universität Münster. His research focuses on the bioinorganic chemistry of nucleic acids, with a particular interest in metal-mediated base pairing. He was Dean of Student Affairs from 2011 to 2014, Chair of the European research initiative COST Action CM1105 ("Functional metal complexes that bind to biomolecules"), and guest Editor of several themed issues of chemistry journals. Since 2018, he has served as Editor of *Inorganica Chimica Acta*. He is the Chair of EuroBIC-17 (2024 in Münster, Germany).

Bernhard Lippert retired in 2011 from Chair of Bioinorganic Chemistry at the Technische Universität Dortmund, Germany. He received his Ph.D. degree from Technische Universität München (TUM), Germany, in 1974. Following a postdoctoral stay with Barnett Rosenberg at the Biophysics Department of Michigan State University, USA, he started his independent research at TUM, which was focused on fundamental aspects of interactions of metal species, notably of Pt, with nucleobases, as well as supramolecular constructs derived from these components. During his career at TUM, the University of Freiburg, Germany, and TU Dortmund, he has trained 70 Ph.D. students and in addition numerous Bachelor and Master students as well as postdoctoral fellows, a fair number of whom eventually earned academic positions. Results of his group's work are documented in over 400 refereed scientific articles and have been communicated at many international conferences and lectureships. He served the community as an Editorial Board member of several journals (*Inorg. Chem.*, *Dalton Trans.*, *Inorg. Chim. Acta*, *J. Biol. Inorg. Chem.*, *Biometals*), and was the Editor of *Inorg. Chim. Acta* from 2008 to 2019. He was (Co)-Editor of a number of themed issues in chemistry journals, and the Editor of the book *Cisplatin: Chemistry and Biochemistry of a Leading Anticancer Drug*, which reviewed the knowledge on Pt antitumor complexes at the turn of the century. He has been involved in the management of European research activities in the COST frame, has been the Secretary of EuroBIC conferences for 11 years, and has organized numerous scientific meetings such as the "EURESCO Research conference on the *Inorganic Side of Molecular Architecture*" (2002), EuroBIC-7 (2004), and "*4th EuCheMS*

Conference on Nitrogen Ligands" (2008), among others. Since 2014, he has been an Honorary Member of the Society of Biological Inorganic Chemistry (SBIC).

Astrid Sigel has studied languages; she was an Editor of the *Metal Ions in Biological Systems* (MIBS) series (until Volume 44) and also of the *Handbook on Toxicity of Inorganic Compounds* (1988), the *Handbook on Metals in Clinical and Analytical Chemistry* (1994; both with H. G. Seiler and H.S.), and the *Handbook on Metalloproteins* (2001; with Ivano Bertini and H.S.). She is also an Editor of the *MILS* series from Volume 1 on, and she co-authored more than 50 papers on topics in Bioinorganic Chemistry.

Helmut Sigel is Emeritus Professor (2003) of Inorganic Chemistry at the University of Basel, Switzerland. He is a Co-editor of the series *Metal Ions in Biological Systems* (1973–2005; 44 volumes) as well as of the Sigels' new series *Metal Ions in Life Sciences* (since 2006). He also co-edited 3 handbooks and published over 350 articles on metal ion complexes of nucleotides, amino acids, coenzymes, and other bio-ligands. Together with Ivano Bertini, Harry B. Gray, and Bo G. Malmström, he founded (1983) the International Conferences on Biological Inorganic Chemistry (ICBIC). He lectured worldwide and was named 'Protagonist in Chemistry' (2002) by *Inorganica Chimica Acta* (issue 339). Among Endowed Lectureships, appointments as Visiting Professor (e.g., Austria, China, Japan, Kuwait, and UK), and further honors, he received the P. Ray Award (Indian Chemical Society, of which he is also an Honorary Fellow), the Alfred Werner Award (Swiss Chemical Society), and a Doctor of Science *honoris causa* degree (Kalyani University, India). He is also an Honorary Member of SBIC (Society of Biological Inorganic Chemistry).

Eva Freisinger is an Associate Professor of Bioinorganic Chemistry and Chemical Biology (2018) at the Department of Chemistry at the University of Zürich, Switzerland. She obtained her doctoral degree (2000) from the University of Dortmund, Germany, working with Bernhard Lippert and spent 3 years as a postdoc at SUNY Stony Brook, USA, with Caroline Kisker. Since 2003, she performs independent research at the University of Zürich where she held a Förderungsprofessur of the Swiss National Science Foundation from 2008 to 2014. In 2014, she received her *Habilitation* in Bioinorganic Chemistry. Her research is focused on the study of plant metallothioneins with an additional interest in the sequence-specific modification of nucleic acids. Together with Roland Sigel, she chaired the 12th European Biological Inorganic Chemistry Conference (2014 in Zürich, Switzerland) as well as the 19th International Conference on Biological Inorganic Chemistry (2019 in Interlaken, Switzerland). She also serves on a number of Advisory Boards for international conference series; since 2014, she is the Secretary of the European Biological Inorganic Chemistry Conferences (EuroBICs), and currently co-Director of the Department of Chemistry. She joined the group of Editors of the *MILS* series from Volume 18 on.

About the Editors

Roland K. O. Sigel is Full Professor (2016) of Chemistry at the University of Zürich, Switzerland. In the same year, he became Vice Dean of Studies (BSc/MSc), and in 2017, he was elected Dean of the Faculty of Science. From 2003 to 2008, he was endowed with a Förderungsprofessur of the Swiss National Science Foundation, and he is the recipient of an ERC Starting Grant 2010. He received his doctoral degree *summa cum laude* (1999) from the University of Dortmund, Germany, working with Bernhard Lippert. Thereafter, he spent nearly 3 years at Columbia University, New York, USA, with Anna Marie Pyle (now Yale University). During the 6 years abroad, he received several prestigious fellowships from various sources, and he was awarded the EuroBIC Medal in 2008 and the Alfred Werner Prize (SCS) in 2009. In 2015–2019, he was the Secretary of the Society of Biological Inorganic Chemistry (SBIC), and since 2018, he is the Secretary of the International Conferences on Biological Inorganic Chemistry (ICBIC). His research focuses on the structural and functional role of metal ions in ribozymes, especially group II introns, regulatory RNAs, and on related topics. He is also an Editor of Volumes 43 and 44 of the *MIBS* series and of the *MILS* series from Volume 1 on.

Historical Development and Perspectives of the Series *Metal Ions in Life Sciences**

It is an old wisdom that metals are indispensable for life. Indeed, several of them, like sodium, potassium, and calcium, are easily discovered in living matter. However, the role of metals and their impact on life remained largely hidden until inorganic chemistry and coordination chemistry experienced a pronounced revival in the 1950s. The experimental and theoretical tools created in this period and their application to biochemical problems led to the development of the field or discipline now known as Bioinorganic Chemistry, Inorganic Biochemistry, or more recently also often addressed as Biological Inorganic Chemistry.

By 1970, *Bioinorganic Chemistry* was established and further promoted by the book series *Metal Ions in Biological Systems* founded in 1973 (edited by H.S., who was soon joined by A.S.) and published by Marcel Dekker, Inc., New York, for more than 30 years. After this company ceased to be a family endeavor and its acquisition by another company, we decided, after having edited 44 volumes of the *MIBS* series (the last two together with R.K.O.S.), to launch a new and broader-minded series to cover today's needs in the *Life Sciences*. Therefore, the Sigels' new series is entitled

"Metal Ions in Life Sciences".

After publication of 22 volumes (since 2006), we are happy to join forces from Volume 23 on in this still-growing endeavor with Taylor & Francis, London, UK, a most experienced publisher in the *Sciences*.

The development of *Biological Inorganic Chemistry* during the past 40 years was and still is driven by several factors; among these are (1) attempts to reveal the interplay between metal ions and hormones or vitamins, etc., (2) efforts regarding the understanding of accumulation, transport, metabolism, and toxicity of metal ions, (3) the development and application of metal-based drugs, (4) biomimetic syntheses with the aim to understand biological processes as well as to create efficient catalysts, (5) the determination of high-resolution structures of proteins, nucleic acids, and other biomolecules, (6) the utilization of powerful spectroscopic tools allowing studies of structures and dynamics, and (7), more recently, the widespread use of macromolecular engineering to create new biologically relevant structures at will. All this and more is reflected in the volumes of the series *Metal Ions in Life Sciences*.

---

* Reproduced with some alterations by permission of John Wiley & Sons, Ltd., Chichester, UK (copyright 2006), from pages v and vi of Volume 1 of the series *Metal Ions in Life Sciences* (MILS-1)

The importance of metal ions to the vital functions of living organisms, hence, to their health and well-being, is nowadays well accepted. However, in spite of all the progress made, we are still only at the brink of understanding these processes. Therefore, the series *Metal Ions in Life Sciences* links coordination chemistry and biochemistry in their widest sense. Despite the evident expectation that a great deal of future outstanding discoveries will be made in the interdisciplinary areas of science, there are still "language" barriers between the historically separate spheres of chemistry, biology, medicine, and physics. Thus, it is one of the aims of this series to catalyze mutual "understanding". It is our hope that *Metal Ions in Life Sciences* continues to prove a stimulus for new activities in the fascinating "field" of *Biological Inorganic Chemistry*. If so, it will well serve its purpose and be a rewarding result for the efforts spent by the authors.

Astrid Sigel and Helmut Sigel
Department of Chemistry, Inorganic Chemistry
University of Basel, CH-4056 Basel, Switzerland

Eva Freisinger and Roland K. O. Sigel
Department of Chemistry
University of Zürich, CH-8057 Zürich, Switzerland

October 2005 and March 2023

Preface to Volume 25
Modern Avenues in Metal-Nucleic Acid Chemistry

Since the days when it became evident that nucleic acids are polyanions and consequently require cations for charge neutralization, interactions between metal ions and DNA, RNA, and their constituents have become a matter of general interest. The original focus on metal-nucleobase chemistry has clearly been on a deeper understanding of the resulting genuine biological functions (e.g. effects on replication processes, structural aspects, mutagenicity, toxicity, degradation, etc.). These scenarios were substantially extended with the discovery of metal-containing anticancer drugs such as Cisplatin, Carboplatin, and Oxaliplatin, their putative interaction with DNA, and their effects on replication. In fact, metal-containing drugs have become a landmark in medicinal chemistry and their successful clinical applications during the past five decades. Numerous monographs, relevant series issues (including in *Metal Ions in Biological Systems* (MIBS) and *Metal Ions in Life Sciences* (MILS)), as well as regular themed issues of chemistry journals have highlighted developments in this field in impressive ways, including progress made in relevant spectroscopic, analytical, computational, and molecular biological techniques.

During the past two to three decades, this field has received new facets, originating from supramolecular coordination chemistry, nanochemistry, and materials science. This volume of MILS aims at pointing out some of these developments in more detail, as well as providing selected aspects related to these.

The first four chapters of this book focus on materials science aspects of metal-nucleobase chemistry. Chapter 1 summarizes efforts to obtain porous materials based on metal ions and nucleobases. Due to the hydrogen-bonding ability of the nucleobases, these metal-organic frameworks are additionally sustained by hydrogen bonds. Chapter 2 showcases polynuclear and extended polymeric structures obtained by combining cytosine, additional auxiliary ligands, and metal ions. Crystal engineering and supramolecular architecture are a particular focus of this chapter. Chapters 3 and 4 highlight coordination polymers based on modified nucleobases and how these can be processed to yield colloids, gels, and aerogels with fascinating applications, with each chapter focusing on different aspects.

Chapters 5 and 6 cover more traditional metal-nucleobase chemistry, but present them from modern standpoints. The relevance of non-covalent interactions such as metallophilic, cation-π and anion-π interactions, and regium bonds are discussed in Chapter 5, whereas Chapter 6 presents a blend of different nucleobase metal complexes and how these interfere with biological processes.

The next three chapters center on the interaction of metal complexes and nucleic acids. Chapter 7 reports how such an interaction can be precisely controlled by endogenous stimuli such as pH changes or external stimuli such as light irradiation. Cationic platinum complexes and how they can be applied to induce higher-order structural changes to genomic DNA represent the focus of Chapter 8. Metal ions and complexes can also be useful in genotyping, as is described in Chapter 9, where the metal is reported to be used either as a contrast-enhancing agent or in the context of an alternate base-pairing pattern.

This theme leads over to the next three chapters, which deal with DNA acting as a template for metal complexes and nanoclusters. In Chapter 10, strategies for the formation of customized metal assemblies at the nanoscale are presented. Artificial metal-mediated base pairs and their application in metal-responsive functional DNA are discussed in detail in Chapter 11. The subsequent Chapter 12 is an authoritative tutorial review on DNA-templated silver nanoclusters as well as their formation, properties, and applications.

Guanine quadruplexes are the common theme of the following two chapters. While Chapter 13 presents an insight into the interaction of such quadruplexes with metal ions from a quantum chemical point of view, Chapter 14 summarizes recent progress in quadruplexes with artificial metal-mediated base tetrads. By introducing metal-based functionality to nucleic acids, such metal-DNA conjugates bear good prospects in DNA nanotechnology.

The final Chapter 15 focuses on a biologically relevant aspect and is the only one in this volume dedicated entirely to RNA. It presents for the first time a detailed overview of the role of metal ions in folding, ligand binding, and functionality of riboswitches.

Overall, this volume showcases the state of the art of metal-nucleobase chemistry beyond medicinal inorganic chemistry and shows that it remains a flourishing and vibrant field of research.

Jens Müller

Bernhard Lippert

Contents

About the Editors iii
Historical Development and Perspectives of the Series vii
Preface to Volume 25 ix
Contributors to Volume 25 xiii
Handbooks and Book Series Published and (Co-)edited by the SIGELs xvii

Chapter 1 Porous Materials Built Up from Metal-Nucleobase Materials 1

Garikoitz Beobide, Oscar Castillo, Antonio Luque, and Sonia Pérez-Yáñez

Chapter 2 Cytosine and Its Derivatives as Useful Tools to Build Unusual and Fascinating Architectures 25

Teresa F. Mastropietro and Giovanni De Munno

Chapter 3 Coordination Polymers with Nucleobase Derivatives: From Electronic Nanodevices to Sensors 51

Noelia Maldonado and Pilar Amo-Ochoa

Chapter 4 Heavy Coinage Metal Nucleobase, Nucleoside and (Oligo) Nucleotide Systems: Recent Developments in Self-Assembly, Opto-Electronics and DNA Integration 79

Andrew Houlton

Chapter 5 Interplay between Noncovalent Interactions and Metal Ions in Nucleic Acids and Their Constituents 105

Miquel Barceló-Oliver, Antonio Frontera, Juan Jesús Fiol, Ángel García-Raso, and Ángel Terrón

Chapter 6 Biological Implications of Metal-Nucleobase Complexes 133

Saurabh Joshi, Ankita Jaiswal, Rajneesh Kumar Prajapati, and Sandeep Verma

Chapter 7 Stimuli-Responsive DNA-Binding Metal Complexes 159

Tim Kench and Ramon Vilar

Chapter 8 How Do Cationic Pt(II) Complexes Modify the Higher-Order Structure of DNA? 189

Seiji Komeda, Masako Uemura, Yuko Yoshikawa, and Kenichi Yoshikawa

Chapter 9 Metals in Genotyping: From SNPs to Sequencing 211

Tuomas Lönnberg

Chapter 10 Nucleic Acids for the Preparation and Control of Continuous Hybrid Metallic Assemblies 229

Miguel A. Galindo, Fátima Linares, Alicia Domínguez-Martín, and Antonio Pérez-Romero

Chapter 11 Recent Advances in the Development of Metal-Responsive Functional DNAs Based on Metal-Mediated Artificial Base Pairing 257

Yusuke Takezawa and Mitsuhiko Shionoya

Chapter 12 Nucleic Acid-Templated Metal Nanoclusters 291

Rweetuparna Guha and Stacy M. Copp

Chapter 13 G-Quadruplex Nucleic Acids and the Role of Metal Ions: Insights from Quantum Chemical Bonding Analyses 343

Celine Nieuwland and Célia Fonseca Guerra

Chapter 14 Transition Metal-Binding G-Quadruplex DNA 373

Lukas M. Stratmann and Guido H. Clever

Chapter 15 Metabolite Regulation by Riboswitches: The Role of Metal Ions in Folding, Ligand Binding and Functionality 399

Maria Reichenbach, Sofia Gallo, and Roland K.O. Sigel

Index 435

Contributors to Volume 25

Pilar Amo-Ochoa
Department of Inorganic Chemistry
Autonomous University of Madrid
E-28049 Madrid, Spain, and Institute
for Advanced Research in Chemistry
at UAM (IAdChem)
Universidad Autónoma de Madrid
E-28049 Madrid, Spain

Miquel Barceló-Oliver
Department of Chemistry
University of the Balearic Islands
E-07122 Palma (Mallorca), Spain

Garikoitz Beobide
Departamento de Química Orgánica
e Inorgánica
Facultad de Ciencia y Tecnología
Universidad del País Vasco/Euskal
Herriko Unibertsitatea
E-48080 Bilbao, Spain
and
BCMaterials, Basque Center
for Materials, Applications, and
Nanostructures
E-48940 Leioa, Spain

Oscar Castillo
Departamento de Química Orgánica
e Inorgánica
Facultad de Ciencia y Tecnología
Universidad del País Vasco/Euskal
Herriko Unibertsitatea
E-48080 Bilbao, Spain
and
BCMaterials, Basque Center
for Materials, Applications, and
Nanostructures
E-48940 Leioa, Spain

Guido H. Clever
Faculty of Chemistry and Chemical
Biology
TU Dortmund University
D-44227 Dortmund, Germany

Stacy M. Copp
Department of Materials Science and
Engineering
University of California
Irvine, CA 92697-2585, USA
and Department of Physics and
Astronomy
University of California
Irvine, CA 92697-4575, USA
and
Department of Chemical and
Biomolecular Engineering
University of California
Irvine, CA 92697-4575, USA

Giovanni De Munno
Dipartimento di Chimica e Tecnologie
Chimiche
Università della Calabria
I-87036 Arcavacata di Rende
(Cosenza), Italy

Alicia Domínguez-Martín
Departamento Química Inorgánica
Universidad de Granada
E-18071 Granada, Spain

Juan Jesús Fiol
Department of Chemistry
University of the Balearic Islands
E-07122 Palma (Mallorca), Spain

Célia Fonseca Guerra
Department of Theoretical Chemistry
Amsterdam Institute of Molecular and
Life Sciences (AIMMS), Amsterdam
Center of Multiscale Modeling
(ACMM)
Vrije Universiteit Amsterdam
NL-1081 HV Amsterdam,
The Netherlands

Antonio Frontera
Department of Chemistry
University of the Balearic Islands
E-07122 Palma (Mallorca), Spain

Miguel A. Galindo
Departamento Química Inorgánica
Universidad de Granada
E-18071 Granada, Spain

Sofia Gallo
Department of Chemistry
University of Zurich
CH-8057 Zurich, Switzerland

Ángel García-Raso
Department of Chemistry
University of the Balearic Islands
E-07122 Palma (Mallorca), Spain

Rweetuparna Guha
Department of Materials Science and
Engineering
University of California
Irvine, CA 92697-2585, USA

Andrew Houlton
Chemistry, School of Natural and
Environmental Sciences
Newcastle University
Newcastle upon Tyne
NE3 1UB, United Kingdom

Ankita Jaiswal
Department of Chemistry
Indian Institute of Technology Kanpur
Kanpur 208016, U. P., India

Saurabh Joshi
Department of Chemistry
Indian Institute of Technology Kanpur
Kanpur 208016, U. P., India

Tim Kench
Department of Chemistry
Imperial College London
London, W12 0BZ, United Kingdom

Seiji Komeda
Faculty of Pharmaceutical Sciences
Suzuka University of Medical Science
Suzuka 513-8670, Japan

Fátima Linares
Centro de Instrumentación
Científica (CIC)
Universidad de Granada
E-18071 Granada, Spain

Tuomas Lönnberg
Department of Chemistry
University of Turku
FI-20500 Turku, Finland

Antonio Luque
Departamento de Química Orgánica
e Inorgánica
Facultad de Ciencia y Tecnología
Universidad del País Vasco/Euskal
Herriko Unibertsitatea
E-48080 Bilbao, Spain
and
BCMaterials, Basque Center
for Materials, Applications, and
Nanostructures
E-48940 Leioa, Spain

Contributors to Volume 25

Noelia Maldonado
Department of Inorganic Chemistry
Autonomous University of Madrid
E-28049 Madrid, Spain

Teresa F. Mastropietro
Dipartimento di Chimica e Tecnologie Chimiche
Università della Calabria
I-87036 Arcavacata di Rende (Cosenza), Italy

Celine Nieuwland
Department of Theoretical Chemistry
Amsterdam Institute of Molecular and Life Sciences (AIMMS), Amsterdam Center of Multiscale Modeling (ACMM)
Vrije Universiteit Amsterdam
NL-1081 HV Amsterdam,
The Netherlands

Antonio Pérez-Romero
Departamento Química Inorgánica
Universidad de Granada
E-18071 Granada, Spain

Sonia Pérez-Yáñez
Departamento de Química Orgánica e Inorgánica
Facultad de Ciencia y Tecnología
Universidad del País Vasco/Euskal Herriko Unibertsitatea
E-48080 Bilbao, Spain
and
BCMaterials, Basque Center for Materials, Applications and Nanostructures
E-48940 Leioa, Spain

Rajneesh Kumar Prajapati
Center for Nanoscience
Indian Institute of Technology Kanpur
Kanpur 208016, U. P., India

Maria Reichenbach
Department of Chemistry
University of Zurich
CH-8057 Zurich, Switzerland

Mitsuhiko Shionoya
Department of Chemistry
Graduate School of Science
The University of Tokyo
Tokyo 113-0033, Japan

Roland K.O. Sigel
Department of Chemistry
University of Zurich
CH-8057 Zurich, Switzerland

Lukas M. Stratmann
Faculty of Chemistry and Chemical Biology
TU Dortmund University
D-44227 Dortmund, Germany

Yusuke Takezawa
Department of Chemistry
Graduate School of Science
The University of Tokyo
Tokyo 113-0033, Japan

Ángel Terrón
Department of Chemistry
University of the Balearic Islands
E-07122 Palma (Mallorca), Spain

Masako Uemura
Faculty of Pharmaceutical Sciences
Suzuka University of Medical Science
Suzuka 513-8670, Japan

Sandeep Verma
Department of Chemistry, Center for Nanoscience, and Mehta Family Center for Engineering in Medicine
Indian Institute of Technology Kanpur
Kanpur 208016, U. P., India

Ramon Vilar
Department of Chemistry
Imperial College London
London W12 0BZ, United Kingdom

Kenichi Yoshikawa
Faculty of Life and Medical Sciences
Doshisha University
Kyotanabe 610-0321, Japan

Yuko Yoshikawa
Faculty of Life and Medical Sciences
Doshisha University
Kyotanabe 610-0321, Japan

Handbooks and Book Series Published and (Co-)edited by the SIGELs

"**Handbook on Toxicity of Inorganic Compounds**" (ISBN: 0-8247-7727-1) Eds H. G. Seiler, H. Sigel, A. Sigel; Dekker, Inc.; New York; 1988; 1069 pp

"**Handbook on Metals in Clinical and Analytical Chemistry**" (ISBN: 0-8247-9094-4) Eds Hans G. Seiler, Astrid Sigel, Helmut Sigel; Dekker, Inc.; New York, Basel, Hong Kong; 1994; 753 pp

"**Handbook on Metalloproteins**" (ISBN: 0-8247-0520-3) Eds I. Bertini, A. Sigel, H. Sigel; Marcel Dekker, Inc.; New York, Basel; 2001; 1182 pp

Metal Ions in Biological Systems
Volumes 1–44
https://www.routledge.com/Metal-Ions-in-Biological-Systems/book-series/IHCMEIOBISY
(see also the website given below)

Metal Ions in Life Sciences
Volumes 1–24
Details about all books (series) edited by the SIGELs, including the Guest Editors, can be found at http://www.bioinorganic-chemistry.org/mils

1 Porous Materials Built Up from Metal-Nucleobase Materials

Garikoitz Beobide, Oscar Castillo, Antonio Luque, and Sonia Pérez-Yáñez
Departamento de Química Orgánica e Inorgánica, Facultad de Ciencia y Tecnología, Universidad del País Vasco/Euskal Herriko Unibertsitatea, UPV/EHU, Apartado 644, E-48080 Bilbao, Spain
BCMaterials, Basque Center for Materials, Applications and Nanostructures, UPV/EHU Science Park, E-48940 Leioa, Spain
garikoitz.beobide@ehu.eus, oscar.castillo@ehu.eus, antonio.luque@ehu.eus, sonia.perez@ehu.eus

CONTENTS

1	Introduction	2
2	Metal-Nucleobase Coordination Bond Sustained MOFs	2
3	Metal-Nucleobase Base-Pairing Assembled SMOFs	10
4	Metal-Nucleobase π-Stacking Assembled SMOFs	15
5	Hybrid Metal-Nucleobase Porous Materials	21
6	General Conclusions	22
	Acknowledgments	22
	Abbreviations and Definitions	23
	References	23

Abstract

This chapter aims to provide an insight into the different approaches that can be applied to obtain porous materials based on metal-nucleobase systems. The rigidity and the multiple donor sites of the nucleobases make them suitable linkers to provide coordination bond sustained metal-organic frameworks (MOFs). Furthermore, the ability of the nucleobases to establish complementary hydrogen-bonding interactions allows for achieving similar metal-nucleobase porous materials but sustained by hydrogen bond pairing interactions between the nucleobases (supramolecular metal-organic frameworks, SMOFs). The latter approach can also be extended to the use of π-stacking interactions between the nucleobases as the driving force for a new family of SMOFs.

KEYWORDS

Metal-Organic Frameworks; Metal-Biomolecule Frameworks; Supramolecular Metal-Organic Frameworks; Porous Materials; Nucleobase; Crystal Engineering; Crystal Structure

1 INTRODUCTION

Nucleobases are one of the key biomolecules that provide unique structural features that have allowed the appearance and evolution of life on Earth [1]. Among these key features, we can easily agree that one of the most important ones is their capacity to establish specific supramolecular interactions through hydrogen-bonding or π-stacking interactions. Another feature not so evident for non-experts is their capacity to coordinate metal centers, although it has been well exploited by the antitumor drug cisplatin and other metallodrugs [2]. The characteristic of the nucleobases that opens the venue to all these very useful properties is the combination of high nitrogen content, rigidity, aromaticity, acid-base equilibria, and the presence of adjacent hydrogen bond donor and acceptor groups.

In this chapter, we will focus on how to obtain the maximum from these features of the nucleobases for the design of porous metal-organic materials [3]. Therefore, the aim is to provide an overview of opportunities that simple, cheap, ubiquitous, and versatile nucleobases offer to the emerging area of extended metal-organic porous materials. This contribution has been arbitrarily restricted to those examples in which the nucleobases play a key role in sustaining the three-dimensional (3D) framework as crucial linkers and not only as mere terminal ligands or tethered substituents. The manuscript is divided into more common coordination bond-based metal-organic frameworks (MOFs) and the emerging hydrogen bond and π-stacking sustained supramolecular metal-organic frameworks (SMOFs). Potential applications and properties that arise from the biological functionality of the nucleobases, such as sensing [4] and gene regulation [5], are beyond the scope of this work.

2 METAL-NUCLEOBASE COORDINATION BOND SUSTAINED MOFs

A subclass of MOFs (the most developed metal-organic porous material) [6] are those built up with biomolecules (MBioFs). They are becoming more and more popular over time as they enhance the biocompatibility of these materials, are relatively cheap and ubiquitous, and provide strong and selective interactions with the adsorbate molecules that penetrate these porous materials. However, it requires the nucleobase to be able to act as a bridging ligand connecting the metal centers and promoting the 3D expansion of the metal-organic structure. Not all the nucleobases share the same capacity to act as that. Although the keto and exocyclic amino groups could in principle be able to coordinate the metal centers, the more favorable positions are those of the endocyclic imine groups containing a lone electron pair (Figure 1).

Porous Materials Built up from Metal-Nucleobase Materials

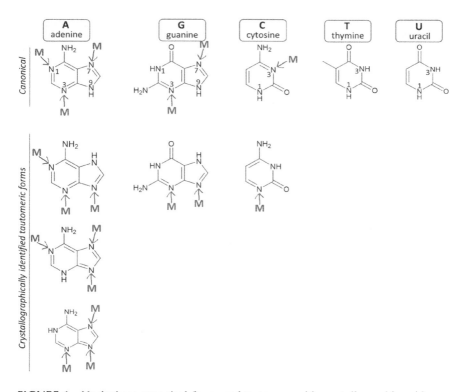

FIGURE 1 Nucleobase canonical forms and tautomers with crystallographic evidence. Metallation positions are highlighted, but it does not imply that all of them are employed simultaneously.

The purinic adenine and guanine nucleobases in their neutral form have three and two endocyclic nitrogen positions, respectively, fulfilling these conditions although their precise positions change depending on their tautomeric form [7]. In the case of the pyrimidinic cytosine, uracil, and thymine nucleobases, in their neutral form, only one nitrogen position of this kind is present for cytosine and none for uracil and thymine. Under these conditions in which the nucleobase molecules are employed in their neutral form, the chances to obtain the expected 3D spreading coordination network are null for the pyrimidinic nucleobases.

In the case of purinic nucleobases, they can behave as bridging ligands according to Figure 1, and this is true especially for adenine. However, adenine's more common coordination mode is through the N3 and N9 positions, which implies that the two coordinated metal centers are close (approximately 3 Å) and more prone to create polynuclear discrete entities than to facilitate a 3D polymerization. In principle, adenine can also behave as a μ_3-bridging ligand, but in its neutral form, it would imply to accumulate an excessively high positive charge in a reduced spatial volume. The latter is better understood if we have in mind that adenine is not an extended molecule, and as a consequence, the coordinated metal centers remain close to each other. This fact is verified when analyzing the Cambridge Structural Database (CSD) [8]. The results indicate that there is only one example of a μ_3-adenine that corresponds to a copper(II)-based MOF in which both adenine and adeninato are present [9]. The formula of this compound, [Cu$_4$(benzene-1,3,5-tricarboxylato)$_2$(adeninato)(adenine)(OH)(H$_2$O)$_3$]· 0.4[Cu(adeninato)$_2$(H$_2$O)$_4$], evidences the complexity of the crystal structure and the fact that the auxiliary bridging ligand benzene-1,3,5-tricarboxylato was needed in addition to adeninato to help achieving the required 3D polymerization. Interestingly, the pores of this compound are partially occupied by mononuclear complexes with the formula of [Cu(adeninato)$_2$(H$_2$O)$_4$]. This feature has been described by the authors as a ship-in-a-bottle structure.

In the case of guanine, a more mundane problem arises, namely the great insolubility it presents in its neutral form. In fact, only two examples of metal-bridging neutral guanine have been found, but the polymerization capacities of guanine without the presence of an auxiliary bridging ligand only provide a one-dimensional (1D) coordination polymer [10]. The crystal structures of these two compounds show the guanine in its canonical form coordinating the metal centers through its N3 and N7 positions to generate cationic [Cu(Hgua)(H$_2$O)$_3$]$_n^{2n+}$ polymeric chains counterbalanced by structurally innocent BF$_4^-$, SiF$_6^{2-}$, and CF$_3$SO$_3^-$ anions.

To overcome the poor bridging capacity of the neutral nucleobases, most researchers have shifted to the use of deprotonated nucleobases which offer a larger number of coordination positions and a negative charge that helps increasing the number of metal centers that can accumulate around the nucleobase (Figure 2) [11, 12].

This new approach was successful especially with purinic nucleobases that offer up to four coordination positions. In fact, the first porous MBioF based on a nucleobase was reported by our research group in 2004 using the deprotonated adenine nucleobase [13]. It consists of a 3D coordination polymer with formula [Cu$_4$(μ_3-adeninato-$\kappa N3$:$\kappa N7$:$\kappa N9$)$_4$(ox)$_2$(H$_2$O)$_4$]$_n$ (ox: oxalate), containing the adenine nucleobase as an anionic N3,N7,N9-bridging ligand. The deprotonation of adenine in the reaction medium promotes the polymerization of the framework by sequentially bridging [Cu$_2$(μ-adeninato)$_4$(H$_2$O)$_2$] paddle-wheel entities through [Cu(ox)(H$_2$O)] units (Figure 3a). The resulting structure, with **nbo** topology, contains 1D tubular channels with a diameter of about 13 Å that represent around a 40% of the total volume.

In 2009, Rosi et al. reported a porous network of formula (Me$_2$NH$_2$)$_2$[Zn$_8$(μ_4-adeninato-$\kappa N1$:$\kappa N3$:$\kappa N7$:$\kappa N9$)$_4$(μ-BPDC-κO:$\kappa O'$)$_4$(μ-BPDC-$\kappa^2 O,O'$:$\kappa^2 O'',O'''$)$_2$ (μ_4-O)] (BPDC: biphenyldicarboxylate; bio-MOF-1) obtained under solvothermal conditions at 130 °C [14]. It consists of infinite zinc-adeninato columnar secondary building units (SBUs) composed of apex-sharing zinc-adeninato octahedral cages with a **pcu** topology (Figure 3b). The zinc-adeninato columns are interconnected via multiple BPDC linkers, giving rise to an anionic network that allows the exchange of the cationic counterions. The authors proved that this compound presents permanent porosity with a BET surface area of 1,700 m^{2}g^{-1}, and additionally,

Porous Materials Built up from Metal-Nucleobase Materials

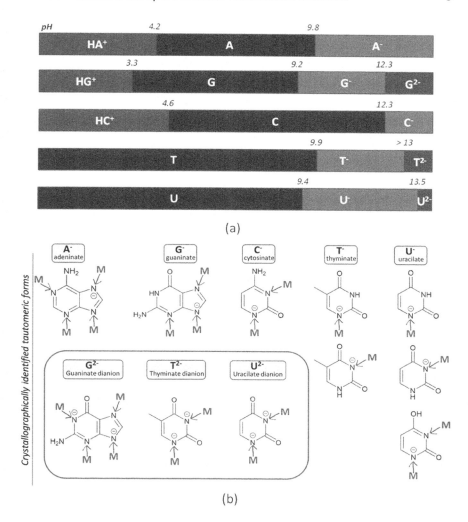

FIGURE 2 (a) pK_a values of the nucleobases. (b) Crystallographically identified tautomers of the nucleobase anions and dianions. Metallation positions are highlighted but do not imply all of them are employed simultaneously.

it is able to store and release cationic drug molecules. Later, in 2012, they published (Me$_2$NH$_2$)$_4$[Zn$_8$(μ$_4$-adeninato-κ$N1$:κ$N3$:κ$N7$:κ$N9$)$_4$(μ-BPDC-κO:κO')$_6$ (μ-O)] (bio-MOF-100) with the same building blocks, but obtained at a lower solvothermal reaction temperature of 85 °C to afford an augmented **lcs** net (Figure 3c). The same components are arranged in such a way that they build up a mesoporous material with a high surface area (4,300 m^{2}g^{-1}) and one of the largest, reported to date, pore volumes (4.3 cm^{3}g^{-1}) for MOFs [15].

Interestingly, although the use of methylated nucleobases usually lowers their chances to develop porous metal-organic materials based on them, it

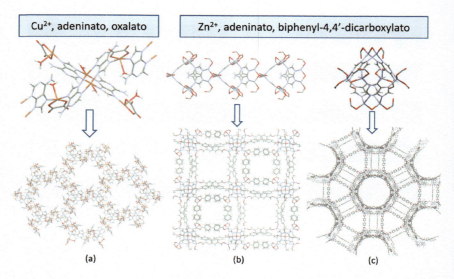

FIGURE 3 SBUs and the resulting crystal structures of (a) {[Cu$_2$(μ-adeninato)$_4$(H$_2$O)$_2$][Cu(ox)(H$_2$O)]$_2$}$_n$ [13], (b) (Me$_2$NH$_2$)$_2$[Zn$_8$(μ$_4$-adeninato)$_4$(μ-BPDC)$_6$(μ$_4$-O)]·8DMF·11H$_2$O [14] and (c) (Me$_2$NH$_2$)$_4$[Zn$_8$(μ$_4$-adeninato)$_4$(μ-BPDC)$_6$(μ-O)]·49DMF·31H$_2$O [15]. Solvent molecules not shown.

was not the case for (Me$_2$NH$_2$)$_2$[Zn$_6$(μ$_3$-N6-butyladeninato-κ*N3*:κ*N7*:κ*N9*)$_4$(μ-BPDC-κ*O*:κ*O′*)$_4$(μ-O)] [16]. In this case, the presence of 1D SBUs comprising [Zn$_8$(adeninato)$_4$(OOC)$_{12}$O] subunits held together by tetracoordinated oxide anions located at opposite vertices implies that the connectivity of this compound is far greater than required to sustain a 3D architecture. Therefore, it is possible to omit some of the metal centers and carboxylato ligands by using an N6-butyladeninato ligand that avoids the coordination through its N1 position. This lower coordination capacity leads to a [Zn$_6$(N6-butyladeninato)$_4$(OOC)$_8$O] subunit for the 1D SBU that still is able to provide a 3D porous architecture closely related to that of the non-methylated adeninato-containing bio-MOF-1 (Figure 4).

In addition to that, the resulting compound (Me$_2$NH$_2$)$_2$[Zn$_6$(μ$_3$-N6-butyladeninato-κ*N3*:κ*N7*:κ*N9*)$_4$(μ-BPDC-κ*O*:κ*O′*)$_4$(μ-O)] seems to be able to release dimethylamine through thermal activation under vacuum at 110 °C with the transfer of a proton from dimethylammonium to the N1 position of two butyladeninato ligands to afford [Zn$_6$(μ$_3$-N6-butyladeninato-κ*N3*:κ*N7*:κ*N9*)$_2$(μ$_3$-N6-butyladenine-κ*N3*:κ*N7*:κ*N9*)$_2$(μ-BPDC-κ*O*:κ*O′*)$_4$(μ-O)] that shows permanent porosity and a Brunauer–Emmett–Teller (BET) surface area of 1,048 m^{2}g^{-1}. This behavior shows us another feature of the nucleobases, which accounts for the fact that when the nucleobases are not employing to the maximum of their coordination capabilities, these uncoordinated positions still play a role in the resulting MBioFs by providing them with additional stability toward pH changes. In other words, the nucleobases are able to accept protons without altering the fundamental structural features of the MBioFs in which they are incorporated.

Porous Materials Built up from Metal-Nucleobase Materials

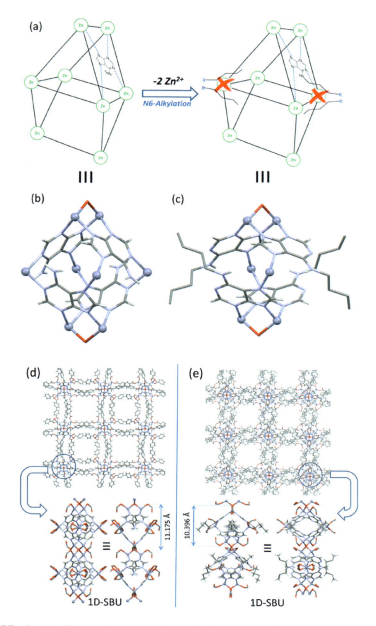

FIGURE 4 (a) Schematic description of the structural changes taking place upon N6-alkylation of the adeninato ligand. Comparative depiction of the [Zn$_8$(adeninato)$_4$(OOC)$_{12}$O] (b) and the [Zn$_6$(N6-alkyladeninato)$_4$(OOC)$_8$O] (c) subunits. Details of the 1D-SBU and coordination framework of (Me$_2$NH$_2$)$_2$[Zn$_8$(μ$_4$-adeninato-κN1:κN3:κN7:κN9)$_4$(μ-BPDC-κO:κO′)$_6$(μ-O)] (bio-MOF-1) (d) and (Me$_2$NH$_2$)$_2$[Zn$_6$(μ$_3$-N6-butyladeninato-κN3:κN7:κN9)$_4$(μ-BPDC-κO:κO′)$_4$(μ-O)] (e). (Reproduced from Ref. [16]; copyright 2020 Royal Society of Chemistry.)

Another family of metal-adenine-carboxylato compounds that has attracted great interest is that of formula [M$_2$(μ$_3$-adeninato-κ*N3*:κ*N7*:κ*N9*)$_2$(μ-OOC(CH$_2$)$_x$ CH$_3$-κ*O*:κ*O'*)$_2$]$_n$ [17–19]. Their crystal structure consists of paddle-wheel-shaped centrosymmetric dimeric units in which two metal(II) ions are bridged by two adeninato ligands coordinated by their N3 and N9 nitrogen atoms and by two carboxylic ligands with a μ-*O,O'* coordination mode. These units are cross-linked through the apical coordination of the imidazole N7 atom of the adeninato ligands in such a way that each paddle-wheel-shaped unit is linked to four adjacent entities (Figure 5). This self-assembling process generates a four-connected uninodal net (**lvt** topology) that exhibits a 3D system of intersecting cavities. The accessible effective volume is directly related to the length of the aliphatic chain, which is pointing toward the inner portion of the channels with free volume that ranges from *ca.* 40% for the acetate analogs and negligible values for pentanoate and longer carboxylates. It is worth mentioning that the synthetic conditions play a relevant role in obtaining the different members of this last family of compounds. In fact, cobalt(II) species are obtained under solvothermal conditions [17], the copper(II) ones using aqueous synthesis under ambient conditions [18], and the nickel(II) and zinc(II) ones employing a less common solvent-free approach under conventional oven or microwave-assisted heating [19]. The presence of highly polar amino groups of the adenine residues in the pore walls provides these compounds with a great adsorption selectivity toward CO_2, especially those with narrower pores [20–22]. Related to this great adsorption selectivity and taking advantage of the retention of the crystal structure even when the carboxylic ligand is changed, core-shell frameworks comprising a porous mixed core (acetato/pentanoato) and a less porous shell (pentanoato) were performed. Thus, the resulting material exhibited 30% higher CO_2 uptake than the pentanoato analog and low N_2 uptake in comparison to the core [23].

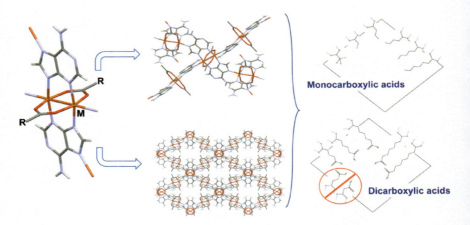

FIGURE 5 Porous crystal structure of [M(μ$_3$-adeninato)(μ-carboxylato)]$_n$ compounds (M being Co^{2+}, Ni^{2+}, Cu^{2+} or Zn^{2+}).

Moreover, this last crystal structure seems to be so robust that it is obtained even when using long-chain aliphatic dicarboxylic acids such as HOOC(CH$_2$)$_n$COOH [n from 3 to 5] [24]. Surprisingly, only one of the two carboxylic groups is deprotonated and coordinated to the metal centers, μ-κ*O1*:κ*O2*, while the other remains protonated inside the channels of the crystal structure in such a way that the dicarboxylic ligands do not join the dimeric fragments as they could, which initially could have been expected. Only when very short-chain dicarboxylic acids are employed (oxalate, malonate, and succinate), a different crystal structure is obtained. In this last case, the great tendency of these acids to chelate metal ions hinders the formation of paddle-wheel-shaped SBUs, providing crystal structures based on discrete complex entities [25].

There are other examples of MOFs sustained by collaborative nucleobase/non-nucleobase bridging ligands, such as the anionic [Cd$_4$(μ-Cl)(μ$_4$-adeninato-κ*N1*:κ*N3*:κ*N7*:κ*N9*)$_2$Cl$_6$]$_n^{n-}$ network, which is counterbalanced by the presence of H$^+$/H$_3$O$^+$ cations in the channels [26]. The small opening of the 1D channels (diameter: ~4 Å) present in this compound precludes the adsorption of N$_2$ but not the adsorption of CO$_2$ (10.5 cm^{3}g^{-1} at 273 K) in a clear example of size-dependent adsorption selectivity.

In 2016, Zhang et al. reported two isostructural and anionic porous MOFs with an **sqc** topology by introducing isophthalato or 2,5-thiophenedicarboxylato ligands to assemble with adenine and cadmium salt [27]. In this case, paddle-wheel-shaped [Cd$_2$(μ-adeninato-κ*N3*:κ*N9*)$_4$Br$_2$] units are attached to monomeric cadmium subunits through their N1 and N7 positions to create a 1D-SBU of formula [Cd$_6$(μ$_4$-adeninato-κ*N1*:κ*N3*:κ*N7*:κ*N9*)$_4$Br$_2$]. These cadmium-adeninato rods are further connected by the rigid dicarboxylato ligands that are coordinated to the cadmium monomeric subunits of the 1D-SBU. Interestingly, the compound containing the isophthalato ligand shows permanent porosity with a Langmuir surface area of 770.1 m^{2}g^{-1} and exhibits high separation capacity on C$_2$/C$_1$ hydrocarbons.

Furthermore, the use of pyridine-4-carboxylato ligands together with deprotonated adenine gave rise as well to zeolitic-type MOFs. In fact, two compounds, showing the same **dmp** topology, were obtained with isonicotinate, [Zn(μ-adeninato-κ*N7*:κ*N9*)(μ-isonicotinato-κ*N*:κ*O*)]$_n$ [28, 29], and 2-aminoisonicotinate, [Zn(μ-adeninato-κ*N7*:κ*N9*)(μ-2-aminoisonicotinato-κ*N*:κ*O*)]$_n$ [30]. The functionalization of the isonicotinato ligand with an amino group resulted in a significant enhancement of the adsorption selectivity toward CO$_2$.

Despite the great success of the strategy to develop porous MBioFs based on the deprotonation of adenine, the success is not further extended to the other purinic nucleobase, and as far as we know, not a single example can be provided for deprotonated guanine. In our opinion, this is only due to synthetic difficulties arising from the great insolubility of neutral guanine. In the case of the deprotonated cytosine, thymine, and uracil nucleobases, most of their compounds are devoted to the formation of metal-organic polyhedra (squares, hexagons, and tetrahedra) with second/third-row transition metal centers such as platinum or rhodium [31–34].

3 METAL-NUCLEOBASE BASE-PAIRING ASSEMBLED SMOFs

These new materials replace the coordination bonds, as builders of the final crystal architecture, with hydrogen bonds, which are also directional and predictable interactions (Figure 6). Although such kinds of alternative materials can arise an alike fascination to that of MOFs, the crystal engineering principles and the synthetic approach are not yet settled, and examples of this kind of materials are rather scarce. In 2015, we reported a successful synthetic approach to achieve this goal based on the following key factors [35]:

i. The use of rigid building units,
ii. The establishment of predictable and rigid synthons between the building units,
iii. The non-coplanarity of functional groups involved in the predictable synthons.

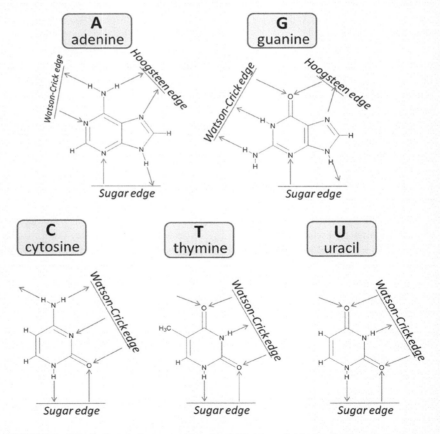

FIGURE 6 Nucleobase edges capable of establishing rigid complementary hydrogen-bonding synthons.

The rigidity of the building units (discrete complexes) can be achieved using rigid ligands bonded through multiple positions. This means, in most common cases, a double anchoring of the ligand by means of two simultaneous coordination bonds or the combination of a coordination bond and an intramolecular hydrogen bond. The predictability and rigidity of the synthons require the presence of adjacent functional groups, incorporated into the rigid ligands, able to establish complementary hydrogen-bonding interactions. Finally, the requisite of a non-coplanar arrangement of the synthons comes from our objective of obtaining 3D extended systems that is achieved by the presence of at least three non-coplanar synthons. The use of complexes with non-planar coordination geometry makes this last condition easy to be accomplished.

Focusing now on the opportunities arising from the five natural nucleobases, the first thing that can be envisaged is that the purinic adenine and guanine offer three sides—Watson-Crick, Hoogsteen, and sugar—to establish rigid complementary hydrogen bonds (the rigid synthons appearing in the second requirement). There are only two edges—Watson-Crick and sugar—for the pyrimidinic nucleobases. On the other hand, in order to get rigid discrete entities as building units, the nucleobases should establish at least two coordination bonds. Purinic nucleobases can accomplish this requirement and still have available edges for complementary hydrogen-bonding interactions. Pyrimidinic ones need to employ both edges for coordination, unless an enolato tautomer allows establishing a chelate with a single metal center and leaves one side available for complementary hydrogen bonding, but this is not common. Finally, the third requirement (at least three non-coplanar synthons) is easier to achieve for the purinic nucleobases, as their three edges depicted in Figure 6 have the capacity of behaving as a rigid synthon, whereas the pyrimidinic ones only present two edges of this kind. The consequence is that most examples that we are going to describe here are devoted to the purinic adenine nucleobase. In principle, examples with guanine should also be relatively common, but the previously mentioned synthetic problems related to its great insolubility in water and most other solvents prevent it from happening.

[Zn$_6$(μ-adeninato-κ$N7$:κ$N9$)$_6$(pyridine)$_6$(dimethylcarbamate)$_6$]·10.5DMF is representative of these compounds since it consists of hexameric Zn-adeninate macrocycles that are connected through the Watson-Crick faces of the nucleobases, giving rise to a 3D supramolecular framework in which the macrocyclic cavities are ordered into 1D channels (Figure 7a) [36]. The entrance to each cavity is occluded by pyridine rings. Therefore, the activation of this compound was achieved under conditions in which a fraction of the coordinated pyridine molecules was removed to widen the cavity aperture. In this way, this compound was able to take up N$_2$ (77 K and 1 bar: ~90 cm^3 g^{-1}), H$_2$ (77 K and 1 bar: ~1 wt%), and CO$_2$ (273 K and 1 bar: ~3.5 mmol g^{-1}).

Apart from the previous compound, the first examples that allowed us to settle the synthetic approach to render SMOFs are based on [Cu$_2$(μ-adenine)$_4$(X)$_2$]$^{2+}$ (X = Cl$^-$, Br$^-$) supramolecular building blocks in which two or more nucleobases are tightly anchored to the metal centers by two donor positions (N3 and

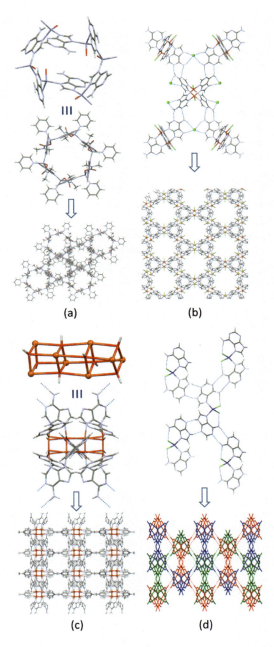

FIGURE 7 Discrete entity and porous supramolecular architecture of (a) [Zn$_6$(μ-adeninato-κ$N7$:κ$N9$)$_6$(pyridine)$_6$(dimethylcarbamate)$_6$] [36], (b) [Cu$_2$(μ-adenine)$_4$Cl$_2$]Cl$_2$ [37], (c) [Cu$_8$(μ$_4$-OH)$_4$(μ$_3$-OH)$_4$(adeninato-κ$N9$)$_4$(μ-adeninato-κ$N3$:κ$N9$)$_4$(μ-adenine-κ$N3$:κ$N9$)$_2$] [35] and (d) [Co(adenine-κ$N7$)$_2$Cl$_2$] [35] (each subnet of this triply interpenetrated crystal structure is represented using a different color).

N9 sites), imposing a rigid building unit [37, 38]. Moreover, this coordination motif imposes a rigid geometrical restraint among the nucleobases providing a set of non-coplanar synthons. As many hydrogen donor/acceptor positions of the nucleobase remain free, these discrete entities are able to self-assemble among them by means of double hydrogen bonds to provide extended supramolecular solids with **reo** topology, in which great channels are present (Figure 7b). These compounds present a surface instability that creates a diffusion barrier permeated only by strongly interacting adsorbate molecules such as CO_2, but not N_2, H_2, and CH_4, which makes them attractive for selective gas adsorption and separation technologies. Zaworotko et al. reported an analogous compound, based on the $[Cu_2(\mu\text{-adenine-}\kappa N3{:}\kappa N9)_4(X)_2]^{2+}$ dinuclear entity, replacing the halides by bulkier TiF_6^{2-} anions that improve the chemical stability of the supramolecular network toward humidity, thus avoiding the surface instability, and therefore, being able to adsorb CO_2, CH_4, and N_2 [39]. These studies also pointed out the relevance of solvent selection, because strong hydrogen bond donor and acceptor solvent molecules such as water could disrupt the direct hydrogen-bonding interactions between the nucleobases, which is one of the key factors to achieve this type of compounds.

There exists an example in which $[Cu_8(\mu_4\text{-OH})_4(\mu_3\text{-OH})_4(\text{adeninato-}\kappa N9)_4(\mu\text{-adeninato-}\kappa N3{:}\kappa N9)_4(\mu\text{-adenine-}\kappa N3{:}\kappa N9)_2]$ octameric clusters are formed by the stacking of four $Cu_2(\mu\text{-OH})_2$ dimers that are rotated by 90° and linked by a semi-coordination to the neighboring Cu(II) ions through hydroxido bridges (Figure 7c) [35]. The resulting aggregate can be described as the stacking of three cubanes (cubes with the vertices alternatively occupied by the metal and the bridging hydroxido ligand). The surface of each octamer is occupied by eight adeninato (four μ-κN3:κN9 bridging ligands and four terminal ones) and two neutral adenine ligands (μ-κN3:κN9). All the adenines, adeninato, and hydroxido ligands are rigidly anchored to the octameric entity because of their multiple coordination bonds (OH/adenine/adeninato) or the combination of a coordination bond and an intramolecular hydrogen bond (terminal adeninato). The interaction of each octamer with the adjacent ones takes place through complementary hydrogen-bonding interactions between the adenine and adeninato ligands to give rise to a 3D supramolecular net with **sqc3** topology with large mono-dimensional channels of *ca.* 4.9 Å diameter that occupy 30% of the unit cell volume.

The final example corresponds to a supramolecular structure containing neutral monomeric $[Co(\text{adenine-}\kappa N7)_2Cl_2]$ units. 9*H*-Adenine acts as a monodentate ligand, and it is coordinated to the Co(II) metal center through the N7 position, but it requires a second anchoring position of the nucleobase to be stiff enough to generate a supramolecular porous structure [35]. Such stiffness is achieved by the presence of intramolecular hydrogen-bonding interactions between the amino hydrogen atom and the chlorido ligand. The adenine also exposes its Watson-Crick and sugar edges to establish intermolecular complementary hydrogen-bonding interactions with adjacent adenine molecules (Figure 7d). These interactions build up a four-connected uninodal 3D supramolecular net with **dia** topology that would represent a new porous material with 67% of void space. Nevertheless, the real crystal structure involves three interpenetrated networks that occupy all the available space, thereby providing a non-porous material. This entanglement problem is also common in MOFs [35]. Moreover, it is worth mentioning that diamondoid nets tend to exhibit interpenetration, so gas adsorption studies with this kind of compounds are scarce. Although this problem can be surpassed in some coordination bond-based interpenetrated MOFs [40–42], it still remains a challenge for SMOFs.

These are successful results in which we achieved the predicted output by using discrete metal-nucleobase entities that fulfill the above-described three conditions, but the validity of these conditions should be checked by analyzing not only the successful cases but also the unsuccessful ones and including non-DNA nucleobases (Table 1) [43].

TABLE 1
Compliance of the Requirements of Each Metal-Nucleobase Entity to Obtain SMOFs

Entity	Rigid Entity?	Rigid Synthons?	Non-coplanar Synthons (≥ 3)?	Porous Structure?	Ref.
[Cu$_2$(μ-adenine-κ$N3$:κ$N9$)$_4$(X)$_2$]$^{2+}$ in MeOH	Yes	Yes	Yes	Yes	[37]
[Cu$_2$(μ-adenine-κ$N3$:κ$N9$)$_4$(X)$_2$]$^{2+}$ in H$_2$O	Yes	No	No	No	[44]
[Co$_3$(μ-adenine-κ$N3$:κ$N9$)$_2$ (μ-Cl)$_2$C$_{12}$(H$_2$O)$_4$]	Yes	No	No	No	[43]
[Cu$_2$(μ-Cl)$_2$Cl$_2$(guanine-κ$N9$)$_2$(guaninium-κ$N9$)$_2$(H$_2$O)$_2$]$^{2+}$	Yes	Yes	No	No	[43]
[Co(9-methyladenine-κ$N7$)$_2$(H$_2$O)$_4$]$^{2+}$	Yes	Yes	No	No	[43]
[Cu$_2$(μ-acetato-κO:κO')$_2$ (μ-9-methyladenine-κ$N1$:κ$N7$)]$_n$	Yes	No	No	No	[43]
[Co(6-chloropurinato-κ$N9$)$_2$(H$_2$O)$_4$]	Yes	No	No	No	[43]
[Co(thioguaninato-κ$S6$,κ$N7$)$_3$]	Yes	Yes	Yes	Yes	[35]
[Co(adenine-κ$N7$)$_2$Cl$_2$]	Yes	Yes	Yes	Yes (interpenetrated)	[35]
[Cu$_4$(μ$_3$-adeninato-κ$N3$:κ$N7$:κ$N9$)$_2$ (μ-adenine-κ$N3$:κ$N9$)$_2$(n-pentylNH$_2$)$_2$ (CH$_3$OH)$_2$(CO$_3$)$_2$(H$_2$O)$_2$]	Yes	Yes	Yes	Yes	[35]
[Cu$_8$(μ$_4$-OH)$_4$(μ$_3$-OH)$_4$(adeninato-κ$N9$)$_4$(μ-adeninato-κ$N3$:κ$N9$)$_4$ (μ-adenine-κ$N3$:κ$N9$)$_2$]	Yes	Yes	Yes	Yes	[35]

Source: Taken with permission from Ref. [43].

4 METAL-NUCLEOBASE π-STACKING ASSEMBLED SMOFs

As we have seen, nucleobases are key structure-directing agents to build up ordered porous structures known as SMOFs. However, the supramolecular recognition capability of the nucleobases does not rely exclusively on hydrogen-bonding interactions but also on their ability to establish π-stacking interactions. These latter interactions are less directional than hydrogen bonds but can play a crucial role in the resulting supramolecular architecture. In fact, calculations on the stability of the DNA indicate that these π-stacking interactions are crucial for providing stability to the double helix [45].

In our studies of the copper(II)-adenine system, we realized the resulting entities were very dependent on the pH of the reaction medium (Figure 8). In fact, it is possible to obtain the previously described paddle-wheel-shaped dinuclear entities both cationic ([Cu$_2$(μ-adenine-κ$N3$:κ$N9$)$_4$(H$_2$O)$_2$]$^{4+}$) and neutral ([Cu$_2$(μ-adeninato-κ$N3$:κ$N9$)$_4$(H$_2$O)$_2$]), a neutral octameric entity ([Cu$_8$(μ$_4$-OH)$_4$(μ$_3$-OH)$_4$(adeninato-κ$N9$)$_4$(μ-adeninato-κ$N3$:κ$N9$)$_4$(μ-adenine-κ$N3$:κ$N9$)$_2$]) and a cationic wheel-shaped heptameric entity ([Cu$_7$(μ-adeninato-κ$N3$:κ$N9$)$_6$(μ$_3$-OH)$_6$(μ-H$_2$O)$_6$]$^{2+}$). The latter is particularly interesting because it crystallizes from aqueous solution to provide a porous SMOF without complementary hydrogen-bonding interactions between the nucleobases, but rather containing π-stacking interactions. Apparently, the Watson-Crick and Hoogsteen edges of the adeninato ligand prefer to establish hydrogen-bonding interactions with water molecules instead of between each other. This fact has been observed also for [Cu$_2$(μ-adenine-κ$N3$:κ$N9$)$_4$Cl$_2$]Cl$_2$ which, depending on the reaction medium, provides a porous supramolecular architecture (when using an alcoholic medium) or an unappealing non-porous structure (when the synthesis is performed in aqueous medium). In the latter, the nucleobase prefers to establish hydrogen bonds with water molecules that do not lead to a rigid synthon [44]. Something similar happens to the heptameric entity with respect to the hydrogen bonds, but in this case, the adeninato ligands arrange themselves to establish π-stacking. Somehow, the supramolecular stabilization of the system is greater when establishing hydrogen bonds with the water molecules and π-staking

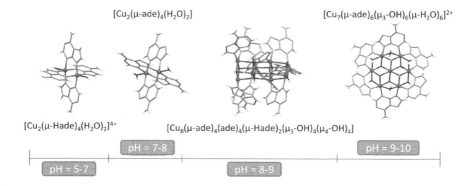

FIGURE 8 pH-driven structural variability in the copper(II)-adenine system.

interactions among them, than establishing only hydrogen-bonding interactions among the nucleobases without π-stacking interactions.

Initially, the heptameric entity was crystallized using sulfate counterions, and the porosity of the resulting supramolecular architecture is reduced because these counterions and in addition co-crystallized $(NHEt_3)_2(SO_4)$ are located inside the channels of the compound (Figure 9a) [46].

In order to avoid this drawback, it was decided to incorporate the counterions within the π-stacking supramolecular architecture instead of locating them inside the pores and channels of the structure. For that purpose, the sulfate counterion was replaced by the planar organic anion theobrominate to afford $[Cu_7(\mu-H_2O)_6(\mu_3-OH)_6(\mu-adeninato-\kappa N3:\kappa N9)_6]$(theobrominate)$_2$ [47]. As expected, the organic counterion was placed between the adeninato ligands, thus extending the previously single π-stacking interaction into a more complex adeninato···theobrominate···theobrominate···adeninato one (Figure 9b). In addition to that, the crystal structure of these compounds is flexible upon the removal of the solvent molecules. This feature has been attributed to the less directional nature of π-stacking interactions because, although the two interacting planar entities must be parallel or almost parallel, usually they are not so well defined with respect to the rotation around this interaction. Therefore, to get a truly rigid synthon, two π-stacking interactions are required between the two interacting discrete entities, as happens for synthon A in Figure 9b. Interestingly, the structural rearrangement that takes place during the solvent removal is completely reversible if the sample is placed in a humidity-saturated atmosphere.

As has become evident, the cationic nature of these heptameric discrete entities provides a rich source for novel compounds by simply replacing the counterion. In the next example, mono- and dicarboxylate counterions were selected, namely benzoate and benzene-1,4-dicarboxylate (terephthalate). π-stacking and hydrogen-bonding interactions can be understood in a simplified ways as the attraction between partial charges of opposite sign. In this sense, it is possible to predict the resulting supramolecular architecture based on the effect of the counterion charge density distribution. In this case, the cationic nature of the discrete heptameric entity imposes a net positive density on the coordinated adeninato ligands (in spite of their formal anionic nature). This fact favors their interaction with the negative charge density of the organic anion, mainly located on the carboxylate groups. Therefore, depending on the presence of two carboxylate groups (terephthalate) or one (benzoate) within the organic anion, these would be able to be sandwiched between π-stacking adenines or not (Figure 10) [48]. Accordingly, the ligand with just one carboxylate would imply for a sandwich-like arrangement such a short distance between the heptameric entities located above and below the carboxylate group that it is sterically forbidden.

As a consequence, the benzoate anions are displaced into the channels, reducing the accessible volume (Figure 11a). On the contrary, the two carboxylate groups located at opposite sites in the terephthalic anion do not present this steric hindrance and allow a sandwich arrangement of the terephthalate anion between the interacting π-stacking adenines (Figure 11b). This arrangement provides a more open

Porous Materials Built up from Metal-Nucleobase Materials 17

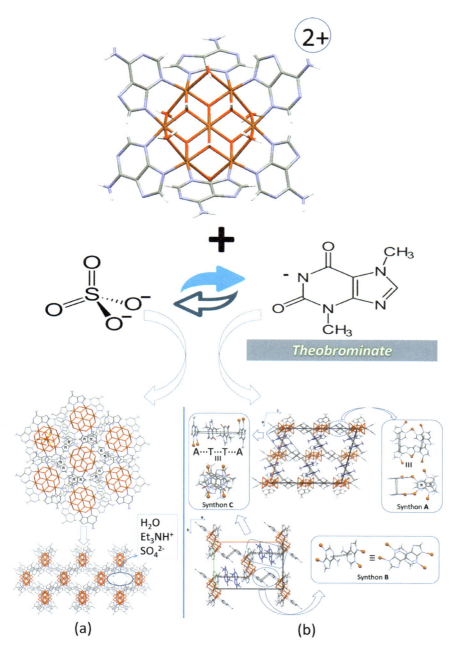

FIGURE 9 Supramolecular building units and the resulting supramolecular architecture based on π-stacking interactions (π sign) of (a) [Cu$_7$(μ-H$_2$O)$_6$(μ$_3$-OH)$_6$(μ-adeninato-κ*N3*:κ*N9*)$_6$](NHEt$_3$)$_2$(SO$_4$)$_2$ and (b) [Cu$_7$(μ-H$_2$O)$_6$(μ$_3$-OH)$_6$(μ-adeninato-κ*N3*:κ*N9*)$_6$](theobrominate)$_2$. The theobrominate anions are highlighted in blue.

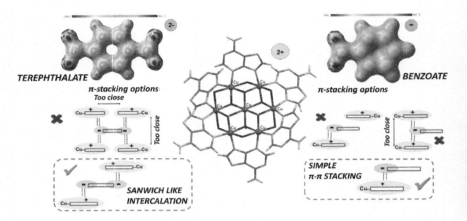

FIGURE 10 Potential supramolecular π-stacking interactions between the adeninato ligands and the carboxylate anions. (Reproduced by permission from Ref. [48]; copyright 2020 Elsevier.)

porous supramolecular structure than that obtained using the benzoate anion, but both of them share the fact that their supramolecular crystal structures are flexible.

Finally, a hallmark feature of the nucleobase-based SMOFs in comparison with MOFs is their facile assembly/disassembly reversibility at room temperature due to the protonation/deprotonation of the nucleobases, which may be used for the fast capture of different species from solution. For this purpose, the chemical stability of the heptameric entities was improved by the incorporation of the kinetically inert Cr(III) ion at the central position [49]. This replacement is relatively easy to accomplish as the central position in the copper(II)-only heptameric species presents a relatively regular MO_6 environment in comparison with the six peripheral ones with a CuO_4N_2 coordination sphere that shows a notable Jahn-Teller tetragonal distortion. In the generated compound [CrCu$_6$(μ-H$_2$O)$_6$(μ$_3$-OH)$_6$(μ-adeninato-κ*N3*:κ*N9*)$_6$](SO$_4$)$_{1.5}$, each heptanuclear entity acts as a four-connected node, in which the π-stacking interactions between adeninato ligands provide a supramolecular porous architecture (44.3% of unit cell volume) with **cds** (CdSO$_4$-like) topology.

The rich acid-base chemistry of the adenine nucleobase allows dissolving the SMOF in acidic aqueous solutions while retaining the molecular structure of the heptameric entities. Note that the bridging μ-κ*N3*:κ*N9* coordination mode leaves the pyrimidine N1 and the imidazole N7 positions of adeninato ligands as suitable acceptor positions for protonation without altering the key features of the wheel-shaped heptamer. This process was previously attempted with the homometallic Cu$_7$ analog, but its lability allows acidic media not only to attack the basic positions of the adeninato ligand but also the hydroxido ligands that bridge the central metal ion to the peripheral ones, leading eventually to the decomposition of the heptameric structure, as clearly deduced from the adeninium sulfate precipitation. However, the presence of the inert chromium(III) ion at the central position plays a crucial role, as it provides kinetic inertness toward protonation

Porous Materials Built up from Metal-Nucleobase Materials

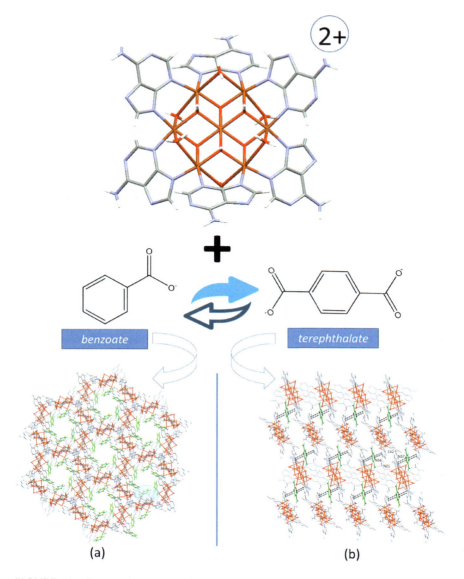

FIGURE 11 Supramolecular building units and the resulting supramolecular architecture of (a) [Cu$_7$(μ-H$_2$O)$_6$(μ$_3$-OH)$_6$(μ-adeninato-κ$N3$:κ$N9$)$_6$](benzoate)$_2$ [48] and (b) [Cu$_7$-(μ-H$_2$O)$_6$(μ$_3$-OH)$_6$(μ-adeninato-κ$N3$:κ$N9$)$_6$](terephthalate) [48]. The benzoate and terephthalate anions are highlighted in green.

of the hydroxido ligands. As a consequence, protonation takes place only at the nucleobases, which are able to deal with it without collapsing the molecular structure of the heptameric entities. This feature allows its complete dissolution, which requires a pH close to 1.8. The obtained solution is stable for a few hours before the thermodynamically favored breakdown of the heptameric unit starts.

This fact confirms the kinetic inertness of the CrCu$_6$ entity in an acidic medium and, if placed in an aqueous medium with pH > 6.5, the starting compound is recovered.

All these features provide a material able to actively entrap drugs of extensive use such as the anionic anti-inflammatory compounds naproxen and ibuprofen, which are nowadays a source of water contamination concern. These drugs have been selected because of their capability to form supramolecular interactions with the heptameric entity, either by hydrogen-bonding or via π-stacking interactions, but also because their anionic nature (pK_a = 4.2 and 5.3, respectively) allows the replacement of the SO$_4^{2-}$ anions to balance the positive charge of the heptameric cluster. For this purpose, an acidic solution of the CrCu$_6$ heptamer was added dropwise into a solution containing these anionic drugs at concentrations of 248, 413, and 826 µM (corresponding to 51, 85, and 170 mg/L for ibuprofen and 57, 95, and 190 mg/L for naproxen). The mixture of the CrCu$_6$ heptamer and the anionic drug led to CrCu$_6$ heptamer:drug ratios of 1:6, 1:10, and 1:20. During the addition of the highly acidic solution of the heptamer, the pH of the solution was kept between pH 7 and 8 by the simultaneous addition of 1 M NaOH in order to prevent the precipitation of the highly insoluble neutral forms of the drugs. As the heptamer was added to the drug, a green suspension appeared, but interestingly the amount of precipitate clearly increased as the concentration of the drug solution increased. The characterization of the resulting precipitates indicated that the amount of drug captured per heptameric entity differs depending on the drug concentration: 1:3 (for naproxen), 1:6 (for ibuprofen and naproxen), and 1:9 (for ibuprofen and naproxen). The incorporation of a maximum of nine monoanionic drug molecules per heptameric entity enabled us to assume that in acidic solution of CrCu$_6$, the heptameric entities are able to incorporate 6 H$^+$, probably located on the non-coordinated endocyclic nitrogen atoms of the adenines in such a way that the discrete entities acquire a 9+ charge, allowing, in turn, to capture up to nine anions of these drugs per formula unit. Apparently, depending on the concentration/ratio of the drug solution, the addition of these highly protonated 9+ entities into a nearly neutral solution leads to two competing processes: (1) the neutralization of these acidic entities and (2) their precipitation in the form of a cationic heptamer–anionic drug adduct, an insoluble compound (Figure 12). At high drug concentrations, the second process takes place before any neutralization process can occur and results in the isolation of H$_6$CrCu$_6$/ibuprofen 1:9 and H$_6$CrCu$_6$/naproxen 1:9 compounds. At intermediate concentrations, partial neutralization takes place before the anionic drug is able to precipitate the adduct, giving rise to samples of the composition H$_3$CrCu$_6$/ibuprofen (1:6) and H$_3$CrCu$_6$/naproxen (1:6). At the lower end of employed concentrations, the neutralization can be completed for CrCu$_6$/naproxen (1:3), but for the ibuprofen analog, a mixture of the apparent 1:3 and 1:6 compounds is obtained.

In summary, making use of the facile reversible assembling/disassembling capacity of SMOF [CrCu$_6$(µ-H$_2$O)$_6$(µ$_3$-OH)$_6$(µ-adeninato-κ$N3$:κ$N9$)$_6$](SO$_4$)$_{1.5}$ made it possible to capture ibuprofen and naproxen with different stoichiometries (1:3, 1:6, and 1:9), depending on the drug concentration. This was enabled by the different protonation states that the CrCu$_6$ building block can display without

Porous Materials Built up from Metal-Nucleobase Materials 21

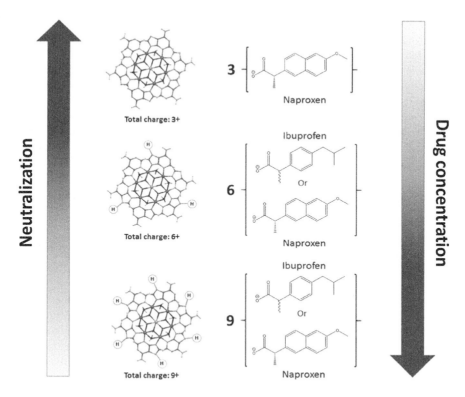

FIGURE 12 Relation between the protonation of the adeninato ligand, the captured drug ratio per heptamer, and the drug concentration in the batch. (Reproduced by permission from Ref. [49]; copyright 2021 Cell Press.)

altering its molecular structure, which is directly related to the presence of multiple donor sites in the adenine nucleobase.

5 HYBRID METAL-NUCLEOBASE POROUS MATERIALS

The goal to obtain metal-nucleobase porous materials can be also achieved by simultaneous and collaborative polymerization through both coordination bond and complementary hydrogen-bonding interactions. This was observed in case of $[Cu_2(\mu\text{–adeninato-}\kappa N3{:}\kappa N9)_2(\mu\text{-adeninato-}\kappa N7{:}\kappa N9)(\mu\text{-OH})(H_2O)(CH_3OH)]_n$ [35]. This compound consists of 1D infinite coordination polymers held together by complementary hydrogen-bonding interactions in a 3D supramolecular porous structure. The coordination polymer can be described as non-centrosymmetric dinuclear units in which two Cu(II) ions are bridged by two adeninate moieties through their N3 and N9 positions and also by one hydroxido ligand. These dinuclear units are connected by additional bridging adeninato ligands that are coordinated to the Cu(II) centers by their N7 and N9 positions to provide a 1D coordination chain. The bridging adeninato ligands inside the dinuclear units are tilted 22°, but they present a wider tilt angle with respect to those connecting the dimeric units (56° and 78°, respectively) in the polymeric chain. This fact, together with the complementary double hydrogen-bonding interactions of the nucleobases, promotes a 3D propagation of the supramolecular structure. The μ-κ*N3*:κ*N9*-adeninato ligands are able to establish double base-pairing synthons through Watson-Crick and Hoogsteen faces. On the other hand, the μ-κ*N7*:κ*N9*-adeninato ligands are hydrogen bonded to the bridging hydroxido ligand and the coordinated aqua ligand of an adjacent polymeric chain through N1 and N6 positions of the Watson-Crick face. The resulting supramolecular crystal structure shows the presence of 1D channels that represent 44% of the total volume.

6 GENERAL CONCLUSIONS

In this chapter, we have paid attention to the suitability of the metal-nucleobase systems to provide porous materials. The molecular stiffness and the multiple coordinating positions of the nucleobases, especially adenine, make them appropriate building blocks to build up 3D porous structures based on the polymerization through coordination bonds (MOFs). Additionally, the well-known ability of the nucleobases to establish complementary hydrogen bond interactions allows generating a new type of porous materials, SMOFs, in which the base-pairing interactions replace the coordination bonds in the role of sustaining the 3D architecture. However, not all discrete metal-nucleobase systems are well suited to provide supramolecular porous materials. They should meet the following requirements: (1) rigid discrete entity, achievable if the nucleobase is anchored to the building unit through multiple positions, usually by two coordination bonds or the combination of a coordination bond and an intramolecular hydrogen bond, (2) rigid and predictable synthons, as those provided by complementary hydrogen-bonding interactions taking place between nucleobases, and (3) a metal coordination geometry that imposes a non-coplanar arrangement of several nucleobases allowing a 3D propagation of the base-pairing interactions. It is also possible to employ π-stacking interactions between the nucleobases for the same purpose, but the lower directionality of these interactions makes the resulting supramolecular architecture flexible upon the removal and adsorption of the water molecules located in the channels. It has been proven that under certain circumstances, it is possible to reversibly assemble/disassemble the SMOF to provide a faster route for the capture of different species from solution than the conventional diffusion-driven adsorption approach. Finally, it should be mentioned that further efforts must be made in order to obtain more examples of porous metal-nucleobase materials based on the guanine nucleobase.

ACKNOWLEDGMENTS

This work has been funded by Eusko Jaurlaritza/Gobierno-Vasco (IT1291-19 and IT1722-22) and Ministerio de Ciencia e Innovación (PID2019–108028GBC21).

ABBREVIATIONS AND DEFINITIONS

Ade   adenine
BET   Brunauer–Emmett–Teller
BPDC   [1,1'-biphenyl]-4,4'-dicarboxylate
CSD   Cambridge structural database
DNA   deoxyribonucleic acid
Hgua   guanine
MBioF   metal-biomolecule framework
MOF   metal-organic framework
ox   oxalate
SBU   secondary building unit
SMOF   supramolecular metal-organic framework

REFERENCES

1. B. Liu, C. G. Pappas, J. Ottelé, G. Schaeffer, C. Jurissek, P. F. Pieters, M. Altay, I. Marić, M. C. A. Stuart, S. Otto, *J. Am. Chem. Soc.* **2020**, *142*, 4184–4192.
2. E. J. Anthony, E. M. Bolitho, H. E. Bridgewater, O. W. L. Carter, J. M. Donnelly, C. Imberti, E. C. Lant, F. Lermyte, R. J. Needham, M. Palau, P. J. Sadler, H. Shi, F.-X. Wang, W.-Y. Zhang, Z. Zhang, *Chem. Sci.* **2020**, *11*, 12888–12917.
3. G. Beobide, O. Castillo, A. Luque, S. Pérez-Yáñez, *CrystEngComm* **2015**, *17*, 3051–3059.
4. A. Shibata, S. L. Higashi, M. Ikeda, *Polym. J.* **2022**, *54*, 751–766.
5. K. Chen, B. S. Zhao, C. He, *Cell Chem. Biol.* **2016**, *23*, 74–85.
6. H. Furukawa, K. E. Cordova, M. O'Keefe, O. M. Yaghi, *Science* **2013**, *341*, 974.
7. M. K. Shukla, J. Leszczynski, *Wiley Interdiscip. Rev. Comput. Mol. Sci.* **2013**, *3*, 637–649.
8. C. R. Groom, I. J. Bruno, M. P. Lightfoot, S. C. Ward, *Acta Cryst.* **2016**, *B72*, 171–179. CSD version 4.52, September 2021.
9. A. Gładysiak, T. N. Nguyen, J. A. R. Navarro, M. J. Rosseinsky, K. C. Stylianou, *Chem. Eur. J.* **2017**, *23*, 13602–13606.
10. T. F. Mastropietro, D. Armentano, E. Grisolia, C. Zanchini, F. Lloret, M. Julve, G. De Munno, *Dalton Trans.* **2008**, 514–520.
11. S. Ganguly, K. K. Kundu, *Can. J. Chem.* **1994**, *72*, 1120–1126.
12. V. Verdolino, R. Cammi, B. H. Munk, H. B. Schlegel, *J. Phys. Chem. B* **2008**, *112*, 16860–16873.
13. J. P. García-Terán, O. Castillo, A. Luque, U. García-Couceiro, P. Román, L. Lezama, *Inorg. Chem.* **2004**, *43*, 4549–4551.
14. J. An, S. J. Geib, N. L. Rosi, *J. Am. Chem. Soc.* **2009**, *131*, 8376–8377.
15. J. An, O. K. Farha, J. T. Hupp, E. Pohl, J. I. Yeh, N. L. Rosi, *Nat. Commun.* **2012**, *3*, 604.
16. A. García-Raso, A. Terrón, Y. Roselló, A. Frontera, O. Castillo, G. Beobide, S. Pérez-Yáñez, E. C. Escudero-Adán, J. J. Fiol, *CrystEngComm* **2020**, *22*, 4201–4205.
17. J. An, S. J. Geib, N. L. Rosi, *J. Am. Chem. Soc.* **2010**, *132*, 38–39.
18. S. Pérez-Yáñez, G. Beobide, O. Castillo, J. Cepeda, A. Luque, A. T. Aguayo, P. Román, *Inorg. Chem.* **2011**, *50*, 5330–5332.
19. M. Lanchas, S. Arcediano, G. Beobide, O. Castillo, A. Luque, S. Pérez-Yáñez, *Inorg. Chem. Front.* **2015**, *2*, 425–443.

20. S. Pérez-Yáñez, G. Beobide, O. Castillo, M. Fisher, F. Hoffmann, M. Fröba, J. Cepeda, A. Luque, *Eur. J. Inorg. Chem.* **2012**, 5921–5933.
21. T. Li, D.-L. Chen, J. E. Sullivan, M. T. Kozlowski, J. K. Johnson, N. L. Rosi, *Chem. Sci.* **2013**, *4*, 1746–1755.
22. Z. Xie, T. Li, N. L. Rosi, M. A. Carreon, *J. Mat. Chem. A* **2014**, *2*, 1239–1241.
23. T. Li, J. E. Sullivan, N. L. Rosi, *J. Am Chem Soc.* **2013**, *123*, 9984–9987.
24. S. Pérez-Yáñez, G. Beobide, O. Castillo, J. Cepeda, A. Luque, P. Román, *Cryst. Growth Des.* **2012**, *12*, 3324–3334.
25. S. Pérez-Yáñez, O. Castillo, J. Cepeda, J. P. García-Terán, A. Luque, P. Román, *Eur. J. Inorg. Chem.* **2009**, 3889–3899.
26. Y. Song, X. Yin, B. Tu, Q. Pang, H. Li, X. Ren, B. Wang, Q. Li, *CrystEngComm* **2014**, *16*, 3082–3085.
27. Y.-P. He, N. Zhou, Y.-X. Tan, F. Wang, J. Zhang, *J. Solid State Chem.* **2016**, *238*, 241–245.
28. F. Wang, Y.-X. 3Tan, H. Yang, H.-X. Zhang, Y. Kang, J. Zhang, *Chem. Commun.* **2011**, *47*, 5828–5830.
29. F. Wang, H. Yang, Y. Kang, J. Zhang, *J. Mater. Chem.* **2012**, *22*, 19732–19737.
30. E. Yang, H.-Y. Li, F. Wang, H. Yang, J. Zhang, *CrystEngComm* **2013**, *15*, 658–661.
31. E. Gil Bardají, E. Freisinger, B. Costisella, C. A. Schalley, W. Brüning, M. Sabat, B. Lippert, *Chem. Eur. J.* **2007**, *13*, 6019–6039.
32. A. Kashima, M. Sakate, H. Ota, A. Fuyuhiro, Y. Sunatsuki, T. Suzuki, *Chem. Commun.* **2015**, *51*, 1889–1892.
33. M. J. Rauterkus, B. Krebs, *Angew. Chem. Int. Ed.* **2004**, *43*, 1300–1303.
34. H. Rauter, E. C. Hillgeris, A. Erxleben, B. Lippert, *J. Am. Chem. Soc.* **1994**, *116*, 616–624.
35. J. Thomas-Gipson, R. Pérez-Aguirre, G. Beobide, O. Castillo, A. Luque, S. Pérez-Yáñez, P. Román, *Cryst. Growth Des.* **2015**, *15*, 975–983.
36. J. An, R. P. Fiorella, S. J. Geib, N. L. Rosi, *J. Am. Chem. Soc.* **2009**, *131*, 8401–8403.
37. J. Thomas-Gipson, G. Beobide, O. Castillo, M. Fröba, F. Hoffmann, A. Luque, S. Pérez-Yáñez, P. Román, *Cryst. Growth Des.* **2014**, *14*, 4019–4029.
38. J. Thomas-Gipson, G. Beobide, O. Castillo, J. Cepeda, A. Luque, S. Pérez-Yáñez, A. T. Aguayo, P. Román, *CrystEngComm* **2011**, *13*, 3301–3305.
39. P. S. Nugent, V. L. Rhodus, T. Pham, K. Forrest, L. Wojtas, B. Space, M. J. Zaworotko, *J. Am. Chem. Soc.* **2013**, *135*, 10950–10953.
40. Y.-N. Gong, D.-C. Zhong, T.-B. Lu, *CrystEngComm* **2016**, *18*, 2596–2606.
41. R. J. Marshall, C. T. Lennon, A. Tao, H. M. Senn, C. Wilson, D. Fairen-Jimenez, R. S. Forgan, *J. Mater. Chem. A* **2018**, *6*, 1181–1187.
42. H.-L. Jiang, T. A. Makal, H.-C. Zhou, *Coord. Chem. Rev.* **2013**, *257*, 2232–2249.
43. J. Thomas-Gipson, G. Beobide, O. Castillo, A. Luque, J. Pascual-Colino, S. Pérez-Yáñez, P. Román, *CrystEngComm* **2018**, *20*, 2528–2539.
44. P. Yakovchuk, E. Protozanova, M. D. Frank-Kamenetskii, *Nucleic Acids Res.* **2006**, *34*, 564–574.
45. P. De Meester, A. C. Skapski, *J. Chem. Soc. A*, **1971**, 2167–2169.
46. R. Pérez-Aguirre, G. Beobide, O. Castillo, I. de Pedro, A. Luque, S. Pérez-Yáñez, J. Rodríguez Fernández, P. Román, *Inorg. Chem.* **2016**, *55*, 7755–7763.
47. J. Pascual-Colino, G. Beobide, O. Castillo, I. da Silva, A. Luque, S. Pérez-Yáñez, *Cryst. Growth Des.* **2018**, *18*, 3465–3476.
48. J. Pascual-Colino, G. Beobide, O. Castillo, P. Lodewyckx, A. Luque, S. Pérez-Yáñez, P. Román, L. F. Velasco, *J. Inorg. Biochem.* **2020**, *202*, 110865.
49. R. Pérez-Aguirre, B. Artetxe, G. Beobide, O. Castillo, I. de Pedro, A. Luque, S. Pérez-Yáñez, S. Wuttke, *Cell Rep. Phys. Sci.* **2021**, *2*, 100421.

2 Cytosine and Its Derivatives as Useful Tools to Build Unusual and Fascinating Architectures

Teresa F. Mastropietro and Giovanni De Munno
Dipartimento di Chimica e Tecnologie Chimiche,
Università della Calabria, I-87036 Arcavacata di Rende,
Cosenza, Italy
giovanni.demunno@unical.it

CONTENTS

1 Introduction 26
2 Metal Ion Coordination with Nucleobases 28
3 Coordination Materials Based on Metal Ions and Cytosine Nucleosides and Nucleotides 28
    3.1 Polynuclear Discrete and Polymeric 3D Compounds with Cytidine 30
    3.2 Polymeric Compounds with Cytidine (or Deoxycytidine) 5′-Monophosphate 32
4 Polymeric Compounds Containing Auxiliary Ligands 38
    4.1 Polymeric Compounds with Bridging Auxiliary Ligands 38
    4.2 Polymeric Compounds with Terminal Auxiliary Ligands 42
5 General Conclusions 45
Acknowledgments 46
Abbreviations and Definitions 46
References 47

Abstract

Nucleobases, nucleosides, and nucleotides are the essential constituents of DNA and RNA. Owing to their several coordination sites, these natural biomolecules have emerged as useful building blocks for the construction of highly ordered nanostructured materials, replacing synthetic organic molecules in the coordination to metal ions. These metal-containing self-assembled biomaterials are simple to prepare, exhibit highly tuneable structures and properties, and present outstanding biocompatibility. Within these bioinspired multi-component assemblies, the biomolecules mainly direct the resultant architecture at the supramolecular scale and are responsible for the chirality delivery. The metal ions, conversely, not only play a structural role, but can also introduce additional functionalities, such as luminescence, magnetism, catalytic activity, etc.

In this review, we chose cytosine and its derivatives as a representative case study. We briefly summarize the metal-binding properties of these biomolecules in simple systems of low nuclearity, focusing on both the coordination binding pattern established upon metal ion coordination and the intermolecular interactions which drive their supramolecular organization. Then, we illustrate how these interactions have been exploited to assemble sophisticated nanostructured and functional architectures, including discrete polynuclear and extended polymeric materials. The discussion will be mainly performed from a crystallographic and supramolecular point of view, through a comprehensive survey of the X-ray single crystal diffraction data reported in the CCDC (Cambridge Crystallographic Data Centre) database. We hope that this review of past and recent results related to metal-cytosine interactions will further stimulate the research in the areas of coordination and supramolecular chemistry, crystal engineering, and material sciences of metal-containing bioinspired systems.

KEYWORDS

Nucleotide; Cytosine; Metal Ions; Self-assembly; Nanostructures

1 INTRODUCTION

"Chemists are builders by nature" is the incipit of the contribution "DNA as clay" of Roald Hoffman in *American Scientist* [1]. Like engineers at a molecular scale endowed with creativity and childish ingenuousness, chemists design modular building units which can be assembled into ordered structures of increased complexity. Countless synthetic organic molecules have been synthesized and exploited as building blocks in this "bottom-up" nanofabrication, with the aim of controlling the structure of the resulting material and directing their functional properties.

This creative effort often takes significant inspiration from nature. Many "biomimetic" or "bioinspired" original systems try to replicate nature with designed synthetic architectures. On the other hand, nature offers numerous biomolecules which, besides being the constituents of life, also represent an excellent source of building blocks for supramolecular chemists, since they intrinsically hold precise instructions that guide their cooperative integration into larger structures. So, why not to use them "*to allow human beings to sculpt something new, perhaps beautiful, perhaps useful, certainly unnatural*" [1]. Indeed, the specific binding properties of biological molecules, optimized over billions of years of evolution, provide a powerful platform that can be used in nanotechnology to direct the assembly of highly ordered structured materials with tailored properties and functions.

Nucleotides, the primary building blocks of nucleic acids, are important biological molecules formed by a nucleobase, a pentose sugar moiety (ribose or 2′-deoxyribose), and one, two, or three phosphate groups [2]. They are also attractive ligands due to their intrinsic chirality, their multiple metal-binding sites characterized by different donor properties and their ability to self-organize in highly ordered self-assembled structures [3–10]. The coordination complexity of the nucleotide ligands mainly derives from their rich structural diversity and the presence of multiple metal-binding sites, whose coordination ability depends on their hard/soft character and differs under different pH conditions. Primarily, nucleobases, nucleosides, and nucleotides have been extensively used for the preparation of metal-containing compounds which have been investigated as artificial biomimetic systems [11, 12]. In this regard, starting with the pioneering work of Sletten in 1967 [13], numerous studies on metal complexes containing natural nucleobases or their biologically more relevant derivatives have been performed over the years, mainly with the aim of understanding the metal ion role in several biological processes, as well as for gaining insight into the mechanism of action of certain metal complexes employed as metallodrugs, and, in particular, as antitumor agents. These studies highlighted the diversities of the coordination modes and the metal-mediated supramolecular assemblies of nucleotides when interacting with metal ions, inspiring researchers in the field of supramolecular and material chemistry to design and investigate functional coordination complexes containing nucleotides for the obtainment of new biomaterials [14–18]. Both discrete nanosized metal complexes and coordination polymers of higher dimensionality (1D–3D) with fascinating solid-state architectures and interesting properties have been reported in the literature. In these systems, the presence of the metal centers mainly accounts for the additional functional properties conferred to these multicomponent molecular-based materials. Moreover, the biocompatibility of nucleotides, their environmental friendliness, and chiral properties make bio-coordination polymers based on nucleotides applicable in biomimetic, medical, chiral, and environmentally friendly materials.

Among nucleosides and nucleotides, during the last decade, cytidine (H_2Cyd) and cytidine 5′-monophosphate (H_2CMP) have attracted the interest of supramolecular and materials chemists. They have been successfully employed as ligands and elegant supramolecular inducers of chirality for the design and synthesis of discrete chiral polynuclear and polymeric transition metal complexes [19–23]. In this chapter, we chose cytosine and its derivatives as a representative case study. We briefly discuss the modes of interaction observed in simple cytosine (or its derivatives)-metal ion systems of low nuclearity. Then, we illustrate how these interactions have been exploited to assemble sophisticated nanostructured and functional architectures, including discrete polynuclear and extended polymeric materials. This chapter will discuss the main results and achievements from crystallographic and supramolecular chemistry viewpoints. We will focus on the design, structural features, and functional properties of complex architectures assembled by using cytosine and its derivatives as ligands towards metal ions through a comprehensive survey of the available crystal structure information registered in the CSD (Cambridge Structural Database). The aspect of chirality and chiral delivery will be also discussed, in terms of nucleoside/nucleotide-metal complex chirality, supramolecular helical chirality, and extended axial chirality. Finally, future research challenges and opportunities in this field will be discussed.

2 METAL ION COORDINATION WITH NUCLEOBASES

Comprehensive reviews have been published that systematically describe metal ion-nucleobase interactions and the authors invite the readers to consult them to acquire more exhaustive information on the subject [11, 24–29].

Focusing on cytosine (cyt) and its derivative 1-methylcytosine (1-Mecyt), the usual modes of binding are *via* N(3) and N(3)-O(2) [30–34]. Examples of coordination *via* O(2) are quite rare and have been observed with Mg(II), Ca(II), Mn(II), Co(II) and Ni(II) metal ions only [35–39]. The simultaneous chelation *via* N(3)-O(2) and the O(2) bridging has been reported in some Ca(II) and Ba(II) compounds [39, 40].

The cyt- and 1-Mecyt-containing compounds are generally mononuclear or polynuclear, depending on whether they use only one or more than one site for coordination, and are not interesting from a structural point of view. Compounds of Ag+ with 1-Mecyt and 1-hexylcytosine, which show a fascinating double-helical motif due to argentophilic and hydrogen-bonding interactions, are noteworthy examples [41, 42]. These compounds are particularly interesting for their similarity with the double-helical DNA containing metal-mediated base pairs as well for their possible technological applications.

The supramolecular assemblies of Mg(II), Mn(II), Co(II) with 1-Mecyt, of formula [M(H$_2$O)$_6$(1-Mecyt)$_6$](ClO$_4$)$_2$·H$_2$O where the nucleobase is not directly bonded to the respective metal ion, are also remarkable (Figure 1a). They present interesting features, not only for their supramolecular architecture, by also because they can be considered precursors of the related compounds containing metal-nucleobase covalent bonds [37, 38]. Indeed, crystals containing the nucleobase directly coordinated to the metal ion are formed in solution over time. Moreover, in the Co(II) case, the compound was also obtained from the supramolecular assembly in the solid state. Noteworthy, the direct coordination between the Mn(II) metal ion and the nucleobase has never been observed.

3 COORDINATION MATERIALS BASED ON METAL IONS AND CYTOSINE NUCLEOSIDES AND NUCLEOTIDES

Concerning the nucleoside H$_2$Cyd (no deoxycytidine metal complexes are known) in its neutral form, it binds metal ions through the nitrogen and oxygen donor atoms on the nucleobase fragment or through the oxygen atoms on the sugar.

Several compounds in which the ligand coordinates *via* N(3) or N(3)-O(2) are known [20, 43, 44]. Remarkably, a compound of Ag+, similar to analogous compounds of 1-Mecyt and 1-hexylcytosine, has been obtained with H$_2$Cyd [45].

Cytosines as Tools to Build Unusual and Fascinating Architectures 29

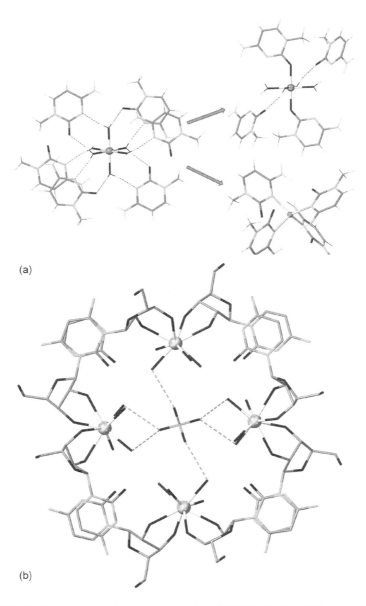

FIGURE 1 Structure of the supramolecular $[M(H_2O)_6(1\text{-Mecyt})_6]^{2+}$ assembly with $M(II) = Mg(II)$ or $Co(II)$ (a), considered as a precursor of the two compounds featuring the direct coordination of two [Mg(II)] and four [Co(II)] cytosine molecules. Perspective view of the supramolecular tetranuclear assembly containing Co(II) ions and H_2Cyd (b). Hydrogen atoms have been omitted for clarity.

The coordination via O(2′)-O(3′) is very unusual and has been found only in two compounds of Ca(II) of formula [Ca(H$_2$Cyd)$_2$(H$_2$O)$_4$](ClO$_4$)$_2$·3H$_2$O and [Ca(H$_2$Cyd)$_2$(H$_2$O)$_4$]Cl$_2$·3H$_2$O, which, though containing the same cationic unit, show a different supramolecular architecture, due to the anion [39]. A supramolecular wheel motif containing four metal ions and eight H$_2$Cyd molecules is formed by π-π interactions between pyrimidine rings, templated by the perchlorate anion (Figure 1b). H$_2$CMP and deoxycytidine 5′-monophosphate (H$_2$dCMP) nucleotides coordinate only in their anionic forms. Due to the involvement of several coordination sites, extended structures have been obtained. Coordination through O(2) of the nucleobase and the O(2′) and O(3′) oxygen atoms of the sugar moiety is rare and was only observed in two dinuclear compounds of Ca(II) [37] and Ba(II) [46]. Surprisingly, in these compounds, phosphate oxygen atoms are not involved in metal ion coordination.

In this section, we will focus on the cooperative interactions occurring with multiple binding sites of anionic cytosine nucleosides and nucleotides which drive the assembly of nanoclusters or coordination polymer materials upon metal ion binding.

3.1 Polynuclear Discrete and Polymeric 3D Compounds with Cytidine

In the monoanionic (HCyd) and dianionic (Cyd) forms, only three compounds with Cu(II) are reported in the CCDC database, that is two polynuclear discrete clusters and a three-dimensional compound. In all these examples, the Cu(II) metal ion binds to both hard and soft sites of the cytidine, including an oxygen atom of the sugar moiety upon *in situ* deprotonation of one or two hydroxyl groups.

A cyclic polynuclear metal complex of formula [Cu(H$_2$O)$_6$][Cu$_8$(HCyd)$_8$(CF$_3$SO$_3$)$_4$](CF$_3$SO$_3$)$_6$·12H$_2$O has been reported with HCyd [19]. The compound crystallizes in the chiral orthorhombic $P2_12_12_1$ space group. It features an octanuclear cationic [Cu$_8$(HCyd)$_8$(CF$_3$SO$_3$)$_4$]$^{4+}$ ring that includes a [Cu(H$_2$O)$_6$]$^{2+}$ cation (Figure 2a). The ring is built up of four dicopper(II) subunits, each one supported by a bis-monodentate O(2′) and a monodentate O(3′) from the ribose moiety, and one O-S-O sulfonato group of the triflate counterion as bridges. Simultaneously, the HCyd links these structural units to each other *via* the pyrimidine N(3) and the exocyclic O(2) atoms. Consequently, the HCyd ligand is coordinated to three copper atoms. An elongated distorted octahedral coordination results around each copper atom. The ring shows receptor properties toward [Cu(H$_2$O)$_6$]$^{2+}$ cations, which bind to the calixarene-like structure by means of multiple hydrogen bonds involving the O(2) atoms of the pyrimidine rings, that point toward the center of the cavities, and four water molecules. A very similar octanuclear motif has been reported in an uridinato-containing compound [47].

A chiral dodecanuclear globular-shaped compound of formula [Cu$_{12}$(HCyd)$_{12}$(CO$_3$)$_2$](ClO$_4$)$_8$·11H$_2$O has been obtained with the cytidine nucleoside in the monoanionic form and a templating carbonate anion [20]. The expansion of nuclearity,

Cytosines as Tools to Build Unusual and Fascinating Architectures

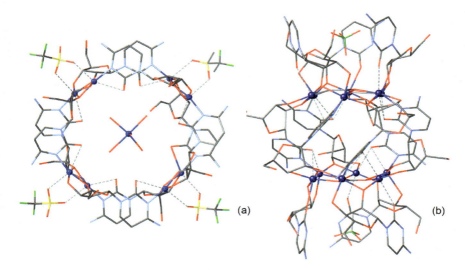

FIGURE 2 Perspective view of the octanuclear (a) and dodecanuclear compounds (b) of formulae [Cu(H$_2$O)$_6$][Cu$_8$(HCyd)$_8$(CF$_3$SO$_3$)$_4$](CF$_3$SO$_3$)$_6$·12H$_2$O and [Cu$_{12}$(HCyd)$_{12}$(CO$_3$)$_2$](ClO$_4$)$_8$·11H$_2$O, respectively, containing mono-deprotonated cytidine. Hydrogen atoms have been omitted for clarity. Color legend for atoms: blue Cu(II), green F (a) and Cl (b), yellow S, grey C, light blue N, red O.

from the previously described octanuclear ring to a dodecanuclear species, and the different topology mainly result from the substitution of the triflate counterion by the perchlorate one, which demonstrated a reduced coordination propensity. It is important to note that, differently from the octanuclear compound, the dodecanuclear species requires the assistance of a coordinated carbonate, generated *in situ* upon atmospheric CO$_2$ uptake. This discrete macromolecule of nanoscopic dimensions features a globular hollow structure hosting water molecules and two distinct basket-like cavities with receptor properties toward ClO$_4^-$ anions (Figure 2b). The hydrophilic cavity is defined by two quasi-planar hexagons of Cu(II) centers assembled by μ$_6$-bridging carbonate ions, held together by six mono-deprotonated HCyd ligands coordinated *via* N(3)-O(2) and O(3′)-O(2′) as unidentate/bis-monodentate bridges, so that the two carbonate ions are perfectly staggered. Six terminal HCyd ligands, three for each Cu$_6$ moiety, complete the structure, shaping the basket-like cavities. The terminal HCyd ligands coordinate two adjacent Cu(II) atoms through O(3′)-O(2′) and O(2) in the monodentate/bis-monodentate bridging coordination mode. The occurrence of both bridging and terminal HCyd ligands is interesting from a coordination chemistry viewpoint, the bridging character of O(2) in the bridging HCyd and the uncoordinated N(3) in the terminal HCyd being unprecedented for a monodeprotonated cytidinato ligand.

Finally, a cytidinato-bridged three-dimensional (3D) coordination polymer of formula {[Cu$_6$(H$_2$O)$_7$(ClO$_4$)$_3$Cu(Cyd)$_4$](ClO$_4$)$_3$}$_n$ [21] was obtained by assembling the chiral multiarmed mononuclear building block [Cu(H$_2$Cyd)$_4$](ClO$_4$)$_2$·5H$_2$O] into an extended structure by further coordination to auxiliary copper ions [20]. This compound is a rare example of the coordination of a nucleoside in its dianionic form. In the mononuclear [Cu(Cyd)$_4$]$^{6-}$ unit four Cyd ligands chelate the metal ion through N(3)/O(2) atoms with a 4+4' coordination around the Cu(II) ion. Upon deprotonation, the O(2'), O(3') oxygen atoms of the ribose bind two different Cu(II) atoms in a bis-monodentate bridging mode. The remaining O(5') atom further binds to another Cu(II) atom. The hyper-coordination of the Cyd ligand, due to the involvement of O(5'), that enables the self-assembling of the 3D structure, is noteworthy.

3.2 Polymeric Compounds with Cytidine (or Deoxycytidine) 5'-Monophosphate

H$_2$CMP and H$_2$dCMP as well as their monomethyl phosphate esters (HCMOMeP and HdCMOMeP), i.e., nucleotides further esterified at the phosphate group with a methyl group, were successfully used as ligands yielding polynuclear compounds of different dimensionality. All these compounds feature common characteristics:

1. The nucleotide is always mono- or dianionic.
2. The phosphate group is always coordinated to the metal center and precludes the involvement of the hydroxyl groups of the sugar moiety in metal binding.
3. The binding sites of the nucleobase can cooperate with the phosphate group for metal coordination and, consequently, the ligands behave like bridges between the metal centers.

They crystallize in chiral space groups, but unfortunately, for most of them, the absolute configuration was not determined. The structural differences (1D, 2D, or 3D) between these compounds can be attributed to the coordination mode of the phosphate group, which could be either monodentate or bridging (μ_2 or μ_3). The monodentate coordination mode was observed for monoanionic nucleotides, while μ_2 and μ_3 are typical of the dianionic form. In addition, the μ_2 coordination is present in both a 2D and a 3D compound, while the μ_3 coordination was found only in 3D compounds.

The monodentate coordination mode of the phosphate group was observed in two isomorphous 1D compounds of Zn(II) and CMOMeP or dCMOMeP (both monoanionic ligands) of formula {[Zn(CMOMeP)$_2$]·9(H$_2$O)}$_n$ and {[Zn(dCMOMeP)$_2$(H$_2$O)$_5$]·11(H$_2$O)}$_n$, crystallizing in the trigonal chiral space group $P3_22_1$. Only one phosphate oxygen atom is available for coordination, since the other is methylated (OCH$_3$) [48]. The ligand behaves as a bridge by means of an oxygen atom of the phosphate group and the N(3) atom of the nucleobase. Two nucleotides coordinate two adjacent Zn metal centers in a "head-to-tail" fashion forming dinuclear subunits, which connect each other assembling a "wave-like" motif along the c axis. Four nucleotides are coordinated to each Zn ion, two of them *via* N(3) and the other two through the phosphate oxygen atoms, in a distorted tetrahedral geometry. However, taking into account the Zn⋯O(2) contacts of 2.70 Å for Zn(CMOMeP)$_2$ and 2.72 Å for Zn(dCMOMeP)$_2$, an approximately 4+2 geometry around the metal atoms could be defined. The μ_2 coordination mode of the phosphate group was found in two isomorphous 2D compounds of Co(II) [49] or Zn(II) [50] and a 3D compound of Cd(II)-dCMP [51].

The cobalt compound of formula {Co(CMP)(H$_2$O)}$_n$ crystallizes in the monoclinic chiral $P2_1$ space group, and the correct chirality was established by repeating the refinement cycles for the two sets of inverted atomic coordinates. The Co(II) atom lies within a distorted tetrahedral environment consisting of the N(3) atom of the cytosine base, one water molecule, and two oxygen atoms, each from a different phosphate group. The exocyclic O(2) atom of the cytosine moiety also interacts with the metal center [2.64(1) Å], defining a 4+1 coordination environment. The bridging coordination of the phosphate groups to the metal ions produces an infinite -Co-O-P-O-Co- helix, wherein each phosphate bridges two Co atoms [Co⋯Co 5.076(2) Å], spiraling in an anti-clockwise manner along the c direction (Figure 3a and b). Each helix is further connected to two other adjacent

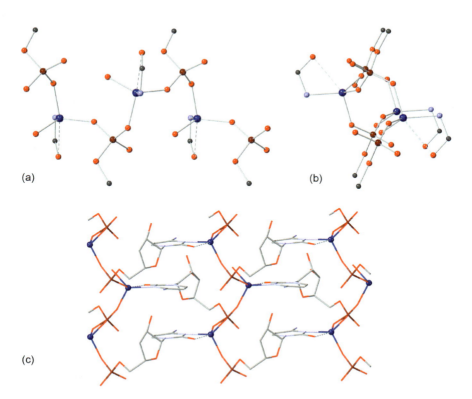

FIGURE 3 Side (a) and perspective view (b) of the helical and view of the 2D motif (c) in the compound of formula {Co(CMP)(H$_2$O)}$_n$. Hydrogen atoms have been omitted for clarity. Color legend for atoms: blue Cu, dark red P, grey C, light blue N, red O.

spirals through the N(3) atoms of the pyrimidine moieties of the nucleotides, which act as bridges between metal ions of different helices. The resulting 2D layer (Figure 3c) lies in the crystallographic bc plane. The H$_2$CMP residues alternate in a head-to-tail fashion along the b direction, establishing stacking interactions between their pyrimidine moieties. Successive layers are held together by hydrogen bond interactions.

Different 3D cadmium-cytidine or H$_2$dCMP compounds have been reported. Interestingly, both the Cd-dCMP and Cd-CMP derivatives have been obtained in two crystalline forms, orthorhombic and monoclinic. The monoclinic Cd-dCMP and Cd-CMP are isomorphous and the presence or absence of the ribose hydroxyl O(2′) exerts little influence on the metal coordination behavior of the nucleotides. In both cases, the phosphate group adopts a μ_3 coordination mode. On the contrary, the orthorhombic forms show different structures, depending on the coordination mode of the phosphate group (μ_2 or μ_3). All the compounds feature common structural characteristics: (1) the chiral nature of the 3D polymeric motif, in which a nucleotide molecule is bonded to metal ions through both the base and phosphate groups, (2) the formation of Cd-phosphate clusters (with some differences in the clustering modes), (3) the absence of metal-sugar bonding.

The orthorhombic dCMP compound has formula {Cd(dCMP)(H$_2$O)$_2$}$_n$ and crystallizes in the chiral $P2_12_12_1$ space group [51].

As already observed in the 2D compound of Co(II), the phosphate group of the nucleotide adopts a μ_2 coordination mode. However, the Co(II) and Cd(II) derivatives differ in the coordination sphere of the metal ion, which increases from 4+1 to 6, due to the presence of an additional water molecule in the Cd(II) derivative. The nucleotide molecule is bonded to one Cd(II) atom through both N(3) and the carbonyl O(2) of cytosine with a longer distance [2.64(1) Å], and to two other Cd(II) atoms through two oxygen atoms of the phosphate group (μ_2-bridging). In turn, each Cd(II) atom is coordinated to three nucleotide molecules (one through the base and two through the phosphate groups) and two water molecules. The coordination geometry is approximately octahedral. Analogously to the Co(II) derivative, the coordination of the phosphate groups to the metal ions produces an infinite -Cd-O-P-O-Cd- helix, wherein each phosphate bridges two Cd(II) atoms [Cd⋯Cd 5.587(2) Å], spiraling along the c axis (Figure 4a and b).

In this case, and different from what is observed in the Co(II) derivative containing CMP, the planes of the cytosine moieties are parallel to the bc plane, and adjacent nucleobases establish hydrogen-bonding interactions involving the exocyclic NH$_2$ and carbonyl groups of neighboring cytosine moieties within the same helix. Each helix is further connected to the other four adjacent spirals *via* nucleotide bridges, involving the N(3) and O(2) atoms of the cytosine moieties linking Cd(II) metal centers of neighboring helices. The resulting 3D structure (Figure 4c) features small slit-like channels along the c direction, defined by nucleotides alternating in a head-to-tail fashion.

The 3D Cd(II) compound containing a μ_3-phosphate coordination mode was obtained with 5′-CMP. The compound of formula {[Cd(CMP)(H$_2$O)]·H$_2$O}$_n$ crystallizes in the chiral space group $P2_12_12_1$. In this case, the absolute configuration

Cytosines as Tools to Build Unusual and Fascinating Architectures

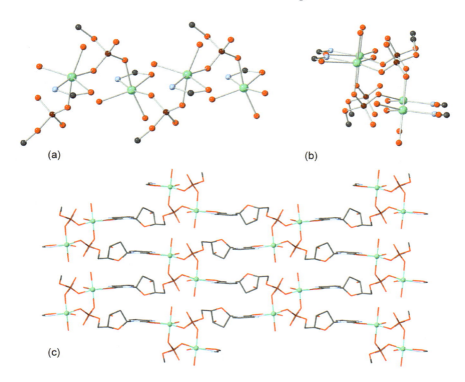

FIGURE 4 Side (a) and perspective (b) view of the helical motif and view of the 3D net (c) in the compound of formula {Cd(dCMP)(H$_2$O)$_2$}$_n$. Hydrogen atoms have been omitted for clarity. Color legend for atoms: cyan Cd, dark red P, grey C, light blue N, red O.

was determined, by repeating the refinement cycles in the two sets of inverted atomic coordinates [49–52]. In contrast to the analogous Cd(II) derivative containing dCMP, each CMP molecule is coordinated to one Cd(II) atom through the N(3) atom of the pyrimidine ring and to three other metal ions, instead of two, through three oxygen atoms of the phosphate group. The change in phosphate coordination from μ_2 to μ_3 is accompanied by the elimination of a water molecule from the coordination sphere of the metal center. Each Cd(II) ion is penta coordinated to one CMP through its cytosine base, to the other three CMP through their phosphate groups and to a one water molecule. The exocyclic O(2) atom of the cytosine moiety and an additional oxygen atom of phosphate group also interact with the metal ion [2.921(1) and 2.932 Å], defining a 5+2 coordination environment. Taking into account these interactions, we can consider each nucleotide bonded to one Cd(II) atom through N(3) and the carbonyl O(2) of the cytosine base and additionally to three other Cd(II) atoms through the phosphate oxygen atoms. In particular, two oxygen atoms belonging to the phosphate are linked to a single metal atom, while the remaining oxygen atom coordinates two metals. This coordination mode of the phosphate is also present in the monoclinic 3D

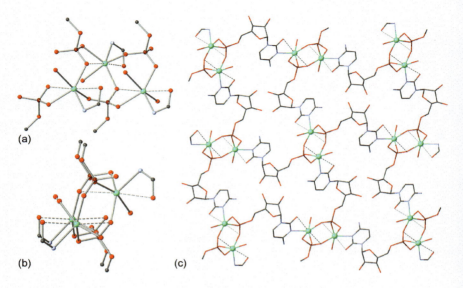

FIGURE 5 Side (a) and perspective (b) view of the spiraling columns and view of the 3D motif (c) in the compound of formula {[Cd(CMP)(H$_2$O)]·(H$_2$O)}$_n$. Hydrogen atoms and non-coordinating water molecules have been omitted for clarity. Color legend for atoms: cyan Cd, dark red P, grey C, light blue N, red O.

compounds (*vide infra*). Spiraling columns of the sequence -Cd$_2$-(O-P-O)$_2$-Cd$_2$ made up of Cd$_2$-(O-P-O)$_2$ units extend throughout *b* axis in an anti-clockwise manner (Figure 5a and b). The main difference between these spiraling motifs and those previously observed in the orthorhombic dCMP derivative consists in the presence of an increased number of atoms of the sequence unit in the former case, resulting in a considerable shortening of the Cd⋯Cd distances [Cd⋯Cd 4.346(2) Å]. The same type of columnar spirals has been found in the monoclinic Cd(II) compounds (*vide infra*). Each column is further cross-linked to four additional adjacent columns, flipped in the opposite direction, through Cd-CMP bridges. A 3D porous structure (Figure 5c) is assembled, with hydrophilic channels running along the crystallographic *c* direction defined by four Cd(II) and four bridging CMP. The channels host crystallization water molecules.

The monoclinic Cd-dCMP [51] compound, of formula {[Cd$_2$(dCMP)$_2$(H$_2$O)$_2$]·3H$_2$O}$_n$, is isomorphic to the Cd-CMP derivative {[Cd$_2$(CMP)$_2$(H$_2$O)$_2$]·3H$_2$O}$_n$ [53], both crystallizing in the chiral space group C_2. The asymmetric unit consists of two non-equivalent Cd(II) ions and, consequently, two different subunits can be defined. Similar to the orthorhombic Cd-CMP compound, spiraling columns of the sequence -Cd$_2$-(O-P-O)$_2$-Cd$_2$ made up of Cd$_2$-(O-P-O)$_2$ units, which extend throughout the *b* axis, were found both in the dCMP and CMP monoclinic compounds. In these cases, the mean Cd⋯Cd distances were in the range between 4.110(2) and 4.335(2) Å. However, differences in the metal-oxygen distances involving both cytosine and phosphate moieties, which shift from regular to longer bond lengths, can be observed in the two subunit spirals of both compounds. Considering these interactions, all Cd(II) atoms could be considered hepta-coordinated with a distorted pentagonal geometry. Each nucleotide is bonded to one Cd(II) atom through N(3) and the carbonyl O(2) of the cytosine base and additionally to three other Cd(II) atoms through the phosphate oxygen atoms with a μ^3-coordination (two oxygen atoms belonging to the phosphate are linked to a single metal ion, while the remaining oxygen coordinates two metals). In turn, each Cd(II) atom is coordinated to three nucleotide molecules (one through the base and two through the phosphate groups) and a water molecule. Each column is further cross-linked to four additional adjacent columns through Cd-CMP bridges, assembling a 3D porous structure (Figure 6). In this case, however, all spirals are oriented in the same manner with respect to the *ac* plane, while, in the previous compound, due to the different symmetry, cross-linked adjacent spirals are oriented into opposite directions alternate within the net. The 3D motif features two structurally different channels running parallel to *b*, larger cylindrical ellipse-shaped and cross-shaped channels. Nucleotide molecules forming the larger cylindrical channels point their -NH$_2$ base moieties into the channel, while those forming the smaller channels point either the exocyclic oxygen atoms or their sugar moieties inwards. Both channels host crystallization water molecules.

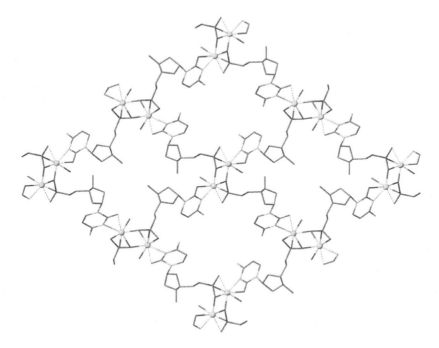

FIGURE 6 3D porous structure in the compound of formula $\{[Cd_2(dCMP)_2(H_2O)_2]\cdot 3H_2O\}_n$. Hydrogen atoms and non-coordinating water molecules have been omitted for clarity.

A manganese H$_2$CMP compound of formula {[Mn(CMP)(H$_2$O)]·1.5H$_2$O}$_n$ was reported [54]. Unfortunately, no crystallographic data are available for this compound, although the corresponding entry is present in the CCDC database. Consequently, we have to rely on and be satisfied with the structural information that the authors provide in their paper. The compound crystallizes in the chiral orthorhombic space group $P2_12_12_1$. Curiously, only the exocyclic O(2) and not the N(3) atom of the pyrimidine ring is involved in the coordination with the metal ion. The coordination geometry around the Mn(II) atom is elongated octahedrally, involving the O(2) atom of the pyrimidine base, a water molecule, and four oxygen atoms of three different phosphate groups, two of which bridge across two manganese ions. A three-dimensional porous network is assembled, composed of cylindrical channels with a helical sequence of -Mn-O-Mn-O- atoms.

A 3D coordination polymer of formula {Ag(HCMP)·H$_2$O}$_n$ was generated as a consequence of the special Ag coordination [55]. It crystallizes in the chiral space group $P2_12_12_1$ of the orthorhombic system. Three symmetrically-equivalent Ag(I) metal centers are coordinated to three different nucleosides via the N(3) and O(2) atoms of the nucleobase and an oxygen atom of the phosphate group of the nucleotide. Moreover, each Ag(I) metal center is connected to two additional Ag(I) atoms via argentophilic interactions, the Ag(I)···Ag(I) distance (2.997(1) Å) being between the sum of the van der Waals radii (3.44 Å) and the distance of a Ag–Ag single bond (2.53 Å). An infinite 1D zigzag chain is formed by Ag(I) ions along the *a* direction, further supported by bridging HCMP coordinating two equivalent Ag(I) metal centers through the N(3) and O(2) atoms. Each chain is further connected to four additional chains by the HCMP ligands through both phosphate oxygen atoms. A 3D polymeric porous structure results in the solid state, which presents channels that incorporate water molecules in their interior.

4 POLYMERIC COMPOUNDS CONTAINING AUXILIARY LIGANDS

Some examples of polymeric structures containing cytidine or deoxycytidine monophosphate and different auxiliary ligands have been reported. We can classify the auxiliary ligands into two main categories, depending on whether they show the bridging or chelating coordination mode. In the first case, they exclusively assure or contribute to the extension of the dimensionality, the nucleotide correspondingly acting as terminal or bridging ligand. On the contrary, in the second case, the chelating ligand behaves as a pure structure "modulator", competing with CMP for metal coordination and thus altering its binding patterns, without contributing to the expansion of the dimensionality.

4.1 POLYMERIC COMPOUNDS WITH BRIDGING AUXILIARY LIGANDS

Examples of polymeric structures, essentially 1D compounds, containing bridging auxiliary ligands have been reported. In most cases, the extension of the dimensionality is entirely due to the auxiliary ligands, while the biomolecules act

Cytosines as Tools to Build Unusual and Fascinating Architectures

as terminal ligands, anchoring to the metal center through the phosphate group. Some examples of 2D compounds obtained with the contribution of CMP acting as a bridging ligand are also reported.

4,4′-bipyridine (4,4′-bipy), 1,2-bis(4-pyridyl)ethane (bpa), bis(4-pyridyl)ethylene (bpe), and azpy have been used as auxiliary N-donor ligands with Mn(II), Co(II), Ni(II), and Cu(II) metal ions and nucleotides such as CMP, dCMP, HCMP, HdCMP, and H$_2$dCMP. For simplicity, we will distinguish five types of compounds:

1. M-L-L′-3H$_2$O   M = Co(II), Ni(II)   L = CMP   L′ = 4,4′-bipy
2. M-L-L′-2H$_2$O/H$_2$O M = Co(II), Cu(II)   L = CMP, dCMP   L′ = 4,4′-bipy
3. M-2L-L′-2H$_2$O   M = Co(II), Mn(II)   L = HCMP   L′ = bpe
4. M-L-L′-L″-2H$_2$O M = Co(II), Mn(II)   L = H$_2$dCMP   L″ = bpe, azpy
                                              L′ = dCMP
5. M[M-L-L′-3H$_2$O]L M = Co(II), Ni(II)   L = HdCMP   L′ = bpa

Two 1D (type 1) and one 2D (type 2) homochiral nucleotide coordination polymers containing CMP-4,4′-bipy-M(II) (M = Cu, Co, Ni) have been reported [23].

The 1D compounds of formula {[M$_2$(CMP)$_2$(4,4′-bipy)$_2$(H$_2$O)$_6$]·11H$_2$O}$_n$ containing Co(II) or Ni(II) are isomorphous (Figure 7a) and crystallize in the

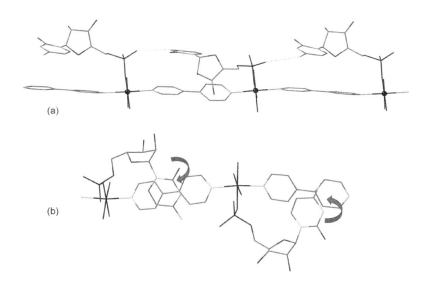

FIGURE 7 1D motif (a) and a fragment (b) of the compound of formula {[M$_2$(CMP)$_2$(4,4′-bipy)$_2$(H$_2$O)$_6$]·11H$_2$O}$_n$ (type 1) showing the anti-clockwise and clockwise oriented nucleotide ligand above the plane of the 4,4′-bipy, resulting in M and P axial chirality of the ligand, respectively. Hydrogen atoms and non-coordinating water molecules have been omitted for clarity.

chiral monoclinic space group $P2_1$. In both compounds, the metal ions are six-fold coordinated by two 4,4'-bipy, one phosphate oxygen atom, and three solvent molecules, with a distorted octahedral geometry. In the asymmetric unit, two CMP ligands coordinate to two crystallographically independent metal ions, arranged in different directions, clockwise and counter clockwise, around the metal-bipy-metal axis, respectively (Figure 7b). This supramolecular orientation results in longer and shorter M(II)⋯M(II) distances alternating along the chain motif and induces the "Extended Axial Chirality" (EAC) of the 1D coordination compounds [56, 57]. The nucleotide acts as a chiral inducer. In particular, through the metal coordination and supramolecular intra-chain interactions (mainly H-bonds and π–π stacking interactions), the chirality of CMP is delivered along the 1D coordination chain, by "locking" the 4,4'-bipy axial conformation. The two different chiral sources, i.e., the inherent chirality of the CMP ligands and the extended axial chirality, coexist in these nucleotide coordination polymers, as evidenced in the solid-state circular dichroism (CD) spectroscopy of the compounds. The resultant overall conformation of the EAC is P, as testified by the solid-state CD spectrum.

Interestingly, the analogous Cu(II) compound of formula $\{[Cu_2(CMP)_2(4,4'$-bipy$)_2(H_2O)_2]\cdot 9H_2O\}_n$ (type 2) is a 2D coordination polymer of Cu(II). It is isomorphous to the compound of formula $\{[Co(dCMP)(4,4'$-bipy$)(H_2O)_2]\cdot 3.5H_2O\}_n$, (type 2) [58], where dCMP, instead of CMP, is present. Different from the previously discussed type 1 Co(II) and Ni(II) compounds, in the Cu(II) derivative, a coordinated water molecule is replaced by an oxygen atom of a phosphate group, which acts as a bridge, thus originating the 2D motif. All Cu(II) ions are six-coordinated with two 4,4'-bipy, two phosphate oxygen atoms, and two solvent water molecules, presenting a distorted octahedral geometry. The EAC existing along the Cu-bipy-Cu chain is similar to that of the previously discussed 1D complexes and is conveyed to the 2D layer through the bonding between Cu(II) ions and phosphate bridging ligands. The configuration of 4,4'-bipy in EAC is P because all CMP ligands surrounding the ligand axis are oriented clockwise. Strong π–π stacking interactions between the pyrimidine bases of nucleotide ligands and the pyridine rings as well as intra-layer H-bondings orient the nucleotide ligands above and below the layer in the same direction.

Two isomorphous 1D compounds of general formula $\{[M(HCMP)_2(bpe)(H_2O)_2]\cdot 3.5H_2O\}_n$ with M=Co(II) or Mn(II) and bpe (type 3) have been reported [59], containing two monoanionic nucleotide molecules (HCMP) coordinated to the metal ion instead of one dianionic (CMP). An isomorphous compound containing Co(II) and dCMP instead of CMP, with the general formula $\{[Co(H_2dCMP)(dCMP)(bpe)(H_2O)_2]\cdot 5.5H_2O\}_n$ has been also described (type 4) [58], together with two additional isomorphous compounds containing Mn(II) and azpy as coligand, having formulae $\{[Mn(H_2CMP)(CMP)(azpy)(H_2O)_2]\cdot 3H_2O\}_n$ and $\{[Mn(H_2dCMP)(dCMP)(azpy)(H_2O)_2]\cdot 5H_2O\}_n$ (both type 4). Within these two series, types 3 and 4, the compounds have been formulated differently, the two nucleotides per unit formula being reported either as monodeprotonated HCMP, the remaining H⁺ being located on one of the phosphate oxygen atoms, or

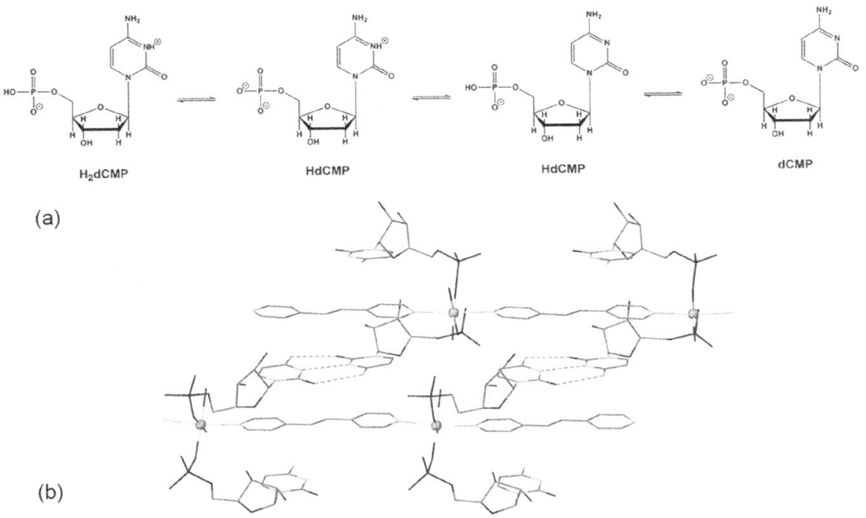

Cytosines as Tools to Build Unusual and Fascinating Architectures 41

FIGURE 8 dCMP equilibria in water (a), the pK_a values of H$_2$dCMP, HdCMP, and dCMP are 1.9, 4.4, and 6.2, respectively; supramolecular 2D motif (b) in the compound of formula {[Mn(HCMP)$_2$(bpe)(H$_2$O)$_2$]·3.5H$_2$O}$_n$; solvent water molecules and hydrogen atoms have been omitted for clarity. The interactions between the atoms involved in the hemiprotonated cytosine:cytosine base pair are represented by dashed lines.

as a mixture of H$_2$CMP/CMP as well as H$_2$dCMP/dCMP. The compounds have been obtained from their respective mother solution at pH in the range of 5–5.36. Considering the equilibria involving dCMP or CMP in water (see Figure 8a as an example) and taking into account the very low pK_a for the first deprotonation step (1.9) [59, 60], we believe that the first formulation, proposing either a protonated phosphate oxygen atom or a protonated pyrimidine ring, can be considered the most likely even in the crystalline solid state. However, the simultaneous occurrence of different species in the solid state cannot be ruled out only on the basis of crystallographic data.

All type 3 and 4 compounds crystallize in the chiral orthorhombic space group P2$_1$2$_1$2$_1$. They are 1D polymers, thanks to the auxiliary bridging ligands, while the CMP or the dCMP ligands coordinate the metal ions as terminal ligands. For all the compounds, EAC can be expected, but we will not discuss this aspect in further detail. On the other hand, the crystal structure analyses reveal the formation of a hemiprotonated cytosine:cytosine base pair, described by the authors as an i-motif (cytosine–cytosine base-pair mismatch) [61–63] in all the compounds although this feature is examined only in one of the two research papers [58]. The hemiprotonated cytosine:cytosine base pair between cytosine and its derivatives appears in several entries of the CCDC databases, the first report going back to 1973 [64–69].

For simplicity, we will refer to the description of all the isomorphous compounds belonging to types 3 and 4 to the Mn(II) derivative containing HCMP and bpe as ancillary ligand of the formula $\{[Mn(HCMP)_2(bpe)(H_2O)_2]\cdot 3.5H_2O\}_n$. Each Mn(II) ion in the asymmetric unit is six-coordinated with two protonated HCMP, two nitrogen atoms from different bpe bridging ligands, and two water molecules. The adjacent Mn(II) ions are linked by the bridging bpe ligands into extended 1D chains (Figure 8b). π–π stacking interactions between cytosine bases and bpe ligands within the same chain restrict the CMP ligands to arrange along the 1D chain in the same direction and hinder the free rotation of the pyridine rings around the C–C bond of the bpe molecules, thus capturing the extended axial chirality (EAC) of bpe. The hemiprotonated cytosine:cytosine base pair is generated by H-bonds between the neighboring cytosine moieties of successive chains and assembles a 2D motif (Figure 8b). The two cytosine rings involved in the base pair are nearly coplanar. It is evident that if the nucleotide is present as HCMP, the two mono-deprotonated forms must alternate along the 1D coordination polymer to enable the hemiprotonated cytosine-cytosine pair interaction.

In the mentioned paper [58], the authors used different co-ligands, bpe and azpy, as well as bpa and 4,4'-bipy, to investigate the effect of the length and flexibility of the organic connector on the hemiprotonated cytosine:cytosine base-pair formation. While azpy (azpy = 4,4'-azopyridine), which has a similar molecular length as bpe, leads to the formation of a similar perfect base pair, the use of the more flexible bpa partially disrupts the base pair. Two 1D isostructural compounds containing either Co(II) or Ni(II) of general formula $\{[M(HdCMP)(bpa)(H_2O)_3]\cdot HdCMP\cdot 3H_2O\}_n$ (type 5) have been reported with bpa. Similar to type 1, in these compounds a water molecule replaces a phosphate group of the nucleotide in the metal coordination sphere, while the other balances the charge as an uncoordinated counterion. The hemiprotonated cytosine:cytosine base pair is formed between the coordinated and uncoordinated HdCMP nucleotides, but it is very distorted, with a high dihedral angle between the cytosine rings (up to 14.3(1)°).

4.2 Polymeric Compounds with Terminal Auxiliary Ligands

In all the previously discussed examples, we have seen how ligands such as 4,4'-bipy or similar, which contain nitrogen atoms "far apart" on the molecular frame, act as a "bridge" between the metal ions, directly leading to the construction of extended one- or two-dimensional architectures when used together with cytidine or deoxycytidine monophosphate. This latter acts either as a terminal ligand in the 1D compounds or as a bridging ligand when assisting the assembly of 2D architectures.

With co-ligands containing nitrogen atoms in a "close" position, namely chelating ligands, such as 2,2'-dipyridylamine (dpa), ethylenediamine (en), 2,2'-bipyridine (bpy) and 1,10-phenanthroline (phen), CMP coordinates metal ions in a bridging fashion.

Cytosines as Tools to Build Unusual and Fascinating Architectures

By using 2,2′-dipyridylamine and ethylenediamine two dinuclear species were obtained, namely a Cu(II) and Pt(II) compound, respectively, of formula [Cu$_2$(CMP)$_2$(dpa)$_2$(H$_2$O)$_2$]·5H$_2$O and [Pt$_2$(CMP)$_2$(en)$_2$]·2H$_2$O. In the first, two CMPs act as μ_2-bridges by coordinating the two metal ions by means of two oxygen atoms of the phosphate group [70]. In the second, two CMP molecules bridge two Pt(II) ions via N(3) and an oxygen atom of the phosphate group [71]. A one-dimensional compound of Cu(II), of formula {[Cu$_2$(en)$_2$(CMP)$_2$]·5H$_2$O}$_n$, where both bridging CMP coordination modes were found it is also known. In these chains, pairs of Cu(II) bridged by oxygen atoms of two CMP in μ_2 mode are connected by means of the N(3) and O(2) atoms of the nucleobase [72].

On the contrary, when using bpy and 1,10-phenanthroline, generally extended structures have been obtained.

Two 1D homochiral helical biopolymers of opposite helicity have been reported in two compounds of Cu(II)-CMP with bpy [22] of formulae {[Cu$_5$(bpy)$_5$(OH)(H$_2$O)$_2$(CMP)$_2$(ClO$_4$)](ClO$_4$)$_4$·9H$_2$O}$_n$ (P) and {[Cu$_{15}$(bpy)$_{15}$(OH)$_3$(H$_2$O)$_7$(CMP)$_6$(CF$_3$SO$_3$)](CF$_3$SO$_3$)$_{14}$·15H$_2$O}$_n$ (M), containing either ClO$_4^-$ (P) or CF$_3$SO$_3^-$ (M) as counterions. Remarkably, the chirality of the two polymers can be rapidly interconverted by exchanging the anions, in a reversible manner. The corresponding inversion of the copper(II) absolute configuration and helicity is also observed. P and M helical compounds crystallize in the chiral space groups $P2_12_12_1$ and $P2_1$ of the orthorhombic and monoclinic systems, respectively. The structure of P consists of single-stranded helices containing the repeating [Cu$_5$(bpy)$_5$(H$_2$O)$_2$(OH)(CMP)$_2$(ClO$_4$)]$^{4+}$ unit (Figure 9a). On the other hand, 15 crystallographically independent copper atoms are present in the cationic unit of M, which could be alternatively formulated as {[Cu$_5$(bpy)$_5$(H$_2$O)$_2$(OH)(CMP)$_2$(CF$_3$SO$_3$)][Cu$_5$(bpy)$_5$(H$_2$O)$_3$(OH)(CMP)$_2$][Cu$_5$(bpy)$_5$(H$_2$O)$_2$(OH)(CMP)$_2$]}$^{14+}$. In both P and M helices, the CMP ligands act as bridges, coordinating the Cu(II) metal centers through the oxygen atoms of the phosphate groups and via N(3) and the exocyclic O(2). Pairs of μ_4-phosphate groups connect four copper(II) ions, assembling a

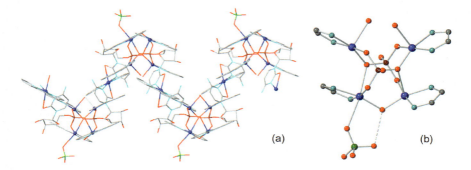

FIGURE 9 Side view (a) of the helical motif based on the [Cu$_5$(bpy)$_5$(H$_2$O)$_2$(OH)(CMP)$_2$(ClO$_4$)]$^{4+}$ unit and (b) view of the tetranuclear core. Hydrogen atoms have been omitted for clarity. Color legend for atoms: blue Cu, green Cl, dark red P, grey C, light blue N, red O.

butterfly-shaped tetranuclear core of the type [Cu$_4$(μ_4-PO$_4$)$_2$(μ-OH)], also supported by a bridging hydroxido group (Figure 9b). Two oxygen atoms of each phosphate are linked to a single metal atom, while the remaining oxygen atom coordinates two metal centers in a μ_2- fashion. This phosphate μ_3-coordination mode is similar to that observed in the orthorhombic and monoclinic 3D compounds of Cd(II) with CMP, although four metal centers instead of three are connected in this case. Three Cu(II) atoms of the core have a square-pyramidal geometry, being also coordinated to a bpy molecule, water molecules, and μ_2-hydroxido groups.

Interestingly, some metal ions are further anion-linked, thus achieving an octahedral geometry. The remaining copper ions, chelated by the cytosine base of CMP and by a bpy, constitute the connectors of the tetranuclear cores and the chiral inducers of the overall helical structure. They exhibit an octahedral geometry in both *P* and *M* but with opposite C(*D*) or A(*L*) chirality [73, 74].

The use of a counterion such as bromide instead of perchlorate or triflate leads to a different architecture. In this case, depending on the different coordinative properties of bromide with respect to perchlorate or triflate anions, a hexameric compound of formula [Cu$_6$(bpy)$_6$(CMP)$_2$(μ-O)Br$_4$]Br$_2$·46H$_2$O compound was formed [75].

Interestingly, the cationic [Cu$_6$(bpy)$_6$(CMP)$_2$(μ-O)Br$_4$]$^{2+}$ hexameric units feature a [Cu$_4$(μ_4-PO$_4$)$_2$(μ-O)] core, very similar to that found in the perchlorate and triflate chain compounds, with a bridging oxido, instead of hydroxido group. As already observed in the previous 1D helical compounds, each Cu(II) atom is also coordinated to a bpy molecule. Water molecules and μ_2-oxido groups complete the square-pyramidal geometry of metal ions. The cytosine moieties of the two crystallographically distinct CMP ligands are bonded *via* N(3)-O(2) to two additional copper ions that complete their distorted octahedral geometry through one bpy and two bromide anions. The coordination of the halogenide prevents the formation of a 1D structure observed in the compounds of perchlorate and triflate.

The terminal copper atoms, chelated by the cytosine base of the nucleotide molecules, constitute the terminal tails of the hexanuclear entities, which allow intermolecular π-π stacking interactions involving the ancillary bipyridine ligands. These interactions are at the origin of the formation of alternating hydrophobic and hydrophilic chiral nanopores, containing either acetal oxygen atoms from the ribose moiety and pyridine ligands or hydroxyl groups of the sugar moiety, respectively.

A different architecture was found in Cu-CMP compounds when phenanthroline was used as coligand with nitrate as counterion. The 3D compound (Figure 10a), of formula {Cu$_7$(phen)$_6$(CMP)$_4$](NO$_3$)$_6$·46H$_2$O}$_n$ [76], crystallizes in the chiral *P*2$_1$ space group of the monoclinic system, and its absolute configuration was reliably assigned. It contains [Cu$_7$(phen)$_6$(CMP)$_4$(H$_2$O)$_4$]$^{6+}$ cationic units made up of hexanuclear cores of the type [Cu$_6$(μ_4-PO$_4$)$_4$(phen)$_6$(H$_2$O)$_4$] and Cu(II) cations. Each hexanuclear core is composed of two trinuclear units, similar to those of the previous compound. Pairs of μ_3-phosphate groups connect three Cu(II) ions within each trinuclear sub-unit, binding the metal centers

Cytosines as Tools to Build Unusual and Fascinating Architectures 45

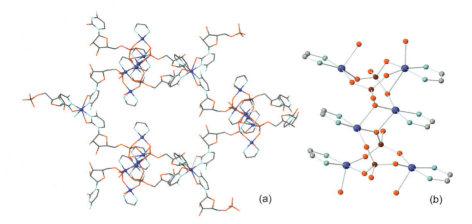

FIGURE 10 Chiral channel (a) in the 3D porous compound of formula {[Cu$_7$(phen)$_6$(CMP)$_4$](NO$_3$)$_6$·46H$_2$O}$_n$ and view of the hexanuclear core (b), formed by two subunits bridged by means of two μ$_2$-oxygens of two different phosphate groups. Hydrogen atoms, solvent water molecules and the phen rings have been omitted for clarity. Color legend for atoms: blue Cu, green Cl, dark red P, grey C, light blue N, and red O.

through monodentate oxygen atoms. The two subunits are bridged by means of two μ$_2$-oxygen atoms of two different phosphate groups. A μ$_4$-coordination mode for the central phosphate groups results (Figure 10b). Each Cu(II) atom is also coordinated to a phen molecule. Water molecules are linked to the peripheral Cu(II) atoms. In the hexameric core, all Cu(II) show a square-pyramidal coordination environment. The cytosine moiety of the four CMP ligands binds via N(3)-O(2) to additional copper ions, which feature an octahedral geometry. A 3D chiral porous network results. The functional channels possess both hydrophilic hydroxyl groups and acetal oxygen atoms from the ribose units, pointing towards the pores, and hydrophobic phenanthroline moieties. Free water molecules and nitrate anions reside within these functional channels. The polar and chiral environment provided by the residues decorating the walls of the pores allows for an efficient chiral recognition process.

5 GENERAL CONCLUSIONS

In this chapter, we tried to lead the readers through a systematic survey of bioinorganic hybrid nanostructured materials obtained by exploiting the metal-binding properties and self-assembling ability of the natural cytosine nucleobase and its derivatives. The studies in this field, originally undertaken with the aim of gaining basic knowledge on the mechanisms underlying metal-nucleic acid interactions, unexpectedly opened up new avenues for materials chemistry. In turn, in combination with materials science, the research on metal coordination to biological ligands has acquired new vitality.

In this chapter, we try to show how advantageous interactions can originate even in simple systems. Intriguing complex architectures have been assembled by harnessing these simple components, proving that nucleobases and their derivatives, despite being constituted by a limited pool of molecules, have the ability to provide a significantly expanded set of polynuclear compounds featuring diverse nanostructures. Here, the biomolecules played a major role in determining both the hierarchical organization in the solid state and the unique properties resulting in these materials, including molecular recognition, chirality delivery, and hydrophilic/hydrophobic functional porosity.

The ability of cytosine and its derivatives, as well as of other nucleobases, nucleosides, and nucleotides, to serve as building blocks for the preparation of new biomimetic systems and bioinorganic hybrid materials certainly deserves to be further explored in the future. New research opportunities can derive from facing the challenges these materials present, including the definition of more rational synthetic strategies aimed to reach a stricter structural and chemical control of the resulting material. The final structural and chemical-physical property can be tailored by changing the nucleoside/nucleotide, the metal ion and their relative ratios as well as by using auxiliary ligands able to influence the self-assembling process. Moreover, the pool of available bioligands can be further expanded by modification of the nucleobase moieties and/or the phosphate groups, in order to modulate the binding preference of the ligands, to introduce additional properties, or to increase the stability and biocompatibility of the material. Finally, in order to fully achieve the great potential of these systems, further efforts need to be directed to exploit their unique properties in real-world applications.

ACKNOWLEDGMENTS

This work was supported by the Ministero dell'Università e della Ricerca (Italy).

ABBREVIATIONS AND DEFINITIONS

1-Mecyt	1-methylcytosine
4,4′-bipy	4,4′-bipyridine
Azpy	4,4′-azopyridine
bpa	1,2-bis(4-pyridyl)ethane
bpe	bis(4-pyridyl)ethylene
bpy	2,2′-bipyridine
CMOMeP	monoanionic cytidine 5′-monophosphate monomethyl phosphate ester
CMP	dianionic cytidine 5′-monophosphate
Cyd	dianionic cytidine
cyt	cytosine
dCMOMeP	monoanionic deoxycytidine 5′-monophosphate monomethyl phosphate ester
dCMP	dianionic deoxycytidine 5′-monophosphate

dpa	2,2'-dipyridylamine
en	ethylenediamine
H₂CMP	cytidine 5'-monophosphate
H₂Cyd	cytidine
H₂dCMP	deoxycytidine 5'-monophosphate
H₂dCyd	deoxycytidine
HCMOMeP	cytidine 5'-monophosphate monomethyl phosphate ester
HCMP	monoanionic cytidine 5'-monophosphate
HCyd	monoanionic cytidine
HdCMOMeP	deoxycytidine 5'-monophosphate monomethyl phosphate ester
HdCMP	monoanionic deoxycytidine 5'-monophosphate
phen	1,10-phenanthroline

REFERENCES

1. R. Hoffmann, *Am. Sci.* **1994**, *82*, 308–311.
2. Eds G. M. Blackburn, M. J. Gait, D. Loakes, D. M. Williams, *Nucleic Acids in Chemistry and Biology: Edition 3*, The Royal Society of Chemistry, Cambridge, **2006**, pp. 1–470.
3. Y. Takezawa, S. Yoneda, J.-L. H. A. Duprey, T. Nakama, M. Shionoya, *Chem. Sci.* **2016**, *7*, 3006–3010.
4. Y. Takezawa, M. Shionoya, *Acc. Chem. Res.* **2012**, *45*, 2066–2076.
5. P. Scharf, J. Müller, *ChemPlusChem* **2013**, *78*, 20–34.
6. Y. Takezawa, K. Nishiyama, T. Mashima, M. Katahira, M. Shionoya, *Chem. Eur. J.* **2015**, *21*, 14713–14716.
7. T. Kobayashi, Y. Takezawa, A. Sakamoto, M. Shionoya, *Chem. Commun.* **2016**, *52*, 3762–3765.
8. S. Johannsen, N. Megger, D. Böhme, R. K. O. Sigel, J. Müller, *Nat. Chem.* **2010**, *2*, 229–234.
9. J. Liu, Y. Lu, *Angew. Chem. Int. Ed.* **2007**, *46*, 7587–7590.
10. S. Liu, G. H. Clever, Y. Takezawa, M. Kaneko, K. Tanaka, X. Guo, M. Shionoya, *Angew. Chem. Int. Ed.* **2011**, *50*, 8886–8890.
11. B. Lippert, *Coord. Chem. Rev.* **2000**, *200–202*, 487–516.
12. K. Aoki, K. Murayama, in Interplay between Metal Ions and Nucleic Acids. Metal Ions in Life Sciences, Vol. 10 of *Metal Ions in Life Sciences*, Eds A. Sigel, H. Sigel, R. Sigel, Springer, Dordrecht, **2012**, pp. 43–102.
13. E. Sletten, *Chem. Commun.* **1967**, 1119–1120.
14. I. Imaz, M. Rubio-Martínez, J. An, I. Solé-Font, N. L. Rosi, D. Maspoch, *Chem. Commun.* **2011**, *47*, 7287–7302.
15. M. J. Rauterkus, B. Krebs, *Angew. Chem. Int. Ed.* **2004**, *43*, 1300–1303.
16. C. S. Purohit, S. Verma, *J. Am. Chem. Soc.* **2006**, *128*, 400–401.
17. J. An, S. J. Geib, N. L. Rosi, *J. Am. Chem. Soc.* **2009**, *131*, 8376–8377.
18. J. An, R. P. Fiorella, S. J. Geib, N. L. Rosi, *J. Am. Chem. Soc.* **2009**, *131*, 8401–8403.
19. D. Armentano, T. F. Mastropietro, M. Julve, R. Rossi, P. Rossi, G. De Munno, *J. Am. Chem. Soc.* **2007**, *129*, 2740–2741.
20. D. Armentano, N. Marino, T. F. Mastropietro, J. Martínez-Lillo, J. Cano, M. Julve, F. Lloret, G. De Munno, *Inorg. Chem.* **2008**, *47*, 10229–10231.
21. N. Marino, D. Armentano, T. F. Mastropietro, M. Julve, F. Lloret, G. De Munno, *Cryst. Growth Des.* **2010**, *10*, 1757–1761.

22. N. Marino, D. Armentano, E. Pardo, J. Vallejo, F. Neve, L. Di Donna, G. De Munno, *Chem. Sci.* **2015**, *6*, 4300–4315.
23. P. Zhou, J. Yao, C. Sheng, H. Li, *CrystEngComm.* **2013**, *15*, 8430–8436.
24. J. A. R. Navarro, B. Lippert, *Coord. Chem. Rev.* **1999**, *185–186*, 653–667.
25. R. K. O. Sigel, H. Sigel, *Acc. Chem. Res.* **2010**, *43*, 974–984.
26. R. K. O. Sigel, *Angew. Chem. Int. Ed.* **2007**, *46*, 654–656.
27. B. Lippert, P. J. Sanz Miguel, *Acc. Chem. Res.* **2016**, *49*, 1537–1545.
28. B. Lippert, P. J. Sanz Miguel, in Supramolecular Chemistry, Vol. 71 of *Advances in Inorganic Chemistry*, Eds R. van Eldik, R. Puchta, Elsevier, **2018**, pp. 277–326.
29. B. Lippert, P. J. Sanz Miguel, *Coord. Chem. Rev.* **2022**, *465*, 214566.
30. R. Bruno, J. Vallejo, N. Marino, G. De Munno, J. Krzystek, J. Cano, E. Pardo, D. Armentano, *Inorg. Chem.* **2017**, *56*, 1857–1864.
31. J. Thomas-Gipson, G. Beobide, O. Castillo, A. Luque, S. Perez-Yanez, P. Roman, *Eur. J. Inorg. Chem.* **2017**, 1333–1340.
32. R. Bruno, N. Marino, R. Adduci, D. Armentano, G. De Munno, *J. Coord. Chem.* **2018**, *71*, 615–632.
33. T. F. Mastropietro, D. Armentano, N. Marino, G. De Munno, J. Anastassopoulou, T. Theophanides, *Cryst. Growth Des.* **2007**, *7*, 609–612.
34. L. Mistry, P. G. Waddell, N. G. Wright, B. R. Horrocks, A. Houlton, *Inorg.Chem.* **2019**, *58*, 13346–13352.
35. G. Cervantes, J. J. Fiol, A. Terrón, V. Moreno, J. R. Alabart, M. Aguilo, M. Gomez, X. Solans, *Inorg. Chem.* **1990**, *29*, 5168–5173.
36. N. Marino, D. Armentano, G. De Munno, *Inorg. Chim. Acta* **2016**, *452*, 229–237.
37. M. A. Geday, G. De Munno, M. Medaglia, J. Anastassopoulou, T. Theophanides, *Angew. Chem., Int. Ed. Engl.* **1997**, *36*, 511–513.
38. G. De Munno, M. Medaglia, D. Armentano, J. Anastassopolou, T. Theophanides, *J. Chem. Soc., Dalton Trans.* **2000**, 1625–1629.
39. N. Marino, D. Armentano, C. Zanchini, G. De Munno, *CrystEngCom.* **2014**, *16*, 8286–8296.
40. N. Marino, R. Bruno, D. Armentano, G. De Munno, *J. Coord. Chem.* **2018**, *71*, 828–844.
41. A. Terrón, B. Moreno-Vachiano, A. Bauzá, A. García-Raso, J. J. Fiol, M. Barceló-Oliver, E. Molins, A. Frontera, *Chem. Eur. J.* **2017**, *23*, 2103–2108.
42. F. Linares, E. García-Fernández, F. J. López-Garzón, M. Domingo-García, A. Orte, A. Rodríguez-Diéguez, M. A. Galindo, *Chem. Sci.* **2019**, *10*, 1126–1137.
43. M. Sabat, K. A. Satyshur, M. Sundaralingam, *J. Am. Chem. Soc.* **1983**, *105*, 976–980.
44. D. J. Szalda, L. G. Marzilli, T. J. Kistenmacher, *Biochem. Biophys. Res. Commun.* **1975**, *63*, 601–605.
45. L. Mistry, O. El-Zubir, G. Dura, W. Clegg, P. G. Waddell, T. Pope, W. A. Hofer, N. G. Wright, B. R. Horrocks, A. Houlton, *Chem. Sci.* **2019**, *10*, 3186–3195.
46. J. Hogle, M. Sundaralingam, G. H. Y. Lin, *Acta Cryst.* **1980**, *B36*, 564–570.
47. J. Galy, A. Mosset, I. Grenthe, I. Puigdomenech, B. Sjoberg, F. Hulten, *J. Am. Chem. Soc.* **1987**, *109*, 380–386.
48. S. K. Miller, L. G. Marzilli, S. Dorre, P. Kollat, R.-D. Stigler, J. J. Stezowski, *Inorg. Chem.* **1986**, *25*, 4272–4277.
49. G. R. Clark, J. D. Orbell, *Acta Cryst.* **1978**, *B34*, 1815–1822.
50. K. Aoki, *Biochim. Biophys. Acta* **1976**, *447*, 379–381.
51. K. Aoki, W. Saenger, *J. Inorg. Biochem.* **1984**, *20*, 225–245.
52. D. M. L. Goodgame, I. Jeeves, C. Reynolds, A. C. Skapski, *Biochem. J.* **1975**, *151*, 467–468.

53. J. K. Shiba, R. Bau. *Inorg. Chem.* **1978**, *17*, 3484–3488.
54. K. Aoki, *J. Chem. Soc., Chem. Commun.* **1976**, 748–749.
55. A. Terrón, L. Tomàs, A. Bauzá, A. García-Raso, J. J. Fiol, E. Molins, A. Frontera, *CrystEngComm* **2017**, *19*, 5830–5834.
56. T. Hashimoto, H. Kimura, H. Nakatsu, K. Maruoka, *J. Org. Chem.* **2011**, *76*, 6030–6037.
57. K. Aikawa, M. Kojima, K. Mikami, *Angew. Chem. Int. Ed.* **2009**, *48*, 6073–6077.
58. Q.-m. Qiu, P. Zhou, L. Gu, L. Hao, M. Liu, H. Li, *Chem. Eur. J.* **2017**, *23*, 7201–7206.
59. P. Zhou, C. Wang, Q-m. Qiu, J.-f. Yao, C.-f. Sheng, H. Li, *Dalton Trans.* **2015**, *44*, 17810–17818.
60. P. Zhou, R. Shi, J.-f. Yao, C.-f. Sheng, H. Li, *Coord. Chem. Rev.* **2015**, *292*, 107–143.
61. B. Yang, R. R. Wu, G. Berden, J. Oomens, M. T. Rodgers, *J. Phys. Chem.* **2013**, *B117*, 14191–14201.
62. O. O. Brovarets, D. M. Hovorun, *Phys. Chem. Chem. Phys.* **2015**, *17*, 21381–21388.
63. C. Chen, *Langmuir* **2012**, *28*, 17743–17748.
64. C. Tamura, S. Sato, T. Hata, *Bull. Chem. Soc. Jpn.* **1973**, *46*, 2388–2394.
65. F. Fujinami, K. Ogawa, K. Arakawa, S. Shirotake, S. Fujii, K. Tomita, *Acta Cryst.* **1979**, *B35*, 968–970.
66. T. J. Kistenmacher, M. Rossi, J. P. Caradonna, L. G. Marzilli, *Adv. Mol. Relaxation Interact. Processes* **1979**, *15*, 119–133.
67. T. J. Kistemacher, M. Rossi, L. G. Marizilli, *Biopolymers* **1978**, *17*, 2581–2585.
68. S. Vijay-Kumar, T. D. Sakore, H. M. Sobell, *Nucleic Acids Res.* **1984**, *12*, 3649–3657.
69. A. Schimanski, E. Freisinger, A. Erxleben, B. Lippert, *Inorg. Chim. Acta* **1998**, *283*, 223–232.
70. K. Aoki, *J. Chem. Soc., Chem. Commun.* **1979**, 589–591.
71. S. Louie, R. Bau, *J. Am. Chem. Soc.* **1977**, *99*, 3874–3876.
72. R. Bruno, T. F. Mastropietro, G. De Munno, E. Pardo, D. Armentano, *J. Coord. Chem.* **2021**, *74*, 200–215.
73. E. C. Constable, *Chem. Soc. Rev.* **2013**, *42*, 1637–1651.
74. Nomenclature of Inorganic Chemistry. IUPAC Recommendations 2005 at http://old.iupac.org/publications/books/rbook/Red_Book_2005.pdf.
75. R. Bruno, T. F. Mastropietro, G. De Munno, D. Armentano, *Molecules* **2021**, *26*, 4594–4606.
76. R. Bruno, N. Marino, L. Bartella, L. Di Donna, G. De Munno, E. Pardo, D. Armentano, *Chem. Commun.* **2018**, *54*, 6356–6359.

3 Coordination Polymers with Nucleobase Derivatives
From Electronic Nanodevices to Sensors

Noelia Maldonado
Department of Inorganic Chemistry, Autonomous University of Madrid, E-28049 Madrid, Spain
noelia.maldonado@uam.es

Pilar Amo-Ochoa
Department of Inorganic Chemistry, Autonomous University of Madrid, E-28049 Madrid, Spain
Institute for Advanced Research in Chemistry at UAM (IAdChem), Universidad Autónoma de Madrid, E-28049 Madrid, Spain
pilar.amo@uam.es

CONTENTS

1	Introduction		52
2	Nucleobase Versatility and Dynamic Coordination Bonds		55
	2.1	Versatility of Nucleobase Derivatives	55
	2.2	Supramolecular Interactions and Molecular Recognition Ability	56
	2.3	Stimulus-Responsive CPs Based on Nucleobase Derivatives	57
3	Additive Properties due to the Presence of Metal Ions		58
	3.1	The Magnetism of CPs Based on Nucleobase Derivatives	59
	3.2	Electrical Conductivity of CPs Based on Nucleobase Derivatives	60
		3.2.1 Electrical Conductivity CPs Using Nucleobase Derivatives as Bridging Ligands	61
		3.2.2 Electrical Conductivity Using Nucleobase Derivatives as Terminal Ligands	63

4   Nano Processing of CPs Based on Nucleobase Derivatives:
     Potential Applications... 65
     4.1   Semiconductors Based on Nano-CPs with Nucleobase
            Derivatives: Electronic Nanodevices.. 66
     4.2   Soft Materials and Composites Based on Nano-CPs with
            Nucleobase Derivatives: Stimulus-Responsive Properties 67
            4.2.1   Colloids and Metal-Organic Gels (MOGs) Based
                     on Nano-CPs with Nucleobase Derivatives for
                     Sensor Applications 67
            4.2.2   MOAs Based on nano-CPs with Nucleobase
                     Derivatives for Selective Separation of Drugs 71
            4.2.3   Composites Based on Nano-CPs with Nucleobase
                     Derivatives as Sensors Devices....................................... 73
5   General Conclusions 74
Acknowledgments.. 75
Abbreviations and Definitions 75
References.. 76

ABSTRACT

This chapter describes how coordination polymers (CPs) based on modified nucleobases constitute a new area of research with interesting ramifications and a growing number of new compounds. The versatility of these ligands, their molecular recognition capability, the metal-ligand dynamic bonds, and the additive properties provided by the metal ions allow creating multifunctional compounds with amazing properties. In addition, their high insolubility in the reaction media enable these CPs to be nanoprocessed and to generate colloids, gels, and metal-organic aerogels through bottom-up approaches. Furthermore, they allow the use of external stimuli such as temperature or ultrasound. Additionally, the modification of the nucleobases permits increasing their versatility, enabling the binding of the metallic centers to positions that do not interfere with the pyrimidine/purine residue, generating infinite entities with magnetic, electrical, or optical properties, and the ability of selective molecular recognition. As a whole, in this chapter, we can see how these new CPs provide interesting applications as materials that respond to stimuli, are useful in the manufacture of sensors that can be printed in 3D such as composite materials, are useful as well as electronic nanodevices, drug nanocarriers, single-chain magnets, light-emitting devices, metal ions detectors, or as stationary phases in high-pressure separation columns for selective separation of drugs, among others.

KEYWORDS

Coordination Polymers; Molecular Recognition; Nanodevices; Nucleobases; Stimulus-Responsive Materials; Metal-Organic Gels; Metal-Organic Aerogels; Sensors

1   INTRODUCTION

For decades, coordination compounds formed by binding metal ions to nucleobases/nucleic acids have attracted significant attention. These compounds can act

Coordination Polymers: From Electronic Nanodevices to Sensors

as biomimetic models used for understanding the biological effect of metal ions. Moreover, they represent an important area of research at the frontiers of bioinorganic chemistry, supramolecular coordination chemistry, and deoxyribonucleic acid (DNA) nanotechnology [1]. Indeed, the systematic studies on metal ion-nucleobase interactions have generated many interesting directions of research [2].

The structural features of nucleobases and their derivatives (Figure 1) have allowed going beyond basic coordination chemistry, achieving more extensive and more complex architectures based on the formation of supramolecules. Selective binding of metal ions to single nucleobases or additional ligands leads to the formation of "infinite" structures, depending on base-pairing interactions and coordination bonds formed. These infinite architectures, whose chemistry dates back to the late 19th century with the so-called Werner complexes [3] and Hofmann clathrates [4], were not defined as "coordination polymers (CPs)" until 1963 [5]. In the subject that concerns us, these ordered infinite structures, formed

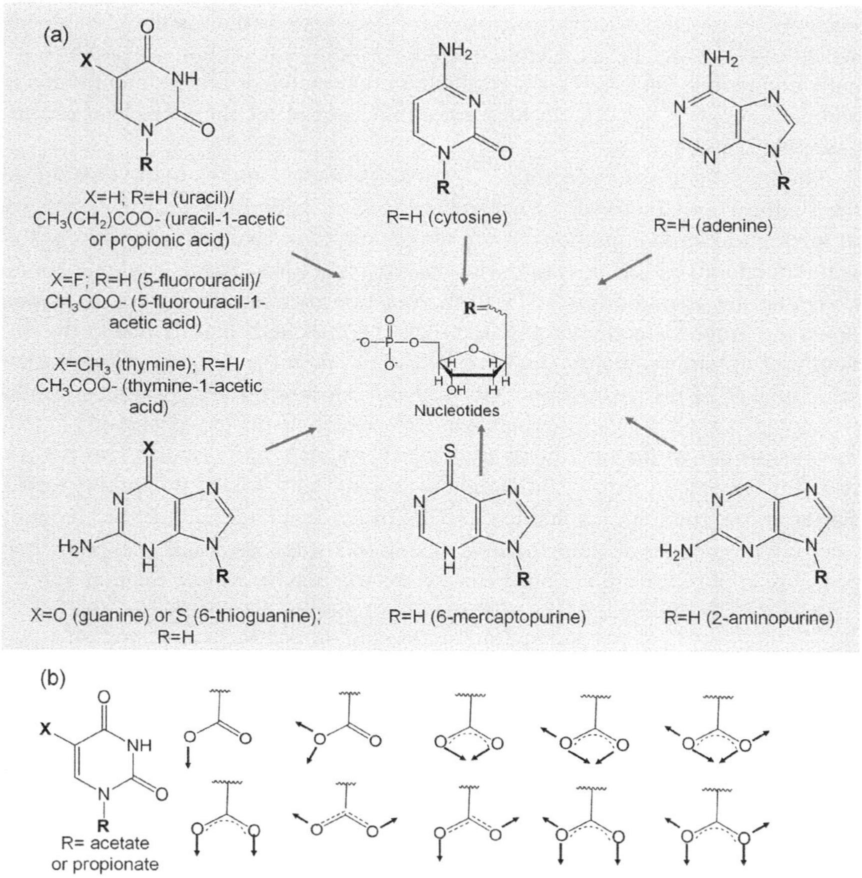

FIGURE 1 The basic structures of pyrimidine and purine nucleobases and their derivatives presented in this chapter (a). General coordination modes of the carboxylate oxygen atoms in modified pyrimidine nucleobases (b).

by nodes (metal ions) and linkers (nucleobases and derivatives), can generate extended networks of different dimensionalities (1D, 2D, or 3D), with numerous supramolecular interactions depending on the selected nucleobase. Moreover, the binding of the building blocks and supramolecular interactions will define the final properties of the CP [6].

By themselves, CPs have interesting characteristics, such as their high insolubility in the reaction media, which facilitates nanoprocessing of these compounds through bottom-up approaches [7, 8]. Additionally, modification of the synthetic conditions for getting CPs facilitates the creation of new phases of the same CP such as the well-known metal-organic gels (MOGs) or the corresponding Metal-Organic Aerogels (MOAs) obtained using supercritical CO_2 [9]. Moreover, their dynamic bonds allow the design of stimulus-responsive CPs [10, 11], and the correct selection of the organic ligands (nucleobases and derivatives) makes it possible to obtain CPs capable of selective molecular recognition [12].

Creating CPs with multidisciplinary applications, with linkers based on nucleobases and their derivatives, can be a great option because nucleobases are structurally diverse, have different metal ion binding sites (Figure 1), are biologically compatible, and are easily available in reasonable quantities and prices. In addition, some of these molecules are chiral, and all of them are able to self-assemble [13–15].

These advantages can facilitate CPs with biological applications. Thereby, in the synthesis of CPs based on nucleobases and their derivatives, it is necessary to work under mild conditions (room temperature), in an aqueous or poorly solvating medium, and, if possible, with one-step reactions. These synthetic conditions and the insolubility of CPs in the reaction medium have initially slowed down the progress in studying these types of compounds mainly due to the difficulty of obtaining quality single crystals that allow the determination of their structures by X-ray diffraction (XRD) [9, 16]. However, the appearance of new technologies such as hydrothermal synthesis, which favors the formation of quality crystals due to the modification of solvent (density and viscosity) properties, or improvements in the crystallization processes, have solved this problem [16]. Furthermore, the high insolubility of CPs in the reaction medium has recently allowed these materials to be nanoprocessed in a single step and to expand their potential applications in various fields, as we will see below (see Section 4).

Along with the application of natural and modified nucleobases, the use of transition metal ions and lanthanoids stands out among the most commonly used metal ions as nodes because they offer a wide variety of oxidation states and coordination numbers. Additionally, their inherent properties, such as magnetism, conductivity, or luminescence, increase the number of possible applications of these CPs [17].

These exciting options have opened up new and more current research paths with fields still little explored despite the long existence of CPs and the many CPs published to date. Currently, the research tries to reduce the gap between academia and business. For this reason, it will combine the exciting properties that custom-designed CPs can present with new methodologies and technologies.

2 NUCLEOBASE VERSATILITY AND DYNAMIC COORDINATION BONDS

2.1 Versatility of Nucleobase Derivatives

The structural versatility of these ligands can offer a variety of interesting molecular structures and supramolecular assemblies. A wide range of nucleobase-derived molecules (Figure 1) emerge that have been designed, synthesized, and functionalized to preserve the specific H-bonds between complementary nucleobases and to increase the stability of the materials containing them [18–20]. Indeed, the modifications of nucleobases would increase the structural possibilities by adding other coordination modes [1] (Figure 1b).

In this regard, the use of uracil- or thymine-1-acetic acid under solvothermal conditions led to the creation of different 1D- and 2D-CPs with formulae $[Cu_2(TAcO)_2(C_2O_4)(4,4'-bipy)]_n \cdot 4nH_2O$ (CP1), $[Cu_2(UAcO)_2(C_2O_4)(4,4'-bipy)]_n \cdot 2nH_2O$ (CP2) and $[Cu_2(TAcO)_2(4,4'-bipy)]_n$ (CP3) (4,4'-bipy = 4,4'-bipyridine; UAcO = uracil-1-acetate; TAcO = thymine-1-acetate; C_2O_4 = oxalate) [21]. In all cases, nucleobases are coordinated to copper ions through the oxygen atoms of the carboxylate group of the pyrimidine residue, leaving the nucleobases free (terminal) along the chains with their molecular recognition capability unaltered. Therefore, in these CPs, the nucleobases can establish complementary H-bonding interactions among themselves (Figure 2) to provide the final 3D crystal structure.

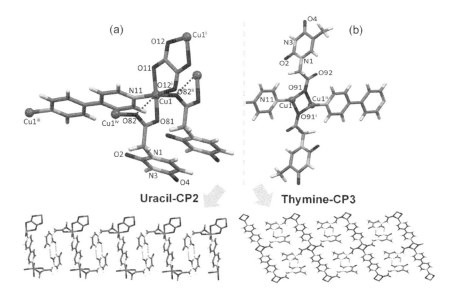

FIGURE 2 Molecular structure of the 2D- and 1D-coordination polymers CP2 (a) and CP3 (b). Copper(II) coordination environment (top) and crystal packing (bottom). Blue dotted lines correspond to nucleobase-nucleobase pairing. (Adapted by permission from Ref. [21]; copyright 2019, Elsevier.)

2.2 SUPRAMOLECULAR INTERACTIONS AND MOLECULAR RECOGNITION ABILITY

This section highlights the importance of combining coordination bonds (dynamic bonds) with non-covalent bonds and the molecular recognition capability of the nucleobases and their derivatives. These characteristics have great relevance in the preparation of complex tunable molecular architectures with stimuli-responsive properties [22]. From hydrogen bonds, through π-π interactions, or purely ionic bonds and hydrophobic effects, the versatility of non-covalent bonds offers differences in strength, bond formation kinetics, and directionality that allow choosing the proper interaction for the desired purpose.

As it is well-known, examples of versatile supramolecular interactions are found in the interaction between the two strands of DNA or ribonucleic acid (RNA). These are essentially mediated by five nucleobases: adenine (A), thymine (T), guanine (G), cytosine (C), and uracil (U), with predominant Watson and Crick-type pairing between the A-T, A-U and C-G bases, and with interactions via two (A-T) or three (G-C) hydrogen bonds. As a result, 28 pairing modes between the five nucleobases that involve two hydrogen bonds at least, including reverse Watson-Crick, Hoogsteen, and "wobble" pairing, are feasible [23]. If metallic entities (e.g., Pt or Ag) and nucleobase derivatives with functional groups (e.g., 9-methylguanine or 9-methyladenine) that allow metal coordination are used [24, 25], the number of new types of supramolecular aggregates can be increased and stabilized by non-traditional H-bond formation [26–28].

One of the main goals in this H-bond formation is to extrapolate the behavior of biological systems to new CPs [12, 28], thereby achieving highly selective and directional-specific interactions. These can be established via molecular recognition to define the supramolecular polymers' size, direction, or dimension and, in turn, interact with host molecules resulting in new materials that may have fascinating applications in drug transport, self-healing response, or elastomeric properties by mimicking biological systems [6, 9, 29]. For this purpose, modified nucleobases have become an exciting option to coordinate directly with metal ions without compromising the nucleobase H-bonding positions. An example of a CP with molecular recognition capability has been obtained using thymine-1-acetic acid (TAcOH) [12]. The authors have presented a new biocompatible Cu(II) 1D-CP, with the formula $[Cu(TAcO)_2(4,4'\text{-bipy})(H_2O)]_n \cdot 2nH_2O$ (CP4). CP4 can recognize adenine oligonucleotide chains selectively and transport them to cells. In this experiment, five different chains, poly(dA), poly(dT), poly(dG), poly(dC), and a scrambled oligonucleotide sequence (SCR) chain were incubated with this CP. As a result, the authors found that the CP4 has a higher affinity to the poly(dA) chain than to any of the other chains (Figure 3a). These results support the potential use of CPs with modified nucleobases as platforms for the interaction with oligonucleotides via Watson-Crick base pairs and/or more complex interactions, such as non-canonical base pairs and metal-nucleobase interactions. To test its biocompatibility, its toxicity was evaluated in different cell lines, such as uveal melanoma pancreatic (C918), pancreatic cancer (Panc-1), and

Coordination Polymers: From Electronic Nanodevices to Sensors

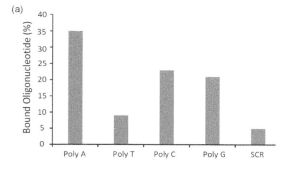

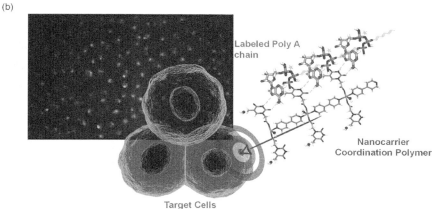

FIGURE 3 (a) Affinity of $[Cu(TAcO)_2(4,4'-bipy)(H_2O)]_n \cdot 2nH_2O$ against different oligonucleotide sequences represented as % of the bound material. (b) Representation of the CP4 transporting the labeled poly(dA) chain into the cell and fluorescence microscopy image of C918 cells treated with the CP4/poly(dA)-fluorescein system. (Adapted by permission from Ref. [12]; copyright 2017 Wiley-VCH Verlag GmbH & Co. KGaA, Weinheim.)

non-tumoral cells (HaCaT), showing some cytotoxicity (80% viability) at a concentration of 200 μm. Given these satisfactory results, this CP was explored as a cellular vehicle for fluorescein-labeled poly(dA) chain to cells (Figure 3b), which were incubated with both labeled poly(dA) chain alone and combined with the CP. The study revealed that the poly(dA) chain alone was not able to interact with the cells, while cells treated with $[Cu(TAcO)_2(4,4'-bipy)(H_2O)]_n \cdot 2nH_2O$ showed a clear fluorescence signal in the cells (Figure 3b).

2.3 Stimulus-Responsive CPs Based on Nucleobase Derivatives

Together with the structural versatility offered by nucleobases, CPs present an additional interest, namely their ability to behave as stimulus-responsive materials as a consequence of their highly dynamic coordination bonds. The structural dynamics of these compounds are influenced by many physical and chemical factors such as the type of solvent, temperature, pH, ligand competition, or stoichiometry [30–37].

The choice of solvent is a crucial factor since the solubilization of the starting reagents and the ease of synthesis under mild conditions depend on it. Still, the solvent molecules can act as ligands, in turn, by forming part of the final structure. This can affect the coordination geometry, modifying the topology or pore size depending on the size and the polarity of the used solvent [35] and, therefore, the final properties of the CP.

In water, the pH is a vital stimulus due to the presence of (1) acidic or basic groups in the nucleobases themselves [36, 37], (2) functional groups in the nucleobase derivatives, and (3) the lability of the coordination bonds as a function of pH. Thus, adjusting and varying the pH of the reaction medium can be a factor to be taken into account to direct the reaction and to obtain the desired products. This idea has been reported in the case of the reaction of TAcOH with copper(II) acetate or chloride, carried out at 25°C and different pHs. The pH variation led to the formation of two one-dimensional (1D) CPs $[Cu(TAcO)_2(H_2O)_2]_n$ (pH 2) and $[Cu_{1.5}(TAcO)_2(H_2O)(OH)]_n \cdot 4nH_2O$ (pH 5), while more forcing reaction conditions (reflux and pH 5) favored the synthesis of a discrete complex $[Cu(TAcO)_2(H_2O)_4] \cdot 4H_2O$ [36].

Besides the pH- and solvent-dependent stimulus response of CPs designed *à la carte,* the correct selection of ligands and ligand competition can also be useful tools to generate new species of high added value. Using these principles, Vegas et al. [37] have designed nucleobase-derived CPs with notable anti-cancer activity. They synthesized in a single step at pH 2.5 two isostructural 1D-CPs of Cu(II). Both compounds, with chemical formulae $[Cu_2(UAcO)_4(4,4'-bipy)_2]_n \cdot 3nH_2O$ (CP5) and $[Cu_2(5\text{-FUAcO})_4(4,4'-bipy)_2]_n \cdot 4nH_2O$ (CP6), were synthesized using uracil-1-acetic acid (UAcOH) and the anti-cancer derivative 5-fluorouracil acetic acid (5-FUAcOH), respectively. Although both CPs are chemically stable in water between pH 4 and 7, with slight morphological modifications, both undergo hydrolysis in biological media (Dulbecco's Modified Eagle Medium, DMEM or Roswell Park Memorial Institute, RPMI, pH=7.2), generating new Cu(II) and Cu(I) species. These biological media are composed of biomolecules that compete with the CP's ligands, giving rise to a mixture of the new species. The newly generated compounds and their proportions are critical for their cytotoxic activity and are also vital to rationalize the different cytotoxicities of both compounds against melanoma (Mel202) and pancreas (Pac-1) cancer cells. CP6 shows a remarkable increase in cell toxicity and reactive oxygen species (ROS) production compared to CP5 (Figure 4), possibly due to the release of the antitumor-active 5-fluorouracil [37].

3 ADDITIVE PROPERTIES DUE TO THE PRESENCE OF METAL IONS

The presence of metal ions as nodes along the CP chains has expanded their stimulus-responsive and molecular recognition properties. Indeed, metal ions can

Coordination Polymers: From Electronic Nanodevices to Sensors 59

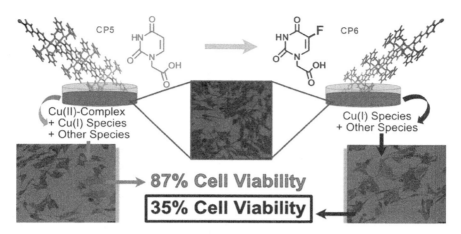

FIGURE 4 Schematic illustration of effects of CP5 and CP6 complexes incubated in biological media at pH 7.2 for treatment of cancer cells. (Reproduced by permission from Ref. [37] (https://doi.org/10.1021/acsami.1c11612); copyright 2021, American Chemical Society. Further permission related to the material excerpted should be directed to the ACS.)

give additional properties such as electrical conductivity, magnetism, or luminescence [17, 38–42], allowing to create multifunctional materials with applications in electronic or sensor devices, among others [43–45]. So, in the design of these types of CPs, the search for synergy in the properties of rationally chosen building blocks should be a major goal.

3.1 The Magnetism of CPs Based on Nucleobase Derivatives

Up to now, studies concerning the magnetism of CPs with nucleobases are mainly based on single-chain magnets [38–42], and superexchange [12, 21, 32, 36, 37], in which strong antiferromagnetic coupling occurs between two nearest-neighbor cations through an anion, or on the direct exchange, which occurs without an intermediate anion, and that in some cases can lead to metamagnetization of the compound [32, 36]. A representative example was the study of the magnetic properties of the 1D thymine- and uracil-modified-Cu(II) CPs, $[Cu_{1.5}(TAcO)_2(H_2O)(OH)]_n \cdot 4nH_2O$ (Figure 5a) and $[Cu_3(UPrO)_2Cl_2(OH)_2(H_2O)_2]_n$ (Figure 5c). Despite presenting very similar chain structures, Cu(II) centers of both CPs showed very different magnetic properties. Moderate-weak antiferromagnetic interactions between Cu(II) atoms were found in compound $[Cu_{1.5}(TAcO)_2(H_2O)(OH)]_n \cdot 4nH_2O$, while a combination of strong and weak antiferromagnetic interactions was found in compound $[Cu_3(UPrO)_2Cl_2(OH)_2(H_2O)_2]_n$. From quantum density functional theory (DFT) calculations, authors estimated the magnetic coupling constants for each magnetic superexchange: $J_1 = +28 \, cm^{-1}$ (weakly ferromagnetic), $J_2 = +36 \, cm^{-1}$, $J_3 = -8 \, cm^{-1}$ (Figure 5b) for compound $[Cu_{1.5}(TAcO)_2(H_2O)(OH)]_n \cdot 4nH_2O$ and $J_1 = -295 \, cm^{-1}$ (strongly antiferromagnetic), $J_2 = -18 \, cm^{-1}$, $J_3 = -27 \, cm^{-1}$ (Figure 5d) for compound $[Cu_3(UPrO)_2Cl_2(OH)_2(H_2O)_2]_n$. In compound $[Cu_{1.5}(TAcO)_2(H_2O)(OH)]_n \cdot$

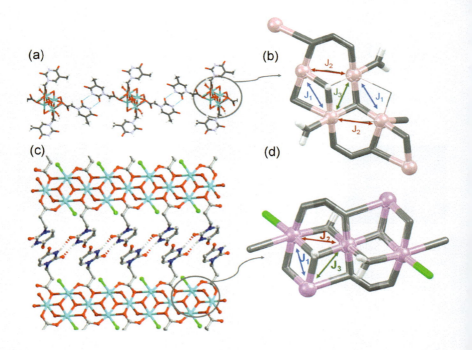

FIGURE 5 Fragments of the polymeric chains of $[Cu_{1.5}(TAcO)_2(H_2O)(OH)]_n \cdot 4nH_2O$ (a) and $[Cu_3(UPrO)_2Cl_2(OH)_2(H_2O)_2]_n$ (c), showing T-T/U-U base pairing between adjacent chains. Proposed magnetic superexchange pathways for $[Cu_{1.5}(TAcO)_2(H_2O)(OH)]_n \cdot 4nH_2O$ (b) and $[Cu_3(UPrO)_2Cl_2(OH)_2(H_2O)_2]_n$ (d). The core is highlighted with different colors (copper ions in pink, ligands in gray; modified thymine has been omitted for clarity). (Adapted by permission from Ref. [36]; copyright 2013, American Chemical Society.)

$4nH_2O$, the carboxylate group is coordinated in a basal (short, 1.945(2) Å)-axial (long, 2.624(2) Å) bridging mode, leading to almost zero overlaps between the two magnetic orbitals centered on the metal, resulting in weak anti- or ferromagnetic coupling [36].

3.2 Electrical Conductivity of CPs Based on Nucleobase Derivatives

In 2012, Givaja et al. carried out an extensive review on CPs with electrical properties [45]. As they described, the CPs exhibit many advantages by offering a wide range of structural binding motifs. Moreover, unlike amorphous organic polymers, the CPs possess long-range crystal order, offering a powerful platform to study the intrinsic properties of charge generation, transport, and recombination. Additionally, that contribution also helped to investigate structure-function relationships to guide the design of new conductive materials and to optimize their performance as electrical or optoelectronic devices. That publication

Coordination Polymers: From Electronic Nanodevices to Sensors 61

already described the first studies of CPs based on nucleobases and their derivatives with electrical properties, with just a couple of examples focused on CPs with nucleobases acting as bridging ligands, yet none with nucleobases acting as terminal ligands. Since that time, new examples have been published showing interest in this subject.

3.2.1 Electrical Conductivity CPs Using Nucleobase Derivatives as Bridging Ligands

The first studies using CPs derived from modified nucleobases as possible conductive materials were published in the 1990s and were based on the intention of generating structurally simplified analogs of the new M-DNA variety previously published [46]. In these systems, electrical conductivity was considered possible as a consequence of the presence of metallic ions along the DNA double helix. The so-called M-DNA (Figure 6a) was formed by divalent ions such as Zn, Co,

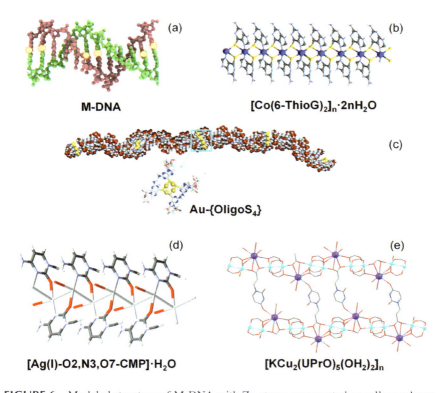

FIGURE 6 Modeled structure of M-DNA with Zn atoms represented as yellow spheres (a); fragment of the polymeric chain in [Co(6-ThioG)$_2$]$_n$·2nH$_2$O, where Co atoms are represented in dark blue and water solvation molecules have been omitted for clarity (b); fragment of DNA-semiconductor strands Au-{oligo-S$_4$} formed by metal-ion-induced self-assembly (c). (Adapted by permission from Ref. [52], copyright 2017, The Author(s).) [Ag(I)-*O2,N3,O7*-CMP]·H$_2$O (d) and [KCu$_2$(UPrO)$_5$(OH$_2$)$_2$]$_n$ (e).

or Ni, and was maintained throughout the DNA structure at pH values above 8. Following this idea, a coordination polymer based on Cd(II) and 6-mercaptopurine $[Cd(6-MP)_2·2H_2O]_n$ (6-MP=6-mercaptopurine) (Figure 8b) had been synthesized, which represented a simplified structural analog of this M-DNA [47]. However, this CP, with M···M distances of 3.918 Å, displayed insulating behavior as explained by the large band gap existing between the HOMO and LUMO levels. The DFT calculations helped to design new isostructural 1D-CPs of formula $[M(6-MP)_2·2H_2O]_n$ where M = Ni(II), Co(II), Cu(II), Fe(II). The band-gap energy values were calculated to predict an improvement in electrical conductivity by modifying the metal center [48]. According to the theoretical results, the corresponding coordination polymer with M = Ni(II) was synthesized ($[Ni(6-MP)_2·2H_2O]_n$), and another analogous CP was synthesized using 6-thioguanine (6-ThioGH) $[Ni(6-ThioG)_2·2H_2O]_n$ [49, 50]. In all of them, the nucleobase is deprotonated, acting as a bridging ligand and connecting the metal centers at short M···M distances (3.677 and 3.646 Å). Their electrical conductivity measurements in single crystals by direct current (DC) gave values of 1.10×10^{-5} and 1.34×10^{-4} S cm^{-1}, respectively. These studies continued with cobalt(II), since it offered interesting possibilities for its inclusion in these thiopurine systems, and resulted in the formation of a CP of composition $[Co(6-ThioG)_2]_n·2nH_2O$ (Figure 6b), with electrical conductivity in the range 10^{-6} to 10^{-7} S cm^{-1} at 400 K [51]. The obtained experimental data agree with the results expected from the DFT calculations.

Later investigations in this area allowed to obtain a metal-organic gel (see Section 4.2.1) based on the spontaneous assembly between Au(I) and a derivative of the nucleoside 6-thioguanosine, 6-thiodeoxyguanosine, which acts as a bridging ligand. This combination results in a gel, composed of luminescent helical chains structurally analogous to DNA. Structural analysis was mainly performed by XRD using a simplified Rietveld method, obtaining bond lengths of 1.87, 2.31, and 3.18 Å, assigned to the C–S, Au–S, and Au···Au distances, respectively, and a larger distance (17.6 Å) that could be interpreted as the diameter of the helix. Modeling of the molecular structure, based on the experimental data, showed a central polymeric Au(I)-thiolate backbone, around which the nucleobase and ribose groups extend, and the resulting helical polymer is strikingly similar in size, topology, and surface functionality to the DNA duplex (Figure 6c). DFT calculations of the electronic structure showed substantial delocalization of the HOMO, including major contributions from the ${Au-\mu-S}_n$ backbone, as well as minor contributions from the π-system of the nucleobase. When a single electron is removed from the system and the spin density is calculated in the same geometry, it also showed delocalization in the ${Au-\mu-S}_n$ chain and in the nucleobase. The changes in the average atomic partial charges are larger for the gold-thiolate backbone, but with some contribution from the nucleobase. Taken together, these results suggested that oxidative doping of the material could produce a conductive material, since this material *per se* did not show any relevant conductivity. Experimentally, this material could be transformed into a conductive stranded species by the oxidative doping method, increasing the conductivity by at least two orders of magnitude after treatment. This semiconducting device could be easily incorporated coaxially into the structural framework of DNA, since the chain assembly occurs by selective coordination of the metal ion with the modified guanine nucleoside. This assembly produces individual structures of Au-{oligo-S$_4$}, which can be concatenated and extended in length to several mm involving thousands of individual DNA duplexes [52].

In addition to guanine derivatives, the use of cytosine derivatives as bridging ligands has been used to assemble metal ions, mainly Ag(I), as they can form continuous helical strands via complementary hydrogen bonding and argentophilic interactions, remarkably similar to those of a DNA-Ag duplex. These compounds are promising in this field, although as above, these types of supramolecular architecture do not appear to be good electrical conductors despite their micrometer lengths and short M···M distances. To try to alleviate this fact, a study focused on the synthesis of a 3D-MOF with the cytidine-5′-monophosphate (CMP) nucleotide, ([Ag-(*O2,N3*-Cyt)]$^+$)$_n$ (Figure 6d), showing that Ag···Ag distances can be modulated by substitution of the solvent occluded in the channels of this compound, and leading to distances within 5% of the metallic distance. However, this structure did not present any conductivity but rather proved to be an effective insulator. The authors found the explanation for this behavior through DFT data when calculating the projected ground-state density of states in the central silver ions and the surrounding organic structure. In this study, it was found that the band-gap energy at the Fermi level was 3.32 eV (373 nm) and that the HOMO state has a large population in the central silver ions, but the LUMO state is mainly distributed in the organic structure. Thus, although the Ag···Ag distances are very short, they are insufficient to produce conductivity since the Ag ions are not populated near the Fermi energy [53].

Otherwise, the recent use of other pyrimidine-derived nucleobases capable of acting both as a bridging ligand and as a terminal ligand, has yielded CPs with interesting conductivity, as in the case of the 2D-CP of formula [KCu$_2$(UPrO)$_5$(OH$_2$)$_2$]$_n$, composed of parallel paddlewheel chains. In this structure, copper dimers are bonded through a bridging carboxylate group of the modified uracil ligands and K$^+$ cations. These chains are linked by neighboring ones via K$^+$ ions, which bridge oxygen groups of the heterocyclic uracil rings, showing a conductivity of 8.3×10^{-7} S cm^{-1} (Figure 6e) [35].

3.2.2 Electrical Conductivity Using Nucleobase Derivatives as Terminal Ligands

As we have already commented, one of the objectives of modifying nucleobases is to provide them with functional groups liable to be coordinated with metal ions to retain the positions of molecular recognition in the basic skeleton of nucleobases. For this purpose, modified pyrimidine bases such as TAcOH and uracil-1-propionic acid (UPrOH) have offered encouraging results with respect to the conductance of the resulting CPs. Using these ligands, the group of Amo-Ochoa and Zamora has been reporting since 2013 a series of novel CPs, where these modified nucleobase ligands form extended networks that connect metal ions via bridging carboxylate groups attached to the nucleobase. These constructs self-assemble through the nitrogenous bases to give their final 3D structures. For instance, 1D-CPs of formulae $[Cu(TacO)_2(H_2O)_2]_n$, $[Cu_{1.5}(TacO)_2(H_2O)(OH)]_n \cdot 4nH_2O$ and $[Cu_3(UprO)_2Cl_2(OH)_2(H_2O)_2]_n$ were designed [36], whose semiconductor behavior and conductivity values (10^{-6} to 10^{-9} S cm^{-1} at 300 K) were analyzed. Compound $[Cu(TAcO)_2(H_2O)_2]_n$ is a double-bridge 1D-polymer, in which TAcO ligands are forced to occupy the empty coordination sites in an elongated octahedral geometry, and its carboxylate groups adopt a μ-1κO:2κO coordination mode (Figure 7a). These ligands are projected outward from the 1D chain which allows the establishment of complementary hydrogen bonding interactions, resulting in 2D supramolecular sheets. Compound $[Cu_{1.5}(TAcO)_2(H_2O)(OH)]_n \cdot 4nH_2O$ is also a 1D polymer in which TAcO ligands bridge adjacent metal centers showing different coordination modes (μ_3-1κO:2κO:3$\kappa O'$ and μ-1κO:2κO). They remain available to establish additional supramolecular interactions (Figure 5a). Unlike these thymine-based CPs, the compound $[Cu_3(UPrO)_2Cl_2(OH)_2(H_2O)_2]_n$ is composed of modified uracil ligands (UPrO), which act as a monoanionic ligand with both carboxylate oxygen atoms coordinated to the copper ions differently. One of them binds in a monodentate fashion to Cu, whereas the other one bridges adjacent copper centers, giving rise to an overall tridentate coordination mode (μ_3-1κO:2κO:3$\kappa O'$) (Figures 5a and 7b).

Apart from functionalizing the nucleobases, another strategy might be the simultaneous use of a second ligand in the reaction that acts as a bridge.

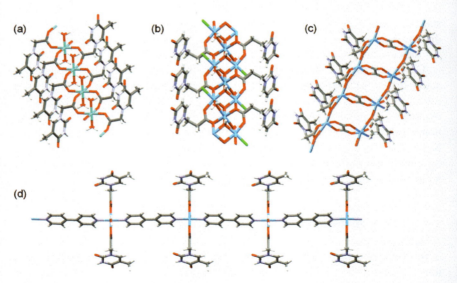

FIGURE 7 Structural chain fragments of CPs $[Cu(TAcO)_2(H_2O)_2]_n$ (a), $[Cu_3(UPrO)_2Cl_2(OH)_2(H_2O)_2]_n$ (b), $[Cu_2(TAcO)_2(C_2O_4)(4,4'\text{-bipy})]_n \cdot 4nH_2O$ (c) and $[Cu(TAcO)_2(4,4'\text{-bipy})(H_2O)]_n \cdot 2nH_2O$ (d). Copper atoms are colored in blue, oxygen atoms in red, nitrogen atoms in violet, chlorine atoms in green, carbon atoms in gray, and hydrogen atoms in white.

This is the case in 1D-CP with the formula [Cu(TAcO)$_2$(4,4′-bipy)(H$_2$O)]$_n$·2nH$_2$O (Figure 7d). Its conductivity was measured in several single crystals, giving values of about 10^{-6} S cm^{-1} [12]. The CP structure shows 4,4′-bipy acting as bridging ligands and the modified thymine residues as lateral ligands, with the peculiarity of being coordinated in a monodentate fashion. Subsequently, three more Cu(II)-CPs with TAcOH and UAcOH, respectively were synthesized [21]. Two of these CPs, [Cu$_2$(TAcO)$_2$(C$_2$O$_4$)(4,4′-bipy)]$_n$·4nH$_2$O and [Cu$_2$(UAcO)$_2$(C$_2$O$_4$)(4,4′-bipy)]$_n$·2nH$_2$O, with analogous two-dimensional structures in which, in addition to the 4,4′-bipy, the oxalate ligand (C$_2$O$_4^{2-}$) is acting as a bridging ligand, exhibited a conductivity of 5.0×10^{-9} and 3.4×10^{-11} S cm^{-1}. In contrast, the third one, a 1D-CP with the formula [Cu$_2$(TAcO)$_2$(4,4′-bipy)]$_n$, showed a conductivity of 1.8×10^{-7} S cm^{-1}. To corroborate the semiconductor behavior of [Cu$_2$(TAcO)$_2$(C$_2$O$_4$)(4,4′-bipy)]$_n$·4nH$_2$O (Figure 7c), a study of conductivity versus temperature (from 300 to 373 K) showed an increase in conductivity from 5.1×10^{-9} to 9.4×10^{-7} S cm^{-1}. The conductivity was evaluated in the presence of a p-type dopant agent such as iodine for 13 h, showing an increase by two orders of magnitude (from 5.1×10^{-9} to 1.1×10^{-7} S cm^{-1}). In this case, it can be assumed that the conductivity enhancement takes place through a mechanism involving an electronic charge transfer from the ligand to the oxidant. In general, when doping with iodine the electrons are removed from the HOMO of the ligand, leaving positive holes with formation of I$_3^-$ as counterions. The authors conclude that the low conductivity values presented by these CPs are a consequence of the Cu···Cu distances (*ca.* 11 Å) produced by the presence of the 4,4′-bipyridine ligands acting as a bridging ligand.

4 NANO PROCESSING OF CPs BASED ON NUCLEOBASE DERIVATIVES: POTENTIAL APPLICATIONS

Coordination polymers in bulk do not always fulfill the needs required for their use in some advanced applications, such as biomedical or optoelectronic applications, due to their incompatible size with respect to proteins, nano-/micrometer-scale cells, and tissues, or due to their tendency to be electrical insulators and to have poor charge transport properties. The chemical and physical properties of solids are primarily subject to their size and shape, being especially true for materials smaller than 100 nm in at least one dimension, where the ratio of surface area to volume increases enormously. For this reason, quantum-mechanical effects start to play an important role and become increasingly relevant when reaching nanometer size [54]. Thus, the miniaturization of CPs to the nanometer scale is a unique opportunity to develop highly tunable functional materials that combine their intrinsic properties with the advantages of nanomaterials. There are two main routes to obtain nanometer materials: the bottom-up and top-down approaches [55].

The first approach involves starting from atoms or molecules to begin building structures by self-assembly. In contrast, the second one consists of miniaturizing the bulk material until a product of reduced shape and size is obtained. The bottom-up approach is the most commonly used one for synthesizing nano-CPs thanks to their insolubility in the reaction media. The direct self-assembly of the building blocks occurs in a one-step reaction, and size modification will depend on the reaction conditions. One of the possible advantages of synthesizing CPs with modified nucleobases is their ability to be nanoprocessed to generate electronic nanodevices with potential molecular recognition capability [27, 56–58].

4.1 Semiconductors Based on nano-CPs with Nucleobase Derivatives: Electronic Nanodevices

Research on CPs as electrically conductive devices for electronic and optoelectronic applications is still in its infancy. The synthesis of conductive CPs is a great challenge since most of these materials are electrical insulators or present low conductivity at room temperature. However, relevant advances have been made in this sense, with CPs involved in creating transistors, chemisorption solar cells, or photodetectors. They allow nowadays to obtain materials with superconductivity and high charge carrier mobility [44].

As mentioned in the introduction, nucleobase-derived ligands make it possible to obtain materials capable of selective molecular recognition (see Section 2.2), which could present a significant advantage over the electronic devices studied to date. Technological advances have made it possible to study CPs derived from nucleobases not only on a micrometer but also on a nanometer scale, opening the door to the possibility of using these materials as electronic nanodevices [59]. Indeed, the nanoprocessing of these CPs with potential optoelectronic applications started in the 2000s with David Olea et al. conducting a detailed analysis of the isolation of a CP as a random distribution of individual chains [57]. In this work, Cd(II)-CP [Cd(6-MP)$_2$·2H$_2$O]$_n$ with a structure analogous to M-DNA (Figure 8a and b), is again the protagonist (see Section 3.2). It had been obtained as single chains from micrometer-sized single crystals. Using a top-down approach, the [Cd(6-MP)$_2$·2H$_2$O]$_n$ crystals were dehydrated at 200°C for 4h and later redispersed in ethanol prior to sonication, thereby favoring exclusively interchain interactions by van der Waals forces. The mixture was deposited by drop-casting on a mica surface and characterized by atomic force microscopy (AFM). This method confirmed the nanoprocessing of the crystals, indicating heights between 0.5 and 15 nm (Figure 8c and d). In the chains obtained this way, electrical transport properties were measured by Electrostatic Force Microscopy (EFM) and conductance AFM. The results indicated that the chains are insulators. Thus, DFT calculations were needed to get further information. The collected data from the large band-gap and small bandwidths (2.30 and 0.23 eV, respectively) showed this structure should be an insulator, refuting the proposal by Lee and co-workers [46] about the original M-DNA with Zn(II) ions as a tentative material for use in electric circuits. The Zn-DNA structure was also subjected to the same calculations, and the results were similar to the Cd(II) structure with an energy gap of 2.33 eV and a HOMO bandwidth of 0.30 eV. These findings thus suggested that M-DNA obtained as nanowires does not necessarily imply conductance. After this work, calculations with other transition metals, Cu(II), Fe(II), Ni(II), and Co(II), as well as the use of another modified nucleobase (6-thioguaninate=6-ThioG) revealed

Coordination Polymers: From Electronic Nanodevices to Sensors

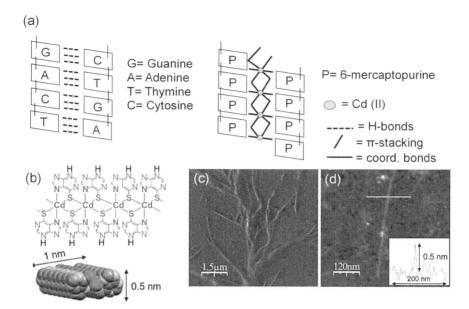

FIGURE 8 Schematic representation [Cd(6-MP)$_2$]$_n$ interactions compared to DNA (a). 2D-structure representation and space-fill-model of [Cd(6-MP)$_2$]$_n$. AFM images of the compound after soft centrifugation upon nanoprocessing (c) and an isolated individual chain after consecutive sonication and centrifugation in the final nanoprocessing stage (d). (Reproduced by permission from Ref. [57]; copyright 2005, Wiley-VCH Verlag GmbH & Co.)

that these could enhance electrical conduction. This led to the synthesis of various CPs, with the exploration of their electrical properties, demonstrating their semiconductivity [49, 51], as has already been detailed in Section 3.2.1.

4.2 Soft Materials and Composites Based on nano-CPs with Nucleobase Derivatives: Stimulus-Responsive Properties

4.2.1 Colloids and Metal-Organic Gels (MOGs) Based on nano-CPs with Nucleobase Derivatives for Sensor Applications

The dynamics that characterize coordination bonds and the molecular recognition capacity provided by this type of bioligands are essential for the formation of colloids and gels, also called "soft materials" [60–72]. At around 2004, reports on gels based on coordination polymers (i.e. coordination polymer gels, CPGs), also called MOGs, started to appear [60–62]. Indeed, colloidal suspensions of nanoparticles, nanofibers, or nanoribbons can be transformed into gels by appropriate incubation times or by the effect of external physical factors such as agitation or temperature. The formation of these supramolecular architectures is dominated by the presence of hydrogen bonds and nanometer particle sizes with fibrillar morphology [64]. However, these phases can be modified by post-synthetic conditions and, hence, they might have stimulus-responsive properties to different external factors such as pH, stirring, pressure, temperature, or the presence of solvents [9]. Thanks to all their properties, MOGs are of great interest in biological applications such as antimicrobial drugs, drug release, and wound healing [37, 65, 67].

Most of the methods used for nanoprocessing CPs with nucleobases employ the bottom-up approach and involve the formation of colloidal suspensions or gels [9, 37, 61, 62]. Furthermore, among the works devoted to synthesizing nano-CPs to form colloids and MOGs with nucleobases and their derivatives with different interesting potential applications, only in two cases the structures described herein have been solved and refined by single-crystal XRD [63, 72].

One of them in which the network structure is known was recently reported by Vegas et al. [63]. Herein, the direct reaction at room temperature at pH 4.5, between 4,4′-bipyridine (4,4′-bipy), dissolved in a small volume of acetic acid, and copper (II) acetate hydrate, UAcOH and NaOH, dissolved in water, was performed. Under those synthetic conditions, a colloidal suspension of a 1D double-chain CP with the formula $[Cu(UAcO)(\mu\text{-}CH_3COO)(\mu\text{-}4,4'\text{-}bipy)]_n \cdot 3nH_2O$ has been obtained. The corresponding MOG was formed by sonication and 24 h of resting at room temperature. The average height of the nanofibers that form the dry hydrogel (xerogel) is around 8 nm, as characterized by AFM (Figure 9a). These authors also subsequently reported the nanoprocessing in colloidal form of $[Cu_2(UAcO)_4(4,4'\text{-}bipy)_2]_n \cdot 3nH_2O$ (CP5n) and $[Cu_2(5\text{-}FUAcO)_4(4,4'\text{-}bipy)_2]_n \cdot 4nH_2O$ (5-FUAcOH = 5-fluorouracil acetic acid) (CP6n) obtained in water by simply lowering the temperature to 5°C. Nanometer-sized crystals with widths of 150 nm and heights between 20 and 40 nm were obtained for CP5n (Figure 9b), while widths of around 284 nm and heights between 40 and 60 nm were observed in CP6n nanocrystals with interesting possible applications as a cytotoxic agent [37] (see Section 2.3).

There are fascinating examples of MOGs based on nucleotides and metal ions such as silver or lanthanoides with selective molecular recognition of fluorescent or colored compounds that allow obtaining new hybrid materials with interesting optical properties [66, 67, 69–71]. For example, Dash et al. reported supramolecular hydrogels composed of 5′-guanosine monophosphate (GMP) and Ag(I) ions. Self-assembly of these two building blocks in water results in helically stacked nanofilaments, which undergo sol-gel transitions between 50 °C and 80 °C. Their rheological properties could be modulated according to the molar ratio between the metal ion and the ligands. Those nanofilaments are adorned with plasmonic silver nanoparticles. The photoreduction of Ag(I) ions resulted in the optical and fluorescent properties of the hydrogel. These series of gels can immobilize proteins such as cytochrome *c* while preserving their function or detecting substances such as Hoechst-33258 (cationic dye) by inducing gel disruption [66].

Another work with Ag(I) showed that its reaction with the commercial nucleotide inosine-5′-monophosphate (IMP) (Figure 9c) produces a multifunctional

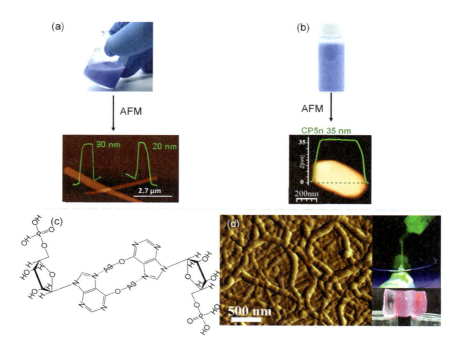

FIGURE 9 AFM images of the nano-CPs [Cu(UAcO)(μ-CH$_3$COO)(μ-4,4'-bipy)]$_n$·3nH$_2$O (a) and [Cu$_2$(UAcO)$_4$(4,4'-bipy)$_2$]$_n$·3nH$_2$O CP5n (b). (Adapted by permission from Ref. [63], copyright 2020, The Royal Society of Chemistry and Ref. [37] (https://doi.org/10.1021/acsami.1c11612), copyright 2021, American Chemical Society (Further permission related to the material excerpted should be directed to the ACS).) Proposed structure for Ag-IMP MOG (c). AFM image (d, left) and photographs of Ag-IMP gel under UV-lamp showing its injectable property (d, right-top), and four blocks of this gel self-healed to give a single block held horizontally (d, right-bottom). (Ref. [67], copyright 2018 American Chemical Society.)

(stimuli-responsive, self-healable, bactericidal) gel formed by 8 nm high fibers, as measured by AFM (Figure 9c). Among other properties, this gel undergoes reversible sol-gel transitions when it is exposed to different substances (sulfate anions, bases, acids…) and a reduction when is exposed to a white LED light source, generating *in situ* Ag nanoparticles inside the gel. Therefore, this nano-CP is interesting as a sensor with luminescent properties and the ability to be injectable (Figure 9d) [67].

Inspired by the use of 2-aminopurine (2-AP) as a probe for the development of biosensors thanks to its luminescent properties [68], Lopez et al. performed a comparative study among 2-AP, adenine and adenosine and different metal ions (Hg(II), Au(III), Ag(I), Fe(III), Zn(II), Mg(II), Tb(III), and Mn(II)) to compare the optical and catalytic properties of the generated CPs. The study took into account that both adenine and 2-AP have four metal coordination sites (Figure 1), while for nucleosides and nucleotides the N9 position is no longer available, which is likely to change the coordination geometry and bond strength, as well as charge. The authors observed that hard metals not having a strong interaction with DNA nucleobases (interacting mainly with the phosphate groups of nucleotides) did not produce any noticeable change in the fluorescence of 2-AP. The best coordination, and thus the formation of CP nanoparticles, occurred with Au(III); so the results showed that at very low concentrations of Au(III) the 2-AP fluorescence was 100% quenched. Once the required Au(III) concentration for total chelation was optimized, fluorescence recovery studies were carried out by adding different molecules that could act as chelators [glutathione (GSH), CN$^-$, I$^-$, and Br$^-$]. In this case, the best results were obtained for KCN recovering the fluorescence completely, while GSH seemed to be the least effective [69].

The search for light-emitting devices for sensing applications is also reflected in the next work, in which *in situ* generated CdS quantum dots (QDts) were integrated during the formation of a series of MOGs composed of Cd(II) ions and nucleobases. Thymine (Cd-T)- and uracil (Cd-U)-based gels were formed spontaneously at alkaline pH, and the addition of Na$_2$S to the reaction mixture led to the growth of quantum dots within the gels, whose emission could be tuned from blue to white and yellow, depending on the concentration of the precursor sulfide. The effect of temperature on the emission of the CdS quantum dots was studied, taking as a model the CdS-Cd-T- hydrogel with yellow emission. At 5°C the emission was maximum, at 25°C it was intermediate, and at 60°C the emission was the least intense. Furthermore, ion detection was explored in the gels with white light emission, which underwent quenching in the presence of Fe(III) and Cu(II) at millimolar concentrations [70].

Besides the development of biosensors, work has been reported whose objectives go further, demonstrating the value of luminescent CPs by attempting to apply them as devices for the execution of computational logic operations. The tuneability of this property employing the implicit and specific response or detection of these compounds against different molecules is key to this approach. To this end, Gao et al. synthesized a series of lanthanoide (Tb(III), Eu(III), and Ce(III))-based nano-CPs, using GMP in an aqueous solution by a simple reaction at room temperature. By modifying the ratio of the different metal ions in the mixture, they achieved white light emission based on the RGB (red-green-blue) color composition scheme. The study of luminescence indicated that this property in Tb(III)-nano-CP can be modified in intensity by adjusting the pH, showing the highest green emission intensity at pH 10. However, weak emission was shown for Ce(III) and Eu(III) nano-CPs, with no remarkable changes at different pH values. In all cases, at acidic pH (below 8) the luminescence contributed by the interaction with the ions disappears, leaving only the blue emission characteristic of the ligand. Considering that GMP could provide blue light, by utilizing Tb(III) ions (green emission) individually doped in it, it could be possible to construct a new white light-emitting material for LED applications by adjusting the pH of the aqueous solution.

Moreover, the photoluminescence can be modified in these CPs by the inclusion of dipicolinic acid (DPA) due to a response of these materials toward this molecule. In the case of the Tb(III)-nano-CP, doping with DPA resulted in a quenching of this property. At the same time, for the compounds formed by Eu(III) and Ce(III), their visible emission was significantly increased in red and blue, respectively. Consequently, it was possible to perform a gradient adjustment of the chromaticity in the visible emission from red to green for a compound with a mixture of Tb(III) and Eu(III) doped with DPA. Subsequently, the synthesis of a material that contains the three ions was carried out by adjusting the proportions of each ion to achieve white light emission. After these tests, the authors decided to build a series of multifunctional devices from these stimulus-responsive materials, based on Boolean logic integration circuits (molecular logic gates) for the execution of non-arithmetic operations that could find their application in the regulation of the encapsulation and switching capabilities of fluorescence in nano-CPs [71].

4.2.2 MOAs Based on nano-CPs with Nucleobase Derivatives for Selective Separation of Drugs

Some barriers related to tailoring the physical and chemical properties of MOGs have yet to be overcome for creating functional materials [9, 73]. For instance, the architecture of these materials must be liquid-free at the macroscale for applications such as catalysis or substance capture. This can be achieved by specific drying methods obtaining the so-called aerogels (MOAs), in which a gas replaces the liquid phase. The fact that the generation of MOAs can provide materials with certain porosity, even starting from structures that lack it, is a considerable advance in materials engineering. In both MOGs and MOAs, there is an added difficulty related to obtaining quality crystals, which is essential to determine the structure of these materials accurately. Therefore, the structures are usually proposed.

Surprisingly, Vegas et al. overcame this barrier with the design of a non-porous 1D-CP based on modified uracil (UAcOH), 4,4′-bipyridine (4,4′-bipy) and copper(II) acetate in water and 1:2:1 stoichiometry under standard conditions. The resulting double-chain compound possesses a "core" of formula [$Cu_2(\mu$-$CH_3COO)_2(\mu$-4,4′-bipy$)_2$], decorated with modified uracil residues along and on both sides of the double chain. The addition of a small amount of acetic acid to the reaction mixture in combination with sonication favors the reticulation process from a colloid to gel within 24 h (Figure 10a). Its drying with supercritical CO_2 gave rise to the corresponding aerogel (Cu(UAcO)@MOA). This ultralight aerogel (density 0.0329 g cm^{-3}) showed astonishing mechanical properties with Young's modulus values between 114 and 171 kPa. The specific surface area of this material was 21 m^{2}g^{-1} and was used as a proof-of-concept for the development of a stationary phase for high-performance liquid chromatography (HPLC). For that, a steel column was filled manually with quartz microparticles and the MOA in a 90:10 w/w proportion. It was preliminarily tested to separate molecules

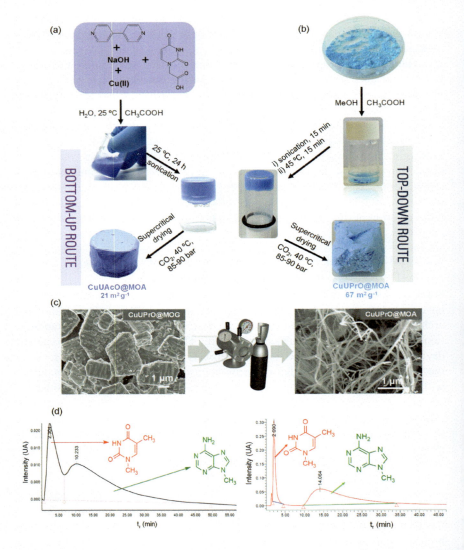

FIGURE 10 Scheme of MOA formation in [Cu(UPrO)$_2$(4,4′-bipy)$_2$(H$_2$O)] (Cu(UPrO)@MOA) via top-down (a) and [Cu(UAcO)(μ-CH$_3$COO)(μ-4,4′-bipy)]$_n$·3nH$_2$O (Cu(UAcO)@MOA) via bottom-up strategies (b). FESEM images of hexagonal platelets of Cu(UPrO)@MOG at the end of the gel formation method and curled and disaggregated nanofibers, after supercritical drying (with CO$_2$ going from liquid to supercritical state (40°C, 80 bar)) (c). Chromatograms obtained following separation of methylated nucleobases from Cu(UAcO)@MOA (d, left) and Cu(UPrO)@MOA (d, right) HPLC columns. (Adapted by permission from Ref. [63], copyright 2020, The Royal Society of Chemistry and Ref. [72], copyright 2022, The Author(s).)

such as methylated nucleobases (Figure 10d – left), offering promising results, even though the signals were not resolved at baseline [63].

Inspired by this work, these properties and applications were improved by Maldonado et al. [72] with the synthesis of a new crystalline MOA (Figure 10b). In this work, the UPrOH replaces the UAcOH to provide a new coordination compound of formula [Cu(UPrO)$_2$(4,4'-bipy)$_2$(H$_2$O)] (CuUPrO). This polycrystalline non-porous material can be transformed into the gel (Cu(UPrO)@MOG) using a top-down approach with ultrasound, temperature, and small amounts of acetic acid. This gel retains the morphology of the quasi-hexagonal micrometric platelets belonging to the material in bulk. This plate-like morphology building up the Cu(UPrO)@MOG was dramatically transformed into very long and relatively homogeneous nanofibers, about 24 nm in diameter (Figure 10c) during its CO$_2$ supercritical drying procedure to provide Cu(UprO)@MOA. The authors carried out a detailed characterization of the different stages in the process by scanning electron microscopy (SEM) and XRD, in an attempt to rationalize the mechanism of this transformation. Cu(UPrO)@MOA triples the surface area of the recently reported Cu(UAcO)@MOA. The porosity studies were completed with the measurements of CO$_2$ adsorption isotherms to estimate the isosteric heats of adsorption (Q_{st}). This value was about 39.6 kJ mol^{-1} and is comparable to those reported for well-known MOFs MIL-101(Cr) (44 kJ mol^{-1}), MOF-74(Ni) (42 kJ mol^{-1}), bioMOF-1(Zn) (35 kJ mol^{-1}), MIL-53(Al) (35 kJ mol^{-1}), and HKUST-1(Cu) (35 kJ mol^{-1}) [74]. Following these results, an exhaustive study was performed to optimize and enhance the use of the aerogel as a stationary phase in an HPLC column. Different loads of Cu(UPrO)@MOA were tested to separate methylated nucleobases, with the perspective of detection and selective separation of drugs of interest such as 5-fluorouracil. An optimum resolution and selectivity were achieved with a 5% load of Cu(UPrO)@MOA (Figure 10d – right) and the elution order of the methylated nucleobases was supported by DFT calculations.

4.2.3 Composites Based on nano-CPs with Nucleobase Derivatives as Sensors Devices

Despite the barriers to overcome, many studies have supported the development of such bioinspired coordination compounds that will lead to the generation of biomimetic and biocompatible materials [73] and will provide innovative applications in fields such as 3D printing [75–77].

3D printing is one of the technologies belonging to the additive manufacturing field that has experienced substantial development in recent years. This technology for printing objects allows obtaining rigid or flexible architectures with sophisticated designs, making its way into the field of chemistry with different applications for sensors [75] or in batteries and supercapacitors [76].

It was only a few years ago that metal-organic compounds started to be explored as composites for new 3D printing inks because of their interest as stimuli-responsive materials and their ability to form gels with rheological and self-healing properties since they can be easily extruded by an injector and give the required shape. The first nano-CP with nucleobases was printed by

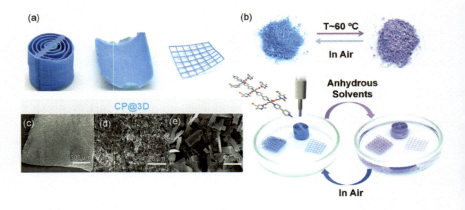

FIGURE 11 Different photographs of 3D printed objects of the [Cu(TAcO)$_2$(4,4'-bipy)(H$_2$O)]$_n$·2nH$_2$O@3D (a). Reversible color change from blue to violet when [Cu(TAcO)$_2$(4,4'-bipy)(H$_2$O)]$_n$·2nH$_2$O is exposed to 60 °C (b, top), and when CP@3D is exposed to anhydrous solvents (b, bottom). SEM images of CP4 crystals 3D printed by extrusion with the polymer matrix (CP@3D). These images correspond to the CP sample with 40 wt%. (Adapted by permission from Ref. [77], copyright 2019, Wiley-VCH Verlag GmbH & Co. KGaA, Weinheim.)

Maldonado et al. [77], using a photopolymerization printing technique known as digital light processing (DLP) (Figure 11a). This non-porous 1D-CP, previously synthesized by Vegas et al. [12] and composed of Cu(II) and thymine-1-acetic acid of composition [Cu(TAcO)$_2$(4,4'-bipy)(H$_2$O)]$_n$·2nH$_2$O (CP4), was used as a water-sensor thanks to its thermo- and solvatochromic properties. This property, related to the loss of coordinated water molecules in the structure of the compound, produces a reversible color change from blue to violet when exposed to a vacuum or 60°C, or in the presence of various dry organic solvents (Figure 11b). To explore the local structural changes caused by dehydration, the authors applied a pair-distribution function (PDF) analysis based on synchrotron X-ray total scattering data. This analysis, which was supported by other complementary techniques such as thermogravimetric analysis and powder XRD, proved that the color change came from the loss of coordinated water molecules rather than of lattice water molecules. To obtain the composite, CP4 nanoribbons were dispersed in a mixture of monomers and photoinitiators, among them dipropylene glycol diacrylate, considered to be biodegradable. Finally, it was printed using two printing formulations, one with 10 wt% of CP4 loading (DLP printer) and another with 40 wt% of CP4 loading (common extruder printer) (Figure 11c–e) preserving the properties of the pristine material.

5 GENERAL CONCLUSIONS

In the early days of coordination chemistry with nucleobases, research focused on a better understanding of the action mechanism of metal ions with biological targets. Nowadays, the research carried out with these types of compounds has been greatly modified and expanded. On the one hand, the nucleobases have been functionalized almost à la carte, creating organic derivatives that maintain their molecular recognition capacity and expand their coordination sites. In addition, coordination with other metallic centers is proposed to generate novel coordination polymeric structures (CPs) with additional and additive properties, thanks to the presence of these metal ions. Eventually, they allow the creation of new semiconductor, magnetic or luminescent materials. On the other hand, there are current approaches that aim to take advantage of the properties of these types of compounds and advance toward areas such as nanoscience, seeking new applications based on the molecular recognition capability and stimuli-responsiveness that these CPs present in their new nano dimensions. This chapter describes how CPs with electrical, magnetic, and optical properties have been designed at both the micro- and nanoscale and how, taking advantage again of their insolubility in the reaction media and their selective molecular recognition, new colloids, gels, and MOAs with nanometric dimensions have been created that further expand their potential applications. Additionally, this chapter shows new trends of these compounds which, together with the use of new technologies, try to reduce the gap between academia and industry. The chapter describes also interesting results leading to the fabrication of electronic nanodevices, light-emitting devices, 3D printable composites that act as sensors, as well as the fabrication and optimization of MOAs that can be used as stationary phases in HPLC columns for selective drug separation.

ACKNOWLEDGMENTS

We thank the grants PID2019–108028GB-C22 and PID2019–108028GB-C21 funded by MCIN/AEI 10.13039/501100011033.

This work is dedicated to all those people who work every day for the common good.

ABBREVIATIONS AND DEFINITIONS

2-AP	2-aminopurine
5-FuAcOH	5-fluorouracil acetic acid
6-MP	6-mercaptopurine
6-ThioG	6-thioguanine
AFM	atomic force microscopy
AMP	adenosine monophosphate
CMP	cytidine-5′-monophosphate
CPGs	coordination polymers gels
CPs	coordination polymers
DFT	density functional theory
DLP	digital light processing
DMEM	Dulbecco's Modified Eagle Medium

DNA	deoxyribonucleic acid
DPA	dipicolinic acid
EFM	electrostatic force microscopy
FESEM	field-emission scanning electron microscopy
GMP	guanosine monophosphate
HPLC	high-performance liquid chromatography
IMP	inosine-5′-monophosphate
MOAs	metal-organic aerogels
MOGs	metal-organic gels
QDts	quantum dots
RNA	ribonucleic acid
ROS	reactive oxygen species
RPMI	Roswell Park Memorial Institute
SEM	scanning electron microscopy
TAcOH	thymine-1-acetic acid
UAcOH	uracil-1-acetic acid
UPrOH	uracil-1-propionic acid
XRD	X-ray diffraction

REFERENCES

1. J. Müller, *Coord. Chem. Rev.* **2019**, *393*, 37–47.
2. B. Lippert, *Coord. Chem. Rev.* **2000**, *200–202*, 487–516.
3. A. Werner, *Z. Anorg. Allg. Chem.* **1893**, *3*, 267–330.
4. Q. Li, X. Sha, S. Li, K. Wang, Z. Quan, Y. Meng, B. Zou, *J. Phys. Chem. Lett.* **2017**, *8*, 2745–2750.
5. R. M. Klein, J. C. Bailar, *Inorg. Chem.* **1963**, *2*, 1190–1194.
6. B. Mohapatra, Pratibah, S. Verma, *Chem. Commun.* **2017**, *53*, 4748–4758.
7. S. R. Batten, S. M. Neville, D. R. Turner, *Coordination Polymers: Design, Analysis and Application*, Royal Society of Chemistry, Cambridge, **2008**, pp. 1–18.
8. V. G. Vegas, M. Villar-Alonso, C. J. Gómez-García, F. Zamora, P. Amo-Ochoa, *Polymers* **2017**, *9*, 565.
9. N. Maldonado, P. Amo-Ochoa, *Nanomaterials* **2021**, *11*, 1865.
10. J. Zhou, H. Han, J. Liu, *Nano Res.* **2022**, *15*, 71–84.
11. M. Mauro, *Eur. J. Inorg. Chem.* **2018**, 2090–2100.
12. V. G. Vegas, R. Lorca, A. Latorre, K. Hassanein, C. J. Gómez-García, O. Castillo, A. Somoza, F. Zamora, P. Amo-Ochoa, *Angew. Chem. Int. Ed.* **2017**, *56*, 987–991.
13. F. Pu, J. Ren, X. Qu, *Chem. Soc. Rev.* **2018**, *47*, 1285–1306.
14. P. Zhou, R. Shi, J. Yao, C. Sheng, H. Li, *Coord. Chem. Rev.* **2015**, *292*, 107–143.
15. J. Li, J. Sun, *Acc. Chem. Res.* **2017**, *50*, 2737–2745.
16. S. Pal, T. K. Pal, P. K. Bharadwaj, *CrystEngComm* **2016**, *18*, 1825–1831.
17. P. Amo-Ochoa, F. Zamora, *Coord. Chem. Rev.* **2014**, *276*, 34–58.
18. J. Li, Z. Wang, Z. Hua, C. Tang, *J. Mater. Chem. B* **2020**, *8*, 1576–1588.
19. P. J. Sanz Miguel, P. Amo-Ochoa, O. Castillo, A. Houlton, F. Zamora, *Metal Complex–DNA Interactions*. Eds N. Hadjiliadis, E. Sletten, John Wiley & Sons, Ltd, Chichester, UK, **2009**, pp. 95–132.
20. S. Bhai, B. Ganguly, *J. Mol. Graph. Model.* **2019**, *93*, 107445.

21. V. G. Vegas, N. Maldonado, O. Castillo, C. J. Gómez-García, P. Amo-Ochoa, *J. Inorg. Biochem.* **2019**, *200*, 110805.
22. E. Moulin, G. Cormos, N. Giuseppone, *Chem. Soc. Rev.* **2012**, *41*, 1031–1049.
23. S. Sivakova, S. J. Rowan, *Chem. Soc. Rev.* **2005**, *34*, 9–21.
24. A. M. Jabgunde, F. Jaziri, O. Bande, M. Froeyen, M. Abramov, H. Nguyen, G Schepers, E. Lescrinier, V. B. Pinheiro, V. Pezo, P. Marliére, P. Herdewjin, *Chem. Eur. J.* **2018**, *24*, 12695–12707.
25. I. B. Rother, E. Freisinger, A. Erxleben, B. Lippert, *Inorg. Chim. Acta* **2000**, *300–302*, 339–352.
26. B. Sreenivasulu, J. J. Vittal, *Angew. Chem. Int. Ed.* **2004**, *116*, 5893–5896.
27. N. Maldonado, P. Amo-Ochoa, *Chem. Eur. J.* **2021**, *27*, 2887–2907.
28. N. Maldonado, P. Amo-Ochoa, *Dalton Trans.* **2021**, *50*, 2310–2323.
29. P. Zhou, R. Shi, J. Yao, C. Sheng, H. Li, *Coord. Chem. Rev.* **2015**, *292*, 107–143.
30. L. Xu, Z. Zhang, X. Fang, Y. Liu, B. Liu, J. Liu, *ACS Appl. Mater. Interfaces* **2018**, *10*, 14321–14330.
31. W. L. Ward, K. Plakos, V. J. DeRose, *Chem. Rev.* **2014**, *114*, 4318–4342.
32. W.-H. Chen, W.-C. Liao, Y. S. Sohn, M. Fadeev, A. Cecconello, R. Nechushtai, I. Willner, *Adv. Funct. Mater.* **2018**, *28*, 1705137.
33. E.-C. Yang, Z.-Y. Liu, Z.-Y. Liu, L.-N. Zhao, X.-J. Zhao, *Dalton Trans.* **2010**, *39*, 8868–8871.
34. A. Lopez, J. Liu, *ChemNanoMat*, **2017**, *3*, 670–684.
35. N. Maldonado, J. Perles, J. I. Martínez, C. J. Gómez-García, M.-L. Marcos, P. Amo-Ochoa, *Cryst. Growth Des.* **2020**, *20*, 5097–5107.
36. P. Amo-Ochoa, O. Castillo, C. J. Gómez-García, K. Hassanein, S. Verma, J. Kumar, F. Zamora, *Inorg. Chem.* **2013**, *52*, 11428–11437.
37. V. G. Vegas, A. Latorre, M. L. Marcos, C. J. Gómez-García, O. Castillo, F. Zamora, J. Gómez, J. Martínez-Costas, M. Vázquez López, A. Somoza, P. Amo-Ochoa, *ACS Appl. Mater. Interfaces* **2021**, *13*, 36948–36957.
38. G. Beobide, O. Castillo, J. Cepeda, A. Luque, S. Pérez-Yáñez, P. Román, J. Thomas-Gipson, *Coord. Chem. Rev.* **2013**, *257*, 2716–2736.
39. H. Miyasaka, M. Julve, M. Yamashita, R. Clérac, *Inorg. Chem.* **2009**, *48*, 3420–3437.
40. A. Caneschi, D. Gatteschi, N. Lalioti, C. Sangregorio, R. Sessoli, G. Venturi, A. Vindigni, A. Rettori, M. G. Pini, M. A. Novak, *Angew. Chem. Int. Ed.* **2001**, *40*, 1760–1763.
41. M. Wang, X. Gou, W. Shi, P. Cheng, *Chem. Commun.* **2019**, *55*, 11000–11012.
42. W.-X. Zhang, T. Shiga, H. Miyasaka, M. Yamashita, *J. Am. Chem. Soc.* **2012**, *134*, 6908–6911.
43. I. Avasthi, Gaganjot, M. Katiyar, S. Vermas. *Chem. Eur. J.* **2020**, *26*, 16706–16711.
44. H. Liu, Y. Wang, Z. Qin, D. Liu, H. Xu, H. Dong, W. Hu, *J. Phys. Chem. Lett.* **2021**, *12*, 1612–1630.
45. G. Givaja, P. Amo-Ochoa, C. J. Gómez-García, F. Zamora, *Chem. Soc. Rev.* **2012**, *41*, 115–147.
46. P. Aich, S. L. Labiuk, L. W. Tari, L. J. T. Delbaere, W. J. Roesler, K. J. Falk, R. P. Steer, J. S. Lee, *J. Mol. Biol.* **1999**, *294*, 477–485.
47. P. Amo-Ochoa, M. I. Rodríguez-Tapiador, O. Castillo, D. Olea, A. Guijarro, S. S. Alexandre, J. Gómez-Herrero, F. Zamora, *Inorg. Chem.* **2006**, *45*, 7642–7650.
48. S. S. Alexandre, J. M. Soler, L. Seijo, F. Zamora, *Phys. Rev. B* **2006**, *73*, 205112.
49. P. Amo-Ochoa, O. Castillo, S. S. Alexandre, L. Welte, P. J. de Pablo, M. I. Rodríguez-Tapiador, J. Gómez-Herrero, F. Zamora, *Inorg. Chem.* **2009**, *48*, 7931–7936.
50. P. Amo-Ochoa, O. Castillo, A. Guijarro, P. J. Sanz Miguel, F. Zamora, *Inorg. Chim. Acta* **2014**, *417*, 142–147.

51. P. Amo-Ochoa, S. S. Alexandre, S. Hribesh, M. A. Galindo, O. Castillo, C. J. Gómez-García, A. R. Pike, J. M. Soler, A. Houlton, F. Zamora, *Inorg. Chem.* **2013**, *52*, 7306–7306.
52. L. L. G. Al-Mahamad, O. El-Zubir, D. G. Smith, B. R. Horrocks, A. Houlton, *Nat. Commun.* **2017**, *8*, 720.
53. L. Mistry, O. El-Zubir, T. Pope, P. G. Waddell, N. Wright, W. A. Hofer, B. R. Horrocks, A. Houlton, *Cryst. Growth Des.* **2021**, *21*, 4398–4405.
54. M. Y. Masoomi, A. Morsali, *Coord. Chem. Rev.* **2012**, *256*, 2921–2943.
55. J. Gómez-Herrero, F. Zamora, *Adv. Mater.* **2011**, *23*, 5311–5317.
56. R. Nishiyabu, N. Hashimoto, T. Cho, K. Watanabe, T. Yasunaga, A. Endo, K. Kaneko, T. Niidome, M. Murata, C. Adachi, Y. Katayama, M. Hashizume, N. Kimizuka, *J. Am. Chem. Soc.* **2009**, *131*, 2151–2158.
57. D. Olea, S. S. Alexandre, P. Amo-Ochoa, A. Guijarro, F. de Jesús, J. M. Soler, P. J. de Pablo, F. Zamora, J. Gómez-Herrero, *Adv. Mater.* **2005**, *17*, 1761–1765.
58. R. K. Saravanan, I. Avasthi, R. K. Prajapati, S. Verma, *RSC Adv.* **2018**, *8*, 24541–24560.
59. L. Wang, H. Xu, J. Gao, J. Yao, Q. Zhang, *Coord. Chem. Rev.* **2019**, *398*, 213016.
60. J. H. Jung, J. H. Lee, J. R. Silverman, G. John, *Chem. Soc. Rev.* **2013**, *42*, 924–936.
61. P. Sutar, T. K. Maji, *Dalton Trans.* **2020**, *49*, 7658–7672.
62. A. Y. Y. Tam, V. W. W. Yam, *Chem. Soc. Rev.* **2013**, *42*, 1540–1567.
63. V. G. Vegas, G. Beobide, O. Castillo, E. Reyes, C. J. Gómez-García, F. Zamora, P. Amo-Ochoa, *Nanoscale* **2020**, *12*, 14699–14707.
64. B. Sharma, A. Mahata, S. Mandani, T. K. Sarma, B. Pathak, *RSC Adv.* **2016**, *6*, 62968–62973.
65. H. Liang, Z. Zhang, Q. Yuan, J. Liu, *Chem. Commun.* **2015**, *51*, 15196–15199.
66. J. Dash, A. J. Patil, R. N. Das, F. L. Dowdall, S. Mann, *Soft Matter* **2011**, *7*, 8120.
67. N. Thakur, B. Sharma, S. Bishnoi, S. K. Mishra, D. Nayak, A. Kumar, T. K. Sarma, *ACS Sustain. Chem. Eng.* **2018**, *7*, 8659–8671.
68. A. C. Jones, R. K. Neely, *Q. Rev. Biophys.* **2015**, *48*, 244–279.
69. A. Lopez, J. Liu, *J. Anal. Test.* **2019**, *3*, 219–227.
70. B. Sharma, S. Mandani, N. Thakur, T. K. Sarma, *Soft Matter* **2018**, *14*, 5715–5720.
71. R.-R. Gao, S. Shi, Y.-J. Li, M. Wumaier, X.-C. Hu, T.-M. Yao, *Nanoscale* **2017**, *9*, 9589–9597.
72. N. Maldonado, G. Beobide, E. Reyes, J. I. Martínez, C. J. Gómez-García, O. Castillo, P. Amo-Ochoa, *Nanomaterials* **2022**, *12*, 675.
73. J. Mu, L. He, P. Huang, X. Chen, *Coord. Chem. Rev.* **2019**, *399*, 213039.
74. S. Saha, S. Chandra, B. Garai, R. Banerjee, *Indian J. Chem. - Sect. A* **2012**, *51*, 1223–1230.
75. H. Ota, S. Emaminejad, Y. Gao, A. Zhao, E. Wu, S, Challa, K. Chen, H. M. Fahad, A. K. Jha, D. Kiriya, W. Gao, H. Shiraki, K. Morioka, A. R. Ferguson, K. E. Healy, R. W. Davis, A. Javey, *Adv. Mater. Technol.* **2016**, *1*, 1600013.
76. U. Gulzar, C. Glynn, C. O'Dwyer, *Curr. Opin. Electrochem.* **2020**, *20*, 46–53.
77. N. Maldonado, V. G. Vegas, O. Halevi, J. I. Martínez, P. S. Lee, S. Magdassi, M. T. Wharmby, A. E. Platero-Prats, C. Moreno, F. Zamora, P. Amo-Ochoa, *Adv. Funct. Mater.* **2019**, *29*, 1808424.

4 Heavy Coinage Metal Nucleobase, Nucleoside and (Oligo) Nucleotide Systems
Recent Developments in Self-Assembly, Opto-Electronics and DNA Integration

Andrew Houlton
Chemistry, School of Natural and Environmental Sciences, Newcastle University, Newcastle upon Tyne, NE31UB, United Kingdom
andrew.houlton@ncl.ac.uk

CONTENTS

1	Introduction	80
	1.1 Overview	80
	1.2 Silver: Basic Coordination Chemistry with Nucleobases	82
	1.3 Gold: Basic Coordination Chemistry with Nucleobases	83
2	Silver-Mediated Base Pair Complexes	84
	2.1 Self-assembly of Small-Molecule Systems	84
	2.2 Electrical Properties and Band Structure of Silver-Nucleobase Chains	87
	2.3 Supramolecular Hydro- and Organogels	89
	2.4 Structures of DNA-Stabilized Silver Nanoclusters	92
3	Thionucleosides	93
	3.1 Coinage Metal-Thiolate Coordination Polymers	93
	3.2 Silver-Thioguanosine: Hierarchical Self-assembly, Gelation, and Circularly Polarized Luminescence	95

DOI: 10.1201/9781003270201-4

3.3   Gold-Thioguanosine: Electrical Conduction and
       Incorporation into DNA Duplex 96
4   Conclusion 99
Acknowledgments 99
Abbreviations and Definitions 99
References 100

ABSTRACT

The heavier congeners of the coinage metals, silver and gold, are not essential elements but do exhibit biomedical activity as antimicrobial, antiarthritic, and anticancer agents. As a result, much early research on the interaction of these metal ions with nucleic acids has focused on this area. However, more recently interest has extended well beyond this field with researchers from supramolecular chemistry, functional materials, and nanotechnology exploring this fascinating area of chemistry. A key aim here has been to introduce new functionality and novel properties into DNA and its component nucleosides ranging from enhancing the thermal stability of DNA duplex, through unique optical features such as photoemission and circularly polarized luminescence to semiconductor-like electrical conduction. This chapter presents aspects of this research along with an overview of the background to the basic underlying coordination chemistry and with a particular focus on the research from our own laboratories.

KEYWORDS

Silver; Gold; Nucleoside; Optoelectronics; DNA; Gels; Thioguanosine

1 INTRODUCTION

1.1 OVERVIEW

DNA, biology's information carrier, is now a well-established constituent of chemistry's arsenal for materials synthesis [1–4]. Its robust nature, reliable synthesis, controllable length, along with sequence-coded self-assembly, address many of the criteria desired for materials design. This is readily seen in the myriad forms of DNA-based architectures and materials produced over the last decades (Figure 1) [1–6].

However, for many areas of technological interest, including the long-sought goal of a DNA-based electronics [7–10], the intrinsic physicochemical properties of the native biopolymer are not optimal. As a result, various strategies have been developed to address this such as the incorporation of pre-synthesized inorganic components, particularly gold nanoparticles [1, 11–13]. So-called DNA-templating [7, 14] is another approach which can integrate technologically useful properties, such as electrical conduction or magnetism, with DNA and is compatible with metals [15–18], binary and tertiary inorganics [19–21] and synthetic polymers [22–26]. The DNA-based nanowires produced *via* this method have

Recent Developments in Self-Assembly and DNA Integration

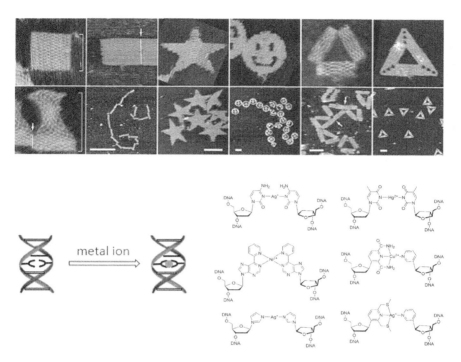

FIGURE 1 Upper. Discrete and extended DNA structures through origami. (Adapted and reproduced from Ref. [4] with permission from Springer Nature.) Lower, left, concept of metal-mediated base pair in duplex DNA and, right, natural and synthetic "ligandoside" examples of MM-bp.

been used to assemble electrical circuits [25, 27] and fabricate ultra-sensitive sensing devices [28]. However, templating loses the structure-building capacity of base-pairing, is not well suited for sequence-specific modification, and lacks the level of control offered by traditional molecular synthesis. So the integration of novel optoelectronic properties, ideally, sequence-specifically into the basic framework of DNA is of great scientific and technological interest but remains challenging.

It is toward addressing this challenge that the field of metal-modified/metal-mediated base pair DNA (MM-bp DNA) has, in large part, developed (Figure 1). For an explanation of the distinction between these types, readers are directed to the recent article by Lippert [29]. Covalent modification of nucleosides is a traditional method by which to introduce new metal-containing functional groups, sequence-specifically, into DNA, and examples of redox and photoactive metal complexes have been demonstrated [30–33]. However, these are generally as pre-synthesized molecular moieties such as ferrocenyl- [34, 35] or tris-phenanthroline type species [36, 37]. In MM-bp-DNA the aim is to use either the *intrinsic* metal-binding properties of natural nucleosides or to design *ligandosides*, capable of providing specific, non-natural, binding modes into the DNA framework (Figure 1) [38–43]. The range of metal ions that have been incorporated into DNA in this way *via* natural nucleosides is Ag, Au, and Hg, while a wider range of transition metal ions, including Mn, Ni, and Cu has been incorporated using synthetic *ligandosides*. This MM-bp approach has been shown to be an especially elegant method for organizing metal ions into homo- and hetero-metallic arrays [39, 44].

This chapter, focused especially on work from our own laboratories, reports on more recent studies on the heavier coinage metals, silver, and gold that relate to this active area of research. Particular emphasis is given to the self-assembly, including gelation, of small-molecule complexes, optoelectronic properties including circularly polarized emission and electrical conductivity, and the integration of functional, electronically delocalized, and coordination polymer motifs into DNA.

1.2 Silver: Basic Coordination Chemistry with Nucleobases

Consideration of the basic coordination chemistry, by way of reviewing the crystallographically characterized [45] complexes of silver and gold ions with nucleobase ligands provides a useful starting point for this chapter [46]. Generally, due to difficulties in crystallizing metal-containing nucleoside/-tide complexes, the majority of these complexes contain substituted-*nucleobase* derivatives and this is true for these elements, too. The parent unsubstituted nucleobases have the potential to bind metal ions at the site of (deoxy)ribose attachment, i.e. N9-purine and N1-pyrimidine. These sites are not available in the corresponding nucleoside or (oligo)nucleotide and so such examples are not considered, unless particularly noteworthy.

Silver was among the first metal ions to be proposed and, later, identified as binding to DNA *via* the nucleobases [47] and has been increasingly explored in this regard ever since. As a monoatomic ion, silver has a single, univalent, oxidation state of relevance and Ag^I complexes are known for all nucleobases. Binding of Ag^I ions has been observed for adenine at N1 [48], N7 [49], and N3 [50] and also includes examples of multiple ions binding to all sites on a single nucleobase [51, 52]. For guanine, only N7 binding has been crystallographically characterized, to date [53]. For T/U, binding has been reported at O2, N3, and O4 with multiple Ag^I ions binding simultaneously to all sites [54–56] or individually to O4 [57]. For C, N3 is the main site of Ag^I binding and this is seen in the principal form of the C–Ag–C MM-bp.

Beyond identifying the site(s) of metal ion binding many of the structurally characterized metal complexes are themselves examples of MM-bp; though often these are part of more extended coordination chains. With this in mind, the following types of Ag-mediated base pairs can be identified in small-molecule complexes; for adenine, *N1*-A–Ag–*N1*-A is found as both discrete molecular complex [58] and extended chain [52, 59] forms, though in all these cases additional ligands are involved in the coordination spheres. A discrete two-coordinate *N1*-A–Ag–*N7*-A complex has been characterized [52] along with *N7*-A–Ag–*N7*-A [52, 59], and *N1*-A–Ag–*N3*-A [59] arrangements as part of extended chains. Lippert has also reported an adenine-containing mismatched base pair in [(*N7*–9-MeA)Ag^I(*N3*-1-MeC)(H$_2$O)]NO$_3$ [60]. For guanine, *N7*-G–Ag–*N7*-G is observed in [Ag^I(*N7*–9-EtA)$_2$]NO$_3$ [53]. For thymine/uracil, extended chains containing Ag-mediated pairings with O2–Ag–O4 and N3–Ag–N3 binding are known [54–56].

A well-established pairing for silver is for *N3*-C–Ag^I–*N3*-C, with crystallographically characterized examples containing the parent nucleobase [61] and alkylated derivatives [62, 63], nucleoside [64] and (oligo)nucleotides [65, 66] and these are discussed in detail below. However, the first reported X-ray structure of a Ag^I–C complex was for a dimer [{Ag^I(*O2,N3*-1-MeC)}$_2$](NO$_3$)$_2$ which featured O2- and N3-binding [67]. This bridging binding mode, which naturally forms a MM-bp arrangement, can also generate true coordination polymers as seen in the recently reported [Ag^I(*O2,N3*-CMP)] [65, 66].

Several oligonucleotides containing Ag-mediated base pairs, either in combination with regular Watson-Crick hydrogen-bonded pairs [68, 69] or as complete replacement to give fully argenated duplex [43, 70] have been structurally characterized by single-crystal XRD. These are of the form; *N3*-C–Ag–*N3*-C [43, 68, 69], *N7*-G–Ag–*N7*-G [43, 69], *N7*-G–Ag–*N3*-U*, *N1*-G–Ag–*N3*-C [43, 70], and *N3*-T–Ag–*N3*-T and are depicted in Figure 2 (U*=5-bromouridine). Incorporation of this type of MM-bp has been shown to enhance the thermal stability of duplex structures [71, 72].

1.3 Gold: Basic Coordination Chemistry with Nucleobases

In comparison to silver, gold is less well-studied. Gold has two relevant oxidation states, d^{10}-Au^I and d^8-Au^{III}, for coordination to nucleobases. These ions present quite differently in HSAB-terms, with the former considerably softer and appearing less well suited to such binding. Examples of nucleobase coordination by Au^I are generally supported by soft phosphine ligands with binding at the N9-purine site. Rare exceptions are for *N3*-T as in [Au^I(*N3*-1-MeT)(PPh$_3$)] [73] and *N3*-G in [Au$_2$(μ^2- *N3,N9*-guanine)(μ^2-DMPE)], for example [74]. For Au^{III}, binding is seen at the typical sites of G-N7, though this is with derivatives 1,9-dimethylguanine or 6-methoxy-9-methylguanine [75], C-N3 [76], and U-N3 [77]. There are also a number of reports of reactions with pyrimidines, such as 1-MeU, yielding non-complexed salts containing the [AuX$_4$]$^-$ anion, as in [Na(1-MeU)$_4$][AuCl$_4$] [78]. No small-molecule Au^{III} adenine-containing complexes have been reported, to date. Interestingly, the serendipitous isolation of a (partially) gold-modified RNA duplex has been reported by Dumas et al. [79]. While initially the G–Au–C site was described as square-planar Au^{III} involving chelation *via* C-N3/O2 and G-N1/N2 [79], this analysis has been questioned and an alternative linear Au^I coordinated by C-N3 and G-N1 has been suggested [44], which is analogous to that seen, subsequently, for silver ions (Figure 2) [43].

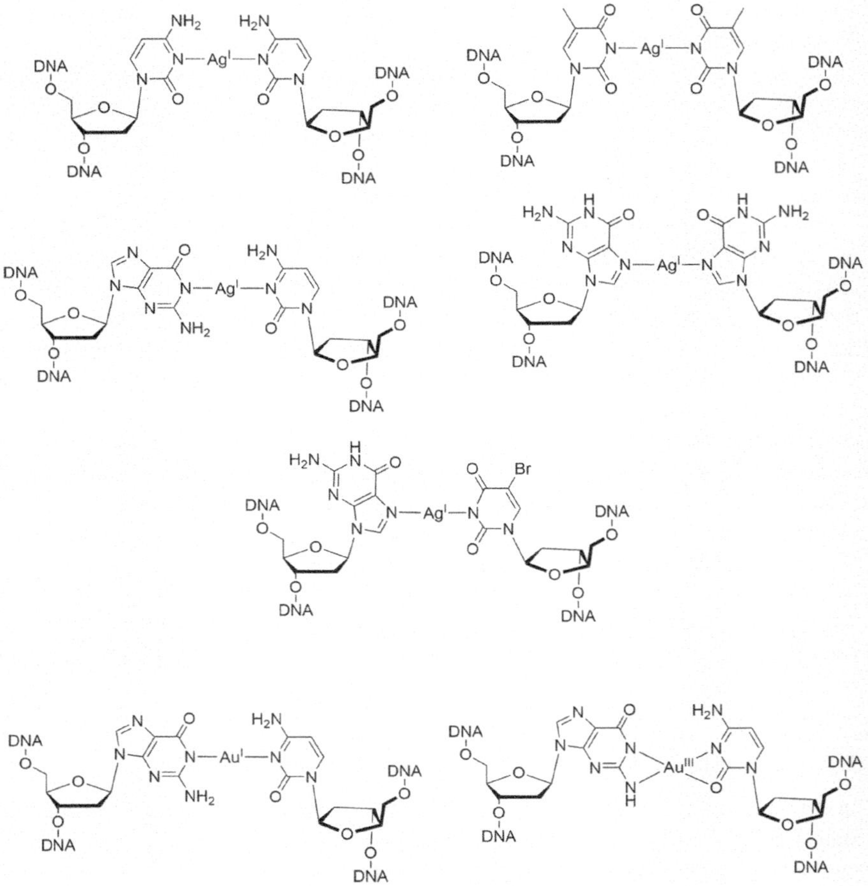

FIGURE 2 Metal-mediated base pairs containing silver and gold ions observed, or proposed, in natural oligonucleotide duplexes by single-crystal X-ray diffraction studies.

2 SILVER-MEDIATED BASE PAIR COMPLEXES

2.1 Self-assembly of Small-Molecule Systems

As well as providing useful models to gain insight into the physiochemical properties of extended MM-bp arrays, small-molecule analogs of MM-bp observed in oligonucleotides are of interest themselves. Surprisingly, it is only recently that the simplest form of the well-established C–Ag–C MM-bp, the parent [Ag^I(*N3*-cytosine)$_2$]$^+$, has been reported [61]. This study on several complex salts identified differences in coordination geometry, molecular conformation, and intermolecular hydrogen-bonding interactions compared to analogs containing N1-functionalized derivatives, such as cytidine [64].

Recent Developments in Self-Assembly and DNA Integration

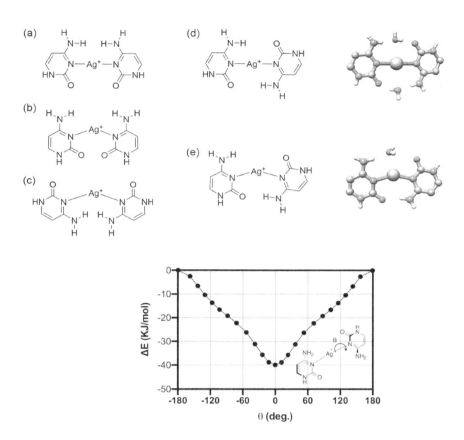

FIGURE 3 Upper left and center. Possible structural variations of *cisoid* (a)–(c) and *transoid* (d)–(e) conformation for the C–Ag^I–C MM-bp for linear or bent coordination geometry and co-planar ligand arrangement. Upper right, molecular structures of the complex cations in *transoid* [Ag^I(*N3*-cytosine)$_2$]PF$_6$·2H$_2$O and *transoid* [Ag^I(*N3*-cytosine)$_2$]NO$_3$·H$_2$O highlighting the intramolecular hydrogen bond in the latter. Lower. Calculated conformational energy against inter-ligand dihedral angle in linearly coordinated [Ag^I(*N3*-cytosine)$_2$]$^+$. *Transoid* conformation corresponds to $\theta=0°$. [61]

From a theoretical viewpoint, for co-planar ligands various conformations of C–Ag–C are possible, based on *cisoid* (**c**) and *transoid* (**t**) arrangements and linear or bent coordination geometry (Figure 3). For linear coordination geometry, the *transoid* arrangement is often cited as preferred due to the favorable orientation of complementary H-bonding sites on the nucleobase. However, as noted [61], typical Ag–N bond lengths locate the respective groups too far apart for such interactions. Despite this, the calculated energies of [Ag^I(*N3*-cytosine)$_2$]$^+$ as a function of the inter-ligand dihedral angle, θ, show that the minimum energy corresponds to the *transoid* ($\theta=0°$) conformation; with the maximum being for the *cisoid* ($\theta = 180°$) arrangement (Figure 3). Experimentally, the former conformation was found in [Ag^I(*N3*-cytosine)$_2$]PF$_6$·2H$_2$O, in which the silver ion occupies an inversion center and so the N–Ag–N angle is strictly 180° by symmetry. As expected from calculations, the O2⋯N4 inter-ligand distance was found to be too long, at 4.43 Å, for direct interaction. Instead, two water molecules bridge these groups through hydrogen bond formation (Figure 3).

When not constrained to linear coordination several bent conformations become possible; **c**$_{bent-OO}$, **c**$_{bent-NN}$, and **t**$_{bent}$ (Figure 3b, c and e, respectively). DFT calculations showed that the last of these corresponds to the minimum global energy conformation with the enhanced stability attributed to the formation of an intramolecular H-bond. This is made possible by a decrease in ∠N–Ag–N to ~156° and this conformation was observed experimentally in the hydrated nitrate salt, [Ag^I(*N3*-cytosine)$_2$]NO$_3$·H$_2$O (Figure 3). These two compounds represent the less common case where the ligands are, essentially, co-planar (twist angle <16°). More typically, C–Ag–C complexes adopt a twisted, non-coplanar ligand arrangement [62–64] which is seen in the anhydrous [Ag^I(*N3*-cytosine)$_2$]NO$_3$ where the inter-ligand plane angle is 47°; this compound features a slightly bent coordination geometry (∠N–Ag–N ~159°) and adopts a **c**$_{bent-OO}$ conformation.

A major finding realized of this work relates to the intermolecular self-assembly in the crystalline state. Compared to analogous complexes containing N1-substituted cytosine all three compounds, [Ag^I(*N3*-cytosine)$_2$]NO$_3$, and the corresponding hydrate and PF$_6^-$ salt, form extended hydrogen-bonded sheets (Figure 4). These sheets are formed through intermolecular hydrogen-bonding interactions that involve all of the donor and acceptor groups in the nucleobase including the donor group on N1H. This group is removed in analogous complexes containing cytidine [64], 1-methyl-C [63], and 1-hexyl-C [62] and a markedly different self-assembled structure is formed in these cases.

In each of these compounds, the C–Ag^I–C units assemble into supramolecular double helical chains *via* a combination of complementary hydrogen-bonding and argentophilic interactions (Figure 4). This type of supramolecular double helical

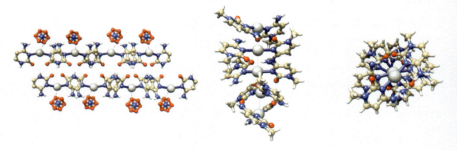

FIGURE 4 Left, a hydrogen-bonded sheet in the solid-state packing of [Ag^I(*N3*-cytosine)$_2$]NO$_3$. Center and right, the right-handed supramolecular duplex found in the solid-state structure of [Ag^I(*N3*-cytidine)$_2$]NO$_3$ sustained through intermolecular hydrogen-bonding and argentophilic interactions. [61, 64]

silver chain now appears to be quite general for small-molecule C–Ag^I–C MM-bp complexes. First reported by Terrón et al. [62] for [Ag^I(N3,N1-hexyl-C)$_2$]$^+$, this self-assembled structure is also noted in the 1-MeC derivative prepared by Galindo et al. [63]. In these cases, a racemic mixture of both right- and left-handed helix is observed.

In contrast, with the ribonucleoside cytidine as a ligand in [Ag^I(N3-cytidine)$_2$]$^+$ only a single, right-handed, double helix is formed [Note: duplex handedness is defined here by the coordinate bond vector, *not* the intermolecular hydrogen bonding] [64]. The single helical orientation observed, in this case, can be attributed to the influence of the chiral nucleoside. The silver ion chain in [Ag^I(N3-cytidine)$_2$]$^+$ forms the core of the duplex which has an ~15 Å helical pitch, as defined by the crystallographic *c*-axis. The chain of Ag atoms is essentially linear, (∠Ag···Ag···Ag range 162°–170°) and the duplex has a diameter similar to that of natural DNA, at 17.5(1) Å. The ligands of individual complex are twisted from co-planarity and generate "strands" of the double helix through NH···O=C hydrogen bonds between adjacent complexes. These are supported by argentophilic interactions with Ag···Ag distances ranging 2.98–3.05 Å; close to the metallic radius of 2.88 Å. Similar structural features are found for the alkylated derivatives [62, 63] though the Ag···Ag distances are typically slightly longer in these cases.

2.2 Electrical Properties and Band Structure of Silver-Nucleobase Chains

The solid-state structures of these small-molecule *N3*-C–Ag^I–*N3*-C complexes bare striking resemblance to the silver array in the fully argenated oligonucleotide duplex of Kondo et al. [43]. On account of the short intermetallic distances and obvious structural resemblance, these systems have been *referred to as nanowires - implying electrical conductivity* [43, 63].

The charge-carrying properties of MM-bp DNA have been of curiosity since Lee et al. reported metallo- or "M-DNA" (M=Co^{II}, Ni^{II} or Zn^{II}) in the late 1990s [80, 81]. Despite conflicting results [82–85], metallo-DNAs remain putative molecular nanowires due to the linear chain of metal atoms produced [43]. Monovalent silver ions' tendency to participate in metallophilic interactions [86] makes these systems especially interesting in this regard. However, there have been rather few reports probing the charge-carrying [87] or electrical properties of Ag^I-DNA chains [63, 87–89].

The structural similarity of [Ag^I(N3-cytidine)$_2$]NO$_3$ to these systems provides a useful model compound for assessing the electrical properties of this type of metallo-DNA assembly. The availability of high-quality crystalline samples in this study allowed electrical conductivity measurements to be performed on oriented single crystals [64]. For these experiments probe contacts were made, either directly or through In-Ga eutectic (to avoid issues of contact resistance), at opposite ends of the long crystallographic *c*-axis that is coincident with the Ag-chain direction (Figure 5). However, current-voltage (I-V) sweep experiments

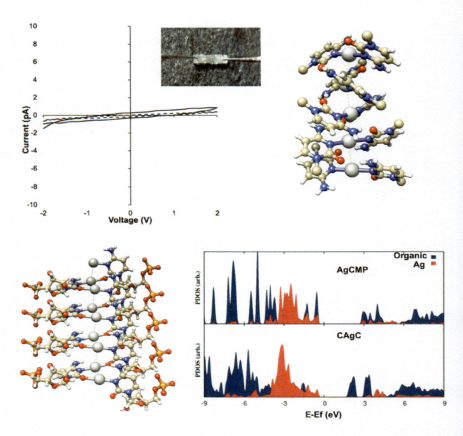

FIGURE 5 Upper left. I-V curves of oriented single crystals of [Ag^I(N3-1-MeC)$_2$]NO$_3$ (dash line) and [Ag^I(O2,N3-CMP)] (solid line) and inset optical image a single crystal of [Ag^I(N3-cytidine)$_2$]NO$_3$ directly contacted to probe needles. Right, molecular structure of the supramolecular helical chain in [Ag^I(N3-cytidine)$_2$]NO$_3$. Lower, left, molecular structure of the coordination chain in [Ag^I(O2,N3-CMP)]. Right, projected density of states in [Ag^I(O2,N3-CMP)] (upper) and [Ag^I(N3-1-MeC)$_2$]$^+$ (lower) showing their similarity in electron density distributions. [64, 66]

over a ±2 V range showed negligible current (<1 pA) indicating the compound was not electrically conducting, but an insulator. These findings of non-conductive behavior are in agreement with conducting-AFM (c-AFM) and scanned conductance microscopy (SCM) experiments on microcrystals of the 1-MeC analog by Galindo et al. [63].

The measured electrical properties for [Ag^I(N3-cytidine)$_2$]NO$_3$ are consistent with calculations of the local density of states for a single-chain [Ag^I(N3-1-MeC)$_2$]$^+$ model [64]. Plots of the ground-state projected density of states on the silver atoms and associated ligands, Figure 5, reveal a band gap at the Fermi energy of 2.502 eV [64] and, hence, the structure would not be expected to be an electrical conductor in the ground state. It was also noted from these calculations that the majority of the electron density in the LUMO states is found on the nucleobase ligands and not the central silver; so even after reduction, or n-doping, such systems would not be expected to be metal-based conductors.

An alternative type of silver chain has been reported for [Ag^I(*O2,N3*-CMP)] [65, 66] which features the *O2,N3*-bridging mode to generate a coordination polymer structure with a zig-zag arrangement of silver ions (Figure 5). These chains are further crosslinked into a porous 3D metal-organic framework (MOF) as the nucleotide phosphate oxygen groups also bind to metal ions. The resulting framework structure is sufficiently flexible to adapt to different solvent molecules, as shown by the isolation of several solvate crystal forms. For the hydrate and methanol solvates, an increase in cell volume of ~8% is noted; the latter being larger [65, 66]. This change in solvent impacts on the intermetallic distance in the coordination chains with Ag$\cdots$Ag distances of 2.959 and 3.140 Å for the hydrate and MeOH solvate, respectively [66]. Electrical conductivity measurements on oriented single crystals of the [Ag^I(*O2,N3*-CMP)]·H$_2$O showed insulating behavior similar to the supramolecular-assembled chains [64]. Band structure calculations for this type of silver coordination chain are also in keeping with this result and show a similar band-gap structure (3.32 eV in [Ag^I(*O2,N3*-CMP)] *vs.* 2.50 eV in [Ag^I(*N3*-1MeC)$_2$]$^+$) and electron density distributions in the ground-state density of states plot. In both the coordination and supramolecular-assembled chains the HOMO states have a large population on the central silver atoms with LUMO states being mostly distributed over the nucleobase ligand [66].

It was highlighted in this work [64] that these findings on conductivity do not necessarily contradict single-molecule STM measurement on Ag^I-polydC structures [88] which show evidence of tunneling current. This is because of the exponential variation of such currents with inter-electrode separation. STM experiments probe electron tunneling over the nanometer range, while SCM and single-crystal I/V measurements are, respectively, concerned with 100 nm and mesoscale distances, and the negligible conductivity in these measurements is unsurprising.

2.3 SUPRAMOLECULAR HYDRO- AND ORGANOGELS

Gelation is a common feature of nucleoside/tide chemistry [90, 91], particularly so for guanosine, and this is often influenced or promoted by metal ions [92, 93]. The resulting complexes act as, so-called, low-molecular-weight gelators [94–96] and, in contrast to traditional chemically crosslinked polymer gels, involve small-molecule self-assembly through supramolecular interactions to form the necessary three-dimensional network for solvent trapping and gelation. Silver-nucleoside/tide complexes have recently shown the ability to act as gelating agents for the formation of hydro- and organogels.

A rather unusual MM-bp has been proposed as responsible for the hydrogel formed by the reaction of silver ions with GMP, Figure 6 [97]. Hydrogels were prepared by reaction of Na$_2$GMP with Ag^I ions with viscosity increasing as the

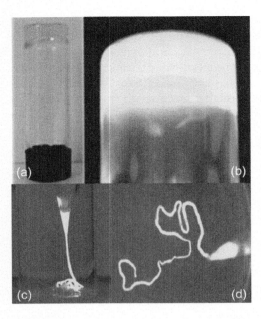

FIGURE 6 Left, optical image of the hydrogel formed by reaction of silver ions and GMP stained with fluorescein under natural light (a) and under UV irradiation (b) and after injection into acetonitrile. Guanosine-based Ag-mediated base pair proposed in the literature. (Reproduced from Ref. [97] with permission from the Royal Society of Chemistry.)

stoichiometry was raised from 1:1 to 1:2. The hydrogels comprised a typical interconnected matrix of nanofilaments, ca. 5 nm diameter, and had a sol-gel transition between 50°C and 80°C, depending on stoichiometry. Analysis by a range of techniques indicated the hydrogels to be constructed of filaments comprising helically stacked arrays of Ag-GMP dimers. These dimers are suggested to feature metal ion binding at N7 and O6 with associated deprotonation of N1 (Figure 6). The DNA-binding dye Hoechst-33258 was shown to bind to these filaments as indicated by chiral induction into the achiral dye by the helical assemblies. Such [(AgGMP)$_2$] dimers have been previously proposed by Petty based on calorimetry and other data (e.g. CD) to explain the increased viscosity of solutions of GMP (10^{-4} M range) upon addition of Ag ions [98].

The resulting Ag^I-GMP hydrogels were shown to be capable of immobilizing biomolecules and even supporting enzymatic transformations, as demonstrated with cytochrome c. Exhaustive washing treatment confirmed the protein to be strongly associated with the Ag^I-GMP matrix and the peroxidase activity of the enzyme was shown to be relatively little affected by immobilization. It was also found that prolonged exposure of the gel to light (12 h) or electron beam produced nanofilaments impregnated with Ag nanoparticles in the 2–4 nm size range with the resulting composite exhibiting the characteristic

Recent Developments in Self-Assembly and DNA Integration

440 nm absorption of the surface plasmon resonance band for metallic silver nanoparticles.

The supramolecular duplex observed in the solid-state for [Ag^{I}(*N3*-cytidine)$_2$]NO$_3$ (Figure 4) was shown to be sufficiently robust to produce alcohol-based organogels, with the formation of an entangled fibrous network of individual ~6.3 nm diameter gel fibers (Figure 7) [64]. The regularity of the fiber diameter is particularly noteworthy, with the size corresponding to 12 individual Ag-duplexes based on the crystal structure analysis. These fibers are seen to assemble into larger bundles in SEM studies (Figure 7). In methanol, the resulting gel is thixotropic i.e. exhibits self-repair, with the gel state collapsing by the application of slight shear force, such as minimal vibration or slow vial inversion, but recovering after ~20 min. Rheological studies showed a shear-thinning behavior with the viscosity reducing by three orders of magnitude as shear rate is increased, in a manner typical for supramolecular gels. Upon addition of 1 M urea, the gel

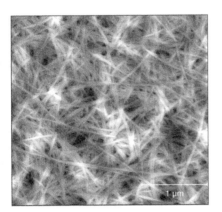
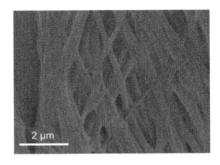
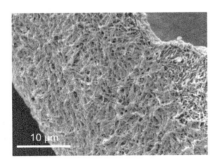
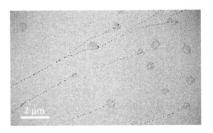

FIGURE 7 Upper, left. AFM image of [Ag^{I}(*N3*-cytidine)$_2$]NO$_3$ xerogel drop-cast onto a silicon wafer highlighting the regular nature of the gel fibers. Upper right lower left, SEM images of the xerogel showing the fiber bundling and the entangled porous matrix formed. Lower, right, TEM bright field image of [Ag^{I}(*N3*-cytidine)$_2$]NO$_3$ xerogel fibers after exposure to ambient light showing the presence of electron-dense silver particles. (Reproduced from Ref. [64] with permission from the Royal Society of Chemistry.)

rapidly collapsed to the solution state. This observation and the self-repair were explained by the reversible nature of the interactions forming the helices and crosslinking interactions between them, with hydrogen bonding being the major contributor to the super-structure of the fibers and gel network.

AFM and TEM of dried xerogel samples showed the presence of silver particles, ranging ~1–4 nm in diameter, rather regularly distributed along fibers (Figure 7). This was explained as arising from their light-sensitive nature, with photoreduction of $Ag^I \rightarrow Ag^0$ occurring in a similar manner to the Ag^I-GMP hydrogels of Mann et al. [97]. In contrast, however, the $[Ag^I(N3\text{-cytidine})_2]NO_3$ organogels exhibit photoemission ($\lambda = 395$ nm), even in freshly-prepared samples [64]. Further UV irradiation, up to 1 h at $\lambda = 300$ nm, showed gel samples to change color, from colorless to red, with an increase in emission intensity. The resulting emission was explained by photoreduction of Ag^I ions forming quantum-confined silver nanoclusters (Ag-NC) of size comparable to the Fermi wavelength for band-gap formation (~5 Å; <30 atoms). Further irradiation >1 h led to a slight decrease in the emission suggesting the formation of some larger, non-emissive, plasmonic nanoparticles over time. Samples remained emissive over weeks indicating the cytidine-bound Ag-NC to be in a highly stabilized coordination environment [64].

2.4 Structures of DNA-Stabilized Silver Nanoclusters

The formation of this type of luminescent Ag-NC on DNA, first reported by Dickson et al. [99, 100], has become one of the most well-studied aspects of silver–DNA chemistry (see also Chapter 12 of this book) [101, 102]. DNA oligonucleotides have been shown to form and stabilize a variety of clusters with different emission profiles, covering the UV–NIR range [102], based on cluster size [103–105], shape [106], and sequence [107, 108]. The importance of Ag^I–cytidine interactions and MM-bp has been noted in the preparations of Ag-NC and homo-C-oligomers have been used to form a variety of emissive materials [106, 109, 110].

Recently details of the nature of the metal–DNA interactions have been revealed by single-crystal samples of DNA-stabilized Ag-NC [104, 105, 111]. The structure by Lieberman et al. [104] features a Ag_8 cluster bound in a stem-like hairpin structure comprised of two 5′-d(AACCCC)-3′ strands (Figure 8). The silver atoms are arranged into two types; a C-rich stem that binds Ag_3 as metal-mediated base pairs involving C-N3 and an A-rich pocket that binds a trapezoidal Ag_5 cluster. In the former, tri-nuclear, grouping the bases are twisted to form hydrogen bonds between adjacent pairs as seen in supramolecular duplex of analogous small-molecule complex, such as $[Ag^I(N3\text{-cytidine})_2]NO_3$ [64]. In the latter grouping, four Ag atoms are co-planar while the fifth is slightly out-of-plane (ca. 12°) to froma Ag_5 core with the closest Ag–Ag distance comparable to that in the metallic element, at 2.9 Å. Each silver has two primary coordinate bonds from the DNA nucleobases which are provided by the endocyclic A-N1/C-N3 and the exocyclic A-N6/C-N4, with the latter sites proposed as deprotonated. It was noted that isolated crystal samples, formed in solution at pH 9.8, could appear colorless or

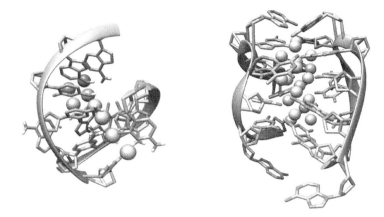

FIGURE 8 Molecular structures of luminescent DNA-stabilized silver clusters. Left, Ag$_8$ and right, Ag$_{16}$ clusters each bound to two, 6-mer and 10-mer, oligonucleotides, respectively.

brown with each showing different emission profiles. Colorless crystals could be converted to the brown by treatment with BH$_4^-$ and all types of crystal-produced superimposable crystal structures [104].

The structure of an NIR-emitting Ag$_{16}$ cluster has been reported by Vosch and Kondo, where the asymmetric unit contains two DNA-Ag$_{16}$ complexes [105]. Each cluster is bound by two DNA decamers with sequence 5'-d(CACCTAGCGA)-3'; a sequence selected from machine learning algorithms designed to predict sequences well-matched for stabilizing Ag-NCs. The Ag$_{16}$ cluster is encapsulated by the two DNA strands each folding in a distorted horseshoe manner and with inter-neighbor Ag–Ag distances typically in the 2.7–2.9 Å range, Figure 8. Distances that lie outside this range (2.6–3.1 Å) are still within the sum of the van der Waals radii (3.44 Å). Coordinate bond formation to the nucleobases involves C-N3 (2.2–2.3 Å), G-N1 (2.4 Å), A-N7 (2.3 Å) and G-O6 (2.3–2.4 Å); longer interactions to C-O2 (2.7–2.9 Å) and A-N1 (2.5 Å) are also noted. The associated ligand binding includes bridging modes involving C-O2/N3 and G-N1/O6. Silver-mediated base pairs, featuring N7-A–Ag^I–N3-A, are also involved in the crystal packing between DNA-Ag$_{16}$ units. While charge assignment of these types of Ag-NC can be difficult, these are generally considered to be quite highly oxidized, containing a mix of Ag^0 and Ag^I. In line with this, Gwinn has previously proposed a core-shell type arrangement for DNA-stabilized Ag-NC with a Ag^0-core and the Ag^I-shell coordinated by the nucleobases [106].

3 THIONUCLEOSIDES

3.1 Coinage Metal-Thiolate Coordination Polymers

Recently, in our efforts to develop methods for the integration of new properties into DNA-based materials and, in particular, to realize extended electronically delocalized states, we have turned to simple thionucleosides, particularly 6-thioguanosine. These are minimally modified mutants of their natural counterparts. Thiopurines and their ribose derivatives are used to treat a variety of medical conditions [112–115] and are rapidly incorporated into nucleic acids as a feature of their mode of action [116]. Their metal ion specificity and binding modes are notably different from the parent nucleosides due to the thione/thiol sulfur functionality [117] which specifies a high affinity for soft metal ions, such as low oxidation state coinage metals. Moreover, it provides the ability to form coordination chains through a single atom thiolate bridge, {-metal-μS-}$_n$ (Figure 9). This linkage can provide delocalization along the resulting metal-sulfur chains and promote effective electronic communication between metal centers. For coinage metals, the resulting thiolate coordination polymers exhibit a range of useful optoelectronic properties such as electrical conductivity [118, 119], tunable luminescence [120] and circularly polarized luminescence (CPL) [121] on account of this delocalized chain structure and, as a class of molecular materials, are increasingly important [122].

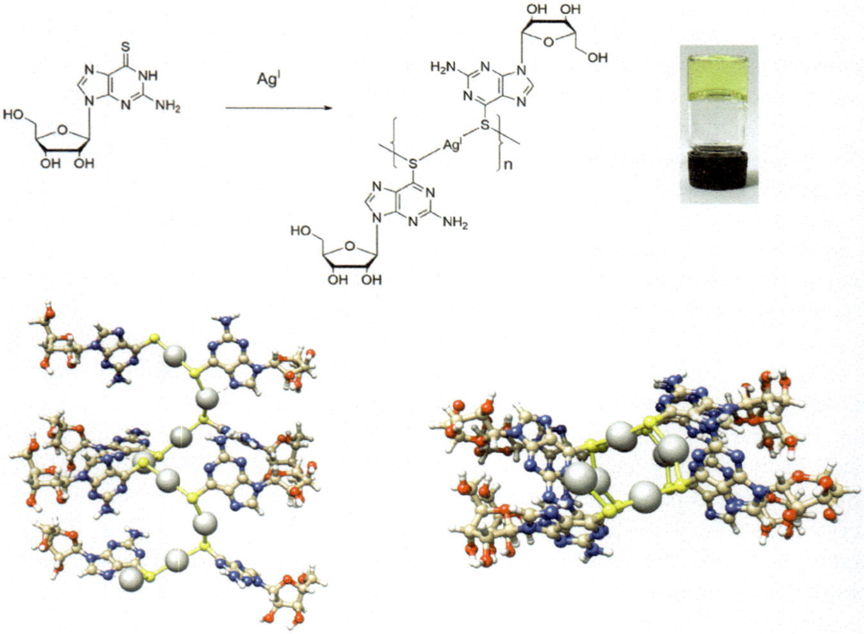

FIGURE 9 Upper, reaction scheme for the formation of Ag-thioguanosine and optical image of vial-inversion test of the resulting hydrogel for samples >15 mmol^{-1}. Lower, a model of the coordination polymer chain of Ag-thioguanosine viewed onto (left) and down (right) the helical axis of 1D supramolecular structure. (Reproduced and adapted from Ref. [121] with permission from the Royal Society of Chemistry.)

3.2 SILVER-THIOGUANOSINE: HIERARCHICAL SELF-ASSEMBLY, GELATION, AND CIRCULARLY POLARIZED LUMINESCENCE

We recently reported on the synthesis of the luminescent chain-like coordination polymer silver-thioguanosine, $\{Ag^I\text{-}\mu S\text{-}tG\}_n$, formed in the aqueous equimolar reaction of Ag^I ions and enantiomerically pure (–)6-thioguanosine (6tGH) (Figure 9) [121]. Formation of the metallo-thiolate polymer chain is indicated by a red-shift in the UV-visible band at longer wavelengths (310 to >338 nm) and an increase in the fluorescence emission lifetime. The increase in fluorescence lifetime was explained by the change in the tautomer equilibrium of 6-tGH from thione to thiolate form upon coordination, along with the stiffening effect of polymerization reducing the non-radiative decay rate.

High-resolution AFM showed the structure to comprise individual [-Ag^I-μS-6tG-]$_n$ chains ~1.9 nm in diameter that are helical and adopt a single, left-handed, sense. Figure 9 shows a model of the structure of an individual [-Ag^I-μS-6tG-]$_n$ polymer strand and highlights the similarity of the central metal-nucleoside arrangement of the coordination chain motif with that of typical MM-bp. The observed homochirality was attributed, at least partly, to the chiral nucleoside directing the metal-ligand self-assembly. The helicity of the chains was further confirmed by CD spectroscopy. This shows a much-increased band intensity compared to the parent ligand indicating a high structural ordering to the nucleobase chromophores. Extended delocalization of the excited state was shown by time-dependent DFT (TD-DFT) calculations. For $\{Ag^I\text{-}\mu S\text{-}6tG\}$ oligomers of increasing length, the CD spectra were shown to converge after 7 units.

The individual $\{Ag^I\text{-}\mu S\text{-}6tG\}_n$ chains were found to be involved in a hierarchical self-assembly process with reactions at higher concentrations ($\geq$15 mmol l^{-1}) forming a hydrogel (Figure 9). These gels contained (super)helical fiber bundles, shown by AFM and SEM/TEM electron microscopy to be several hundred nanometer in diameter and to retain the helicity of the component chains (Figure 10). Hydrophobic base stacking was found to be important in this hierarchical assembly process, as indicated by the appearance of a new, broad, red-shifted luminescence band (~550 nm). This band was ascribed to, approximate, head-to-tail exciton coupling of the organic fluorophores [121]. Gel samples had the ability to self-repair from the sol state; a feature that was explained by the non-covalent nature of the inter-chain interactions and dynamic change to strand length through reversibility of intrachain metal-ligand bonding.

As a result of the chiral nature and inherent photoemission, the $\{Ag^I\text{-}\mu S\text{-}thioG\}_n$ hydrogel was found to directly generate circularly polarized light in the form of circularly polarized luminescence (CPL). The luminescence dissymmetry factor (g_{lum}) was -0.04 ± 0.02 at 600 nm and -0.07 ± 0.01 at 735 nm; by comparison, neither solutions of 6-thioguanosine (6tG) nor $\{Ag^I\text{-}\mu S\text{-}thioG\}_n$ at concentrations <15 mmol^{-1} showed significant CPL. The high CPL emission for the hydrogel was explained by the delocalization of the excited state in a rigid, self-assembled, (super)structure, though a contribution from chiral scattering effects owing to the

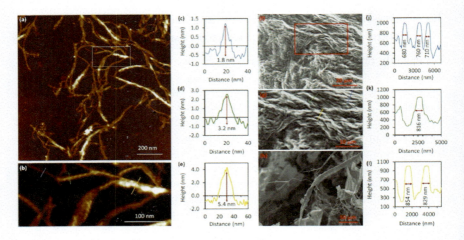

FIGURE 10 AFM and SEM images of Ag-thioguanosine xerogel drop-cast onto a silicon wafer. Large-scan area (a) of AFM height image of the Ag-6tG xerogel. (b) A zoom area of the AFM image (a) shows individual molecular and helical, bundle structures of multi-molecular chains. The associated cross-sections along the blue (c), green (d) and yellow (e) lines in the AFM image (b). (f) SEM images of Ag-thioguanosine xerogel film showing the microscopic metallo-thiolate structures entangled to form the gelating network. (g) and (h) zoom areas of the SEM image (f) showing the entangled fiber and helical structure of the xerogel. The associated cross-sections along the blue (j), green (k) and yellow, (l) lines in the SEM image (g). (Reproduced from Ref. [121] with permission from the Royal Society of Chemistry.)

handedness of the fibers of the gel could not be ruled out. This was the first report of a metallo-nucleoside system to directly exhibit CPL.

3.3 Gold-Thioguanosine: Electrical Conduction and Incorporation into DNA Duplex

We have also demonstrated that the equivalent reaction between Au^I ions and (−)6-tGH yields an analogous chain-like coordination polymer, [Au^I-μS-6-tG]$_n$ [123]. This too forms as a luminescent, sample-spanning, hydrogel with gelation rapidly occurring. Analysis of the corresponding xerogel by AFM reveals micron-long, helically twisted, strands with individual width similar to the case for the silver analog and duplex DNA at ~2 nm (Figure 11). The Au^I-thiolate backbone of the polymer chain was shown to be helical due to the appearance of long wavelengths CD bands (>380 nm) which were assigned to metal-ligand charge transfer.

As was seen in the silver analog, DFT calculations of the electronic structure of individual coordination chains show substantial delocalization of the HOMO. This includes significant contributions from the {Au-μS}$_n$ backbone as well as smaller contributions from the nucleobase π-system. Furthermore, calculations

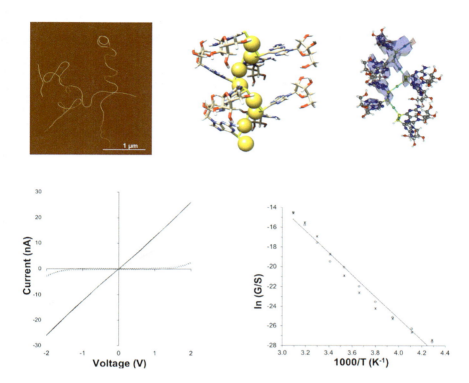

FIGURE 11 Upper. Left AFM image of Au-thioguanosine coordination polymer chains. Molecular model of a single helical coordination polymer chain highlighting the central gold-thiolate backbone (center) and a spin-density map of a {Au^I-μ-6-tG}$_8$ oligomer showing the delocalization of spin density after one-electron oxidation. Lower, I/V curves for Au-thioguanosine xerogel before (....) and after oxidative doping with tris-(4-bromophenyl)ammoniumyl hexachloroantimonate (—) and iodine (---), left and an Arrhenius plot for the zero-bias conductance of the I$_2$-doped Au-thioguanosine showing heating (x) and cooling cycles (o), right. (Reproduced with permission from [123].)

on [Au^I-μS-6-tG] 8-mers after one-electron removal showed residual spin density to be delocalized predominantly along the metal-sulfur chain direction indicating that a *conductive material may be produced by oxidative doping* (Figure 11).

This switching of gold-thioguanosine from an electrically insulating to conducting form by partial oxidation was demonstrated for the corresponding xerogel. While the as-prepared, neutral form, of the material was effectively insulating, after oxidative doping using iodine samples showed a marked increase in electrical conductivity (Figure 11). Variable temperature I/V measurements showed Arrhenius behavior characteristic of a thermally-activated hopping with an activation barrier of 94 kJ mol^{-1}. The use of alternative oxidants, such as tris-(4-bromophenyl) ammoniumyl hexachloroantimonate (magic blue), showed similar behavior confirming electric conduction to be associated with the coordination

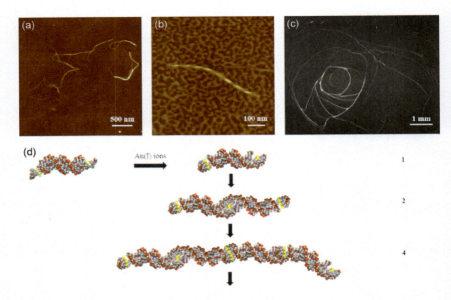

FIGURE 12 Au-thiolate-DNA concatemers. Upper, AFM height images showing the one-dimensional nature of Au-[OligoS$_4$]$_n$ concatemer structures (a) and highlighting the helicity of a single structure (b). Fluorescence image of Au-[OligoS$_4$]$_n$ revealing the macroscopic nature of the fibers (c). Lower, Schematic illustrating the formation of DNA-Au-thiolate sequenced duplex formed by metal-ligand bond self-assembly (d). (Reproduced with permission from Ref. [123].)

polymer and not polyiodide species (Figure 11). The doped material was found to be stable up to at least 50°C.

A particularly significant finding in this work was the compatibility of the metal-ligand bond-forming reaction with thioguanosine-modified oligonucleotides [123]. This then provided a means to integrate the highly functional {Au-μS}$_n$ coordination motif site-specifically into a DNA duplex. This was shown for an 18-mer oligonucleotide, [OligoS$_4$], containing a self-complementary 14-base sequence and a 5'-terminus of four consecutive 6-deoxythioguanosines. This was designed so as to form concatemers upon reaction with Au^I ions through binding and crosslinking of terminal thioguanosine regions. Annealing the self-complementary oligonucleotide was shown to form the regular B-type duplex structure presenting thioG terminal sections. Upon reaction with Au^I ions, a more A-type DNA conformation was adopted and the resulting Au^I-DNA complex exhibited the characteristic orange luminescence of oligomeric Au^I-thiolate species. This resulting emission confirmed the formation of the coordination chain motif at sequence-specific locations generating an alternating {metallo-thiolate/DNA} structure (Figure 12). AFM studies showed the formation of one-dimensional structures extending up to several microns in length, much longer than the parent oligonucleotide duplex, as expected for a concatemeric reaction (Figure 12).

4 CONCLUSION

The coordination chemistry of the heavier coinage metals with DNA and its constituents offers exciting possibilities for future development. While copper is well-studied in this context, silver and gold are now being explored with far more vigor, due to the unique properties that these metal ions can bring to DNA-based materials. Undoubtedly, the discovery of DNA-stabilized Ag-NC [99], the ability to tune their emission [103], and the realization that fully argenated DNA duplex [43, 70] can be prepared have been significant drivers for this. An increased understanding of this chemistry, aided by state-of-the-art structural studies [104, 105, 111, 124], will undoubtedly provide new optically-active probes and tools for a variety of applications [102].

Metallo-gels [93, 125] are an increasingly explored material type that combines the soft-matter properties of traditional gels along with the additional features only offered by metal ions. That silver [97, 121] and gold [123] can provide nucleoside-based gel systems offers yet further avenues to be explored.

Finally, the realization of *electronically delocalized metal-nucleoside chains* with thionucleoside-based coordination polymers provides a range of novel optoelectronic properties for incorporation into DNA [121, 123]. The first report of a metallo-nucleoside system to display circularly polarized luminescence, as with silver-thioguanosine, extends the range of optical properties now available from metallo-DNA complexes and such materials are increasingly sought for applications in displays, lighting, and optical quantum memory [121]. The observation of electrical conduction in the gold-analog [123] delivers on a long-sought challenge for metallo-DNA to develop a DNA-based electronics. That the underlying metal-thiolate self-assembly can be integrated with DNA provides a novel route for the site-specific incorporation of semiconducting regions into duplex DNA. It is interesting to note that the possibility to introduce new types of coordination motif into DNA using thionucleotides has also been demonstrated with 4-thiothymidine with the corresponding base pair mismatch shown to coordinate *pairs of silver ions* [126]. The exploration and development of the above findings provide much opportunity for exciting developments in the future.

ACKNOWLEDGMENTS

Dr Osama El-Zubir is thanked for his assistance in preparing figures for this chapter.

ABBREVIATIONS AND DEFINITIONS

AFM   atomic force microscopy
CMP   5′-cytidine-monophosphate
CPL   circularly polarized luminescence
DMPE   1,2-bis(dimethylphosphino)ethane-P, P′
GMP   5′-guanosine monophosphate
I/V   current/voltage

SCM   scanned conductance microscopy
TEM   transmission electron microscopy

REFERENCES

1. M. R. Jones, N. C. Seeman, C. A. Mirkin, *Science* **2015**, *347*, 1260901.
2. W. J. Meng, R. A. Muscat, M. L. McKee, P. J. Milnes, A. H. El-Sagheer, J. Bath, B. G. Davis, T. Brown, R. K. O'Reilly, A. J. Turberfield, *Nat. Chem.* **2016**, *8*, 542–548.
3. Eds E. Stulz, G. H. Clever, *DNA in Supramolecular Chemistry and Nanotechnology*, John Wiley & Sons, Chichester, **2015**, pp. 1–500.
4. P. W. K. Rothemund, *Nature* **2006**, *440*, 297.
5. T. Tørring, N. V. Voigt, J. Nangreave, H. Yan, K. V. Gothelf, *Chem. Soc. Rev.* **2011**, *40*, 5636–5646.
6. A. Rangnekar, T. H. LaBean, *Acc. Chem. Res.* **2014**, *47*, 1778–1788.
7. E. Braun, K. Keren, *Adv. Phys.* **2004**, *53*, 441–496.
8. J. F. Liu, Y. L. Geng, E. Pound, S. Gyawali, J. R. Ashton, J. Hickey, A. T. Woolley, J. N. Harb, *ACS Nano* **2011**, *5*, 2240–2247.
9. B. Uprety, T. Westover, M. Stoddard, K. Brinkerhoff, J. Jensen, R. Davis, A. T. Woolley, J. Harb, *Langmuir* **2017**, *33*, 726–735.
10. A. Houlton, S. M. D. Watson, *Annu. Rep. Prog. Chem. A* **2011**, *107*, 21–42.
11. K. L. Young, M. B. Ross, M. G. Blaber, M. Rycenga, M. R. Jones, C. Zhang, A. J. Senesi, B. Lee, G. C. Schatz, C. A. Mirkin, *Adv. Mater.* **2014**, *26*, 653–659.
12. D. J. Park, C. Zhang, J. C. Ku, Y. Zhou, G. C. Schatz, C. A. Mirkin, *Proc. Natl. Acad. Sci. U. S. A.* **2015**, *112*, 977–981.
13. Y. Kim, R. J. Macfarlane, C. A. Mirkin, *J. Am. Chem. Soc.* **2013**, *135*, 10342–10345.
14. S. M. D. Watson, A. R. Pike, J. Pate, A. Houlton, B. R. Horrocks, *Nanoscale* **2014**, *6*, 4027–4037.
15. H. A. Becerril, R. M. Stolenberg, D. R. Wheeler, R. C. Davis, J. N. Harb, A. T. Woolley, *J. Am. Chem. Soc.* **2005**, *127*, 2828–2829.
16. J. Richter, M. Mertig, W. Pompe, I. Mönch, H. K. Schackert, *Appl. Phys. Lett.* **2001**, *78*, 536–538.
17. S. M. D. Watson, N. G. Wright, B. R. Horrocks, A. Houlton, *Langmuir* **2009**, *26*, 2068–2075.
18. Y. L. Geng, A. C. Pearson, E. P. Gates, B. Uprety, R. C. Davis, J. N. Harb, A. T. Woolley, *Langmuir* **2013**, *29*, 3482–3490.
19. L. Dong, T. Hollis, B. A. Connolly, N. G. Wright, B. R. Horrocks, A. Houlton, *Adv. Mater.* **2007**, *19*, 1748–1751.
20. H. D. A. Mohamed, S. M. D. Watson, B. R. Horrocks, A. Houlton, *Nanoscale* **2012**, *4*, 5936–5945.
21. R. Hassanien, S. A. F. Al-Said, L. Siller, R. Little, N. G. Wright, A. Houlton, B. R. Horrocks, *Nanotechnology* **2012**, *23*, 075601.
22. L. Dong, T. Hollis, S. Fishwick, B. A. Connolly, N. G. Wright, B. R. Horrocks, A. Houlton, *Chem. Eur. J.* **2007**, *13*, 822–828.
23. S. Pruneanu, S. A. F. Al-Said, L. Dong, T. A. Hollis, M. A. Galindo, N. G. Wright, A. Houlton, B. R. Horrocks, *Adv. Funct. Mater.* **2008**, *18*, 2444–2454.
24. R. Hassanien, M. Al-Hinai, S. A. Farha Al-Said, R. Little, L. Siller, N. G. Wright, A. Houlton, B. R. Horrocks, *ACS Nano* **2010**, *4*, 2149–2159.
25. S. M. D. Watson, J. H. Hedley, M. A. Galindo, S. A. F. Al-Said, N. G. Wright, B. A. Connolly, B. R. Horrocks, A. Houlton, *Chem. Eur. J.* **2012**, *18*, 12008–12019.

26. S. M. D. Watson, M. A. Galindo, B. R. Horrocks, A. Houlton, *J. Am. Chem. Soc.* **2014**, *136*, 6649–6655.
27. E. P. Gates, A. M. Dearden, A. T. Woolley, *Crit. Rev. Anal. Chem.* **2014**, *44*, 354–370.
28. M. N. Al Hinai, R. Hassanien, N. G. Wright, A. B. Horsfall, A. Houlton, B. R. Horrocks, *Faraday Discuss.* **2013**, *164*, 71–91.
29. B. Lippert, *J. Biol. Inorg. Chem.* **2022**, *27*, 215–219.
30. J.-L. H. A. Duprey, J. Carr-Smith, S. L. Horswell, J. Kowalski, J. H. R. Tucker, *J. Am. Chem. Soc.* **2016**, *138*, 746–748.
31. E. Stulz, *Acc. Chem. Res.* **2017**, *50*, 823–831.
32. J. Manchester, D. M. Bassani, J.-L. H. A. Duprey, L. Giordano, J. S. Vyle, Z.-Y. Zhao, J. H. R. Tucker, *J. Am. Chem. Soc.* **2012**, *134*, 10791–10794.
33. H. Yanga, K. L. Meterab, H. F. Sleiman, *Coord. Chem. Rev.* **2010**, *254*, 2403–2415.
34. A. R. Pike, L. C. Ryder, B. R. Horrocks, W. Clegg, M. R. J. Elsegood, B. A. Connolly, A. Houlton, *Chem. Eur. J.* **2002**, *8*, 2891–2899.
35. A. R. Pike, L. C. Ryder, B. R. Horrocks, W. Clegg, B. A. Connolly, A. Houlton, *Chem. Eur. J.* **2004**, *17*, 344–353.
36. D. J. Hurley, Y. Tor, *J. Am. Chem. Soc.* **1998**, *120*, 2194–2195.
37. D. J. Hurley, Y. Tor, *J. Am. Chem. Soc.* **2002**, *124*, 3749–3762.
38. G. H. Clever, C. Kaul, T. Carell, *Angew. Chem. Int. Ed.* **2007**, *46*, 6226–6236.
39. G. H. Clever, M. Shionoya, *Coord. Chem. Rev.* **2010**, *254*, 2391–2402.
40. Y. Takezawa, M. Shionoya, *Acc. Chem. Res.* **2012**, *45*, 2066–2076.
41. P. Scharf, J. Müller, *ChemPlusChem* **2013**, *78*, 20–34.
42. N. Santamaría-Díaz, J. M. Méndez-Arriaga, J. M. Salas, M. A. Galindo, *Angew. Chem. Int. Ed.* **2016**, *55*, 6170–6174.
43. J. Kondo, Y. Tada, T. Dairaku, Y. Hattori, H. Saneyoshi, A. Ono, Y. Tanaka, *Nat. Chem.* **2017**, *9*, 956–960.
44. J. Müller, *Coord. Chem. Rev.* **2019**, *393*, 37–47.
45. F. H. Allen, O. Kennard, *Chem. Des. Autom. News* **1993**, *8*, 31–37.
46. P. J. Sanz Miguel, P. Amo-Ochoa, O. Castillo, A. Houlton, F. Zamora, in Metal Complex–DNA Interactions, Eds N. Hadjiliadis, E. Sletten, Blackwell Publishing Ltd, Chippenham, **2009**, pp. 95–132.
47. G. L. Eichhorn, J. J. Butzow, P. Clark, E. Tarien, *Biopolymers* **1967**, *5*, 283–296.
48. M. A. Galindo, D. Amania, A. Martinez Martinez, W. Clegg, R. W. Harrington, V. Moreno Martinez, A. Houlton, *Inorg. Chem.* **2009**, *48*, 10295–10303.
49. P. C. Gagnon, A. L. Beauchamp, *Acta Crystallogr. B* **1977**, *33*, 1448–1454.
50. M. D. Pandey, A. K. Mishra, V. Chandrasekhar, S. Verma, *Inorg. Chem.* **2010**, *49*, 2020–2022.
51. C. S. Purohit, A. K. Mishra, S. Verma, *Inorg. Chem.* **2007**, *46*, 8493–8495.
52. J. Kumar, Pratibha, S. Verma, *Inorg. Chim. Acta* **2016**, *452*, 214–221.
53. S. Menzer, E. C. Hillgeris, B. Lippert, *Inorg. Chim. Acta* **1993**, *210*, 167–171.
54. F. Guay, A. L. Beauchamp, *J. Am. Chem. Soc.* **1979**, *101*, 6260–6263.
55. K. Aoki, W. Saenger, *Acta Cryst. C* **1984**, *40*, 775–778.
56. M. Barceló-Oliver, B. A. Baquero, A. Bauzá, A. García-Raso, R. Vich, I. Mata, E. Molins, A. Terrón, A. Frontera, *Dalton Trans.* **2013**, *42*, 7631–7642.
57. M. Barceló-Oliver, C. Estarellas, A. Terrón, A. García-Rasoa, A. Frontera, *Chem. Comm.* **2011**, *47*, 4646–4648.
58. A. K. Mishra, R. K. Prajapati, S. Verma, *Dalton Trans.* **2010**, *39*, 10034–10037.
59. C. S. Purohit, S. Verma, *J. Am. Chem. Soc.* **2007**, *129*, 3488–3489.
60. S. Menzer, M. Sabat, B. Lippert, *J. Am. Chem. Soc.* **1992**, *114*, 4644–4649.

61. L. Mistry, P. G. Waddell, N. G. Wright, B. R. Horrocks, A. Houlton, *Inorg. Chem.* **2019**, *58*, 13346–13352.
62. A. Terron, B. Moreno-Vachiano, A. Bauza, A. Garcia-Raso, J. J. Fiol, M. Barceló-Oliver, E. Molins, A. Frontera, *Chem. Eur. J.* **2017**, *23*, 2103–2108.
63. F. Linares, E. García-Fernández, F. J. López-Garzón, M. Domingo-García, A. Orte, A. Rodríguez-Diéguez, M. A. Galindo, *Chem. Sci.* **2019**, *10*, 1126–1137.
64. L. Mistry, O. El-Zubir, G. Dura, W. Clegg, P. G. Waddell, T. Pope, W. A. Hofer, N. G. Wright, B. R. Horrocks, A. Houlton, *Chem. Sci.* **2019**, *10*, 3186–3195.
65. A. Terrón, L. Tomàs, A. Bauzá, A. García-Raso, J. J. Fiol, E. Molins, A. Frontera, *CrystEngComm* **2017**, *19*, 5830–5834.
66. L. Mistry, P. G. Waddell, N. G. Wright, B. R. Horrocks, A. Houlton, *Cryst. Grow. Des.* **2021**, *21*, 4398–4405.
67. T. J. Kistenmacher, M. Rossi, L. G. Marzilli, *Inorg. Chem.* **1979**, *18*, 240–244.
68. J. Kondo, Y. Tada, T. Dairaku, H. Saneyoshi, Y. Okamoto, K. Tanaka, A. Ono, *Angew. Chem. Int. Ed.* **2015**, *54*, 13323–13326.
69. H. Liu, F. Shen, P. Haruehanroengra, Q. Yao, Y. Cheng, Y. Chen, C. Yang, J. Zhang, B. Wu, Q. Luo, R. Cui, J. Li, J. Ma, J. Sheng, J. Gan, *Angew. Chem. Int. Ed.* **2017**, *56*, 9430–9434.
70. T. Atsugi, A. Ono, M. Tasaka, N. Eguchi, S. Fujiwara, J. Kondo, *Angew. Chem. Int. Ed.* **2022**, *61*, e202204798.
71. S. M. Swasey, L. E. Leal, O. Lopez-Acevedo, J. Pavlovich, E. G. Gwinn, *Sci. Rep.* **2015**, *5*, 1016310.
72. S. M. Swasey, E. G. Gwinn, *New J. Phys.* **2016**, *18*, 045008.
73. R. R. Faggiani, H. E. Howard-Lock, C. J. L. Lock, M. A. Turner, *Can. J. Chem.* **1987**, *65*, 1568–1575.
74. E. Colacioa, O. Crespo, R. Cuesta, R. Kivekäs, A. Laguna, *J. Inorg. Biochem.* **2004**, *98*, 595–600.
75. A. Schimanski, E. Freisinger, A. Erxleben, B. Lippert, *Inorg. Chim. Acta* **1998**, *283*, 223–232.
76. M. S. Holowczak, M. D. Stancl, G. B. Wong, *J. Am. Chem. Soc.* **1985**, *107*, 5789–5790.
77. W. Micklitz, B. Lippert, *Inorg. Chim. Acta* **1989**, *165*, 57–64.
78. B. Fischer, H. Preut, B. Lippert, H. Schöllhorn, U. Thewalt, *Polyhedron* **1990**, *9*, 2199–2204.
79. E. Ennifar, P. Walter, P. Dumas, *Nucl. Acid Res.* **2003**, *31*, 2671–2682.
80. P. Aich, S. L. Labiuk, L. W. Tari, L. J. T. Delbaere, W. J. Roesler, K. J. Falk, R. P. Steer, J. S. Lee, *J. Mol. Biol.* **1999**, *294*, 477–485.
81. A. Rakitin, P. Aich, C. Papadopoulos, Y. Kobzar, A. S. Vedeneev, J. S. Lee, J. M. Xu, *Phys. Rev. Lett.* **2001**, *86*, 3670–3673.
82. F. Moreno-Herrero, P. Herrero, F. Moreno, J. Colchero, C. Gómez-Navarro, J. Gomez-Herrero, A. M. Baró, *Nanotechnology* **2003**, *14*, 128–133.
83. B. Liu, A. J. Bard, C.-Z. Li, H.-B. Kraatz, *J. Phys. Chem. B* **2005**, *109*, 5193–5198.
84. K. Mizoguchi, S. Tanaka, T. Ogawa, N. Shiobara, H. Sakamoto, *Phys. Rev. B* **2005**, *72*, 033106.
85. B. Q. Spring, R. M. Clegg, *J. Phys. Chem. B* **2007**, *111*, 10040–10052.
86. H. Schmidbaur, A. Schier, *Angew. Chem. Int. Ed.* **2015**, *54*, 746–784.
87. J. C. Léon, Z. She, A. Kamal, M. H. Shamsi, J. Müller, H.-B. Kraatz, *Angew. Chem. Int. Ed.* **2017**, *56*, 6098–6102.
88. E. Toomey, J. Xu, S. Vecchioni, L. Rothschild, S. J. Wind, G. E. Fernandes, *J. Phys. Chem. C* **2016**, *120*, 7804–7809.
89. G. Ban, R. Dong, K. Li, H. Han, X. Yan, *Nano. Res. Lett.* **2009**, *4*, 321–326.

90. J. T. Davis, G. P. Spada, *Chem. Soc. Rev.* **2007**, *36*, 296–313.
91. F. Carducci, J. S. Yoneda, R. Itri, P. Mariani, *Soft Matter* **2018**, *14*, 2938–2948.
92. G. M. Peters, J. T. Davis, *Chem. Soc. Rev.* **2016**, *45*, 3188–3206.
93. H. Liang, Z. Zhang, Q. Yuan, J. Liu, *Chem. Commun.* **2015**, *51*, 15196–15199.
94. M.-O. M. Piepenbrock, G. O. Lloyd, N. Clarke, J. W. Steed, *Chem. Rev.* **2010**, *110*, 1960–2004.
95. E. R. Draper, D. J. Adams, *Chem* **2017**, *3*, 390–410.
96. X. Du, J. Zhou, J. Shi, B. Xu, *Chem. Rev.* **2015**, *115*, 13165–13307.
97. J. Dash, A. J. Patil, R. N. Das, F. L. Dowdalla, S. Mann, *Soft Matter* **2011**, *7*, 8120–8126.
98. K. Loo, N. Degtyareva, J. Park, B. Sengupta, M. Reddish, C. C. Rogers, A. Bryant, J. T. Petty, *J. Phys. Chem. B* **2010**, *114*, 4320–4326.
99. J. T. Petty, J. Zheng, N. V. Hud, R. M. Dickson, *J. Am. Chem. Soc.* **2004**, *126*, 5207–5212.
100. C. I. Richards, S. Choi, J.-C. Hsiang, Y. Antoku, T. Vosch, A. Bongiorno, Y.-L. Tzeng, R. M. Dickson, *J. Am. Chem. Soc.* **2008**, *130*, 5038–5039.
101. S. Choi, R. M. Dickson, J. Yu, *Chem. Soc. Rev.* **2012**, *41*, 1867–1891.
102. A. Gonzàlez-Rosell, C. Cerretani, P. Mastracco, T. Vosch, S. M. Copp, *Nanoscale Adv.* **2021**, *3*, 1230–1260.
103. S. M. Copp, D. Schultz, S. M. Swasey, E. G. Gwinn, *ACS Nano* **2015**, *9*, 2303–2310.
104. D. J. E. Huard, A. Demissie, D. Kim, D. Lewis, R. M. Dickson, J. T. Petty, R. L. Lieberman, *J. Am. Chem. Soc.* **2019**, *141*, 11465–11470.
105. C. Cerretani, H. Kanazawa, T. Vosch, J. Kondo, *Angew. Chem. Int. Ed.* **2019**, *58*, 17153–17157.
106. D. Schultz, K. Gardner, S. S. Oemrawsingh, N. Markesevic, K. Olsson, M. Debord, D. Bouwmeester, E. G. Gwinn, *Adv. Mater.* **2013**, *25*, 2797–2803.
107. S. M. Copp, P. Bogdanov, M. Debord, A. Singh, E. G. Gwinn, *Adv. Mater.* **2014**, *26*, 5839–5845.
108. S. M. Copp, S. M. Swasey, A. Gorovits, P. Bogdanov, E. G. Gwinn, *Chem. Mater.* **2020**, *32*, 430–437.
109. C. M. Ritchie, K. R. Johnsen, J. R. Kiser, Y. Antoku, R. M. Dickson, J. T. Petty, *J. Phys. Chem. C* **2007**, *111*, 175–181.
110. J. C. Léon, D. González-Abradelo, C. A. Strassert, J. Müller, *Chem. Eur. J.* **2018**, *24*, 8320–8324.
111. C. Cerretani, J. Kondo, T. Vosch, *CrystEngComm* **2020**, *22*, 8136–8141.
112. G. B. Elion, *In Vitro Cell. Dev. Biol.* **1989**, *25*, 321–330.
113. M. Freund, H. Poliwoda, H. Bodenstein, R. Eisert, *Onkologie* **1985**, *8*, 150–152.
114. J. C. Dabrowiak, *Metals in Medicine*, John Wiley & Sons, Chichester, UK, pp. 191–217.
115. B. O. Leung, F. Jalilehvand, V. Mah, M. Parvez, Q. Wu, *Inorg. Chem.* **2013**, *52*, 4593–4602.
116. J. Aarbakke, G. Janka-Schaub, G. B. Elion, *Trends Pharmacol. Sci.* **1997**, *18*, 3–7.
117. P. D. Cookson, E. R. T. Tiekink, *Aust. J. Chem.* **1994**, *47*, 577.
118. H. Yan, J. N. Hohman, F. H. Li, C. Jia, D. Solis-Ibarra, B. Wu, J. E. P. Dahl, R. M. K. Carlson, B. A. Tkachenko, A. A. Fokin, P. R. Schreiner, A. Vailionis, T. R. Kim, T. P. Devereaux, Z.-X. Shen, N. A. Melosh, *Nat. Mater.* **2017**, *16*, 349–357.
119. H. Yan, F. Yang, D. Pan, Y. Lin, J. N. Hohman, D. Solis-Ibarra, F. H. Li, J. E. P. Dahl, R. M. K. Carlson, B. A. Tkachenko, A. A. Fokin, P. R. Schreiner, G. Galli, W. L. Mao, Z.-X. Shen, N. A. Melosh, *Nature* **2018**, *554*, 505–510.
120. O. Veselska, C. Dessal, S. Melizi, N. Guillou, D. Podbevšek, G. Ledoux, E. Elkaim, A. Fateeva, A. Demessence, *Inorg. Chem.* **2019**, *58*, 99–105.

121. O. El-Zubir, P. Rojas Martinez, G. Dura, L. L. G. Al-Mahamad, T. Pope, T. J. Penfold, L. E. Mackenzie, R. Pal, J. Mosely, L. F. McGarry, B. R. Horrocks, A. Houlton, *J. Mater. Chem. C* **2022**, *10*, 7329–7335.
122. O. Veselska, A. Demessence, *Coord. Chem. Rev.* **2018**, *335*, 240–270.
123. L. L. G. Al-Mahamad, O. El-Zubir, D. G. Smith, B. R. Horrocks, A. Houlton, *Nat. Comm.* **2017**, *8*, 720.
124. C. Cerretani, J. Kondo, T. Vosch, *RSC Adv.* **2020**, *10*, 23854–23860.
125. J. Zhang, C.-Y. Su, *Coord. Chem. Rev.* **2013**, *257*, 1373–1408.
126. J. Kondo, T. Sugawara, H. Saneyoshi, A. Ono, *Chem. Commun.* **2017**, *53*, 11747–11750.

5 Interplay between Noncovalent Interactions and Metal Ions in Nucleic Acids and Their Constituents

Miquel Barceló-Oliver, Antonio Frontera*,
Juan Jesús Fiol, Ángel García-Raso,
and Ángel Terrón*

Department of Chemistry, University of the Balearic
Islands, Bldg. Mateu Orfila i Rotger, Carretera
Valldemossa km 7.5, E–07122 Palma (Mallorca), Spain
miquel.barcelo@uib.es, toni.frontera@uib.es,
jfa950@uib.es, angel.garcia-raso@
uib.es, angel.terron@uib.es

CONTENTS

1	Introduction	106
2	Examples of Recognition in the Metal–Nucleotide System	107
	2.1 The Metal Ion Instead of Hydrogen	107
	2.2 Using Polynucleotides or Bases to Produce Argentophilic and Aurophilic Interactions	116
	2.3 Regium Bonds in the Nucleotide World	122
	2.4 Cation–π Interactions	122
	2.5 Anion–π Interactions	123
3	Concluding Remarks and Future Directions	128
Acknowledgments		128
Abbreviations and Definitions		128
References		129

---

[*] Corresponding authors

Abstract

This chapter describes the influence of metal coordination to nucleobases, nucleosides, and nucleotides (and their derivatives) upon their ability to establish a variety of noncovalent interactions. Upon coordination, the electronic density of the nucleobases change drastically, increasing their ability to establish certain interactions like H-bonding, anion–π, lone pair–π, and anti-parallel π-stacking among others. Concurrently, the metal coordination affects the ability of the metal itself to participate in weak interactions like metallophilic, regium bonding, etc. This chapter describes the recent literature on this topic, without the intention to be comprehensive. For this purpose, selected and relevant examples are described in detail to illustrate the ability of the nucleobase to participate in anion–π and cation–π interactions and the metal center in metallophilic, regium bonding interactions or substituting a hydrogen atom.

KEYWORDS

Nucleosides; Nucleotides; Nucleobases; Ion–π; Regium Bonds; DFT Calculations

1 INTRODUCTION

The importance of noncovalent interactions is enormously relevant in many fields related to chemistry and biochemistry. They dictate the geometry of molecules and macromolecules both in the solid state and in solution, their reactivity, and the formation of supramolecular assemblies. In recent times, it has been well-documented that not only hydrogen bonds and π-stacking interactions have a significant role in supramolecular chemistry and crystal engineering [1]. Other less recognized interactions like regium (or coinage) bonds, cation–π, and anion–π, among others, are emerging as important players in the (bio) chemistry world. In addition, cooperative effects are very common in most recognition patterns, where two or more interactions are acting simultaneously and lead, in many cases, to synergistic effects, reinforcing the assemblies [2]. Cooperative effects have been analyzed in the literature for almost all combinations of noncovalent forces [3], as for instance π-stacking and hydrogen bonds. In this sense, the combination of X-ray diffraction analysis and theoretical calculations has granted big advances in this field. The large amount of geometrical information included in the X-ray structure databases combined with the theoretical analysis of the noncovalent forces has allowed the detection of a great deal of interactions, the analysis of their geometrical preferences, and their mutual influence. Nowadays, the scientific community is aware of the relevance of the noncovalent interactions like anion–π [4] or cation–π [5] and that their profound understanding is fundamental to make progress in Chemistry, Biology, and Material Science, among others.

Sigel and co-workers have published general reviews [6, 7] focusing on the coordination/interaction of metals with nucleotides and nucleic acids both in solution and in the solid state. Apart from the dominant Mg^{2+} and K^+ as interacting metals, the authors also described the interaction of nucleobases with most of the first-row transition metals, Na^+ and Ca^{2+}. Other authors [8, 9] have analyzed the interaction of lanthanoides with DNA focusing on the understanding of basic coordination structures, rational design of coordination materials, and the expansion of lanthanoide-based DNA catalytic reactions. Interestingly, DNA sequences can be screened to sensitize luminescence of both Tb^{3+} and Eu^{3+} lanthanoides. Moreover, coordination polymers formed by mixing lanthanoides and nucleotides are especially interesting because nanoparticles, fibers, and hydrogels can be easily afforded.

The development of optical probes for nucleotides has a huge biological significance. In this sense, Haynes et al. [10] have reviewed the current state of the art regarding the application of supramolecular coordination complexes as optical sensors, including a section devoted to nucleotides. Most of the optical sensors developed so far are supramolecular assemblies (metallocages or metallocycles) constructed using Pd^{2+}, Co^{2+}, Zn^{2+}, or Fe^{2+} ions incorporating a fluorescent group for sensing. Qu et al. have recently reviewed how the incorporation of relevant biomolecules (nucleobases, nucleosides, and nucleotides) into nanomaterials can generate functional nanosystems with novel and advanced properties, such as sensing, bioimaging, and drug delivery. The utilization of nucleobases, nucleosides, and nucleotides provides unique properties to the functional nanomaterials, like biocompatibility and chirality, among others [11].

Keeping in mind that other chapters of the present volume focus on the importance of hydrogen bonding and $\pi-\pi$ stacking, this chapter is mainly focused on cation–π, anion–π interactions, regium bonds, metallophilic and other unconventional interactions and their importance in the solid-state architectures of nucleobases, nucleosides, nucleotides, and their derivatives. This chapter is not intended to be comprehensive; instead representative examples have been carefully selected to illustrate relevance of the aforesaid interactions, as described in the following sections. First, examples where the metal center plays the role of hydrogen are emphasized (Section 2.1). Second, the utilization of polynucleotides or bases to produce argentophilic and aurophilic interactions is highlighted in Section 2.2. Third, structures exhibiting regium bonding interactions are described in Section 2.3, which has not, as far as our knowledge extends, been reviewed before. In the final Sections 2.4 and 2.5, structures where ion–π interaction plays a crucial role in the solid state are explained and rationalized.

2 EXAMPLES OF RECOGNITION IN THE METAL–NUCLEOTIDE SYSTEM

2.1 THE METAL ION INSTEAD OF HYDROGEN

The coordination of a metal ion to a puric or pyrimidinic base strongly affects the acidity/basicity of the base permitting in some cases the stabilization of unexpected tautomers [12]. A remarkable example is the imino tautomer of 9-methyladenine (9MeA) in a mixed nucleobase complex of mercury (see Figure 1a) [13]. The geometry of this rare tautomer in its non-complexed form is expected to be very similar to that found in the metal complex by Lippert's group [13].

Different strategies have been carried out to introduce a metal between complementary base pairs. Such studies are important since metal ions are known to be involved in RNA folding. Poor results have been obtained so far for the pairs

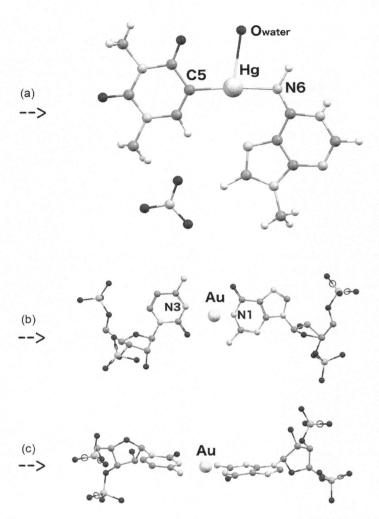

FIGURE 1 (a) View of the complex unit [(1,3-DiMeU-*C5*)Hg(9MeA-*N6*)]NO$_3$·H$_2$O [13] showing the mercury atom coordinated to the imino tautomer of adenine via N6 (hydrogen atoms for the water molecule were not included in the original paper). (b) Zenithal view of the base pair (linear coordination) and (c) lateral view of the base pair in Au^{3+} bound to cytosine and deprotonated guanine, from a Watson–Crick accessible base pair in a 23-mer RNA duplex [14].

guanine–cytosine or adenine–thymine or uracil. In the case of gold, an interesting structure has been reported where a Au^{3+} ion coordinates the deprotonated N1 of a guanine base and the N3 of the complementary cytosine. Despite gold was simply used as a heavy metal stain to resolve the structure, it ended up in an unexpected position. That is, when RNA is soaked with a Au^{3+} salt, a pair is formed with an atom of gold instead of hydrogen, but neither the coordination nor

Interplay between Noncovalent Interactions and Metal Ions 109

the final state of oxidation of gold is completely clear (see Figure 1b and c) [14]. It should be emphasized that the assembly depicted in Figure 1b and c was the first nucleic acid structure in a complex with Au[3+] and the first one with such a cation-modified G–C base pair. Meanwhile, also an analogous Ag[+]-modified pair has been reported [15].

Lippert's group has used *trans*-platinum complexes to generate well-defined model compounds that crystallized with G–Pt–C and A–Pt–U base pair interactions, modified by linear trans-(NH$_3$)$_2$Pt^{2+} units [16–18]. In the first case (see Figure 2a) [16], the Pt^{2+} is bonded to the N3 atom of 1-methylcytosine (1MeC)

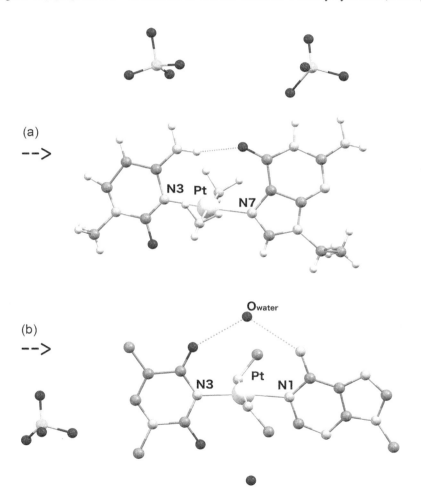

FIGURE 2 (a) *trans*-[Pt(NH$_3$)$_2$(1MeC-*N3*)(9EtGH-*N7*)](ClO$_4$)$_2$ [16] with the intramolecular hydrogen bond between O6 of guanine and N4 of cytosine (donor···acceptor distance: 3.005 Å) clearly visible. (b) *trans*-[Pt(CH$_3$NH$_2$)$_2$(1MeT-*N3*)(9MeA-*N1*)](ClO$_4$)·3.25H$_2$O with the water molecule, which forms H bonds with O4 of thymine and N6 of adenine [19].

and the N7 atom of 9-ethylguanine (9EtGH) leaving both molecular planes in an almost coplanar conformation (dihedral angle 6.3°). An expected feature is the presence of a hydrogen bond between the exocyclic O atom of 9EtGH and one H atom belonging to the NH_2 group of 1MeC. Therefore, this arrangement can be deemed as a metal analog of a Hoogsteen pair between cytosinium and guanine, where the cytosinium proton at N3 is substituted by the *trans*-diammine-Pt^{2+} entity. In the second example, two Watson-Crick metal-modified 9-ethyladenine (9EtA)/1-methyluracilate pairs are cross-linked by additional 9EtA–Pt^{2+}–9EtA bonds via available N7 sites, thereby forming a characteristic Z-shape of the four nucleobases in solid state [17]. This compound crystallizes with the four bases being nearly coplanar, but solution NMR experiments demonstrate the coexistence of a second, U-shaped conformation, which appears to be responsible for an extreme acidification of the adenine amino group through formation of a $NH^-\cdots H_2N$ hydrogen bond. Another significant example is represented in Figure 2b. The Pt^{2+} ion is coordinated to N3 atom of 1-methylthymine (1MeT) and N1 atom of 9MeA and a co-crystallized water molecule bridges both bases by hydrogen bonding interactions [19].

Even nowadays it is quite difficult to obtain well-defined compounds where the metal ion substitutes a hydrogen atom in a DNA base pair scheme. In fact, very few examples have been obtained using modified nucleobases, and for real DNA or polynucleotide decamers or hexamers, no examples are available in the literature, suggesting that this is a very challenging task. The reason for that remains largely unclear, at present. A likely explanation is that the great stability of the Watson-Crick hydrogen bonds markedly hinders the substitution of a proton by a metal center. In this sense, the influence of metal coordination to N7 of guanine on the intermolecular proton-transfer reaction in guanine–cytosine base pairs has been analyzed theoretically. DFT calculations on M^{n+}–GC (M=Cu^+, Ca^{2+}, and Cu^{2+}) suggested that the interaction of divalent metal cations stabilizes the ion pair structure derived from the N1–N3 single-proton-transfer reaction, turning this process from unfeasible to thermodynamically favorable [20]. On the other hand, many examples have been described in the literature of metal ions connecting pyrimidine base derivatives [21]. Many works have exploited the special affinity of Hg^{2+} for uracil and thymine and that of Ag^+ for cytosine to generate a considerable number of compounds and assemblies with applications in nanomaterials [21].

In the case of cytosine, it is known that DNA sequences rich in this base have the tendency to fold into two intertwined parallel-stranded duplexes (structures called i-motifs) under acidic pH, due to the formation of strong C–H^+–C pairs stabilized by three strong H bonds each [22–24]. It is known that i-motif-forming sequences are present in several GC-rich promoter oncogenes and telomeres. It has been suggested that i-motif structures are involved in a variety of biological processes, such as telomere maintenance, regulation of oncogene expression, and DNA repair [22–24]. There is a considerable number of X-ray crystal structures available, where this pair cytosine–cytosinium is present, as the pioneering work from Marzilli et al. [25, 26] for instance

Interplay between Noncovalent Interactions and Metal Ions   111

with the model bases 1MeCH[+]–1MeC that has been confirmed by other authors [27]. In this case, the *trans*-form is observed, exhibiting two N–H⋯O hydrogen bonds between amino and carbonyl groups of the cytosine molecules and the additional N–H⋯N hydrogen bond. The nature of hydrogen bonds in cytidine⋯H[+]⋯cytidine DNA base pairs has been analyzed by Schwalbe and collaborators [28] by combining NMR spectroscopy and DFT calculations and demonstrated that the proton is able to hop between both nucleobases at room temperature. This recognition pattern has been exploited by other authors to design DNA nanomachines [29, 30].

By using the Hg^{2+} ion, different structures of pairs T–Hg^{2+}–T or U–Hg^{2+}–U have been obtained and characterized by X-ray diffraction analysis. In case of using the 1MeT base, the arrangement of the molecules is *transoid*, whereas in the DNA dodecamer the *cisoid* orientation is present owing to the backbone restrictions (see Figure 3) [31–33]. The formation of this type of assembly (T–Hg^{2+}–T) has been also demonstrated in solution by ^{1}H NMR spectroscopy [34] in DNA duplexes with two T–T mispairs. The characteristic signal of the imino proton in T disappears upon the addition of two equivalents of Hg^{2+} [34, 35]. Recently, Nehzati et al. have applied a combination of small molecule X-ray diffraction,

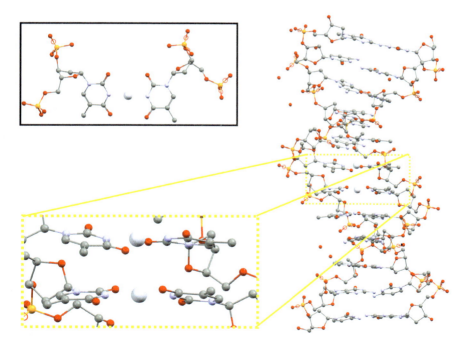

FIGURE 3 Crystal structure of a metallo-DNA duplex containing two consecutive Watson-Crick-like T–Hg–T base pairs and magnification of the coordination sphere (color code: C, dark gray; H, white; O, red; N, blue; Hg, light gray) [32]. In the black box, one of the T–Hg–T base pairs is showing the *cisoid* conformation.

X-ray spectroscopy, and computational chemistry to study the interactions of Hg^{2+} with thymine to disclose that the energetically preferred mode of thymine binding in DNA is through the N3 atom. They have also predicted only minor distortions of the DNA structure on binding one Hg^{2+} to two cross-adjacent thymine nucleotides. The preferred geometry is predicted to be twisted away from coplanar through a torsion angle of between 32° and 43°. Finally, bis-thymine coordination of Hg^{2+} is found to give a highly characteristic X-ray spectroscopic signature [36].

As RNA models, several examples of X-ray crystal structures with 5'-fluorouracil are known [37]. The X-ray crystal structure of one example is presented in Figure 4a [37], which consists of a complex between Hg^{2+} and two 1-hexyl-5-fluorouracilato ligands. The uracil rings are twisted, forming a dihedral angle of 32.9° between the mean planes. The *cisoid* arrangement of both 5'-fluorouracil moieties observed in the solid is due to additional interactions of fluorine with the adjacent bases.

Another RNA model involving Hg^{2+} and uracil is the one indicated in Figure 4b [38]. In this example, the Hg^{2+} ion is coordinated to the N3 atoms of two 1-(3-hydroxypropyl)-5-fluorouracilato ligands in a linear geometry. In addition, the mercury ion also presents a short interaction with the O4 atoms of the uracil rings that enhances the stability of the assembly. These O atoms, belonging to the 3-hydroxypropyl side chain that are weakly bound to Hg^{2+} in an apical fashion, leading to the generation of a coordination polymer in the solid state.

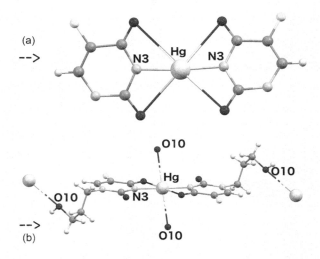

FIGURE 4 (a) Structure of the monomeric unit [Hg(1-hexyl-5-fluorouracilato)$_2$] where the *cisoid* conformation of the nucleobases can be clearly seen (the aliphatic chains have been omitted for clarity) [37]. In the crystal structure, four units form the tetrameric complex [Hg(1-hexyl-5-fluorouracilato)$_2$]$_4$·6H$_2$O thanks to π-stacking interactions and ancillary Hg–O secondary interactions. (b) Linear structure of complex [Hg(1-(3-hydroxypropyl)-5-fluorouracilato)$_2$] [38].

These Hg⋯nucleobase interactions have been also used for the detection of Hg^{2+} as a contaminant by fluorescence, owing to the high specificity and the attenuation of the fluorescence signal intensity by alteration of DNA after coordination with the metal ion [39].

For the Ag$^+$ ion, different motifs have been described for base-pairing interactions with pyrimidine bases in the solid state (Figure 5) [21]. Among them, the interaction C–Ag$^+$–C is very relevant and of interest because this type of base pairing can be accompanied by argentophilic interactions, which will be treated in more detail in the following section. This metal ion, in combination with several nucleic acid systems and models, has been used to construct complex supramolecular assemblies based on this C–Ag$^+$–C motif, especially to build 1D-conductors [21]. Apart from cytosine, the ability of silver to coordinate to uracil is also well known, forming chains with Ag–Ag argentophilic interactions [38, 40]. Analogously, the crystal structure of the complex between 1MeT and silver [15] shows a linear coordination N3–Ag$^+$–N3, where the thymine rings are coplanar and the Ag$^+$ occupies the inversion center. Moreover, the 1MeT rings are further connected by additional Ag$^+$ ions via Ag–O coordinate bonds. Overall, an optimum use is made of the three donors N3, O2, and O4 on each methylthymine.

DNA or polynucleotides with cytosine bases in the same position of the chain have been used to generate cytosine–silver–cytosine assemblies [41]. For instance, Kondo et al. have obtained a metallo-DNA nanowire with uninterrupted one-dimensional (1D) silver arrays. It consists of dodecamer duplexes held together by four different metal-mediated base pairs C–Ag$^+$–C, G–Ag$^+$–G, G–Ag$^+$–C, and T–Ag$^+$–T. Only the first base pair C–Ag$^+$–C was observed prior to Kondo's publication [42]. Furthermore, Liu et al. have reported for the first time a DNA structure containing a G–Ag$^+$–G pair in a short octamer DNA strand that also includes two C–Ag$^+$–C pairs in its structure. This interesting assembly is also the first non-helical DNA structure driven by heavy metal ions, thus further contributing to the structural diversity of DNA [43]. Another interesting work was reported by Nakagawa et al. focusing on the sugar conformation in duplexes. They reported a crystal structure of the non-canonical DNA/DNA duplex containing a 2′-O, 4′-C-methylene bridged nucleic acid that was obtained in the presence of Ag$^+$ ions. Remarkably, it showed a novel type of Ag$^+$-mediated base pair between the N1 positions of the adenines, presenting an *anti*-conformation in the duplex [44].

Unusual dimeric Zn^{2+} cytosine complexes and other Zn^{2+}-mediated nonlinear base pairing have been also described, including AA, CC, GG, and UU pairs that can be connected via coordination to N or O atoms of the nucleobases [45]. For manganese, an external base pair that does not modify the hydrogen bonds of the helix has been found with DNA [46]. In Figure 6, the interaction mode in guanine–Mn^{2+}–guanine of two different helices is depicted. Other interactions with phosphate groups are also present in the X-ray crystal structure. The double helices show end-to-end interactions, in a manner that the terminal guanines interact with the minor groove of the neighboring duplex. The manganese ion is able to cross-link the DNA duplexes by connecting the N7 atoms of the terminal guanines and also by connecting the phosphate oxygen atoms [46].

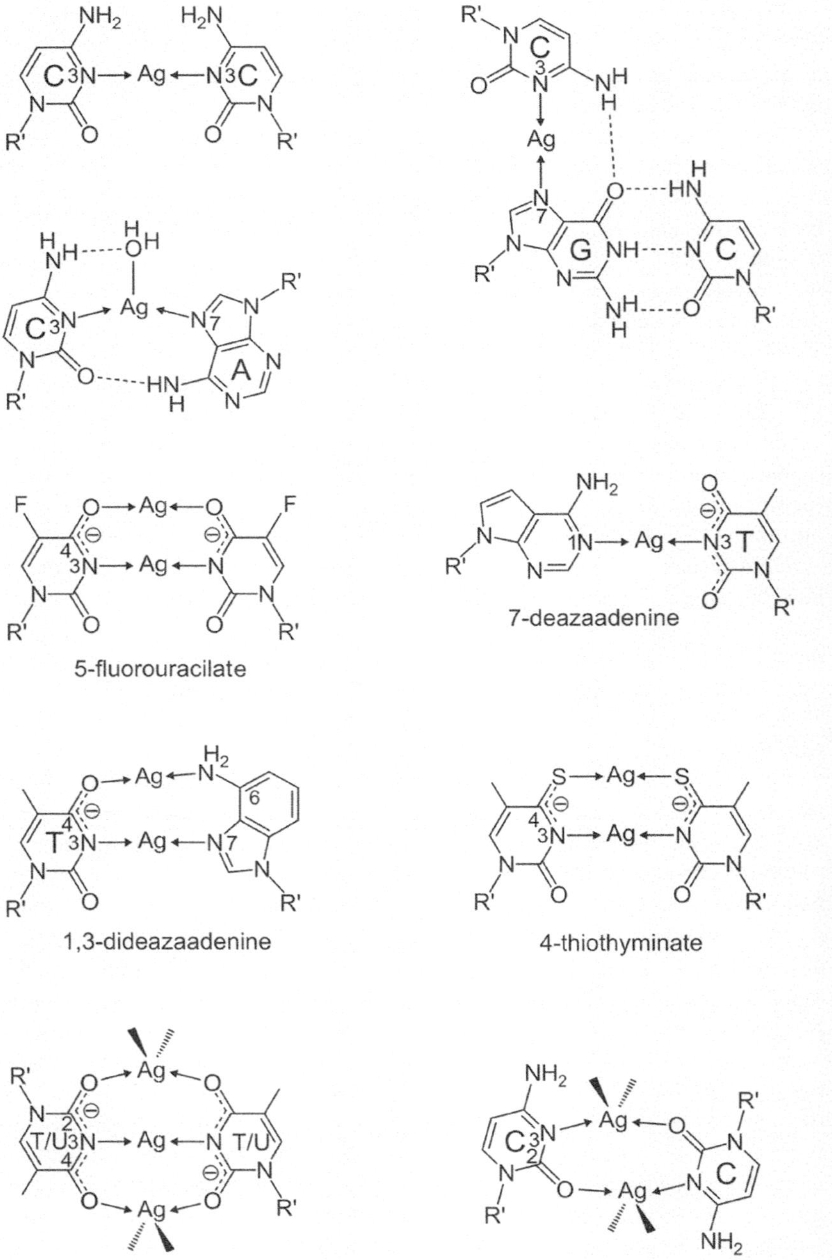

FIGURE 5 Pyrimidine-containing Ag⁺ complexes in models, RNA and DNA [21]. (Adapted with permission from B. Lippert, P. J. Sanz Miguel, *Acc Chem. Res.* **2016**, *49*, 1537–1535. Copyright 2016 American Chemical Society.)

Interplay between Noncovalent Interactions and Metal Ions 115

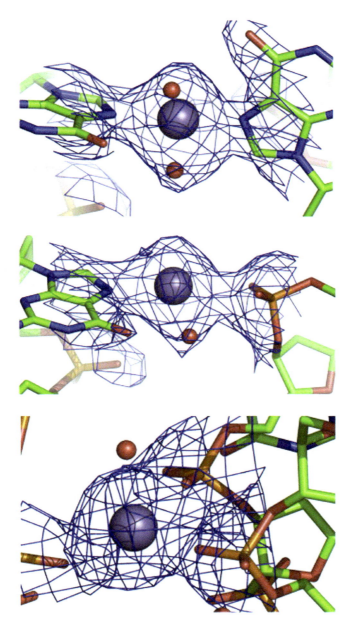

FIGURE 6 View of the different interactions of manganese ions binding to the external part of two DNA duplexes, shown as violet spheres. Adjacent water molecules are shown as small red spheres. The local $2F_o-F_c$ electron density map is represented at 1σ level [46]. (Reprinted from Journal of Inorganic Biochemistry, 103(6), H. Millonig, J. Pons, C. Gouyette, J. A. Subirana, J. L. Campos, *The interaction of manganese ions with DNA*, pp. 876–880, Copyright 2009, with permission from Elsevier.)

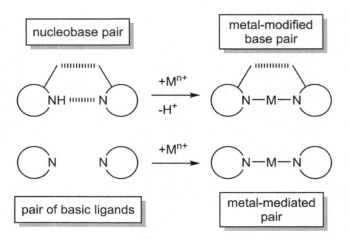

FIGURE 7 Definition of base pairs proposed by Lippert [49]. (Reproduced from Journal of Biological Inorganic Chemistry, 27, B. Lippert, *"Metal-modified base pairs vs. metal-mediated pairs of bases: not just a semantic issue"*, pp. 215–219, 2022, licensed under CC BY-SA 4.0 http://creativecommons.org/licenses/by-sa/4.0/.)

Base pairing in oligonucleotides promoted by Pd^{2+} ion has been also described in short glycol nucleic acid (GNA) oligonucleotides, having either a terminal or an intra-chain nucleobase replaced by pyridine-2,6-dicarboxamide [47]. Moreover, pairs of Cu^{2+}, Hg^{2+}, and Ag^+ have been described using the base 5-carboxyuracil, as demonstrated by duplex melting analysis and mass spectrometry [48]. There are also different kinds of geometries for the metal base complexes that are not linear, which are not described in this chapter, since in our opinion they are less relevant. A more comprehensive description can be found in the excellent review published recently by Müller [39].

Lippert [49] has proposed a distinction between the terms "metal-modified base pairs" and "metal-mediated pairs of bases". The nuance is important since, in the former, the metal ion substitutes a hydrogen of the normal hydrogen bonds. In the latter, the metal "creates" the pair interacting with the two ligands, which would not form a hydrogen bonding network in the absence of the metal (see Figure 7).

The metal-modified base pair must retain the planar configuration and the H-bonding pattern recognition of the natural bases. This is not the case in the metal-mediated base pair where the nucleobases are not necessarily coplanar and, in some cases, not complementary.

2.2 Using Polynucleotides or Bases to Produce Argentophilic and Aurophilic Interactions

The argentophilic and aurophilic interactions have led to a growing interest by the scientific community and they are becoming relevant actors in several chemistry fields, like crystal engineering, supramolecular chemistry, nanodevices, and computational chemistry [50, 51]. The metal ion-nucleic acid system has been shown to act as a good matrix to develop this kind of interactions, especially the possibility to construct 1D conductors. The trend of the uracil [40], 5-fluorouracil [38], or thymine [15] silver complexes to crystallize by forming chains with different types of Ag–Ag interactions is well known. In the case of 5-fluorouracil, a chain of Ag$^+$ ions formed via argentophilic interactions appears with Ag···Ag distances ranging from 3.1 to 3.2 Å [38], which is below the sum of their van der Waals radii (3.44 Å) [52].

Two different strategies have been followed to generate argentophilic interactions in nucleic acids or polynucleotides. The first one consists of the utilization of DNA or polynucleotides with cytosine bases in the same position of the chain to generate a C–Ag$^+$–C assembly [41], as performed by Kondo et al. [43] (described in the previous section). This strategy has been also followed by Galindo's group using DNA sequences comprising non-canonical 7-deazaguanine and canonical cytosine that are able of forming Watson-Crick base pairs via hydrogen bonds as well as Ag$^+$-mediated base pairs [53, 54].

The second strategy consists of taking advantage of the high affinity of Ag$^+$ ions for the N3 atom of cytosine-producing C–Ag$^+$–C synthons that can interact via Ag$^+$···Ag$^+$ argentophilic contacts to produce a linear column of silver [55–60]. This type of columnar assemblies has been obtained by three different research groups, using 1MeC [60], cytidine [58], and 1-hexylcytosine [55]. All three structures are similar, and they consist of a column of Ag$^+$ ions connected through argentophilic interactions assisted by π-stacking interactions involving the cytosine rings, which are not coplanar in the C–Ag$^+$–C synthon [39, 49], thus inducing the formation of helical assemblies. The assemblies are reinforced by hydrogen bonds (carbonyl group–amino group) involving bases of the next C–Ag$^+$–C pair. The conformation of the base pairs within the C–Ag$^+$–C synthon is *transoid*, as shown in Figure 8a. The X-ray diffraction data reveal a structure like a double helix that resembles a DNA, as described in detail by the original authors [55].

The formation of the helical structure depicted in Figure 8a is quite remarkable, as it is similar to DNA, without the support of a backbone. This double-helical structure is also observed with other ligands like 1MeC or cytidine. This suggests that the formation of the C–Ag$^+$–C motif and its supramolecular polymerization via an intricate and cooperative combination of noncovalent interactions (argentophilic, hydrogen bonds, and π-stacking interactions) is a relevant recognition pattern that must be emphasized. Theoretical calculations have permitted to understand the relevance of hydrogen bonds, π-stacking, and other ancillary bonds [55]. Moreover, an important factor is an argentophilic interaction, which was rationalized in terms of orbital donor–acceptor interactions. The latter is likely the most important driving force for the formation of the supramolecular polymer, while the π-stacking and hydrogen bonds between consecutive C–Ag$^+$–C motifs are responsible for the helical pattern.

It is interesting and inspiring to compare DNA and the C–Ag$^+$–C assembly with classical architectural staircases. Leonardo da Vinci constructed a double-helical

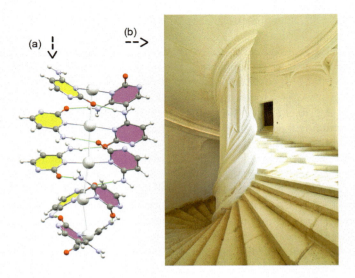

FIGURE 8 (a) Complex unit from the X-ray crystal structure of [Ag(1-hexylcytosine)$_2$]$_5$(SbF$_6$)$_5$·2CH$_3$OH (color code: C, dark gray; H, white; O, red; N, blue; Ag, light gray). Hexyl chains have been omitted for clarity [55]. The hydrogen bond interactions indicated in the figure present values between 2.889 and 3.055 Å (donor⋯acceptor). (b) Photo of the double-helical staircase of the Castle of Rochefoucauld, designed by Leonardo da Vinci. (Photo from René Mattes, reproduced with permission from the copyright holder Hemis/Alamy photo stock.)

staircase in the castle of Rochefoucauld in France (see Figure 8b). In this building, the importance of an axis in the central part of the staircase is relevant, the steps are inserted into the central column (the C–Ag–C metal-mediated pair), and each step is supported by the previous one (stacking between the bases), and a helical vault where each step is implicated (the hydrogen bonds between the bases). Like in the helical and classical iron cast staircases, there is no need of external walls to generate a solid construction.

In DNA structures three principal recognition patterns are involved. The first one is the phosphate-deoxyribose backbone, which permits a proximity between the bases, that facilitates the stacking (second factor); and finally, a third factor, which is the hydrogen bonds within the base pairs. A classical Bramante-Momo staircase in the Vatican Museum would be a good analog (see Figure 9a). In this case, there is a great hole in the center. The need of a cylindrical wall where the steps are inserted is essential (the backbone). Each step is reinforced by the previous one (stacking) and finally, a helical vault is generated by the steps in the central hole that in the case of DNA would be the hydrogen bonds between the pairs.

In the case of the beautiful structure reported by Kondo et al. (Figure 9b), a mixture of the two situations is present. On one hand, a cylindrical wall is the phosphate backbone that forces a *cisoid* conformation of the bases. On the other hand, the central quasi-linear Ag⋯Ag interactions generate a nanowire with a

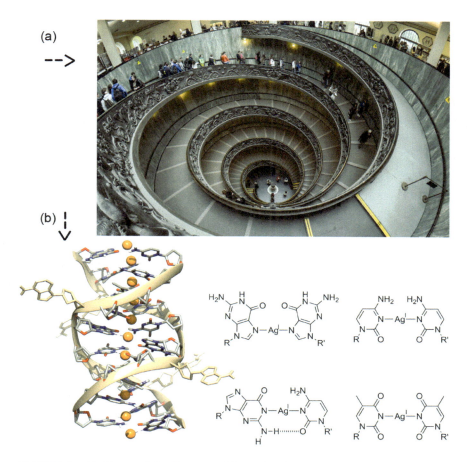

FIGURE 9 (a) Photo of the Bramante-Momo double helix staircase in the Vatican Museums by Colin, https://commons.wikimedia.org/wiki/File:Vatican_Museums_Spiral_Staircase_2012.jpg, licensed under CC BY-SA 3.0 http://creativecommons.org/licenses/by-sa/3.0/. (b) X-ray crystal structure of a DNA containing different Ag^+-mediated base pairs [39]: $G-Ag^+-G$, $G-Ag^+-C$, $C-Ag^+-C$, and $T-Ag^+-T$ pairs, PDB ID 5IX7 [41]. Silver(I) ions are shown as orange spheres. (Reprinted from Coordination Chemistry Reviews, 393, J. Müller, *Nucleic acid duplexes with metal-mediated base pairs and their structures*, pp. 17–47, Copyright 2019, with permission from Elsevier.)

very narrow helicoidal disposition, resembling a Solomonic column, which is characterized by a spiraling twisting shaft. Different combinations of metal-modified or -mediated base pairs are present in this structure, which are (1) a modified $G-Ag^+-C$ base pair with coplanar bases and hydrogen bonds and (2) $G-Ag^+-G$, $C-Ag^+-C$ and $T-Ag^+-T$ mediated base pairs [41]. In this particular case, both the backbone and the central axis of silver ions reinforce the stability and facilitate the formation of such a combination of rare base pairs. In solution, the existence of this kind of rare base pairing was also demonstrated [61] by NMR experiments.

The interest to build 1D nanowires (i.e., 1D silver arrays) is increasing due to their potential applications in nanotechnology. In this sense, Houlton's group has checked the electrical conductivity of the Ag–cytidine coordination polymer chain [58], showing that the material is electrically insulating. Attempts to make this material an electrical conductor upon reduction of Ag⁺ were not successful, since the compound readily deposits silver in form of silver nanoparticles [58]. Although the metallic chain was not electrically conducting, it could provide useful routes to new optical nanomaterials [59], for instance by interchanging the solvent, which has provided a means to modulate the intermetallic distance of the Ag ion chains in solvated structures of [Ag(cytidine-5′-monophosphate)]. This 3D-coordination polymer features the less common O2,N3-binding mode for the nucleobase, which was first described by Marzilli et al. [62]. In this line, several investigations have been reported where new hybrid materials were synthesized consisting of silver nanoparticles encapsulated by DNA that have interesting photophysical properties [39, 63–66].

Theoretical calculations have analyzed the interaction between gold and silver metal ions and DNA/RNA nucleobases [67]. For silver, the more stable metal base pairs are GC and AT where the silver ion is located between the two bases. Other external interactions, in hybrid metal base pair structures, were also analyzed, showing that the stability follows the Ag–GC > Ag–AT trend, allowing the stabilization of the canonical base pairing. For gold, a similar result was obtained revealing that its interaction with the canonical GC pair is more stable than that with the AT pair [67].

Lippert's group has also reported the interaction of Au^{3+} with the C5 atom of 1,3-dimethyluracil (1,3-diMeU) [68]. This organometallic bond cannot be disregarded in future research with nucleic acids. To date, the only known gold-mediated base pair is a pair G–Au–C in an RNA complex [14] where possibly the gold was reduced to Au⁺ during the soaking of the Au^{3+} salt in the RNA crystal.

The question that arises is if aurophilic interactions could be comparable to the argentophilic ones and would be capable to dictate the formation of infinite 1D-chains. To the best of our knowledge, there are very few X-ray crystal structures exhibiting Au⋯Au aurophilic interactions in nucleobase derivatives. One of these consists in an Au⁺–isonitrile derivative of guanosine that was demonstrated to be a reliable scaffold forming tetramers or octamers via self-assembly in the presence or absence of potassium ions, respectively. It also exhibits a switchable emission based on the Au⁺⋯Au⁺ aurophilic interaction [69] that is only present in the octameric assembly.

Another example was reported by Blasco et al., where they synthesized two new [Au(adeninate-*N*9)(PR₃)] (PR₃ = PMe₃ or 1,3,5-triaza-7-phosphaadamantane) complexes which present Au⁺⋯Au⁺ aurophilic interactions (Au⋯Au distances 3.208 and 3.0942 Å, see Figure 10a) [70]. Depending on the phosphine co-ligand used in water, the authors observed either the formation of ultrathin nanowires leading to a blue-luminescent hydrogel (PMe₃) or single crystals (1,3,5-triaza-7-phosphaadamantane).

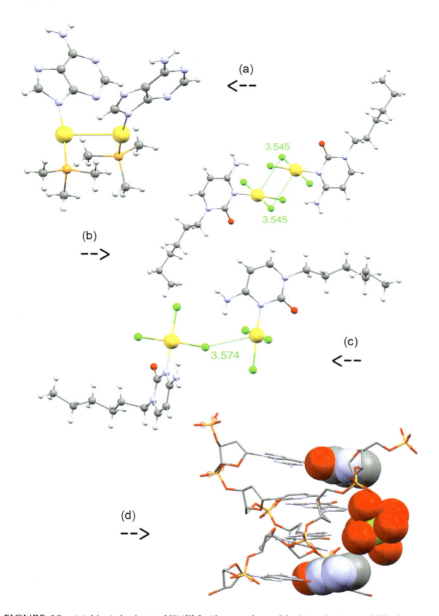

FIGURE 10 (a) [Au(adeninate-N9)(PMe$_3$)]$_2$ complex with Au$^+$⋯Au$^+$ aurophilic interactions [70] (color code: C, dark gray; H, white; P, phosphor; N, blue; Au, yellow). (b) and (c) Regium bonding in two polymorphs of the complex trichlorido-(1-hexylcytosine)gold(III) [72, 73] (color code: C, dark gray; H, white; O, red; N, blue; Cl, green; Au, yellow). (d) Partial view of the DNA crystal structure of PDB: 355B (NDB: BDL084) showing the lateral cation–π interaction of [Mg(H$_2$O)$_6$]$_2$ with two cytosine units [80]. The interacting parts have been depicted using spacefill representation.

2.3 Regium Bonds in the Nucleotide World

The terms regium bond and coinage bond have been used indistinctly to describe noncovalent interactions involving elements belonging to group 11 (Cu, Ag, and Au) [71] acting as Lewis acids. These terms have been used to define the contacts between group 11 elements with electron-rich atoms located at distances that are longer than the sum of covalent radii and shorter than the sum of van der Waals' radii. Therefore, the regium bonding term is intended to differentiate coordination bonds (strong covalent character) from noncovalent interactions (van der Waals force).

The regium bond could play a role in the interaction between metal ions belonging to group 11 and the nucleic acid system [1]. In fact, a bond of this type was first described in the trichloridogold(III) complex of N3-coordinated 1-hexylcytosine (Figure 10b) [72]. The $AuCl_3N$ complex units stack on top of each other by reciprocal [Au···Cl] noncovalent contacts that can be classified as π–hole regium bonds. In fact, these contacts are relevant to rationalize the packing of this compound in the solid state, as can be deduced from the dimerization energies. The formation of the self-assembled dimers is further assisted by exocyclic NHCl hydrogen bonds, which are energetically less important than the regium bonds, as deduced by comparing the dimerization energy of the unmutated and mutated dimers. Moreover, in Figure 10c a regium bond observed in a different polyform of the Au-(1-hexylcytosine) complex [73] is depicted, showing an electron-rich chlorido ligand pointing to the Au^{3+} atom of the adjacent molecule.

A search in the Cambridge Structure Database (version 5.41, with updates until November 2019) has been performed to investigate if this type of regium bonds in tetra-coordinated gold complexes is common and potentially important in crystal engineering. The results of this search confirm that this type of bonds is common in X-ray crystal structures and has remained basically unnoticed likely due to the underestimated van der Waals radius value that is tabulated for gold [72].

2.4 Cation–π Interactions

The cation–π interaction is very important in structural biology [74]. The outstanding importance of this interaction in determining the structure and function of supramolecular assemblies has been reviewed [5]. The putative roles of cation–π interactions along with H bonds and π-stacking interactions between loop residues and the outer G-quartets have been emphasized in the formation and stability of dimeric DNA G-quadruplexes [75]. Theoretical studies based on X-ray structural data have suggested the existence of relevant cation–π interactions between hydrated magnesium and cytosine in a B-DNA [76]. In principle, hydrated metal cations can interact with nucleobases establishing a cation–π contact. The stabilization energy of such complexes would be large and comparable to a cation–π complex with benzene. However, in contrast to the benzene–cation complexes, the cation–π configurations are less preferred in nucleobases due to the competition of the conventional in-plane binding of hydrated cations to the acceptor sites on the nucleobase, which is strongly preferred. Several theoretical DFT studies have also analyzed the binding of nucleobases with alkaline and alkaline earth metal ions [77, 78]. Interestingly, a detailed theoretical case study of the DNA/RNA nucleobases has demonstrated that the nucleobase π-systems are promiscuous ion–π binders with the ability to interact favorably with biologically relevant Li$^+$/Na$^+$ cations and F$^-$ and Cl$^-$ anions [78].

Stewart et al. [79] have analyzed in detail how the conformation of DNA structure modulates many fundamental cellular processes, which are mostly affected by specific DNA sequences. In addition, cation–π interactions between cations or their first hydration shell water molecules and the faces of DNA are also importantly affecting the conformation. The authors characterized the binding patterns found in cation–π interactions between solvated cations and DNA bases in a set of high-resolution X-ray crystal structures. They found that monovalent cations (Tl$^+$) and the polarized first hydration shell water molecules of divalent cations (Mg^{2+}, Ca^{2+}) form cation–π interactions with DNA bases stabilizing unstacked conformations. Moreover, the combination of cation–π interactions with electrostatic interactions creates a pattern of specific binding motifs within the grooves [79].

Zarić has reviewed a special type of cation–π interactions, where ligands coordinated to a metal ion interact with aromatic groups. These interactions are common in metalloproteins, biomimetic metal complexes, and when either DNA or RNA interacts with metal cations. The binding energy associated to this type of contacts varies from 1 to 30 kcal mol^{-1}, depending on the nature and charge of the cation and the electronic nature of the π-system. For instance, a hydrated magnesium located in the major groove and interacting with the π-system of a cytosine unit (Figure 10d) has a calculated energy of 20.2 kcal mol^{-1} [80]. Such large binding energy is likely influenced by the electrostatic attraction with the anionic phosphate groups.

Direct metal ion-nucleobase interactions (without coordinated waters) have been also observed in X-ray crystal structures. For instance, (hexaammine) cobalt(III) shows inner-sphere binding of a (tetraammine)cobalt cation to N7 of a guanine ring and to the phosphate of a bulged-out adenine in the subtype-A DIS duplex [14]. Distances between the cation and RNA ligands lie within 1.9–2.4 Å. This implies that two ammines from the original hexaammine shell were displaced. In that example, K$^+$ cations form cation–π interactions with some of the guanine rings, like those presented by Stewart et al. [79].

2.5 Anion–π Interactions

Since their discovery in 2002, anion–π interactions have attracted increasing attention in many fields, including enzymatic chemistry and nucleic acids [4]. A pioneering study was reported in 2004 describing the interaction of anions with nucleic acids [81]; however, the study did not consider the anion–π interaction mode. Very recently, a theoretical study has highlighted the importance of anion–π interactions in RNA. In particular, it shed light on the interaction between a phosphate group and guanine residues and demonstrated that this anion–π interaction is involved in the stabilization of GAAA and GGAG RNA tetraloops [82]. Previously, Kozelka investigated the importance of the closely related lone pair–π interactions in the biological world, remarking on the influence of such interaction in the stabilization of Z-DNA. In particular, the stabilizing interaction between an electron lone pair belonging to an oxygen atom of a ribose and a guanine ring, and the interaction of chloride and water molecules with uracils [83].

Stacking interactions, where one of the aromatic rings (or π-system) is anionic, can be also considered as a special class of anion–π interactions (also denoted in the literature as π⁻···π). An interesting example of this situation was reported by Rak et al. in 2008 [84], who demonstrated that an adiabatically unstable anionic thymine becomes bound when incorporated into the DNA π-stack. The stabilization of the anionic form of thymine is most likely due to the formation of a π⁻···π stack, which was stronger in the 5'-d(CTC)-3' sequence in DNA compared to other sequences like 5'-d(GTG)-3'.

Anion–π interactions involving metal ions have been reported and they are normally produced with d^{10} metal halido complexes of the type [MCl$_4$]$^{2-}$, where M=Hg^{2+} or Zn^{2+}. In other cases, the metal is coordinated to the nucleobase in a zwitterionic form, thus adequate to self-assemble forming dimers. Several examples illustrating this interesting behavior can be found in a review reported by Fiol et al. in 2013 [85]. Figure 11a depicts one of such complexes where two Zn^{2+} ions are directly coordinated to two adeninium moieties via their N7 atoms [86]. The adenine bases are protonated at N1 and connected by a propylene chain via the exocyclic N6 atoms. The conformation adopted by this dinuclear complex is governed by the formation of two symmetrically equivalent anion–π interactions, where one chlorido ligand points to the center of the six-membered ring of the adenine. This ring is the most π-acidic part due to the protonation of N1.

Anion–π interactions are also possible with planar anions like [AuX$_4$]$^-$, where the anion is stacked over the nucleobase. A nice example of this behavior can be found in Salas' and Beauchamp's work [87] where the X-ray crystal structure of inosinium tetrabromidoaurate(III) was reported, showing the [AuBr$_4$]$^-$ anion located over the center of the hypoxanthine ring (Figure 11b).

Using theoretical models, it has been demonstrated that either adenine or hypoxanthine (even in their neutral forms) are well suited for interacting favorably with anions via both six- and five-membered rings. In adenine, the interaction with chloride is more favorable with the imidazole moiety than with the pyrimidine ring, which has been rationalized using the molecular electrostatic potential (MEP) calculations [86]. They showed that the MEP value over the five-membered ring is more positive than that over the six-membered ring, likely due to the presence of an electron-donating amino group in the latter. The opposite behavior is observed for the interaction of chloride with hypoxanthine where the interaction is stronger over the six-membered ring. This is due to the presence of an electron-withdrawing carbonyl group in hypoxanthine instead of the electron-donating amino group in adenine.

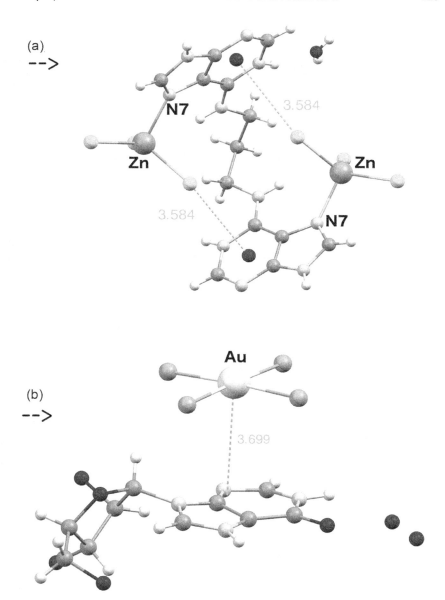

FIGURE 11 (a) X-ray crystal structure of {[(6AH)$_2$C$_3$](ZnCl$_3$)$_2$}·2H$_2$O [86] with symmetric anion–π interactions between chlorido ligands and the six-membered rings which are represented by centroids (distances in Å). (b) Example of an anion–π interaction present in the X-ray crystal structure of inosinium tetrabromido aurate(III) [87], showing the [AuBr$_4$]$^-$ anion located over the center of the hypoxanthine ring.

TABLE 1
Interaction Energies (ΔE in kcal/mol) and Geometric Parameters (Anion to Ring Centroid Distances in Å) Computed for Several Anion-π Complexes. See Original Publication for the Level of Theory [85]

Type	Base	Distance Å	ΔE	Reference
Br$^-$···π	Cytosinium	3.58	−21.7	[88]
Cl$^-$···π	Adeninium	3.48	−15.6	[89]
Cl$^-$···π	Adeninium	3.45	−25.2	[89]
[ZnCl$_4$]$^{2-}$···π	Adeninium (6R)	3.58	−77.8	[86]
[ZnCl$_4$]$^{2-}$···π	Adeninium (5R)	3.32	−83.7	[86]
[ZnCl$_4$]$^{2-}$···π	Hypoxanthine (6R)	3.20	−82.4	[86]
[HgCl$_4$]$^{2-}$···π	Adeninium (6R)	3.29	−83.4	[86]

6R and 5R stand for six- and five-membered rings, respectively.

Table 1 compiles the interaction energies of some representative anion–π complexes available in the literature. The anion–π assemblies used to compute the interaction energies were extracted directly from X-ray crystal structures without further optimization. The energies summarized in Table 1 evidence that the anion–π interaction energies are largely due to the protonation of the base and confirm the energetic relevance and structure-directing role of this interaction in the crystal packing of these salts. For monoanionic anions, the binding energies are similar to those reported for cation–π interactions by Zarić [80]. The energies are larger for the [MCl$_4$]$^{2-}$ dianions due to the stronger Coulombic electrostatic attraction.

Examples with other metal ions like Cd^{2+}, Pt^{2+}, and Pd^{2+} can also be found in the literature [90–92]. An interesting example is shown in Figure 12a [92], where the two 9MeA molecules are coordinated to both Pd^{2+} and Pt^{2+} ions. That is, the Pd^{2+} ions are coordinated to N6 and N1, bridging both adenine moieties, and ethylenediamine was used to complete their square-planar coordination sphere. Moreover, Pt^{2+} ions are mono-coordinated to the adenine rings by N7 and their coordination sphere is completed by ammonia ligands. The coordination of each adenine to three metal atoms increases dramatically the π-acidity of adenine, facilitating the formation of two anion–π contacts (see Figure 12a).

A very significant metal complex has been obtained with a non-canonical base, caffeine in its carbene form (9-methylcaffein-8-yliden) (Figure 12b and c). This caffeine carbene readily reacts with Au$^+$ salts to yield the stable cationic gold-bis(caffein-8-ylidene) complex [93]. In the solid state, the BF$_4^-$ counterion forms several anion–π contacts with the π-acidic surface of caffeine (three fluorine atoms of the anion are pointing to the base). The gold-bis(caffein-8-ylidene) complex adopts a completely planar conformation. It is worthy to comment that

Interplay between Noncovalent Interactions and Metal Ions 127

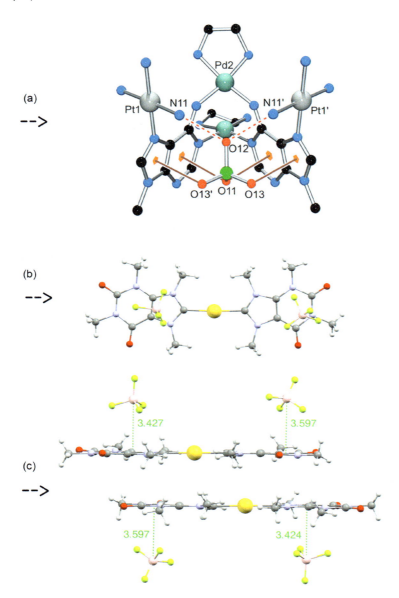

FIGURE 12 (a) View of the interactions of cation *hh*-[{(en)Pd}$_2${(*N1*,*N6*-9MeA$^-$-*N7*)Pt(NH$_3$)$_3$}$_2$] with ClO$_4$ [92]. (Reprinted with permission from S. Ibáñez, F. M. Albertí, P. J. Sanz Miguel, B. Lippert, Inorg. Chem. **2011**, *50*, 10439–10447. Copyright 2011 American Chemical Society.) (b) Zenithal view of the complex unit (where the BF$_4^-$ anion sits on top of the caffeine ring) and (c) lateral view (a set of piled interaction is observed) for the crystal structure of [Au(TMX)$_2$]BF$_4$, where TMX is 1,3,7-trimethylpurine-2,6-dione or caffeine [93] (color code: C, dark gray; H, white; O, red; N, blue; F, light green; B, pink; Au, yellow).

the metal ion drains electronic density off the bases and permits not only the anion–π interaction with BF_4^- but also to target DNA quadruplexes. Its affinity for G-quartet is due to (1) its planar conformation; (2) its cationic nature (attractive electrostatic interaction with DNA), (3) the presence of two aromatic arms ideally suited to interact with the guanines via π-stacking interactions, and (4) the centrally positioned metal atom can interact with the four carbonyl groups of the accessible G-quartet, over the central cation channel.

3 CONCLUDING REMARKS AND FUTURE DIRECTIONS

In the first part of this chapter, the ability of some metal ions to play the role of a hydrogen atom and form base pairs has been described, focusing on the most relevant cases. In case of silver, the formation of these metal-modified pairs or synthons has been used to generate 1D polymers where argentophilic interactions are crucial. The strategy to combine H bonds, π-stacking, and Ag⋯Ag interactions to construct 1D supramolecular assemblies has a bright future since a new family of hybrid nanomaterials can be obtained by modifying the nucleobases with promising and intriguing new photophysical properties.

In the second part, the importance of non-conventional interactions in the solid state of nucleobase derivatives has been emphasized, focusing on cation–π and especially anion–π interactions that are quite common due to the ability of the nucleobases to be protonated. Consequently, the counterion has a strong tendency to establish anion–π interactions with the acidic π-systems. This can be exploited in crystal engineering and supramolecular chemistry, especially anion recognition and sensing. Finally, some examples have been described emphasizing the role of the regium bond in some bases coordinated to Au^{3+} ion. It is expected that this interaction will inspire researchers working on Au-nucleobase complexes. The π-hole regium bonds highlighted in this chapter, involving Au^{3+} derivatives, are an important extension of gold interactions, which are currently dominated by aurophilic bonds, involving Au^+ derivatives.

ACKNOWLEDGMENTS

AF thanks the MICIU/AEI of Spain (project PID2020–115637GB-I00 FEDER funds) for financial support.

ABBREVIATIONS AND DEFINITIONS

1D	one-dimensional
1MeC	1-methylcytosine
1MeCH⁺	1-methylcytosinium
1MeT	1-methylthymine
1,3-diMeU	1,3-dimethyluracil
(6AH)₂C₃	6,6′-trimethylenbisadeninium
9EtA	9-ethyladenine

9EtGH	9-ethylguanine
9MeA	9-methyladenine
A	adenine
B-DNA	B-form of DNA
C	cytosine
C–H⁺–C	hemiprotonated cytosine–cytosine pair
CMP	cytidine 5′-monophosphate
DFT	density functional theory
DIS duplex	duplex form of the HIV-1 RNA dimerization initiation site
DNA	deoxyribonucleic acid
en	ethylenediamine
G	guanine
GNA	glycol nucleic acid
MEP	molecular electrostatic potential
NMR	nuclear magnetic resonance
PMe$_3$	trimethylphosphine
RNA	ribonucleic acid
T	thymine
TMX	1,3,7-trimethylpurine-2,6-dione or caffeine
U	uracil
Z-DNA	Z-form of DNA

REFERENCES

1. I. Alkorta, J. Elguero, A. Frontera, *Crystals* **2020**, *10*, 180.
2. A. S. Mahadevi, G. N. Sastry, *Chem. Rev.* **2016**, *116*, 2775–2825.
3. I. Alkorta, F. Blanco, P. M. Deyà, J. Elguero, C. Estarellas, A. Frontera, D. Quiñonero, *Theor. Chem. Acc.* **2010**, *126*, 1–14.
4. M. Giese, M. Albrecht, K. Rissanen, *Chem. Commun.* **2016**, *52*, 1778–1795.
5. A. S. Mahadevi, and G. N. Sastry, *Chem. Rev.* **2013**, *113*, 2100–2138.
6. *Structural and Catalytic Role of Metal Ions in RNA*, Vol. 9 of *Metal Ions in Life Sciences*, Eds A. Sigel, H. Sigel, R. K. O. Sigel, De Gruyter, Berlin DE, **2011**.
7. *Interplay between Metal Ions and Nucleic Acids*, Vol. 10 of *Metal Ions in Life Sciences*, Eds A. Sigel, H. Sigel, R. K. O. Sigel, Springer, Dodrecht, UK, **2012**.
8. Y. He, A. Lopez, Z. Zhang, D. Chen, R. Yabg, J. Liu, *Coord. Chem. Rev.* **2019**, *387*, 235–248.
9. P. Zhou, R. Shi, J. Yao, C. Sheng, H. Li, *Coord. Chem. Rev.* **2015**, *291*, 107–143.
10. N. Dey, C. J. E. Haynes, *ChemPlusChem* **2021**, *86*, 418–433.
11. F. Pu, J. Ren, X. Qu, *Chem. Soc. Rev.* **2018**, *47*, 1285–1306.
12. B. Lippert, *Coord. Chem. Rev.* **2000**, *200–202*, 487–516.
13. F. Zamora, M. Kunsman, M. Sabat, B. Lippert, *Inorg. Chem.* **1997**, *36*, 1583–1587.
14. E. Ennifar, P. Walter, P. Dumas, *Nucleic Acids Res.* **2003**, *31*, 2671–2682.
15. F. Guay, A. L. Beauchamp, *J. Am. Chem. Soc.* **1979**, *101*, 6260–6263.
16. A. Erxleben, S. Metzger, J. F. Britten, C. J. L. Lock, A. Albinati, B. Lippert, *Inorg. Chim. Acta* **2002**, *339*, 461–469.
17. M. S. Lüth, M. Willermann, B. Lippert, *Chem. Commun.* **2001**, 2058–2059.

18. R. Faggiani, B. Lippert, J. L. Lock, A. Speranzini, *Inorg. Chem.* **1982**, *21*, 3216–3225.
19. O. Krizanovic, M. Sabat, R. Beyerle-Pfnür, B. Lippert, *J. Am. Chem. Soc.* **1993**, *115*, 5538–5548.
20. M. Noguera, J. Bertran, M. Sodupe, *J. Phys. Chem. A* **2004**, *108*, 333–341.
21. B. Lippert, P. J. Sanz Miguel, *Acc. Chem. Res.* **2016**, *49*, 1537–1535.
22. K. Guo, A. Pourpak, K. Beetz-Rogers, V. Gokhale, D. Sun, L. H. Hurley, *J. Am. Chem. Soc.* **2007**, *129*, 10220–10228.
23. M. Debnath, K. Fatma, J. Dash, *Angew. Chem. Int. Ed.* **2019**, *58*, 2942–2987.
24. M. Zeraati, D. B. Langley, P. Schofield, A. L. Moye, R. Rouet, W. E. Hughes, T. M. Bryan, M. E. Dinger, D. Christ, *Nat. Chem.* **2018**, *10*, 631–637.
25. T. J. Kistenmacher, M. Rossi, L. G. Marzilli, *Biopolymers* **1978**, *17*, 2581–2585.
26. T. J. Kistenmacher, M. Rossi, C. C. Chiang, J. P. Caradonna, L. G. Marzilli, *Adv. Mol. Relax. Interact. Processes* **1980**, *17*, 113–134.
27. A. Schimanski, E. Freisinger, A. Erxleben, B. Lippert, *Inorg. Chim. Acta* **1998**, *283*, 223–232.
28. A. L. Lieblein, M. Krümer, A. Dreuw, B. Fürtig, H. Schwalbe, *Angew. Chem. Int. Ed.* **2012**, *51*, 4067–4070.
29. Y. Dong, Z. Yang, D. Liu, *Acc. Chem. Res.* **2014**, *47*, 1853–1860.
30. H. Liu, D. Liu, *Chem. Commun.* **2009**, 2625–2636.
31. H. Torigoe, A. Ono, T. Kozasa, *Chem. Eur. J.* **2010**, *16*, 13218–13225.
32. J. Kondo, T. Yamada, C. Hirose, I. Okamoto, Y. Tanaka, A. Ono, *Angew. Chem. Int. Ed.* **2014**, *53*, 2385–2388.
33. A. Ono, H. Torigoe, Y. Tanaka, I. Okamoto, *Chem. Soc. Rev.* **2011**, *40*, 5855–5866.
34. Y. Miyake, H. Togashi, M. Tashiro, H. Yamaguchi, S. Oda, M. Kudo, Y. Tanaka, Y. Kondo, R. Sawa, T. Fujimoto, T. Machinami, A. Ono, *J. Am. Chem. Soc.* **2006**, *128*, 2172–2173.
35. T. Dairaku, K. Furuita, H. Sato, J. Sebera, K. Nakashima, A. Ono, V. Sychrovsky, C. Kojima, Y. Tanaka, *Inorg. Chim. Acta* **2016**, *452*, 34–42.
36. S. Nehzati, A. O. Summers, N. V. Dolgova, J. Zhu, D. Sokaras, T. Kroll, I. J. Pickering, G. N. George, *Inorg. Chem.* **2021**, *60*, 7442–7452.
37. M. Barceló-Oliver, B. A. Baquero, A. Bauzá, A. García-Raso, R. Vic, I. Mata, E. Molins, A. Terrón, A. Frontera, *Dalton Trans.* **2013**, *42*, 7631–7642.
38. A. Bauza, A. Terrón, M. Barceló-Oliver, A. Garcia-Raso, A. Frontera, *Inorg. Chim. Acta* **2016**, *452*, 244–250.
39. J. Müller, *Coord. Chem. Rev.* **2019**, *393*, 17–47.
40. K. Aoki, W. Saenger, *Acta Crystallogr.* **1984**, *C40*, 775–778.
41. J. Kondo, Y. Tada, T. Dairaku, Y. Hattori, H. Saneyoshi, A. Ono, Y. Tanaka, *Nat. Chem.* **2017**, *9*, 956–960.
42. J. Kondo, Y. Tada, T. Dairaku, H. Saneyoshi, I. Okamoto, Y. Tanaka, A. Ono, *Angew. Chem. Int. Ed.* **2015**, *54*, 13323–13326.
43. H. Liu, F. Shen, P. Haruehanroengra, Q. Yao, Y. Cheng, Y. Chen, C. Yang, J. Zhang, B. Wu, Q. Luo, R. Cui, J. Li, J. Ma, J. Sheng, J. Gan, *Angew. Chem. Int. Ed.* **2017**, *56*, 9430–9434.
44. O. Nakagawa, H. Aoyama, A. Fujii, Y. Kishimoto, S. Obika, *Chem. Eur. J.* **2021**, *27*, 3842–3848.
45. P. Amo-Ochoa, O. Castillo, P. J. Sanz Miguel, F. Zamora, *J. Inorg. Biochem.* **2008**, *102*, 203–208.
46. H. Millonig, J. Pons, C. Gouyette, J. A. Subirana, J. L. Campos, *J. Inorg. Biochem.* **2009**, *103*, 876–880.
47. O. Golubev, G. Turc, T. Lönnberg, *J. Inorg. Biochem.* **2016**, *155*, 36–43.

48. Y. Takezawa, A. Suzuki, M. Nakaya, K. Nishiyama, M. Shionoya, *J. Am. Chem. Soc.* **2020**, *142*, 21640–21644.
49. B. Lippert, *J. Biol. Inorg. Chem.* **2022**, *27*, 215–219.
50. H. Schmidbaur, A. Schier, *Angew. Chem. Int. Ed.* **2015**, *54*, 746–784.
51. H. Schmidbaur, A. Schier, *Chem. Soc. Rev.* **2012**, *41*, 370–412.
52. D. A. Megger, C. Fonseca Guerra, J. Hoffman, B. Brutschy, F. M. Bickelhaupt, J. Müller, *Chem. Eur. J.* **2011**, *17*, 6533–6544.
53. N. Santamaria-Díaz, J. M. Méndez-Arriaga, J. M. Salas, M. A. Galindo, *Angew. Chem. Int. Ed.* **2016**, *55*, 6170–6174.
54. J. M. Méndez-Arriaga, C. R. Maldonado, J. A. Dobado, M. A. Galindo, *Chem. Eur. J.* **2018**, *24*, 1–8.
55. A. Terrón, B. Moreno-Vachiano, A. Bauzá, A. García-Raso, J. J. Fiol, M. Barceló-Oliver, E. Molins, A. Frontera, *Chem. Eur. J.* **2017**, *23*, 2103–2108.
56. A. Terrón, L. Tomàs, A. Bauzá, A. García-Raso, J. J. Fiol, E. Molins, A. Frontera, *CrystEngComm* **2017**, *19*, 5830–5854.
57. L. Mistry, P. G. Waddell, N. G. Wright, B. R. Horrocks, A. Houlton, *Inorg. Chem.* **2019**, *58*, 13346–13352.
58. L. Mistry, O. El-Zubir, G. Dura, W. Clegg, P. G. Waddell, T. Pope, W. A. Hofer, N. G. Wright, B. R. Horrocks, A. Houlton, *Chem. Sci.* **2019**, *10*, 3186–3195.
59. L. Mistry, O. El-Zubir, T. Pope, P. G. Waddell, N. Wright, W.A. Hofer, B. R. Horrocks, A. Houlton, *Cryst. Growth Des.* **2021**, *21*, 4398–4405.
60. F. Linares, E. García-Fernández, F. J. López-Garzón, M. Domingo-García, A. Orte, A. Rodríguez-Diéguez, M. A. Galindo, *Chem. Sci.* **2019**, *10*, 1126–1137.
61. T. Dairaku, K. Furuita, H. Sato, J. Sebera, K. Nakashima, J. Kondo, D. Yamanaka, Y. Kondo, I. Okamoto, A. Ono, V. Sychrovsky, C. Kojima, Y. Tanaka, *Chem. Eur. J.* **2016**, *22*, 13028–13031.
62. T. J. Kistenmacher, M. Rossi, L. G. Marzilli, *Inorg. Chem.* **1979**, *18*, 240–244.
63. C. Cerretani, H. Kanazawa, T. Vosch, J. Kondo, *Angew. Chem. Int. Ed.* **2019**, *58*, 17153–17157.
64. D. J. E. Huard, A. Demissie, D. Kim, D. Lewis, R. M. Dickson, J. T. Petty, R. L. Lieberman, *J. Am. Chem Soc.* **2019**, *141*, 11465–11470.
65. X. Xing, Y. Feng, Z. Yu, K. Hidaka, F. Liu, A. Ono, H. Sugiyama, M. Endo, *Chem. Eur. J.* **2019**, *25*, 1446–1450.
66. S. Vecchioni, M. C. Capece, E. Toomey, L. Nguyen, A. Ray, A. Greenberg, K. Fujishima, J. Urbina, I. G. Paulino-Lima, V. Pinheiro, J. Shih, G. Wessel, S. J. Wind, L. Rothschild, *Sci. Rep.* **2019**, *9*, 6942.
67. L. A. Espinosa, O. Lopez-Acevedo, *Nanotechnol. Rev.* **2015**, *4*, 173–191.
68. F. Zamora, E. Zangrando, M. Furlan, L. Randaccio, B. Lippert, *J. Organomet. Chem.* **1998**, *552*, 127–134.
69. X. Meng, T. Moriuchi, M. Kawahata, K. Yamaguchi, T. Hirao, *Chem. Commun.* **2011**, *47*, 4682–4684.
70. D. Blasco, J. M. López-de-Luzuriaga, M. Monge, M. E. Olmos, D. Pascual, M. Rodríguez-Castillo, *Inorg. Chem.* **2018**, *57*, 3805–3817.
71. M. N. Piña, A. Frontera, A. Bauzá, *J. Phys. Chem. Lett.* **2020**, *11*, 8259–8263.
72. A. Terrón, J. Buils, T. J. Mooibroek, M. Barceló-Oliver, A. García-Raso, J. J. Fiol, A. Frontera, *Chem. Commun.* **2020**, *56*, 3524–3527.
73. J. Buils, Synthesis and characterization of gold–nucleic base complexes, Master's Degree in Chemical Science and Technology, Universitat de les Illes Balears, ES, **2021**.
74. J. P. Gallivan, D. A. Dougherty, *Proc. Natl. Acad. Sci. USA* **1999**, *96*, 9459–9464.
75. X. Yao, D. Song, T. Qin, C. Yang, Z. Yu, X. Li, K. Liu, H. Su, *Sci. Rep.* **2017**, *7*, 10951.

76. J. Šponer, J. Leszczynski, P. Hobza, *Biopolymers* **2002**, *61*, 3–31.
77. W. Zhu, X. Luo, C. M. Puah, X. Tan, J. Shen, J. Gu, K. Chen, H. Jiang, *J. Phys. Chem. A* **2004**, *108*, 4008–4018.
78. B. G. Ernst, K. U. Lao, A. G. Sullivan, R. A. DiStasio Jr., *J. Phys. Chem. A* **2020**, *124*, 4128–4140.
79. M. Stewart, T. Dunlap, E. Dourlain, B. Grant, L. McFail-Isom, *PLoS One* **2013**, *8*, e71420.
80. S. D. Zarić, *Eur. J. Inorg. Chem.* **2003**, 2197–2209.
81. P. Auffinger, L. Bielecki, E. Westhof, *Structure* **2004**, *12*, 379–388.
82. R. Esmaeeli, M. N. Piña, A. Frontera, A. Pérez, A. Bauzá, *J. Chem. Theory Comput.* **2021**, *17*, 6624–6633.
83. J. Kozelka, *Eur Biophys J.* **2017**, *46*, 729–737.
84. M. Kobyłecka, J. Leszczynski, J. Rak, *J. Am. Chem. Soc.* **2008**, *130*, 15683–15687.
85. J. J. Fiol, M. Barceló-Oliver, A. Tasada, A. Frontera, A. Terron, A. García-Raso, *Coord. Chem. Rev.* **2013**, *257*, 2705–2715.
86. A. García-Raso, F. M. Albertí, J. J. Fiol, A. Tasada, M. Barceló-Oliver, E. Molins, D. Escudero, A. Frontera, D. Quiñonero, P. M. Deyà, *Inorg. Chem.* **2007**, *46*, 10724–10735.
87. J. M. Salas, M. Quirós, M. P. Sánchez, A. L. Beauchamp, *Acta Crystallogr.* **1989**, *C45*, 1874–1877.
88. M. Barceló-Oliver, B. A. Baquero, A. Bauzá, A. García-Raso, A. Terrón, I. Mata, E. Molins, A. Frontera, *CrystEngComm* **2012**, *14*, 5777–5784.
89. A. García-Raso, F. M. Albertí, J. J. Fiol, Y. Lagos, M. Torres, E. Molins, I. Mata, C. Estarellas, A. Frontera, D. Quiñonero, P. M. Deyà, *Eur. J. Org. Chem.* **2010**, 5171–5180.
90. R. Pons, C. Ibáñez, A. B. Buades, A. Franconetti, A. García-Raso, J. J. Fiol, Terrón, E. Molins, A. Frontera, *Appl Organomet. Chem.* **2019**, *33*, e4906.
91. B. García, J. García-Tojal, R. Ruiz, R. Gil-García, S. Ibeas, B. Donnadieu, J. M. Leal, *J. Inorg. Biochem.* **2008**, *102*, 1892–1900.
92. S. Ibáñez, F. M. Albertí, P. J. Sanz Miguel, B. Lippert, *Inorg. Chem.* **2011**, *50*, 10439–10447.
93. L. Stefan, B. Bertrand, P. Richard, P. Le Gendre, F. Denat, M. Picquet, D. Monchaud, *ChemBioChem* **2012**, *13*, 1905–1912.

6 Biological Implications of Metal-Nucleobase Complexes

Saurabh Joshi and Ankita Jaiswal
Department of Chemistry, Indian Institute of Technology
Kanpur, Kanpur 208016, Uttar Pradesh, India
saurabhj@iitk.ac.in, ankitaj@iitk.ac.in

Rajneesh Kumar Prajapati
Center for Nanoscience, Indian Institute of Technology
Kanpur, Kanpur 208016, Uttar Pradesh, India
rajkp@iitk.ac.in

Sandeep Verma[*]
Department of Chemistry, Center for Nanoscience,
and Mehta Family Center for Engineering
in Medicine, Indian Institute of Technology
Kanpur, Kanpur 208016, Uttar Pradesh, India
sverma@iitk.ac.in

CONTENTS

1	Introduction	134
2	Metal-Purine Chemistry	136
3	Silver	137
	3.1 Silver Complexes with Nucleobase Derivatives	137
	3.2 Silver-Mediated Base Pairing	138
4	Platinum	139
	4.1 Platinum Complexes	139
5	Gold Cluster Stabilization with Purine Derivatives	142
6	Copper	144
	6.1 Copper Complexes	144
7	Mercury-Mediated Base Pairing	145
8	Zinc	147

[*] Corresponding author

	8.1	Zinc Interaction with Purine Derivatives	147
9	Ruthenium and Osmium Complexes	148
10	Iridium Complexes	150
11	Quartet Self-assembly of Guanine Derivatives by Metal Ions	151
12	Conclusions	152
Acknowledgments	153
Abbreviations and Definitions	153
References	154

Abstract

Nucleobases are heterocyclic biological building blocks that support the foundation of life. These nitrogen-rich molecules play vital roles in biological systems ranging from storage of genetic information, protein synthesis, serving as essential cofactors in enzymatic transformations, signal transduction pathways, facilitation of metabolic pathways, etc. Notably, the purine scaffold presents multiple sites for metal ion coordination affording formation of architecturally challenging metal-bound complexes for biological and therapeutic purposes. In addition to metal coordination, inherent sites for hydrogen bonding further augment the stability of such complexes and support a vast array of three-dimensional structures in the solid state and in solution. In the recent times, metal-mediated base pairing has not only opened up new horizons in artificially coded information, but also expedited the development of biophysical and visualization tools for biochemical processes taking place inside the cells. From a material science standpoint, directional hydrogen bonding in nucleobases and suitably disposed imino nitrogen atoms have been shown to support supramolecular structures, with meticulous recognition abilities, for creating adaptive functional materials. Herein, we focus on the advances in metal-purine coordination, complexation, and systematic synthetic modifications with an emphasis on biological relevance. Different facets of nucleobase coordination to diverse metal ions have been critically reviewed along with selected features and applications such as anticancer activity, antibacterial action, and biological sensing, to name a few. This chapter will provide an understanding of structural aspects of nucleobase-metal coordination, the design of non-natural scaffolds for specific processing, and relevant biological applications.

KEYWORDS

Purines; Metal-Purine Interactions; Biological Applications; Base Pairing; Nucleobase Complexes with Metals

1 INTRODUCTION

Nucleobases are nitrogenous heterocycles that are part of fundamental bioessential substructures supporting coded genetic information of the living systems. Nucleobases are inextricable components present in nucleic acids, nucleosides, enzyme cofactors, and signaling pathway molecules [1]. Nucleobases, when attached to pentose sugars, are called nucleosides, and when attached to sugar and phosphate group(s), are called nucleotides (Figure 1). The latter, when suitably polymerized, support formation of elegant self-assembled biological macromolecular structures, via conventional and non-cognate base-pairing mechanisms.

Biological Implications of Metal-Nucleobase Complexes 135

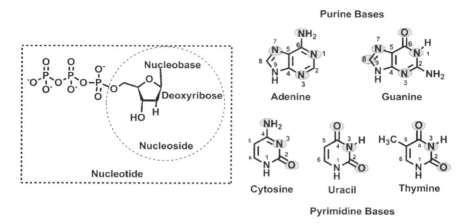

FIGURE 1 General structure of nucleotide and nucleoside along with natural purine and pyrimidine bases. The gray circles denote the preferred potential metal-binding sites.

The resultant nucleic acid biopolymers are able to store genetic information and afford flawless read-out for replication and protein synthesis [2]. Their ability to engage in hydrogen bonding, their multiple coordinating sites for metal ions, their π-π stacking for stabilization of higher-order structures, and their self-assembly supports structural diversity and functional applications [3]. The presence of ring imino nitrogen atoms along with electron-rich cyclic cores (Figure 1) facilitates interactions with different substrates and metal ions to yield supramolecular architectures for surface patterning, deoxyribonucleic acid (DNA) nanotechnology, rapid analyte detection and biochip technology [4, 5]. There are opportunities to modify these molecules through directed chemical synthesis to evolve tuneable architectures for functional applications [3, 5]. Such chemically modified nucleobases could also serve as suitable probes to unravel and understand biochemical mechanisms at the molecular level. Thus, it is widely accepted that understanding nucleobase and nucleic acid chemistry could help with many unresolved challenges of biological relevance, disease diagnosis, and therapeutics.

The negatively charged backbone of nucleic acids offers a strong affinity toward positively charged metal ions and protonated polyamines [6]. Such nucleic acid-metal ion interactions serve, beyond charge neutralization, to accomplish modulation of biochemical processes, structural stability, and support conformational changes. Thus, metal-nucleobase interaction models are excellent biomimetic models to understand gross features of metal-nucleic acid interaction under physiological conditions and its further use to design useful therapeutic agents [7]. A classical example of metal-DNA interaction, onward to commercially viable therapeutics, has been the discovery of the anticancer drug cisplatin by Rosenberg [8]. It was identified that guanine N7 coordination of Pt^{2+} causes crosslinked DNA adducts and distortion in DNA helical structure, thus hindering its replication and promoting apoptosis [9, 10].

Interactions of nucleic acids with different metal ions induce architectural shift and allow for the evolution of interesting structural motifs [11]. This approach has been useful for the advances made in nucleic acid-based functional materials, through nanotechnology manipulations, which have utilized metal ions to arrive at adaptive structures for advanced applications. A bottom-up approach has been successfully employed for preparing metal-templated DNA nanomaterials, for a wide range of biologically relevant targets [11]. However, ribonucleic acid (RNA) templates are yet to receive due attention for advanced nanostructural preparations. Some examples have proven the capability of RNA to help produce functional nanomaterials such as quantum dots [12].

Biocompatible nucleic acid-based hydrogelation, induced by metal coordination, has attracted attention due to significant potential applications in fields such as drug delivery, tissue engineering, and sensing. Guanosine quartet-driven assembly, in the presence of monovalent cations, induces formation of super-assembled hydrogels with practical uses [13]. A recent application in the field of metal ion-nucleic acid interactions is biocomputing at the molecular level [3,14]. The conformational changes in nucleic acid structure upon metal coordination can be used as a signal to trigger different cascades of logic operations in biological systems. The conceptual understanding of implementing chemical interactions into logic circuits has been applied in biosensing and in bioanalyte detection [15].

As mentioned, purines and other modified nucleobases offer multiple sites for metal ion coordination and can be further chemically modified to engineer metal ion binding sites in order to achieve specific interactions for a desired effect or application (Figure 1) [16]. The purine derivatives are synthesized in a straightforward manner, easily equipped with reactive handles, and are cost-effective as compared to whole DNA or RNA modifications. Inevitably, many synthetic purine analogs have been successfully designed and synthesized to interact with different metal ions like Cu^{2+}, Ru^{2+}, Pt^{2+}, Ag^+, and Hg^{2+} for multiple applications.

2 METAL-PURINE CHEMISTRY

Metal ions have diverse roles in biological systems: ferric/ferrous ions are required in oxygen transport, Cu^{2+}, Zn^{2+}, and Co^{2+} are important cofactors in enzymatic catalysis, and Na^+/K^+ ion transport generates electrochemical gradients across cell membranes [17, 18]. Although both amino and imino groups can interact with metal ions, the pK_a of exocyclic amino groups usually renders them less favorable for metal binding in their major tautomeric form (i.e., amino form) at physiological pH [17,19]. However, metal coordination to the exocyclic amino group is possible in its deprotonated or rare tautomeric form (proton shifted from exocyclic to imino N1 atom) [20,21]. In addition, chelation or a bidentate coordination mode of metal ions has been reported for the involvement of the exocyclic amino group in adenine nucleobases [22,23]. Purine-N7 nitrogen atoms are frequently favored for metal interactions since these sites are exposed in the major groove of the DNA duplex, as has been well established in numerous studies [24]. It has been evident that the N7 binding of purine nucleobase to a metal further reinforces non-covalent interactions [25] and offers this possibility to both hard and soft metal ions [22]. The basicity order of adenine nitrogen donor sites is N1 > N7 > N3, but in DNA, N7 is the preferred metal-binding site. This preference

Biological Implications of Metal-Nucleobase Complexes

responds to change in pH, where a lowering of the pH decreases binding at the N1 site due to its protonation, thus pushing metal binding selectively toward N7 [26]. N3 is considered to be in the minor groove of the DNA helix and has a lower affinity for metal ion binding due to steric restrictions. Meiser et al. showed N3 metal binding is possible if N1 and N7 become sterically inaccessible due to steric blockage by dimethylation of the N6 amino group of adenine [27].

Similarly, in case of guanine, it is well established that N1 metal coordination in 9-substituted guanine is kinetically unfavorable at physiological pH, whereas N7 remains unprotonated over a wide pH range and is also highly susceptible for metal ion coordination in the DNA major groove [28]. Although N1 metal coordination in guanine derivatives has been reported numerously [29–31], it was observed that simultaneous coordination of a metal ion to N3 and N7 of guanine enhances the acidity of N1, enabling its deprotonation at neutral pH, which subsequently facilitates metal binding to this position [32]. While N3 metal coordination in adenine nucleobases augmented the generation of aesthetically pleasing macrostructures, the formation of a molecular square was observed with guanine derivatives via N3 coordination [33]. O6 of guanine is also reported to interact with metal ions like K^+ in G-quartet assembly, Na^+/Mg^{2+} in RNA [as suggested by density functional theory (DFT) calculations], and with other metal centers [34–37].

3 SILVER

3.1 Silver Complexes with Nucleobase Derivatives

An *N7,N9*-disubstituted N6-methoxyadenine derivative as a rare purine tautomer was reported for the generation of a metal ion-stabilized carbene at the C8 position (**1**) (Figure 2a). The possible structure was deduced via DFT calculations and the silver-carbene complex showed a cytotoxic effect in A549 lung cancer and

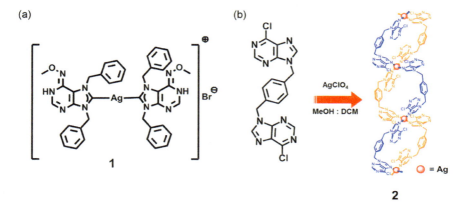

FIGURE 2 (a) Molecular structure of silver-carbene complex. (b) Ag-mediated luminescent double-helical structure of antibacterial purine-silver complex. (Modified by permission from Ref. [40]; Copyright 2016, Wiley-VCH Verlag GmbH & Co. KGaA, Weinheim.)

MCF7 breast cancer cell lines comparable to that of curcumin used as a control [38]. It was observed that the microtubule network, an important cytoskeleton filament responsible for maintaining cell shape [39], and its dynamics were drastically perturbed in the presence of 1.

The silver complex of another designed purine derivative, 1,4-bis((6-chloropurine-9-yl)methyl)benzene, exhibited formation of a luminescent double-helical structure 2 (Figure 2b) with antibacterial activity toward *E. coli* [minimum inhibitory concentration (MIC)—7.8 μg mL^{-1}]. The proposed mechanism of action involves purine-mediated cellular uptake, followed by the slow release of silver ions [40]. A similar antibacterial action was observed by Verma et al. using silver-bispurine metallogels against nosocomial antibiotic-resistant bacterial pathogens. The silver gel showed potent broad-spectrum antibacterial activity against both gram-positive and gram-negative pathogens with MIC in the range of 2–8 μg mL^{-1}, and purine-facilitated uptake of silver ions across the bacterial membrane was proposed as the possible mechanism. A composite polymer film prepared from the mixture of the silver gel with a polyethylene glycol (PEG) and polycaprolactam (PCL) polymer, when spin-coated over a glass surface, exhibited antifouling activity against *S. aureus* through the inhibition of biofilm growth [41].

3.2 Silver-Mediated Base Pairing

Transition metal-mediated base pairs are stabilized by coordination strategies and they circumvent hydrogen bond-supported structural stabilization. Natural bases exhibit metal ion preference for binding, while artificial nucleobases and nucleosides are rather promiscuous toward metal-mediated interactions [42]. Müller and co-workers described Ag$^+$-mediated base pairing of 1,N^6-ethenoadenine (εA), leading to formation of a synthetic DNA duplex comprising an εA:εA dinuclear metal-mediated homo purine base pair, which was used to pattern a two-dimensional adlayer on graphite substrate [43]. In a significant advance, it was possible to engineer the polymerase-driven formation of C–Ag$^+$–A as a novel strategy to gain access to synthetic nucleic acid sequences and the use of metal-supported unnatural base pairs in experiments to generate functional nucleic acids [44,45].

Metal-mediated base pairing has been extensively used to support unnatural base pairs in oligonucleotides. Müller et al. showed that Ag$^+$ mediates three consecutive base pairs of artificial imidazole nucleosides incorporated in a DNA sequence that adopts a duplex structure with these unnatural modifications. It was proposed that the N3 atom of imidazole coordinates the Ag$^+$ to form an imidazole–Ag$^+$–imidazole complex (3) (Figure 3a) [46]. Later on, Galindo and co-workers used the modified nucleobase 7-deazaadenine (^{7C}A) to form its canonical base pair (4) with thymine through silver ion coordination via N1 of deazaadenine and N3 of thymine (Figure 3b) [47]. Similarly, DNA structure engineering was also accomplished via silver-mediated base pairing of 7-deazaguanine with cytosine, where DNA molecules consisting of contiguous

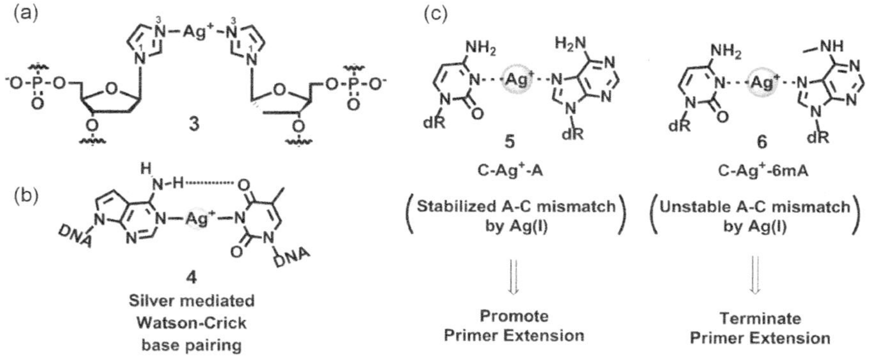

Biological Implications of Metal-Nucleobase Complexes 139

FIGURE 3 (a) Chemical structure of a silver-mediated base pair of the artificial imidazole nucleotide. (b) Chemical structure of metal-mediated base pairing of ^{7C}A-T. (c) Structural difference and discrimination of 6mA and adenine for silver-mediated base pairing by a polymerase. C–Ag$^+$–A base pair stabilized by Ag$^+$ is recognized by the polymerase and promotes primer extension; 6mA-C mismatch not stabilized by Ag$^+$ leading to termination of primer extension.

metalated base pairs were able to support a B-type DNA conformation [48]. Hong et al. exploited the silver-mediated selective stabilization of an A-C mismatch (**5**) to detect N6-methyladenine (6mA), a potential epigenetic marker in eukaryotic genomes, as this modified base was unable to interact with cytosine in the presence of silver ions in a stable manner. Thus, the 6mA–Ag$^+$–cytosine mismatch (**6**) was not recognized by DNA polymerases, thereby resulting in the termination of primer extension (Figure 3c) [49].

4 PLATINUM

Chemotherapeutically active platinum complexes have been successful in the treatment of various cancers, thus revolutionizing the field of medical oncology [50, 51]. Mechanistically, these Pt drugs interact with DNA nucleobases through the formation of inter- and intra-strand crosslinks, followed by helical structure distortion and eventual cell death. It is well established that nucleobases interact preferentially with Pt^{2+} through purine-N7 sites of guanine and adenine to form crosslinked adducts: for example, the cisplatin-DNA interaction results in ~90% intra-strand crosslinking, 6% inter-strand crosslinking and ~4% monofunctional adducts [52, 53]. In the following, selected examples of Pt-nucleobase complexes will be discussed.

4.1 Platinum Complexes

Despite the clinical success of the by now classical platinum-based therapeutics, their off-target cytotoxicity and emergence of drug resistance limit their prolonged applicability. Štarha et al. designed and synthesized

2-chloro-N6-(benzyl)-9-isopropyladenine derivatives to make complexes with Pt^{2+} oxalate, and explored their potency as anticancer agents for osteosarcoma (HOS) and breast adenocarcinoma (MCF7) human cancer cell lines (Figure 4a). The crystal structure of the platinated purine derivatives showed N7 coordination in a 2:1 ligand-to-metal stoichiometry. The *in vitro* cytotoxicity profile of these complexes was compared with the established anticancer drugs cisplatin and oxaliplatin. Complex **7** showed anticancer potency with IC_{50} values of 3.6 and 4.3 µM, while complex **8** showed IC_{50} values of 5.4 and 3.6 µM, for HOS and MCF7 cell lines, respectively (Figure 4a). Moreover, the observed activity was superior to that of cisplatin (IC_{50} = 34.2 and 19.6 µM) and oxaliplatin ($IC_{50} \geq 50$ and >50 µM) [54].

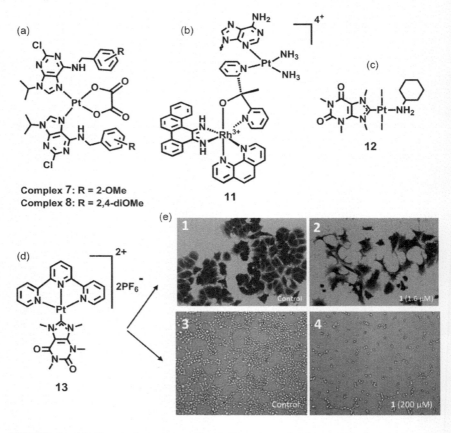

FIGURE 4 (a) Chemical structure of a platinum complex bearing oxalato and purine ligands. (b) Rare N3 coordination of adenine with platinum in a bimetallic complex. (c) Carbene complex based on methylated caffeine with C8 metalation in a square planar geometry. (d) Pt^{2+} terpyridine complex with a caffeine-derived N-heterocyclic carbene ligand. (e) (1–2) Differentiation-like morphological changes of MCF-7 cells treated with complex **13**. (3–4) Anti-angiogenic property of complex **13** in the tube-formation assay using MS-1 cells. (Adapted by permission from Ref. [58], Copyright 2014, Elsevier B.V.)

Recently, Trávníček and co-workers explored the anticancer efficacy of two roscovitine derivatives, i.e. 2-(1-ethyl-2-hydroxyethylamino)-N6-(4-methoxybenzyl)-9-isopropyladenine (**L1**) and 2-chloro-N6-(2,4-dimethoxybenzyl)-9-isopropyladenine (**L2**), coordinated to Pt^{2+}. The *in vivo* evaluation of a tumor-bearing mouse model with complex **9** [**L1**-Pt^{2+}], complex **10** [**L2**-Pt^{2+}], and cisplatin (as control drug) revealed that complex **9** showed better survival of mice as compared to complex **10** and cisplatin (Table 1). The survivability was calculated as %T/C, where T denotes the average survival (in days) for the respective treated group and C represents the average survival (in days) for the control group. Moreover, the side effects of cisplatin like apathy, loss of appetite, tachypnea, etc. were prominent in the mice treated with cisplatin, but mice treated with complex **9** showed fewer side effects, with no eating and neurological disorder. In addition, the antitumor action of complex **9** follows a mechanism of action that is via the activation of Casp-3, which is different from that of cisplatin, which activates the transcription factor p53 [55]. Although the N7 site is preferred in the case of purine nucleobases binding to platinum drugs in the major groove of DNA, there are also examples of N3 binding to Pt drugs in the minor groove. Barton et al. synthesized a rhodium and platinum bimetallic complex (**11**) that binds to the N3 position of adenine, rather than guanine, and displays enhanced anticancer activity in mismatch repair-deficient and proficient human colorectal carcinoma cell lines (Figure 4b). The observed cytotoxicity was attributed to complex-triggered apoptosis. The *in vitro* studies revealed that the complex was bonded preferably to mismatched DNA rather than matched one [56].

Another interesting platinum-purine complex was synthesized by Mailliet, Marinetti et al. by exploiting purine-carbene chemistry at the C8 position. Initially, a Ag^+-stabilized carbene was generated at the C8 position of methylated caffeine, followed by the exchange of Ag^+ by Pt^{2+} to afford a C8 platinated purine (**12**) (Figure 4c). Increased cytotoxicity was observed for this complex, compared to cisplatin, when it was used in two cells lines. Moreover, enhanced antitumor potency for cisplatin-resistant human ovarian cancer cell lines

TABLE 1
Pt^{2+}-Oxalato Complexes of Roscovitine Derivatives Show Different Cellular Effects and Fewer Adverse Effects in Mouse Lymphoma Model Than Cisplatin

Compound	Untreated Control	Complex 9	Complex 10	Cisplatin
Average body weight ± SE (g)	24.7 ± 1.3	21.8 ± 1.2	22.4 ± 0.7	14.8 ± 0.4
Average tumor weight ± SE (g)	5.1 ± 0.6	5.0 ± 0.3	5.0 ± 0.46	1.5 ± 0.1
Mean survival time ± SE (days)	18.2 ± 0.8	19.8 ± 1.9	17.0 ± 1.2	17.0 ± 1.4
% T/C (%)	100.0	108.7	93.3	93.3

Source: Taken with permission from Ref. [55].

(A2780/DDP and CH1/DDP cell lines) was also observed *in vitro*. The purine-Pt^{2+} complex **12** showed potency at micromolar concentrations (IC$_{50}$ = 1.4 µM for A2780/DDP and 2.1 µM for CH1/DDP) and outperformed oxaliplatin (IC$_{50}$ = 17.3 µM for A2780/DDP and 6.2 µM for CH1/DDP) [57].

Ott et al. studied anticancer properties of platinum terpyridine complexes with a caffeine-derived N-heterocyclic carbene (NHC) ligand. The cytotoxic effect of these complexes was determined for different cell lines such as MCF-7, MDA-MB-231, and HT-29. Complex **13** showed promising anti-proliferative activity at sub-micromolar concentrations (IC$_{50}$ = 0.35–0.41 µM), which were lower than for cisplatin (IC$_{50}$ = 2–10 µM) (Figure 4d). This complex also showed indication of neural cell differentiation, since MCF-7 cells were elongated on treatment with this complex as a feature of the neural differentiation (Figure 4e). The tube inhibition assay concluded that the complex possessed anti-angiogenic activity (Figure 4e) and inhibited the thioredoxin reductase (TrxR) enzyme [58].

5 GOLD CLUSTER STABILIZATION WITH PURINE DERIVATIVES

Bioinspired metal nanoclusters play a critical role in sensing, therapeutics, delivery, and imaging applications [59–62]. It is anticipated that these clusters could have potential applications in the construction of hierarchical assemblies, logic gates, enzyme mimetics, and the *de novo* synthesis of metal-based nanoclusters, for applications in various fields of analytical science. Verma and co-workers designed and synthesized C8 thiol-modified adenine analogs to synthesize capped, highly photostable, and biocompatible gold nanoclusters (AuNCs) (**14**) (Figure 5a). Briefly, a C8-modified thioadenine ligand was reacted with chloroauric acid to form a thiolate complex of Au$^+$, followed by its reduction to form highly stable bright green fluorescent AuNCs [63]. The as-synthesized AuNCs (**14**), which possess appreciable fluorescence emission lifetimes, were tested in four different types of cancerous cell lines for cell uptake and biocompatibility studies. Fluorescence microscopy confirmed localization of bright green fluorescence of AuNCs in the cell nucleus, which suggested specific staining (Figure 5a). Focused cellular uptake studies revealed that purine-capped AuNC internalization occurred via the macropinocytosis pathway.

Flexible substrates with desired properties exhibit applications in biomedical technology, energy storage devices, electronics, and sensing [64–67]. Appropriate functionalization of flexible substrates, with various biological materials and biomolecules, offers significant applications in drug delivery, tissue engineering, and biosensing [68]. In particular, electro-spun nanofibers and processed flexible mats possess a large surface-to-volume ratio, high porosity and mechanical strength to be used as flexible platforms [69]. In this context, Verma et al. combined a C8-thiol derivative of adenine (**L**) with a polyacrylonitrile (PAN) polymer blend to obtain electro-spun nanofibrous mats, containing different ligand concentrations. Subsequently, these nanofibrous mats were decorated with gold

Biological Implications of Metal-Nucleobase Complexes 143

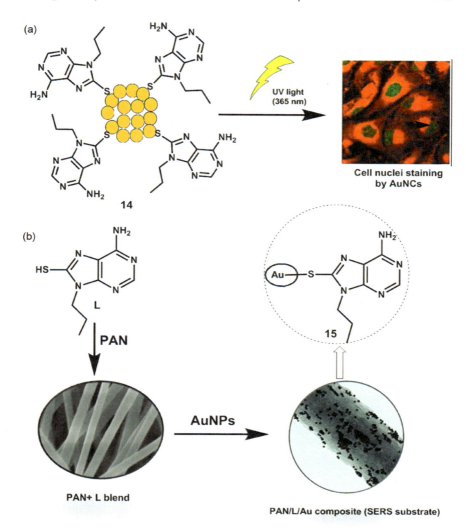

FIGURE 5 (a) C8 thiol-modified adenine-capped AuNCs for specific staining of cell nuclei. (Adapted by permission from Ref. [63]; Copyright 2014 American Chemical Society.) (b) Schematic representation of the synthesis of the L/PAN/AuNPs-based sensor. (Adapted by permission from Ref. [70]; Copyright 2020, Royal Society of Chemistry.)

nanoparticles (AuNPs) by the dipping method and the as-synthesized L/PAN/AuNPs flexible substrate (15) was applied for the detection of uric acid, a major biomarker of gout, kidney disease, cardiovascular diseases, and preeclampsia (Figure 5b) [70]. From the surface-enhanced Raman spectroscopy (SERS) analyses, it was proposed that higher concentrations of modified adenine ligands in the mats will afford better attachment of AuNPs, resulting in a greater number of "hotspot" areas for the attachment of uric acid, thereby leading to enhanced SERS sensitivity.

6 COPPER

The physiological roles of copper and its association with various pathologies urge the controlled regulation of copper in a biological environment [71]. Engineered copper complexes are emerging scaffolds for target-specific advanced therapeutics. There are several copper complexes reported in the literature with a chemotherapeutic success better than that of cisplatin, as these complexes have shown good biocompatibility with fewer side effects [72]. Cu^{2+} complexes have been reported to interact with DNA and are widely explored for imagining probes and diagnostic tools [73].

6.1 COPPER COMPLEXES

Nucleobases are fascinating molecules to scrutinize copper coordination for biological and material applications [16]. Copper clusters have been reported for multipurpose applications in modern science [74]. About a decade ago, Verma et al. designed and synthesized an adenine derivative, 9-(2-thiocyanatoethyl) adenine, and explored its interaction with Cu^+ to yield a rare hexagonal prismatic cuprous iodide cluster **16** (Figure 6a). It was found that the Cu_6I_6 clusters are formed by combination of two chair-shaped trinuclear Cu_3I_3 units where six Cu ions are bonded to six iodido ligands (Figure 6a) [75].

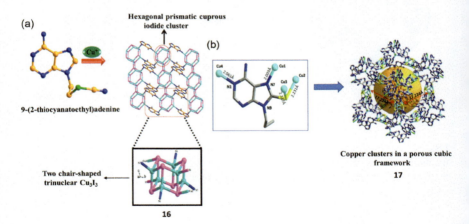

FIGURE 6 (a) Formation of hexagonal prism-shaped Cu_6I_6 unit arrangement. (Adapted by permission from Ref. [75]; Copyright 2011, American Chemical Society.) (b) Asymmetric unit of copper-8-mercaptoadenine derivative and Cu^+ cluster-based porous cubic framework. (Adapted by permission from Ref. [79]; Copyright 2014, Wiley-VCH Verlag GmbH & Co. KGaA, Weinheim.)

In an interesting example, Müller and co-workers reported Cu^+-mediated base pairing in a nucleic acid duplex. The metal coordination in the artificial nucleobase-containing DNA oligonucleotide was found to facilitate the stabilization of the duplex structure. This study also opens up new avenues for metal-mediated base pairing, as Cu is the only metal that can form such pairs in two different oxidation states [76].

In another approach, Shionoya and co-workers developed a Cu^{2+}-responsive DNAzyme based upon a Cu^{2+}-mediated artificial base pair (Im^C–Cu^{2+}–Im^C) (Im^C = carboxyimidazole) into an RNA-cleaving DNAzyme. The excellent and sharp switching ability of the DNAzyme was very selective for Cu^{2+} [77].

Another important aspect of life is the essence of water, and water harvesting is a current need of the hour. Copper-based metal-organic frameworks (MOFs) are important hybrid materials that have proved their utility in environmental applications [78]. Verma and co-workers synthesized an 8-mercaptoadenine derivative and studied its interaction with Cu^+. A discrete tetranuclear copper complex with distorted square planar geometry with C8S and N7 coordination was obtained. Notably, N1 did not participate in coordination in the tetranuclear complex, which was later exploited for additional coordination at elevated Cu^+ concentration to result in the formation of Cu-MOFs (**17**). The highly porous Cu-MOF was then subjected to gas adsorption and solvent adsorption (water and alcohols) studies (Figure 6b). The Cu-MOF has a cuboidal framework structure with 62% solvent accessible voids and shows a maximum 3.02 mmol g^{-1} CO_2 adsorption at a pressure of 1 atm. With respect to the solvent adsorption capacity, the Cu-MOF showed the following size-dependent adsorption order: water > methanol > ethanol > *n*-propanol > *n*-butanol > isopropanol [79].

Likewise, Wang et al. developed a Cu^{2+}-based MOF using an adenine and succinic acid scaffold [Cu_2(adenine)$_2$(SA)] for water harvesting applications. The synthesized MOF revealed high hydrolytic stability and moderate porosity with a Brunauer-Emmett-Teller (BET) surface area of 651 $m^2 g^{-1}$ and a pore volume of 0.34 $cm^3 g^{-1}$. This MOF showed high water-adsorption capacity and balanced working capacity at low humidity. The observed water adsorption was due to hydrogen bonding between the water molecules and uncoordinated N sites of adenine [80].

7 MERCURY-MEDIATED BASE PAIRING

It has been reported that Hg salts affect the stability of DNA and could lead to a denaturation of the duplex form. Contrary to this observation, Ono and co-workers found that Hg^{2+} can specifically support thymine-thymine mispairing to augment the stability of the DNA duplex. They established Hg^{2+} binding at the N3 position of thymidine, where it serves as a bridge to afford Hg^{2+}-mediated thymine–Hg^{2+}–thymine (T–Hg^{2+}–T) base pairs [81]. The crystal structure of DNA duplexes in the presence and absence of mercury ions revealed that T–Hg^{2+}–T pairing nominally distorts the B-DNA structure, while maintaining thermal stability similar to that of native base pairing in duplexes [82]. Due to its structural resemblance with native base pairing, T–Hg^{2+}–T could also mimic a T-A base pair, through T-T mismatch stabilization, during DNA primer extension [83]. The kinetic stability of the T–Hg^{2+}–T base pair inhibits DNA repair and completion of the DNA-lagging strand by inhibiting DNA polymerase activity. This could be a possible reason for the observed cytotoxic effects of Hg on nucleic acid metabolism [84]. Though the thermal stability of duplexes containing T–Hg^{2+}–T base pairing is high, Hg^{2+} was also found to support C-T mispairing, as the rate of Hg^{2+} association and dissociation was determined to be ten times faster for the C-T mispair [85].

Müller and co-workers used an artificial N^6-ethenoadenine derivative to prepare the first Hg^{2+}-mediated base pair where a dinuclear metal center involving a divalent metal ion was incorporated into a base pair (**18**) through an almost parallel alignment of the N–Hg bonds (Figure 7a). This binding arrangement was stabilized through thymine deprotonation to compensate charge accumulation due to the presence of two metal centers in close proximity [86].

Verma et al. showed an interesting example of a metal-mediated pair of a $N7,N9$-dibenzyl purine derivative, supported by Hg^{2+} interactions, through the generation of nearly linear (C8–Hg–C8′ bond angle = 170.62°) NHC species at C8 position as confirmed by density functional theory calculations. This complex (**19**) showed anticancer activity against A549 and MCF-7 cell lines (Figure 7b). This biological activity was attributed to the disruption of the microtubule network through non-covalent interactions at the tubulin binding site [38]. Further modeling studies suggested that such derivatives exhibit a propensity to bind close to the Asn117 residue of β-tubulin, which is a site proximal to the guanosine triphosphate/guanosine diphosphate (GTP/GDP)-binding pocket of β-tubulin.

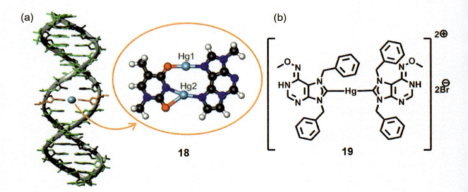

FIGURE 7 (a) Dinuclear mercury-mediated base pair of T–Hg^{2+}–εA derivative. (Reproduced by permission from Ref. [86]; Copyright 2016, Wiley-VCH Verlag GmbH & Co. KGaA, Weinheim.) (b) Chemical structure of a mercury carbene complex with a purine derivative.

Biological Implications of Metal-Nucleobase Complexes   147

8 ZINC

Zn^{2+} is ubiquitously present in the body and considered the second-most abundant metal in biological systems, where it plays a crucial role in enzyme catalysis and gene transcription. Primarily, almost all Zn^{2+} ions present in biosystems are bound to proteins and concentrations of labile Zn are low [87]. Zn homeostasis is believed to be critical for human health. Its disturbance may be the reason for severe neurological disorders like Alzheimer, Parkinson, sclerosis, impaired body growth, and infections [87,88]. From a chemical point of view, Zn^{2+} has a d^{10} configuration, is redox-inactive, Lewis-acidic, and diamagnetic in nature. It coordinates with N, O, and S donors in flexible coordination geometries. In proteins, it generally adopts a tetrahedral geometry, but occasionally also a trigonal bipyramidal one [89].

8.1 ZINC INTERACTION WITH PURINE DERIVATIVES

Due to the significant role of zinc in biosystems, numerous Zn complexes have been developed for pathophysiological diseases or molecular scaffolds that can sense or chelate Zn^{2+} ions [89]. One such example is an adenine derivative to sense extracellular Zn^{2+} ions in cytoplasm and nucleoli of the cell, reported by Verma and co-workers. The dipolar imine-methoxyphenol adenine Schiff base compound selectively chelates Zn^{2+} ions using the N3 position and forms a dimer structure (20) which enhances the green fluorescence of complex (Figure 8a). The sensing property of the ligand was demonstrated in the HeLa cancer cell line and further, the localization of the ligand was confirmed by a ribonuclease (RNase) digestion test [90].

Rosi and co-workers' pioneering work led to the development of many adenine-based bio-MOFs that were employed for drug delivery, sensing, and adsorption studies [91–93] (see also Chapter 1 in this book). MOFs are porous coordination polymers and considered to be non-biocompatible for cellular studies. However, bio-MOFs have shown great promise in recent years for biomedical applications [94]. Recently, Chand et al. synthesized the adenine-based Zn^{2+}-binding DNA-mimicking bio-MOFs KBM-1 and KBM-2 (Figure 8b), which showed good biocompatibility with accessible adenine faces in the framework for base pairing. Furthermore, they showed effective ssDNA loading via the virtue of adenine-thymine base pairing and are protected from enzymatic degradation. Their cytotoxicity profile showed high IC_{50} values of 190 and 155 µM for KBM-1 and KBM-2, respectively, in cancer cells. KBM-2 effectively gets localized in the cell nucleus and delivers ssDNA (fluorescently labeled) without causing any cytotoxicity [95]. Another interesting example is the formation of the first adenine- and Zn^{2+}-based nano-bio-MOF by Jiang et al. for *in vitro* and *in vivo* biological evaluation. The nano-bio-MOF has shown good biocompatibility with a high IC_{50} value of 599.3 µg mL^{-1}, which was far better than the other Zn-based MOFs (ZIF, IC_{50} = 100 µg mL^{-1}). At the lower dose, the nano-bio-MOF showed less toxicity, good cell adhesion, intact morphology, less reactive oxygen species (ROS) production, and mild renal toxicity [96].

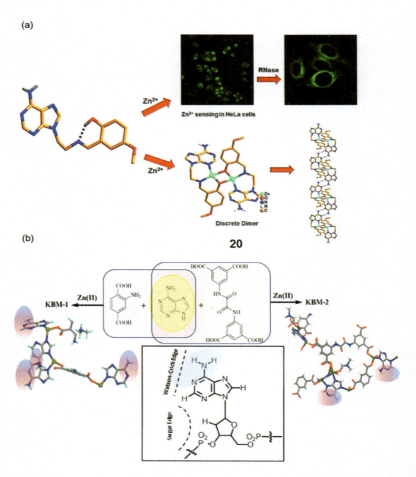

FIGURE 8 (a) N3 coordination complex of Zn^{2+} with a purine derivative and its sensing application in HeLa cells. (Reproduced by permission from Ref. [90]; Copyright 2017, Wiley-VCH Verlag GmbH & Co. KGaA, Weinheim.) (b) Formation of KBM-1 (asymmetric unit at left) and KBM-2 (asymmetric unit at right). Carbon-gray; hydrogen-cyan/white; oxygen-red; nitrogen-blue; zinc-dark yellow. Depiction of Watson-Crick and sugar edge present in a DNA. (Modified with permission from Ref. [95]; Copyright 2022, Chand et al.)

9 RUTHENIUM AND OSMIUM COMPLEXES

Efforts to explore and synthesize ruthenium complexes have been made in the biological and non-biological contexts. Renfrew and co-workers developed a Ru-purine-based photolabile system that delivers the anticancer agent 6-mercaptopurine in the presence of visible light (465 nm) by exploiting the labile Ru^{2+}–N7 purine bond. One of the complexes, **21**, showed DNA binding after release of the

Biological Implications of Metal-Nucleobase Complexes 149

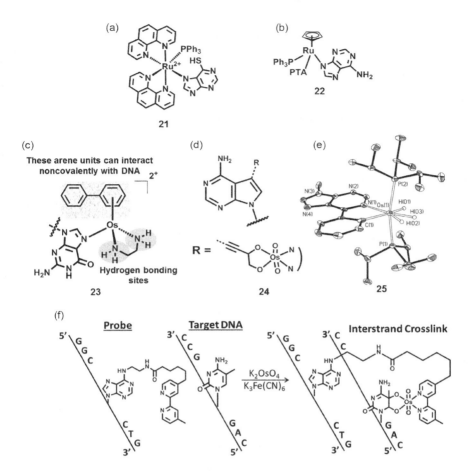

FIGURE 9 (a) Ru-purine complex 21 as photolabile delivery system. (b) N9 adenine-based Ru^{2+} complex 22. (c) N7 guanine binding in osmium complex 23 with anticipated H-bonding and arene-DNA interactions, in gray. (d) Chemical structure of the Os^{6+} DNA complex 24 containing a 7-deazaadenine derivative. (e) Crystal structure of Os complex 25 with 6-phenylpurine derivative. (Reproduced with permission from Ref. [103]; Copyright 2020, American Chemical Society.) (f) Depiction of inter-strand crosslinking of adenine derivative and 5mC via Os complexation. (Modified with permission from Ref. [105]; Copyright 2007, American Chemical Society.)

purine molecule (Figure 9a). Among the synthesized complexes, only complex 21 showed a significant toxicity difference under light and dark conditions [97]. Hajji et al. designed and synthesized purine-based Ru^{2+} complexes having PPh$_3$ and PTA derivatives as ligands. PPh$_3$ was selected for the necessary lipophilicity for effectively crossing the cell membrane and PTA for hydrophilicity. The crystal structure of the complex [RuCp(adeninate-N9)(PPh$_3$)(PTA)] (22) showed that the deprotonated adenine is coordinated through its N9 position to the metal center instead of N7 (Figure 9b). The complex (**22**) showed good stability and its antiproliferative potency was checked for cisplatin-sensitive T2 and SKOV3 human cancer cell lines. It showed an IC$_{50}$ value of ~2 µM for T2 cells, which was better than that of cisplatin. Against SKOV3 cells the complex also showed better activity than cisplatin. It was hypothesized that the activity was due to hydrogen bond formation between DNA bases and the adenine ligand of the complex, analogous to the situation with the free complex, which dimerizes via hydrogen bonds involving solvent molecules and non-coordinated nitrogen atoms [98]. Later the same group synthesized adenine-, guanine- and theophylline-based complexes of ruthenium. The guanine complex [RuCp(G-N9)(PPh$_3$)(mPTA)](CF$_3$SO$_3$) showed potent activity against T2 and SKOV3 cell lines. From all purine-based complexes made by this group, only this guanine-Ru complex showed potent activity against cisplatin-sensitive SKOV3 cells, with an IC$_{50}$ value of 2–10 µM [99].

Osmium has the ability to support the formation of interesting architectures and its versatile oxidation states could be helpful for regulating redox properties inside cells [100]. Brabec and co-workers developed half-sandwich Os^{2+} complexes with activity equipotent to that of cisplatin and carboplatin. The reported complexes showed binding with DNA via N7 position of guanine, through H-bonds and arene-DNA interaction that induces unwinding of DNA structure. Figure 9c illustrates N7 guanine coordination with potential sites for hydrogen bonding and arene-DNA interactions for one of the complexes (**23**) [101]. Hocek and Havran developed a simple protocol for enzymatic polymerase synthesis of cyclic vicinal diol-linked 2′-deoxyribonucleoside triphosphates (**24**) (Figure 9d) to prepare vicinal diol-linked DNA, which was eventually converted to Os-labeled DNA. Osmium specifically interacts with vicinal diols and affords site specificity for labeling purposes [102]. Osmium complexes promote metal-carbon bond formation via σ-bond activation as shown in the case of a 9-methyl-6-phenyl purine derivative (**25**), and this method could further be used to label the DNA (Figure 9e) [103]. 5-Methylcytosine (5mC) detection was selectively achieved by mismatch pairing with an adenine base, bearing a pendant bipyridyl ligand that formed inter-strand crosslinks in the presence of Os (Figure 9f). Mismatch causes oxidation of 5mC at the C5=C6 double bond, thereby allowing the formation of a cross-link for sequence-selective labeling and polymerase chain reaction (PCR) amplification. This methodology was used for the detection of DNA methylation [104, 105].

10 IRIDIUM COMPLEXES

Non-toxic Ir^{3+} complexes of adenine derivatives with amino acids as substituents at N6 (**26**) were reported, in which the metal was coordinated to N9 of the adenine residue, displaying a slightly distorted octahedral geometry (Figure 10a). The complexes showed low cellular uptake and possessed moderate DNA cleaving activity [106]. The endoplasmic reticulum (ER) plays an important role in calcium storage, protein formation, and transportation, and it is known that its viscosity changes under stress-like conditions. Liu et al. designed and

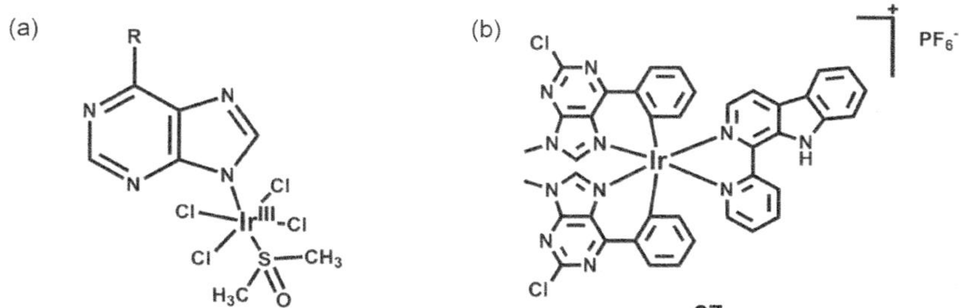

Biological Implications of Metal-Nucleobase Complexes 151

(a)

R = Amino acids (glycine, β-alanine and γ-butyric acid)

26

27

FIGURE 10 (a) Chemical structure of 6-amino acid purine-Ir^{3+} complex **26**. (b) Purine-based Ir^{3+} complex **27** for sensing endoplasmic reticulum (ER) viscosity.

synthesized purine-based Ir^{3+} complexes for sensing the viscosity of the ER [107]. The purine molecule is coordinated through N7 (Figure 10b). The formed Ir^{3+} complex (**27**) was able to accumulate selectively in ER. Tunicamycin, a glycosylation inhibitor, was employed to increase ER stress, resulting in enhanced ER viscosity, followed by a change in fluorescence intensity inside the cells [107]. Structural features of novel heteroleptic phosphorescent Ir^{3+} complexes, derived from 6-phenylpurine nucleosides and nucleotides, were also reported, possessing excellent photophysical properties in films as well as in solution, with good quantum yields [108].

11 QUARTET SELF-ASSEMBLY OF GUANINE DERIVATIVES BY METAL IONS

Guanosine has a unique ability to form a self-assembled structure by the arrangement of four guanine molecules through H-bonding. It is known that cations significantly contribute toward the stability of G-quartet structures and K$^+$ ions have been known to afford the most stable G-quadruplexes, followed by Rb$^+$, Na$^+$, Cs$^+$, and Li$^+$ [109,110]. The ability of a guanine quartet to self-assemble in the presence of metal ions has been exploited in hydrogel formation. Hydrogels are networks that preserve their structure through chemical or physical cross-linking of individual polymer chains, and are able to trap copious volumes of water within the confines of the network. Hydrogels can respond to physical and chemical stimuli to exhibit gel-sol phase or volume phase transitions, thus making them useful for many applications. Nucleobase-containing hydrogels are also expected to possess similar properties (see also Chapter 4 in this book). For example, G$_4$ hydrogels have been investigated and employed for numerous applications in the biomaterial domain [111,112]. Venkatesh et al. conjugated a photoactive dopamine-Pt^{4+} anticancer drug conjugate [platinum-dopamine (Pt-DA)] with the G_4K^+ borate to give the Pt-G_4K^+ borate hydrogel. It showed excellent antiproliferative potency under dark conditions, but under blue light irradiation the hydrogel-drug conjugate displayed superior activity. These results confirmed the beneficial role of the G_4K^+ hydrogel in enhancing the cytotoxic effect of Pt-DA, upon conjugation [113]. Feng et al. studied the crystallization process of a 2′-deoxy-2′-fluoroguanosine hydrogel mediated by K^+ ions, resulting in an unstable hydrogel. Subsequently, addition of Ag^+ ions into the hydrogel resulted in high stability (>6 months) and a silver-mediated base-pairing motif was suggested for stable gel formation. The gel showed excellent antibacterial activity against *Fusobacterium nucleatum*, a gram-negative bacterium, with minimum bactericidal concentration (MBC) = 31.25 μg mL^{-1} [114]. Rowan and co-workers developed a guanosine derivative, 8-methoxy-2′,3′,5′-tri-*O*-acetylguanosine, which formed a gel in the presence of K^+ ions through a continuous helical assembly. This guanosine derivative turned out to be a versatile hydrogelator that can form a gel at physiological salt concentrations and even in cell media, without causing any cytotoxicity [115]. Another study by Rotaru et al. showed the use of two metal ions in G_4 hydrogels for cell adhesion and proliferation of human dermal fibroblast cells. K^+ ions were used to induce gel formation and use of 1,4-diboronic acid added further stability to the hydrogels [116].

12 CONCLUSIONS

Nucleobases are known as versatile templates for metal ion coordination leading to interesting three-dimensional (3D) architectures, for their excellent chemical tunability and application-oriented focus, and for interesting biological and material questions. Their metal-coordinating ability has been translated to the fundamentals of essential therapeutic outcomes, such as Pt-based anticancer drugs. Suitably predisposed nitrogen atoms in nucleobases allow for metal interactions which could be directed with the help of pK_a modulation and by substituents. Although purine N7-coordination in the major groove is preferred, minor groove N3-coordination could also be invoked in new design paradigms for crafting interesting architectures and for the development of various DNA targeting agents [117, 118]. Innumerable nucleobase scaffolds have been described to arrive at novel metal complexes for therapeutic discovery, imaging toolbox, and molecular level understanding of biological pathways. Many metal ions have supported purine coordination networks consisting of complex geometries for specific functions and there is renewed interest to apply metal-nucleobase complexes for emerging applications as dry batteries and supercapacitors [119–121]. Finally, the ability to engender and explore non-covalent interactions has enabled the use of nucleobase-containing systems in creating adaptive functional materials [122], such as porous materials, materials with adhesive or self-healing ability [123], and charge transport, to name a few.

ACKNOWLEDGMENTS

S.V. would like to thank the J. C. Bose Fellowship (SERB, India) for financial support. S.J. thanks MHRD, India. A.J. thanks CSIR, India for senior research fellowships.

ABBREVIATIONS AND DEFINITIONS

εA	1,N^6-ethenoadenine
3D	three-dimensional
5mC	5-methylcytosine
6mA	6-methyladenine
^{7C}A	7-deazaadenine
A	adenine
Asn	asparagine
AuNCs	gold nanoclusters
AuNPs	gold nanoparticles
BET	Brunauer-Emmett-Teller
C	cytosine
Casp3	caspase-3
Cp	cyclopentadienyl ligand
DCM	dichloromethane
DFT	density functional theory
DNA	deoxyribonucleic acid
E. coli	*Escherichia coli*
ER	endoplasmic reticulum
FAD	flavin adenine dinucleotide
FDA	Food and Drug Administration
G	guanine
G_4	guanine quadruplex
GDP	guanosine diphosphate
GTP	guanosine triphosphate
IC_{50}	half-maximal inhibitory concentration
Im^C	carboxyimidazole
MBC	minimum bactericidal concentration
MIC	minimum inhibitory concentration
MOF	metal-organic framework
NHC	N-heterocyclic carbene
PAN	polyacrylonitrile
PCL	polycaprolactam
PCR	polymerase chain reaction
PEG	polyethylene glycol
PPh$_3$	triphenylphosphine

PTA	N-methyl-1,3,5-triaza-7-phosphaadamantane
Pt-DA	platinum-dopamine
RNA	ribonucleic acid
RNase	ribonuclease
ROS	reactive oxygen species
SA	succinic acid
S. aureus	Staphylococcus aureus
SERS	surface-enhanced Raman spectroscopy
ssDNA	single-stranded DNA
T	thymine
TrxR	thioredoxin reductase

REFERENCES

1. K. F. Jensen, G. Dandanell, B. Hove-Jensen, M. Willemos, V. Stewart, *EcoSal Plus* **2008**, *3*, 1–68.
2. J.-F. Lutz, *ACS Macro Lett.* **2020**, *9*, 185–189.
3. F. Pu, J. Ren, X. Qu, *Chem. Soc. Rev.* **2018**, *47*, 1285–1306.
4. R. K. Saravanan, I. Avasthi, R. K. Prajapati, S. Verma, *RSC Adv.* **2018**, *8*, 24541–24560.
5. B. Mohapatra, Pratibha, S. Verma, *Chem. Commun.* **2017**, *53*, 4748–4758.
6. J. Müller, *Metallomics* **2010**, *2*, 318–327.
7. E. Freisinger, R. K. O. Sigel, *Coord. Chem. Rev.* **2007**, *251*, 1834–1851.
8. B. Rosenberg, L. VanCamp, J. E. Trosko, V. H. Mansour, *Nature* **1969**, *222*, 385–386.
9. D. Wang, S. J. Lippard, *Nat. Rev. Drug Discov.* **2005**, *4*, 307–320.
10. H. Zorbas, B. K. Keppler, *ChemBioChem* **2005**, *6*, 1157–1166.
11. L. Zhou, J. Ren, X. Qu, *Mater. Today* **2017**, *20*, 179–190.
12. T. Lee, A. K. Yagati, F. Pi, A. Sharma, J.-W. Choi, P. Guo, *ACS Nano* **2015**, *9*, 6675–6682.
13. J. Li, L. Mo, C.-H. Lu, T. Fu, H.-H. Yang, W. Tan, *Chem. Soc. Rev.* **2016**, *45*, 1410–1431.
14. J. Li, A. A. Green, H. Yan, C. Fan, *Nat. Chem.* **2017**, *9*, 1056–1067.
15. J. Zhang, Y. Lu, *Angew. Chem. Int. Ed.* **2018**, *57*, 9702–9706.
16. S. Verma, A. K. Mishra, J. Kumar, *Acc. Chem. Res.* **2010**, *43*, 79–91.
17. M. H. Shamsi, H.-B. Kraatz, *J. Inorg. Organomet. Polym. Mater.* **2013**, *23*, 4–23.
18. D. O. M. Bonsu, D. Higgins, J. J. Austin, *Sci. Justice* **2020**, *60*, 206–215.
19. V. Singh, B. I. Fedeles, J. M. Essigmann, *RNA* **2015**, *21*, 1–13.
20. T. Mihály, M. Garijo Añorbe, F. M. Albertí, P. J. Sanz Miguel, B. Lippert, *Inorg. Chem.* **2012**, *51*, 10437–10446.
21. B. Lippert, *Chem. Biodivers.* **2008**, *5*, 1455–1474.
22. B. Lippert, *Coord. Chem. Rev.* **2000**, *200–202*, 487–516.
23. R. Silaghi-Dumitrescu, B. Mihály, T. Mihály, A. A. A. Attia, P. J. Sanz Miguel, B. Lippert, *J. Biol. Inorg. Chem.* **2017**, *22*, 567–579.
24. B. Song, J. Zhao, R. Griesser, C. Meiser, H. Sigel, B. Lippert, *Chem. Eur. J.* **1999**, *5*, 2374–2387.
25. J. Šponer, J. V. Burda, M. Sabat, J. Leszczynski, P. Hobza, *J. Phys. Chem. A* **1998**, *102*, 5951–5957.
26. L. E. Kapinos, B. P. Operschall, E. Larsen, H. Sigel, *Chem. Eur. J.* **2011**, *17*, 8156–8164.

27. C. Meiser, B. Song, E. Freisinger, M. Peilert, H. Sigel, B. Lippert, *Chem. Eur. J.* **1997**, *3*, 388–398.
28. B. Lippert, in *Nucleic Acid Metal Ion Interactions*, Ed. N.V. Hud, RSC, Cambridge, **2009**, pp. 39–74.
29. B. Müller, W.-Z. Shen, P. J. Sanz Miguel, F. M. Albertí, T. van der Wijst, M. Noguera, L. Rodríguez-Santiago, M. Sodupe, B. Lippert, *Chem. Eur. J.* **2011**, *17*, 9970–9983.
30. S. Zhu, A. Matilla, J. M. Tercero, V. Vijayaragavan, J. A. Walmsley, *Inorg. Chim. Acta* **2004**, *357*, 411–420.
31. P. Brandi-Blanco, P. J. Sanz Miguel, B. Müller, E. Gil Bardají, M. Willermann, B. Lippert, *Inorg. Chem.* **2009**, *48*, 5208–5215.
32. M. Morell Cerdà, D. Amantia, B. Costisella, A. Houlton, B. Lippert, *Dalton Trans.* **2006**, 3894–3899.
33. C. Price, M. A. Shipman, N. H. Rees, M. R. J. Elsegood, A. J. Edwards, W. Clegg, A. Houlton, *Chem. Eur. J.* **2001**, *7*, 1194–1201.
34. X. Li, A. Sánchez-Ferrer, M. Bagnani, J. Adamcik, P. Azzari, J. Hao, A. Song, H. Liu, R. Mezzenga, *Proc. Natl. Acad. Sci.USA* **2020**, *117*, 9832–9839.
35. S. K. Kolev, P. St. Petkov, T. I. Milenov, G. N. Vayssilov, *ACS Omega* **2022**, *7*, 23234–23244.
36. D. Cozak, A. Mardhy, M. J. Olivier, A. L. Beauchamp, *Inorg. Chem.* **1986**, *25*, 2600–2606.
37. R. K. O. Sigel, H. Sigel, *Acc. Chem. Res.* **2010**, *43*, 974–984.
38. S. Khanna, B. Jana, A. Saha, P. Kurkute, S. Ghosh, S. Verma, *Dalton Trans.* **2014**, *43*, 9838–9842.
39. C. Dumontet, M. A. Jordan, *Nat. Rev. Drug Discov.* **2010**, *9*, 790–803.
40. V. Venkatesh, M. D. B. Kumaran, R. K. Saravanan, P. T. Kalaichelvan, S. Verma, *ChemPlusChem* **2016**, *81*, 1266–1271.
41. Pratibha, M. Shukla, G. Kaul, S. Chopra, S. Verma, *ChemistrySelect* **2019**, *4*, 1834–1839.
42. Y. Takezawa, A. Suzuki, M. Nakaya, K. Nishiyama, M. Shionoya, *J. Am. Chem. Soc.* **2020**, *142*, 21640–21644.
43. S. Mandal, C. Wang, R. K. Prajapati, J. Kösters, S. Verma, L. Chi, J. Müller, *Inorg. Chem.* **2016**, *55*, 7041–7050.
44. A. W. Feldman, F. E. Romesberg, *Acc. Chem. Res.* **2018**, *51*, 394–403.
45. T. Funai, Y. Miyazaki, M. Aotani, E. Yamaguchi, O. Nakagawa, S.-i. Wada, H. Torigoe, A. Ono, H. Urata, *Angew. Chem. Int. Ed.* **2012**, *51*, 6464–6466.
46. S. Johannsen, N. Megger, D. Böhme, R. K. O. Sigel, J. Müller, *Nat. Chem.* **2010**, *2*, 229–234.
47. N. Santamaría-Díaz, J. M. Méndez-Arriaga, J. M. Salas, M. A. Galindo, *Angew. Chem. Int. Ed.* **2016**, *55*, 6170–6174.
48. J. M. Méndez-Arriaga, C. R. Maldonado, J. A. Dobado, M. A. Galindo, *Chem. Eur. J.* **2018**, *24*, 4583–4589.
49. T. Hong, Y. Yuan, T. Wang, J. Ma, Q. Yao, X. Hua, Y. Xia, X. Zhou, *Chem. Sci.* **2017**, *8*, 200–205.
50. A. Khoury, K. M. Deo, J. R. Aldrich-Wright, *J. Inorg. Biochem.* **2020**, *207*, 111070.
51. L. Kelland, *Nat. Rev. Cancer* **2007**, *7*, 573–584.
52. L. Cai, C. Yu, L. Ba, Q. Liu, Y. Qian, B. Yang, C. Gao, *Appl. Organomet. Chem.* **2018**, *32*, e4228.
53. A. M. J. Fichtinger-Schepman, J. L. Van der Veer, J. H. J. Den Hartog, P. H. M. Lohman, J. Reedijk, *Biochemistry* **1985**, *24*, 707–713.
54. P. Štarha, Z. Trávníček, I. Popa, *J. Inorg. Biochem.* **2010**, *104*, 639–647.

55. J. Vančo, P. Štarha, J. Hošek, M. Chalupová, P. Suchý, Z. Trávníček, *J. Biol. Inorg. Chem.* **2020**, *25*, 67–73.
56. A. G. Weidmann, J. K. Barton, *Inorg. Chem.* **2015**, *54*, 9626–9636.
57. M. Skander, P. Retailleau, B. Bourrié, L. Schio, P. Mailliet, A. Marinetti, *J. Med. Chem.* **2010**, *53*, 2146–2154.
58. J.-J. Zhang, C.-M. Che, I. Ott, *J. Organomet. Chem.* **2015**, *782*, 37–41.
59. K. S. Park, H. G. Park, *Curr. Opin. Biotechnol.* **2014**, *28*, 17–24.
60. Y. Tao, M. Li, J. Ren, X. Qu, *Chem. Soc. Rev.* **2015**, *44*, 8636–8663.
61. Y. Yu, B. Y. L. Mok, X. J. Loh, Y. N. Tan, *Adv. Healthcare Mater.* **2016**, *5*, 1844–1859.
62. R. Jin, C. Zeng, M. Zhou, Y. Chen, *Chem. Rev.* **2016**, *116*, 10346–10413.
63. V. Venkatesh, A. Shukla, S. Sivakumar, S. Verma, *ACS Appl. Mater. Interfaces* **2014**, *6*, 2185–2191.
64. Y. Liu, M. Pharr, G. A. Salvatore, *ACS Nano* **2017**, *11*, 9614–9635.
65. K. K. Fu, J. Cheng, T. Li, L. Hu, *ACS Energy Lett.* **2016**, *1*, 1065–1079.
66. E. Singh, M. Meyyappan, H. S. Nalwa, *ACS Appl. Mater. Interfaces* **2017**, *9*, 34544–34586.
67. D. Vilela, A. Romeo, S. Sánchez, *Lab Chip* **2016**, *16*, 402–408.
68. M. Magliulo, M. Y. Mulla, M. Singh, E. Macchia, A. Tiwari, L. Torsi, K. Manoli, *J. Mater. Chem. C* **2015**, *3*, 12347–12363.
69. J. Xue, T. Wu, Y. Dai, Y. Xia, *Chem. Rev.* **2019**, *119*, 5298–5415.
70. R. K. Saravanan, T. K. Naqvi, S. Patil, P. K. Dwivedi, S. Verma, *Chem. Commun.* **2020**, *56*, 5795–5798.
71. R. Giampietro, F. Spinelli, M. Contino, N. A. Colabufo, *Mol. Pharm.* **2018**, *15*, 808–820.
72. S. Zehra, S. Tabassum, F. Arjmand, *Drug Discov. Today* **2021**, *26*, 1086–1096.
73. N. Shahabadi, M. Falsafi, N. H. Moghadam, *J. Photochem. Photobiol. B, Biol.* **2013**, *122*, 45–51.
74. D. Su, L. Gao, F. Gao, X. Zhang, X. Gao, *Chem. Sci.* **2020**, *11*, 5614–5629.
75. R. K. Prajapati, S. Verma, *Inorg. Chem.* **2011**, *50*, 3180–3182.
76. B. Jash, J. Müller, *Angew. Chem. Int. Ed.* **2018**, *57*, 9524–9527.
77. Y. Takezawa, L. Hu, T. Nakama, M. Shionoya, *Angew. Chem. Int. Ed.* **2020**, *59*, 21488–21492.
78. A. Sultana, R. A. Omar, N. Talreja, D. Chauhan, R. V. Mangalaraja, M. Ashfaq, in *Copper Nanostructures: Next-Generation of Agrochemicals for Sustainable Agroecosystems*, Ed. K. A. Abd-Elsalam, Elsevier, **2022**, pp. 701–717.
79. V. Venkatesh, P. Pachfule, R. Banerjee, S. Verma, *Chem. Eur. J.* **2014**, *20*, 12262–12268.
80. L. Wang, K. Wang, H.-T. An, H. Huang, L.-H. Xie, J.-R. Li, *ACS Appl. Mater. Interfaces* **2021**, *13*, 49509–49518.
81. Y. Miyake, H. Togashi, M. Tashiro, H. Yamaguchi, S. Oda, M. Kudo, Y. Tanaka, Y. Kondo, R. Sawa, T. Fujimoto, T. Machinami, A. Ono, *J. Am. Chem. Soc.* **2006**, *128*, 2172–2173.
82. J. Kondo, T. Yamada, C. Hirose, I. Okamoto, Y. Tanaka, A. Ono, *Angew. Chem. Int. Ed.* **2014**, *53*, 2385–2388.
83. K. S. Park, C. Jung, H. G. Park, *Angew. Chem. Int. Ed.* **2010**, *49*, 9757–9760.
84. O. P. Schmidt, G. Mata, N. W. Luedtke, *J. Am. Chem. Soc.* **2016**, *138*, 14733–14739.
85. O. P. Schmidt, A. S. Benz, G. Mata, N. W. Luedtke, *Nucleic Acids Res.* **2018**, *46*, 6470–6479.
86. S. Mandal, M. Hebenbrock, J. Müller, *Angew. Chem. Int. Ed.* **2016**, *55*, 15520–15523.

87. H.-J. Kim, in *Comprehensive Supramolecular Chemistry II*, Ed. J.L. Atwood, Elsevier, Oxford, **2017**, pp. 107–127.
88. N. Roohani, R. Hurrell, R. Kelishadi, R. Schulin, *J. Res. Med. Sci.* **2013**, *18*, 144.
89. M. Porchia, M. Pellei, F. Del Bello, C. Santini, *Molecules* **2020**, *25*, 5814.
90. Pratibha, S. Singh, S. Sivakumar, S. Verma, *Eur. J. Inorg. Chem.* **2017**, *2017*, 4202–4209.
91. J. An, O. K. Farha, J. T. Hupp, E. Pohl, J. I. Yeh, N. L. Rosi, *Nat. Commun.* **2012**, *3*, 604.
92. J. An, C. M. Shade, D. A. Chengelis-Czegan, S. Petoud, N. L. Rosi, *J. Am. Chem. Soc.* **2011**, *133*, 1220–1223.
93. T. Li, J. E. Sullivan, N. L. Rosi, *J. Am. Chem. Soc.* **2013**, *135*, 9984–9987.
94. H.-S. Wang, Y.-H. Wang, Y. Ding, *Nanoscale Adv.* **2020**, *2*, 3788–3797.
95. S. Chand, O. Alahmed, W. S. Baslyman, A. Dey, S. Qutub, R. Saha, Y. Hijikata, M. Alaamery, N. M. Khashab, *JACS Au* **2022**, *2*, 623–630.
96. S. Jiang, J. Wang, Z. Zhu, S. Shan, Y. Mao, X. Zhang, X. Pei, C. Huang, Q. Wan, *Microporous Mesoporous Mater.* **2022**, *334*, 111773.
97. H. Chan, J. B. Ghrayche, J. Wei, A. K. Renfrew, *Eur. J. Inorg. Chem.* **2017**, *2017*, 1679–1686.
98. L. Hajji, C. Saraiba-Bello, G. Segovia-Torrente, F. Scalambra, A. Romerosa, *Eur. J. Inorg. Chem.* **2019**, *2019*, 4078–4086.
99. L. Hajji, C. Saraiba-Bello, F. Scalambra, G. Segovia-Torrente, A. Romerosa, *J. Inorg. Biochem.* **2021**, *218*, 111404.
100. P. Zhang, H. Huang, *Dalton Trans.* **2018**, *47*, 14841–14854.
101. H. Kostrhunova, J. Florian, O. Novakova, A. F. A. Peacock, P. J. Sadler, V. Brabec, *J. Med. Chem.* **2008**, *51*, 3635–3643.
102. P. Havranová-Vidláková, M. Krömer, V. Sýkorová, M. Trefulka, M. Fojta, L. Havran, M. Hocek, *ChemBioChem* **2020**, *21*, 171–180.
103. M. Valencia, A. D. Merinero, C. Lorenzo-Aparicio, M. Gómez-Gallego, M. A. Sierra, B. Eguillor, M. A. Esteruelas, M. Oliván, E. Oñate, *Organometallics* **2020**, *39*, 312–323.
104. A. Okamoto, *ChemMedChem* **2014**, *9*, 1958–1965.
105. K. Tanaka, K. Tainaka, T. Umemoto, A. Nomura, A. Okamoto, *J. Am. Chem. Soc.* **2007**, *129*, 14511–14517.
106. A. García-Raso, A. Terrón, J. Ortega-Castro, M. Barceló-Oliver, J. Lorenzo, S. Rodríguez-Calado, A. Franconetti, A. Frontera, E. M. Vázquez-López, J. J. Fiol, *J. Inorg. Biochem.* **2020**, *205*, 111000.
107. X. Liu, K. Li, L. Shi, H. Zhang, Y.-H. Liu, H.-Y. Wang, N. Wang, X.-Q. Yu, *Chem. Commun.* **2021**, *57*, 2265–2268.
108. C. Lorenzo-Aparicio, M. Gómez Gallego, C. Ramírez de Arellano, M. A. Sierra, *Dalton Trans.* **2022**, *51*, 5138–5150.
109. T. M. Bryan, P. Baumann, *Mol. Biotechnol.* **2011**, *49*, 198–208.
110. L. Stefan, D. Monchaud, *Nat. Rev. Chem.* **2019**, *3*, 650–668.
111. G. M. Peters, J. T. Davis, *Chem. Soc. Rev.* **2016**, *45*, 3188–3206.
112. Y. Zhang, L. Zhu, J. Tian, L. Zhu, X. Ma, X. He, K. Huang, F. Ren, W. Xu, *Adv. Sci.* **2021**, *8*, 2100216.
113. V. Venkatesh, N. K. Mishra, I. Romero-Canelón, R. R. Vernooij, H. Shi, J. P. C. Coverdale, A. Habtemariam, S. Verma, P. J. Sadler, *J. Am. Chem. Soc.* **2017**, *139*, 5656–5659.
114. H. Feng, Y. Du, F. Tang, N. Ji, X. Zhao, H. Zhao, Q. Chen, *RSC Adv.* **2018**, *8*, 15842–15852.

115. L. E. Buerkle, H. A. von Recum, S. J. Rowan, *Chem. Sci.* **2012**, *3*, 564–572.
116. A. Rotaru, G. Pricope, T. N. Plank, L. Clima, E. L. Ursu, M. Pinteala, J. T. Davis, M. Barboiu, *Chem. Commun.* **2017**, *53*, 12668–12671.
117. M. A. Galindo, D. Amantia, A. Martinez Martinez, W. Clegg, R. W. Harrington, V. Moreno Martinez, A. Houlton, *Inorg. Chem.* **2009**, *48*, 10295–10303.
118. R. Oun, Y. E. Moussa, N. J. Wheate, *Dalton Trans.* **2018**, *47*, 6645–6653.
119. D. Dutta, N. Nagapradeep, H. Zhu, M. Forsyth, S. Verma, A. J. Bhattacharyya, *Sci. Rep.* **2016**, *6*, 24499.
120. I. Avasthi, M. M. Kulkarni, S. Verma, *Chem. Eur. J.* **2019**, *25*, 6988–6995.
121. I. Avasthi, Gaganjot, M. Katiyar, S. Verma, *Chem. Eur. J.* **2020**, *26*, 16706–16711.
122. A. del Prado, D. González-Rodríguez, Y.-L. Wu, *ChemistryOpen* **2020**, *9*, 409–430.
123. S. Joshi, G. Mahadevan, S. Verma, S. Valiyaveettil, *Chem. Commun.* **2020**, *56*, 11303–11306.

7 Stimuli-Responsive DNA-Binding Metal Complexes

Tim Kench and Ramon Vilar
Department of Chemistry, Imperial College London, White City Campus, 82 Wood Lane, London W12 0BZ, United Kingdom
t.kench17@imperial.ac.uk, r.vilar@imperial.ac.uk

CONTENTS

1 Introduction 160
2 Endogenous Stimuli 161
    2.1 Redox Responsive Metal Complexes 161
        2.1.1 Platinum(IV) Complexes 161
        2.1.2 Non-platinum Complexes 164
    2.2 pH Responsive 166
    2.3 Enzyme Responsive 167
3 Exogenous Stimuli 168
    3.1 Photoactivation 168
    3.2 Activation Modulated by Metal Ions 172
        3.2.1 Metal-Mediated Peptide Organization 172
        3.2.2 Deactivation of DNA Binders by Metal Ions 175
    3.3 Metal-Catalyzed Activation 177
4 General Conclusions 183
Acknowledgments 183
Abbreviations 183
References 185

ABSTRACT

DNA is a recognized target for several anticancer and antibacterial drugs among others. Since the clinical approval of cisplatin and its analogs as anticancer agents, DNA-binding metal complexes have received a great deal of attention. In addition to their pharmacological properties, the interaction of metal complexes with DNA has also been of interest in sensing and imaging. In spite of the great advances in this area, there is still a need to develop systems where the DNA-binding properties of metal complexes can be controlled by specific stimuli. This could lead to metallopharmaceuticals that are more effective, with improved bioavailability

DOI: 10.1201/9781003270201-7

and decreased unwanted toxicity. The focus of this review is to explore different approaches that have been used to regulate the activity of metal-based DNA binders. The review is divided into two main sections: the first one covers endogenous stimuli (i.e., triggers that occur *in vivo* such as redox and pH changes as well as enzyme activity), while the second one focuses on the use of external stimuli (e.g., light irradiation or addition of a metal catalyst) to regulate the DNA-binding properties of metal complexes.

KEYWORDS

Metal Complexes; Medicinal Inorganic Chemistry; DNA; Prodrugs; Hypoxia; Photoactivation; pH Trigger; Metal Regulated

1 INTRODUCTION

Since the discovery over 50 years ago of the anticancer properties of cisplatin and its analogs, there has been enormous development in medicinal inorganic chemistry. Considering that DNA is recognized to be the main biomolecular target of these platinum-based drugs, thousands of metal complexes have been developed as DNA binders and their cellular and *in vivo* properties studied. In spite of the great progress seen in this area, metal-based drug candidates often have shortcomings, such as poor bioavailability, unwanted toxicity, poor selectivity, and off-target effects. Therefore, several strategies have been studied to improve the efficacy and biocompatibility of metallopharmaceuticals. One of these strategies is to design metal complexes that are only activated, or in some cases deactivated, by a given stimulus [1, 2].

This review covers stimuli-responsive DNA binders based on metal complexes and has been divided into two broad sections based on whether the stimuli that trigger the response of the metal complexes are endogenous (i.e., enzymes, pH, and redox environment) or exogenous (i.e., modulation by light irradiation and addition of metal ions as catalysts or structural regulators). A schematic overview of the different approaches discussed in this review is shown in Figure 1.

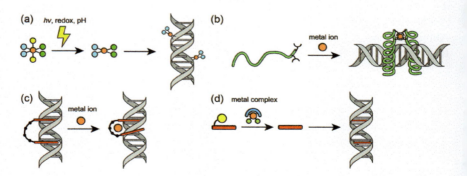

FIGURE 1 Schematic representation of the different strategies discussed in this review to modulate the activity of metal complexes.

2 ENDOGENOUS STIMULI

This section will cover examples where the DNA-binding properties of metal complexes are regulated by conditions found endogenously in living organisms (e.g., redox and pH) or by the activity of enzymes. These changes are often associated with diseased cells/tissues and therefore have attracted significant interest to activate the activity of a prodrug only where it is needed.

2.1 Redox Responsive Metal Complexes

Due to the variable oxidation state of transition metals, they are particularly well suited for the development of prodrugs that are activated by changes in the redox properties of the environment. It is well established that regions of low oxygen (hypoxia) are a common feature of solid tumors which arise from the limited and aberrant angiogenesis during tumor growth. Oxygen deprivation in tumors increases their invasiveness, metastasis, genomic instability, and the suppression of apoptotic signaling. In addition, hypoxic tumors are resistant to standard therapies. Therefore, there has been great interest in developing prodrugs that get activated under reducing conditions.

2.1.1 Platinum(IV) Complexes

Platinum(II) complexes such as cisplatin, carboplatin, and oxaliplatin are the most successful metallodrugs used in the clinic for the treatment of various cancers. While the mode of action of these platinum-based compounds is significantly more complex than initially thought, it is well established that one of their key biological targets is DNA with which they mainly form 1,2-intrastrand d(GpG) links. Platination leads to structural changes in DNA affecting the way it is processed which in turn dictates the biological and pharmacological effects of these metallodrugs. However, platinum(II) complexes have shortcomings such as a broad range of side effects, low bioavailability, intravenous administration (rather than oral), and acquired resistance. Several strategies have been investigated to address these limitations and deliver better and more efficient platinum-based anticancer agents [3]. One of these strategies is based on substitutionally inert platinum(IV) complexes that are only activated under reducing conditions found in the hypoxic tumor environment. In this approach, the octahedral platinum(IV) prodrug undergoes a two-electron reduction releasing two axial ligands and the corresponding square planar platinum(II) species that can then bind to DNA (and other biomolecules) displaying their pharmacological effects. Several comprehensive and critical reviews in this area have been previously published by Gibson [4], Zhu [5], Sadler [6], and Osella [7], among others. Therefore, in this section, we will only present a brief overview of the area and show selected examples.

The nature of the axial ligands that are released from the platinum(IV) prodrugs upon reduction plays an important role in defining the biological properties of the system (Figure 2a). They are key in defining the redox potential of

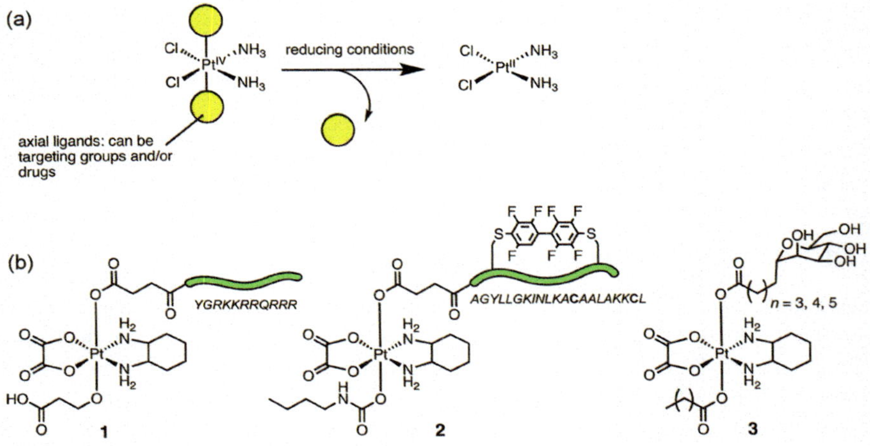

FIGURE 2 (a) Schematic representation of the activation of platinum(IV) prodrugs upon reduction to the corresponding platinum(II) complex and the release of two axial ligands. (b) Selected examples of platinum(IV) prodrugs containing ligands used for targeting.

the platinum(IV) center and therefore its stability *in vivo* (both in normoxic and hypoxic conditions). Pioneering work by Hambley showed that the reduction of Pt^{IV} to Pt^{II} depends mainly on the nature of the axial ligand and follows the order Cl$^-$ > CH$_3$COO$^-$ > OH$^-$ [8]. These mechanistic studies have indicated that linking axial ligands via a carboxylate group seems to provide the best balance between *in vivo* stability and ease of reduction under hypoxic conditions. Consequently, a significant proportion of axial ligands in platinum(IV) prodrugs are bound to the metal center via carboxylates. The axial ligands on the platinum(IV) prodrug can also be used to target tumor tissues by either adding groups that recognize overexpressed receptors in cancer cells or by increasing cellular uptake of the prodrug (Figure 2b). Several compounds including peptides in the axial position of the prodrug have been developed. For example, Keppler reported a platinum(IV) analog (**1**) of oxaliplatin containing the cell-penetrating TAT-peptide fragment (YGRKKRRQRRR) to be more cytotoxic against cancer cells than the parent platinum(II) complex [9]. More recently, Lippard and Pentelute reported a platinum(IV) prodrug (**2**) containing a perfluoroaryl macrocyclic peptide. This compound showed efficacy against glioma stem-like cells, as well as improved serum stability and brain uptake *in vivo* [10]. There are also examples where carbohydrates have been coordinated to the axial positions of the platinum(IV) complex (**3**, [11]).

Another important feature of platinum(IV) prodrugs is that they can be designed to contain axial ligands which are themselves active drugs (Figure 3). Ideally, the released drugs and the reduced platinum(II) species should act synergistically to improve the efficacy and selectivity of the prodrug. Early examples of this multi-action prodrugs approach include ethacraplatin [12] (**4** – with

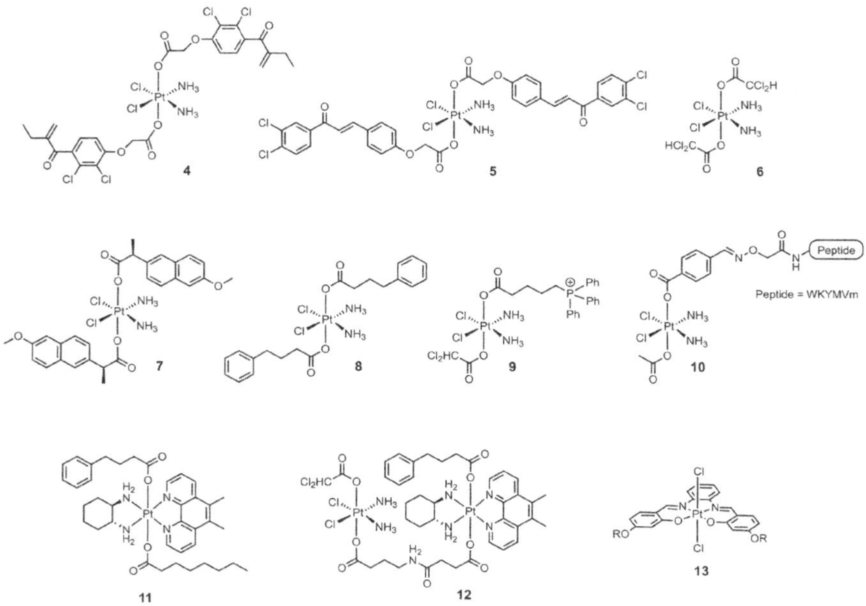

Stimuli-Responsive DNA-Binding Metal Complexes 163

FIGURE 3 Selected examples of platinum(IV) prodrugs containing as axial ligands another drug (**4–12**). Example of a non-active platinum(IV) complex (**13**) that upon reduction releases the corresponding platinum(II) complex which displays a high binding affinity for G-quadruplex DNA.

glutathione-S-transferase inhibitors in the axial positions), chalcoplatin [13] (**5** – with p53 inhibitors in the axial position), and mitaplatin [14] (**6** – containing dichloroacetate axial ligands which is known to reverse the Warburg effect in cancer cells by inhibiting pyruvate dehydrogenase kinase). Several other platinum(IV) prodrugs have been reported containing inhibitors for different enzymes such as cyclooxygenase [15] (**7**) and histone deacetylase [16] (**8**). Other recent studies have focused on targeting mitochondrial DNA [17]. In one study, platinum(IV) complex **9** was encapsulated inside liposomes to deliver it to cancer cells where a proportion of the complex is directed to mitochondria via the phosphonium ligand. Upon intracellular reduction, the prodrug releases two active components: cisplatin (which was found to target mitochondrial DNA) and dichloroacetate, the latter restoring normal mitochondrial-induced apoptotic signaling.

More recently, there has been increased interest in using platinum(IV) multidrug approaches for immune chemotherapy. An example of this approach is compound **10** reported by Ang, which induces cancer cell death via two different pathways: direct cytotoxicity by the reduced platinum(II) species and activation of innate immune cells (induced by the released axial ligand) which generates cell-mediated cytotoxicity [18].

In most of the cases discussed above, the platinum(IV) prodrugs display higher cytotoxicity against a range of cancer cell lines than the parent platinum(II) complex (and/or the drugs in the axial positions). However, as has been documented in several critical reviews [19, 20], the increased cytotoxicity of the resulting compounds is not always a result of simple synergistic effects between the generated platinum(II) drugs and the released axial ligands. In some cases, the increased cytotoxicity is simply due to enhanced cellular uptake of the platinum(IV) prodrug as compared to the parent platinum(II) complexes. In other examples, the released axial ligands are not present in sufficiently high concentration to inhibit their proposed target; yet, they might be involved in other pathways that enhance the activity of the platinum(II) drugs. Therefore when developing platinum(IV) complexes as multiple-action prodrugs, it is essential that detailed cellular studies are carried out with the aim of disentangling the mechanism of action.

While the literature related to platinum(IV) prodrugs is dominated by systems where the released platinum(II) complex is one of the clinically approved drugs (i.e., cisplatin, carboplatin, or oxaliplatin), other platinum systems exploiting this approach have been reported. For example, Aldrich-Wright has studied a number of phenanthroline diamine platinum(IV) complexes as prodrugs, some of which have displayed very high anticancer properties [21]. Recent studies by Gibson and Brabec [22] have shown that this type of compound (e.g., compound **11** – Figure 3) can lead to a range of cellular changes including modification of nuclear DNA (with evidence that it only happens after reduction of the platinum(IV) prodrug), changes in the architecture of cytoskeleton networks, reduction of the mitochondrial membrane potential, and induction of epigenetic processes.

An interesting example by the same authors where two different platinum(IV) complexes are activated under reducing conditions releasing four different active drugs is the dinuclear complex **12**. This compound has very high activity against cancer cells and the proposed mode of action, when the platinum(IV) centers are reduced, involves DNA damage by cisplatin, HDAC inhibition by phenylbutyric acid, and interference with mitochondrial activity likely to be caused by the combined action of dichloroacetate and the platinum(II)-phenanthroline complex [23].

To explore the possibility of targeting different DNA topologies, our group developed a platinum(IV) complex (**13**) which showed poor DNA-binding affinity. However, upon reduction with glutathione or ascorbic acid the corresponding platinum(II)-salphen complex was formed, displaying high affinity and selectivity for G-quadruplex DNA via π–π end-stacking interactions [24].

2.1.2 Non-platinum Complexes

While the area of redox-activated prodrugs that target DNA is overwhelmingly dominated by Pt^{IV}/Pt^{II} systems, there are examples that involve other metals such as Ru^{III}/Ru^{II}, Cu^{II}/Cu^{I}, Fe^{III}/Fe^{II}, and Co^{III}/Co^{II}. However, in most of these cases, the activated (reduced) metal complex does not generally target DNA (particularly in cells); several of these prodrugs either release a known DNA-targeting drug (see cobalt(III) prodrugs below) or localize in the nucleus and upon reduction generate reactive oxygen species (ROS) that subsequently damage DNA (e.g., Cu^{II}/Cu^{I}, Fe^{III}/Fe^{II} pairs). The latter approach is not within the scope of this review and therefore will not be discussed further.

In the 1980s Clarke studied ruthenium(III) complexes as possible prodrugs that would be activated by reduction to generate the kinetically more labile ruthenium(II) species which would in turn metallate DNA [25].

Complexes **14** and **15** (Figure 4) are among the most successful ruthenium-based chemotherapeutics [26]. These complexes have excellent antiproliferative properties against a range of cancer cells and they were assessed in clinical trials – although they have not progressed to their clinical use. While the exact mode of action of these complexes is still not completely understood, it was initially shown *in vitro* that DNA was one of their targets (although recent evidence points to other biomolecular targets as their main mode of action) [27]. It was also shown that the ruthenium(III) center in both these compounds is readily reduced under physiological conditions suggesting that the corresponding ruthenium(II) complexes are the active species in cells. Even though the *in vivo* mode of action for these compounds does not seem to be driven by reduction followed by DNA binding, they serve as inspiration for other ruthenium complexes to be developed using this initially proposed strategy.

In general, cobalt(III) complexes are inert, adopt an octahedral geometry, and can be reduced under hypoxic conditions to the more labile cobalt(II) species. Therefore, such cobalt(III) complexes have been studied as prodrugs to deliver and release pharmacologically active compounds. An early example of this approach was cobalt(III) complex **16** (Figure 4) which under reducing conditions releases a nitrogen mustard ligand known to target DNA [28]. It was shown that this complex was cytotoxic against cancer cells and there was clear evidence of DNA cross-linking by the released nitrogen mustard ligand. A similar approach was used in complex **17** which contains as a ligand a highly toxic DNA minor-groove alkylator [29]. While the complex displayed attenuated cytotoxicity in normoxic cells, under hypoxic conditions it displayed significantly higher activity. In a more recent example, Suntharalingam reported the cobalt(III)-cyclen

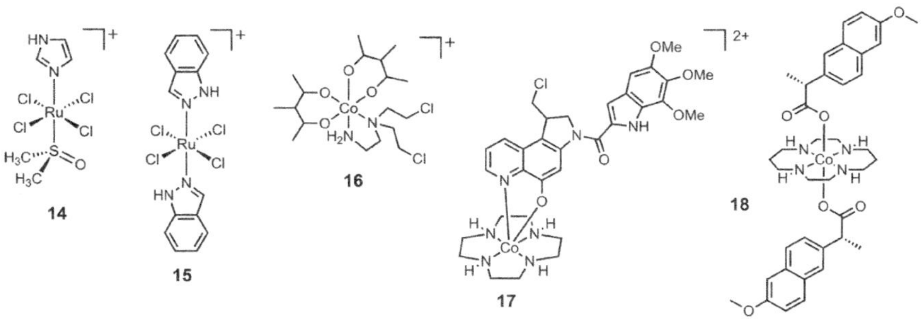

FIGURE 4 Selected examples of ruthenium(III) and cobalt(III) prodrugs that are activated under reducing conditions.

complex **18** bearing two naproxen moieties. This compound was shown to have high cytotoxicity against breast cancer stem cells by inducing a double effect involving DNA damage and inhibition of COX-2 activity [30].

2.2 pH Responsive

In living organisms, there are pH gradients between the extracellular environment and some intracellular compartments (e.g., lysosomes can have pH values as low as 4.5) as well as between healthy and some pathological tissue (e.g., the pH of tumors and inflammatory tissues is generally lower – at around 6.5 – than that of normal tissues at the typical physiological pH of 7.4). Therefore, changes in pH have been studied as triggers for the activation of prodrugs, including some metal complexes. Most examples of this approach include platinum(II) complexes coordinated to ligands that are pH-sensitive. One of the first document examples was complex **19** which contains O-thiocarbonic acid ligands (Figure 5) [31]. At physiological pH, the ligands are deprotonated, coordinating to the platinum in a bidentate fashion; however, at slightly acidic pH values, the ligands are protonated, becoming mono-dentate and hence increasing the ability of the resulting complex to interact with DNA. Similar approaches have been used with other ligands such as amino-alcohols (complex **20** – with various different R groups) to activate the coordinatively saturated platinum(II) complex at slightly acidic pH values by protonating the alkoxide groups [32, 33]. These studies showed that the amino-alcohol platinum(II) complexes displayed higher antiproliferative activity against cancer cells at pH 6.0, which was linked to the larger extent of DNA platination.

Another interesting approach has been taken by Access Pharmaceuticals. They conjugated a diaminocyclohexane platinum(II) complex to a hydroxypropylmethacrylamide (HPMA) polymer (AP5346, **21**). The authors showed that the polymer released a seven-fold higher amount of oxaliplatin at pH 5.4 compared to pH 7.4. This pattern was also seen *in vivo*, in which experiments showed that

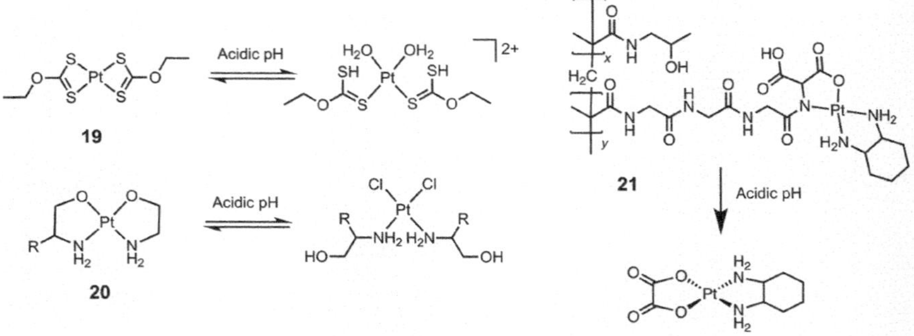

FIGURE 5 Selected examples of platinum complexes that are activated at acidic pH values.

a much higher degree of platinum could be delivered to tumors. AP5346 entered Phase II clinical trials [34].

2.3 ENZYME RESPONSIVE

While many organic drugs have been modified to include enzymatic triggers activated by phosphatase, nitroreductase, and others [35], few enzymatically activated metallodrugs have been investigated. Two relatively recent examples of these build on the previously discussed platinum(IV) to platinum(II) reduction mechanism of activation, adding additional layers of control. For example, Li and co-workers utilized supramolecular self-assembly (compound **22** – Figure 6) to control the uptake and release of a platinum(IV) complex which is a cisplatin prodrug [36]. They attached a hydrophobic peptide with a phosphate group to a mono-carboxylate-functionalized Pt^{IV} complex. The charged phosphate group prevented the self-assembly of the complex. However, upon treatment with alkaline phosphatase and the subsequent conversion of the phosphate to an alcohol group, the self-assembled prodrug could be taken up by cancer cells. Once internalized, cisplatin release can occur in a sustained and

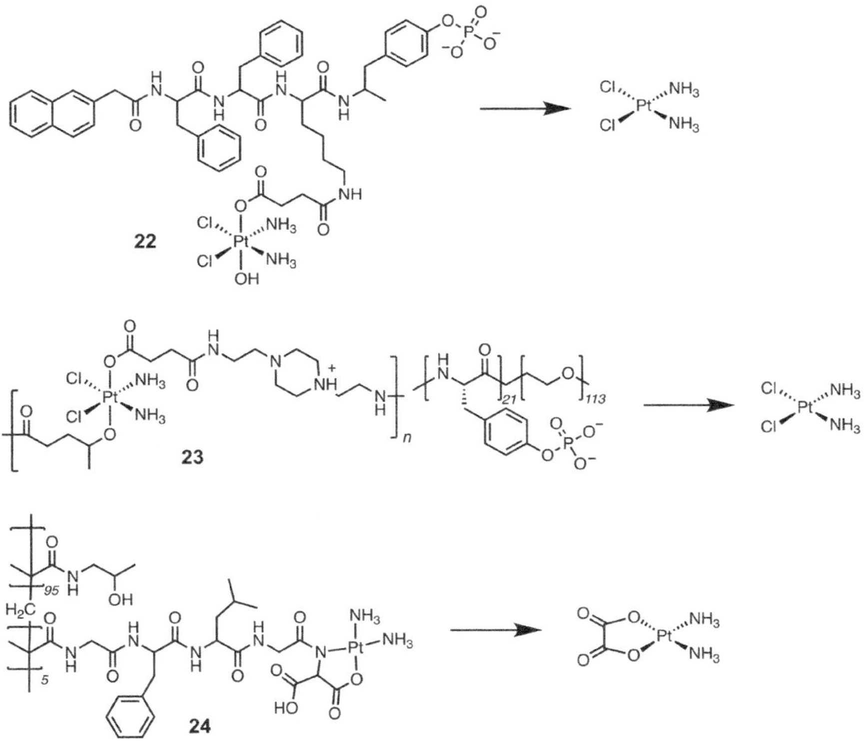

FIGURE 6 Selected examples of platinum complexes that are activated by enzymes.

controlled manner. *In vivo* studies showed that the phosphatase-activated self-assembled prodrug has lower toxicity, better bioaccumulation in the tumor, and less organ damage.

Lu and co-workers developed a phosphatase-triggered polyion micelle encapsulated with platinum(IV) prodrug **23** [37]. Their results indicated that the *in vitro* cellular uptake of this compound was dependent on surface alkaline phosphatase. In order to maximize the loading of the micelle with the prodrug, they used a diaminoethylpiperazine moiety to form a positively charged platinum(IV)-containing polymer which could interact electrostatically with a phosphate-functionalized polymer. Upon cellular uptake and dephosphorylation, these interactions are weakened, allowing for the release of the platinum(IV) polymer and subsequent reduction and cisplatin release. The cytotoxicity of the micelles was shown to be dependent on surface alkaline phosphatase expression across a range of cell lines.

The incorporation of cisplatin and carboplatin into enzyme-cleavable polymers is another interesting approach. AP5280 (**24**) is a water-soluble peptide developed by Access Pharmaceuticals (which entered Phase I clinical trials), which can be cleaved by cathepsin B (a lysosomal cysteine protease) in cells to release the active Pt^{II} complex [38].

3 EXOGENOUS STIMULI

3.1 PHOTOACTIVATION

Metal-based photoactivatable agents can be divided into two broad classes depending on their mode of action: photodynamic therapy (PDT) and photoactivated chemotherapy (PACT). In the former, the metal complex (i.e., the photosensitizer) absorbs light to generate an excited singlet state which, by intersystem crossing, can convert to a long-lived triplet state. This excited-state species can then be quenched by either biomolecules or by molecular oxygen (i.e., $^3O_2$) which in turn generates reactive oxygen species (i.e., oxygen radicals and singlet oxygen,$^1O_2$). These two PDT processes lead to significant oxidative damage to biomolecules such as DNA. In contrast, PACT follows a different mode of action: upon irradiation, an otherwise inert metal complex gets activated producing cytotoxic species. The photoactivation can follow different mechanisms as proposed by Sadler in a recent review [39]: (1) photo-induced electron transfer – inert metal centers are activated by light leading to a transfer of electrons from the ligand to the metal center. This in turn leads to ligand dissociation generating cytotoxic species, namely the activated metal complex and/or the released ligand; (2) photosubstitution – similarly to the previous mechanism, in this process an inert metal complex is activated by light generating an excited metal-to-ligand charge-transfer triplet state (^{3}MLCT). This can then interconvert to an excited metal-centered triplet state (^{3}MC) which in turn leads to metal-ligand dissociation and the concomitant formation of cytotoxic species; (3) bioactive ligand release – this class of PACT agents relies on the release of known bioactive molecules (e.g., NO, CO or enzyme inhibitors) upon irradiation; (4) ligand photocleavage – in this case, the photoactive component is a ligand which can either be photocleaved or photoswitched to generate active species.

Since PDT is a very extensive area of research that has been covered in many other reviews, it will not be covered further herein. Therefore, in this section, we will only cover examples where metal complexes are photoactivated via PACT mechanisms generating species that interact with DNA as the main mode of action. A number of reviews covering PACT have been published by Sadler [40], Gasser [41], Bonnet [42], and Turro [43], among several others.

The initial work on photoactivatable metal complexes for biological applications dates back to the 1980s and 1990s. Initial studies by Morrison showed that irradiation of [M(phen)$_2$Cl$_2$]Cl (where M=Cr^{III}, Rh^{III}; phen=1,10-phenanthroline) led to cleavage of the M–Cl bonds and subsequent metalation of ct-DNA; in the dark, the complexes are stable and minimal DNA metalation was observed [44, 45]. A similar approach was subsequently used by Turro and co-workers [46], who demonstrated that [Ru(bpy)$_2$(NH$_3$)$_2$]$^{2+}$ (bpy=bipyridine) can be activated by irradiation and the resulting [Ru(bpy)$_2$]$^{2+}$ species rapidly coordinates to ct-DNA – while the control [Ru(bpy)$_2$(en)]$^{2+}$ complex (where no photodissociation occurs) does not bind to DNA. Further studies by Glazer showed that the nature of the ligands around ruthenium(II) complexes can dictate the photochemical processes they undergo in the presence of DNA [47]. The three complexes **25**, **26**, and **27** are stable in the dark; under irradiation, complex **25** is stable, but complexes **26** and **27** undergo a photoejection of the N-N ligands yielding [Ru(bpy)$_2$]$^{2+}$. Interestingly, complex **25** leads to DNA photocleavage, complex **26** displays DNA photobinding (i.e., coordination of the generated [Ru(bpy)$_2$]$^{2+}$ species) and complex **27** exhibits a combination of the two mechanisms.

A related approach for the photogeneration of DNA-binding metal complexes is based on the light-induced reductive elimination in platinum(IV) complexes. Initial studies in this area by Bednarski showed that *trans,cis*-[Pt(en)I$_2$(OH)$_2$] and *trans,cis*-[Pt(en)I$_2$(OAc)$_2$] can be rapidly photolyzed using visible light yielding platinum(II) complexes which in turn coordinate to ct-DNA [48]. A subsequent mechanistic study by Sadler and Bednarski confirmed the species formed upon photoreduction and the resulting Pt^{II}-nucleotide adducts [49].

One of the challenges in this approach is for the platinum(IV) complexes to remain stable under physiological conditions in the absence of light. As discussed in the previous section, there has been significant research directed at activating platinum(IV) complexes endogenously by reduction (e.g., in hypoxic cells). Thermal stability is also important for the controlled photoreduction of platinum(IV) complexes. To address this challenge, Sadler and co-workers have developed a series of platinum(IV) complexes containing azido ligands which are stable under physiological conditions unless they are photoactivated. An initial study published in 2007 showed that *trans,trans,trans*-[Pt(N$_3$)$_2$(NH$_3$)(OH)$_2$(py)] was highly stable in the dark, but readily undergoes photoreduction when irradiated with UVA light (365 nm) [50]. This study also showed that the DNA platination levels in cells by the species generated from the photoactivation of *trans*,

trans,trans-[Pt(N$_3$)$_2$(NH$_3$)(OH)$_2$(py)] are similar to those found with cisplatin. A limitation of this first platinum(IV) di-azido complex was the need to use UVA light for photoactivation. This was addressed in a subsequent study that showed that the dipyridine derivative *trans,trans,trans*-[Pt(N$_3$)$_2$(OH)$_2$(py)$_2$] can be photo-reduced by irradiating with visible blue and green light [51].

More recently, detailed single-cell studies with this complex as well as *trans,trans,trans*-[Pt(coumarin-3-carboxylate)(N$_3$)$_2$(OH)(pyridine)$_2$] were reported [52]. The authors used cryosoft X-ray tomography (Cryo-SXT), nanofocused X-ray fluorescence (XRF), and X-ray absorption near edge structure (XANES) spectroscopy to provide a detailed picture of the photoactivation process at a single-cell level. These studies allowed mapping the oxidation state of the platinum centers and their distribution across the cell.

An interesting approach to achieve the photoreduction of platinum(IV) species has been reported by Sessler [53] in which a stable platinum(IV) complex was attached to motexafin gadolinium(III) fragment (known to accumulate in cancer cells) resulting in the mono- and di-platinum(IV) complexes **28** and **29**. Upon irradiation with visible light (or under reducing conditions), these compounds get reduced, releasing the motexafin gadolinium(III) fragment and active Pt^{II} species which bind to DNA. When exposed to visible light, mono-platinum complex **28** displayed *ca.* 8.5 times more DNA platination than when kept in the dark, indicating the importance of the photoactivation process.

Zhu has reported the rhodamine-substituted platinum(IV) complexes **30** and **31** as prodrugs, which upon irradiation undergo the expected photoreduction process liberating platinum(II) species known to interact with DNA [54]. The direct coordination of rhodamine to the platinum(IV) center allowed for a much higher photoconversion of Pt^{IV} to the corresponding Pt^{II} complexes. Cellular work showed these complexes (in particular **31**) to have high phototoxicity against several cancer cell lines. Interestingly, it was shown that **31** accumulates in mitochondria leading to extensive mitochondrial DNA damage, which is likely to be the cause of its high phototoxicity. More recently, the same group reported the photocaged platinum(IV) complex **32** which accumulates preferentially in the nucleoli and, following irradiation, undergoes reduction to yield oxaliplatin [55]. Interestingly, it was found that this prodrug is two times more cytotoxic after irradiation than the parent platinum(II) complex; furthermore, it was reported that it has enhanced tumor penetration properties and a distinct mode of action that overcomes drug resistance.

In an alternative approach, Sadler reported a platinum(IV) diazido complex, where one of the ligands contains N-(carboxymethyl)-1,8-naphthalimide derivatives (for example complex **33** in Figure 7), which are good DNA intercalators [56]. Therefore, these complexes pre-intercalate into DNA in the dark and when irradiated with visible light generate platinum(II) species which lead to interstrand crosslinks.

The photoactivation of metal-containing systems has also been achieved via uncaging self-assembled systems. A recent report by Xiao and co-workers in this area is based on platinum(IV) nanoparticles that can be excited in the

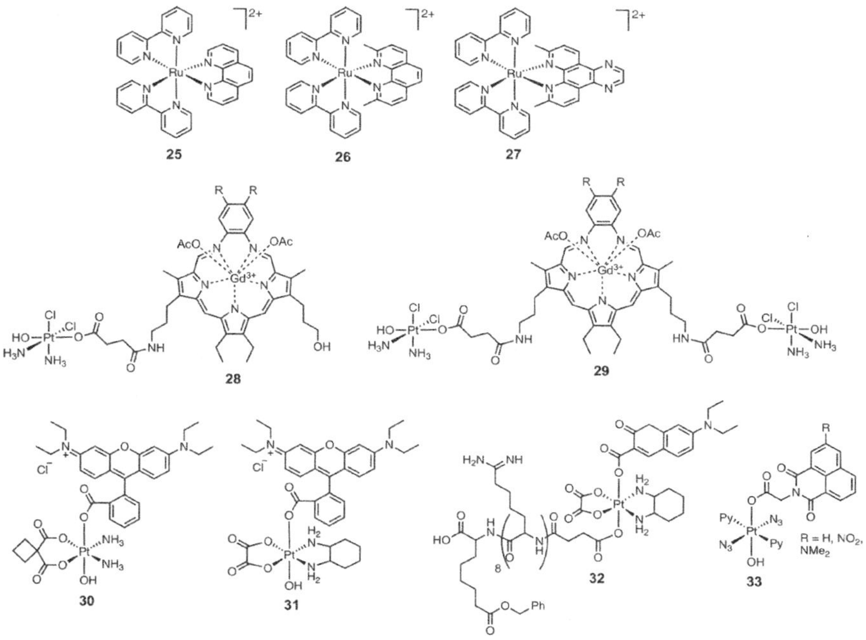

Stimuli-Responsive DNA-Binding Metal Complexes 171

FIGURE 7 Selected examples of metal complexes that upon light irradiation are activated, generating compounds that bind to DNA.

NIR region (at 880 nm) to release DNA-binding platinum(II) complexes [57]. This system is based on polymer chains that include a nuclear targeting peptide, oxaliplatin, and a photosensitizer with known properties in aggregation-induced emission (AIE) photodynamic therapy. These polymer chains self-assemble into nanoparticles which, upon irradiation in the NIR region lead to the reduction of the platinum(IV) center to platinum(II) species and disassembly of the nanoparticle. Besides the cancer and nuclear targeting properties of the peptides included in the nanoparticles, this approach is attractive since the activation takes place in the NIR region overcoming some of the limitations (e.g., lack of depth penetration for clinical translation) of most previously reported photoactive platinum(IV) complexes.

An alternative approach to uncaging metal-based DNA binders relies on the formation of interlocked species; our group has recently reported a rotaxane that contains a platinum(II) complex known to interact with DNA (in particular with G-quadruplex DNA structures) [58]. When incorporated into rotaxane **34** (Figure 8), the DNA-binding properties and cytotoxicity of this platinum-salphen complex were suppressed. However, upon irradiation one of the stoppers is removed, leading to the rotaxane's disassembly and release of complex **35** restoring its DNA-binding properties. It was also shown that this platinum-containing rotaxane is not cytotoxic in the dark, but when irradiated, its cytotoxicity against osteosarcoma cells increased significantly.

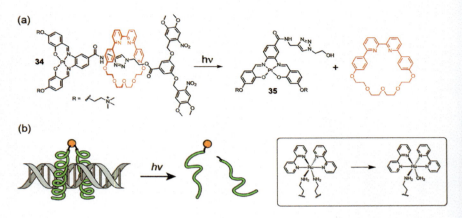

FIGURE 8 (a) Use on a rotaxane to 'cage' a platinum(II) complex known to bind to DNA. (b) A di-peptide ruthenium(II) complex with high affinity to DNA; upon irradiation the assembly is cleaved and generates a ruthenium mono-peptide complex which does not bind to DNA.

Mascareñas and Vázquez have reported an interesting approach to photo-deactivating the DNA-binding properties of peptide dimer [59]. A ruthenium(II) complex containing two brC peptides (Figure 8b) was shown to have high affinity for a specific dsDNA sequence. Upon irradiation with visible light (in the absence and presence of DNA) almost complete photolysis of this Ru-peptide assembly was observed yielding the free brC-NH$_2$ fragment and a mono-peptide ruthenium(II) complex. Interestingly, the latter does not bind to dsDNA, demonstrating that it is possible to control at will the dissociation of the Ru-peptide system with DNA by irradiation.

3.2 Activation Modulated by Metal Ions

The following examples involve systems with DNA-binding properties that are modulated by metal ions, and can be divided into two broad categories. The first group contains compounds based around short peptide sequences which have been modified to incorporate metal-coordinating motifs. The addition of metal ions or complexes with available coordination sites is generally used to assemble multiple units together and induce peptide folding, at which point the resulting hybrid structures can interact and stabilize dsDNA. The second category consists of small molecules which contain polyamines and can already stabilize various nucleic acid structures. In these cases, the addition of metal ions leads to the formation of a 'closed' structure, and binding is switched off.

3.2.1 Metal-Mediated Peptide Organization

Much of the first group of systems is based around basic peptides, which can bind to dsDNA. As these types of activatable basic peptides have been extensively reviewed elsewhere [60], only a selection of examples encompassing a range of activation methods are listed here.

The pioneering work in this field was carried out by Cuenoud and Schepartz in 1993 [61]. In this work they modified the bZIP protein motif, which is characterized by a leucine zipper region and a basic domain, in which the zipper region mediates dimerization between two units and the basic domain can interact with duplex DNA, folding into an α-helix upon insertion into the major groove. The pre-organization of the two basic regions by the zipper region plays a key role in the binding of bZIP proteins to DNA, as it has been shown that monomeric bZIP peptides cannot overcome the entropic cost of folding into an α-helix [62–64].

The authors started from the general control transcription factor GCN4, which is a transcription activator protein, and modified the ZIP domain to contain a transition metal-binding motif. In this system, two terpyridine moieties bind to an octahedrally coordinating metal center in a kinetically inert and well-defined manner. Furthermore, these ligands could be attached to the peptides via disulfide bonds. The terpyridyl substitution pattern was used to control the relative flexibility and orientation of the two basic domains (Figure 9a). Via CD spectroscopy and gel mobility shift assays, the authors were able to show that binding

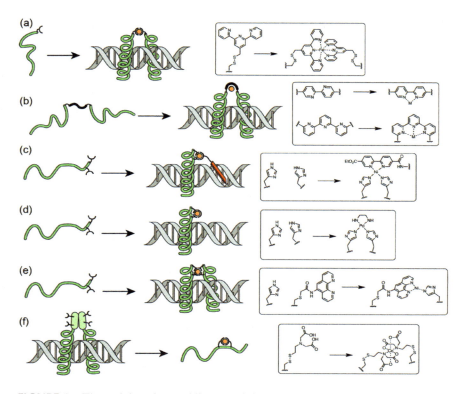

FIGURE 9 The activity of assemblies containing DNA-binding peptides can be regulated by addition of metal ions.

occurred only in the presence of Fe^{III} and when a short linker orientated at 180° was used, due to the necessity of simultaneous interaction of both basic domains. Since then, this concept has been extended in various directions.

Peacock and co-workers replaced the leucine zipper region with bipyridine and terpyridine linkers [65]. Rather than have the metal ion bring together two disconnected GCN4 domains, the metal was used to lock the orientation of the GCN4 domains relative to one another (Figure 9b). In the case of the bipyridine motif, the GCN4 domains would be kept the same distance apart regardless of metal coordination, whereas for the terpyridine they would switch from transoid to cisoid. Using CD spectroscopy and UV-vis spectroscopic titrations, the authors were able to show that the terpyridine-linked GCN4 dimer showed the greatest enhancement of binding upon metal coordination. Furthermore, they demonstrated that this enhancement could be reversed via the addition of EDTA to sequester the metal ions.

As discussed above, the monomeric GCN4 peptide has minimal interaction with DNA as it does not fold into an α-helix. Mascareñas, Vázquez, and co-workers, therefore, investigated various ways to induce α-helix formation in monomeric GCN4 peptides. Having previously shown that this could be achieved by tethering a groove binder to a monomeric peptide unit [66], they next investigated whether a metal-mediated approach could be used to both promote the folding of the peptide into an α-helix and bring together the disparate components [67]. They, therefore, synthesized a peptide in which two residues on two consecutive helical turns were mutated into histidines, along with a bipyridine-functionalized bis(benzamide) unit, which can groove-bind to dsDNA (Figure 9c). The addition of Ni^{II} ions led to the supramolecular assembly of the units via the formation of a square planar complex. They showed that both the metal and an appropriate DNA sequence with both a GCN4 and minor-groove binder site were required for α-helix formation and that the system could be disassembled via the addition of EDTA to sequester the Ni^{II} ion. They then extended this concept even further to include multiple peptide fragments and a groove binder [68].

Mascareñas and Vázquez subsequently investigated whether the modification of the monomeric peptide could lead to DNA binding without the requirement of the minor-groove binding unit [69]. Indeed, by including two histidines, four amino acid residues apart, they were able to induce the assembly of the α-helix via the addition of a Pd^{II} complex and of a dsDNA sequence via the formation of a metal-peptide complex in which the histidines replaced two labile sites in the square planar Pd^{II} complex (Figure 9d). Unlike a covalently stapled peptide, their metal-peptide complex was mostly unstructured, requiring the dsDNA to form the helix. This meant that they could reversibly switch between the folded and unfolded peptide via the addition of Pd^{II}-sequestering species. Importantly, they also demonstrated that the non-coordinated peptide had poor cell uptake but could be efficiently internalized by the addition of their Pd^{II} reagent.

Tezcan and co-workers took an alternative approach, in which they synthesized short, modified peptides named hybrid coordination motifs (HCMs) that included a histidine and phenanthroline unit seven residues apart as well as two salt-bridging side chains [70]. They firstly demonstrated that they could induce α-helix formation via the addition of various metal ions to form a tridentate complex and that this resulting complex had higher thermal stabilization and resistance to proteolytic cleavage. Having previously shown that a protein functionalized with a histidine/quinolate pair could be induced to form a dimer via metal complexation [71], they could apply a similar approach using their metal-coordinated peptide. Thus, they linked their short peptide sequence to a GCN4 peptide and subsequently showed that the introduction of Ni^{II} could induce helicity in their HCM, followed by dimerization and DNA binding (Figure 9).

While all the previous examples have shown how metal ions can be used to trigger basic peptides to bind to dsDNA, Futaki and co-workers took the opposite approach. They modified the zipper region to contain pairs of iminodiacetic acid (IDA motifs) through disulfide bond formation [72]. The addition of Co^{III} led to coordination of two IDA units and the destabilization of the zipper region (Figure 9f). This effect was large enough that it caused disassembly of the dimer and a loss of DNA stabilization. The addition of EDTA to sequester the Co^{III} reversed this effect and completely restored DNA binding.

3.2.2 Deactivation of DNA Binders by Metal Ions

The second group of systems where addition of metal ions can change their DNA-binding properties is based on small molecules (Figure 10 – compounds **36–40**). The ability of polyamine complexes to coordinate metal ions is well established and several groups have utilized this to build metal-mediated DNA binders. In 2002, Luis and co-workers combined two naphthyl units (**36**) capable of DNA intercalation and then linked with polyamines of various lengths [73]. Taking advantage of the moderate binding strength of naphthyl units (as compared to other stronger intercalators), they showed that the conformational distortion upon Cu^{I} addition could switch some systems from a bis-intercalation to mono-intercalation. This led to a switch in the thermal stability trend between DNA and RNA interacting with the complex as the RNA stabilization was affected to a greater extent than the DNA stabilization, which the authors hypothesized to be due to the narrower RNA groove. This work was subsequently extended by Verdejo and García-España to study a wide variety of amine-linked intercalators, including a tripodal system in which two Cu^{I} ions could bind [74].

García-España and co-workers also investigated a metal-mediated conformational switch for dsDNA. They utilized 'scorpiand' ligands, which contain a macrocyclic core appended with an arm containing additional donor groups. They synthesized a small library of compounds in which the scorpiand tail included an anthracene or pyrene unit (**37**), both of which can intercalate into dsDNA [75]. This intercalation is accompanied by a 'switch-on' effect, allowing for this interaction to be followed by fluorescence microscopy. Using a range of techniques, they showed that the free ligand could bind via intercalation, but the addition of Cu^{II} or Zn^{II} led to a conformational change which dramatically decreased binding due to the formation of a more 'closed' structure. Fascinatingly, this change

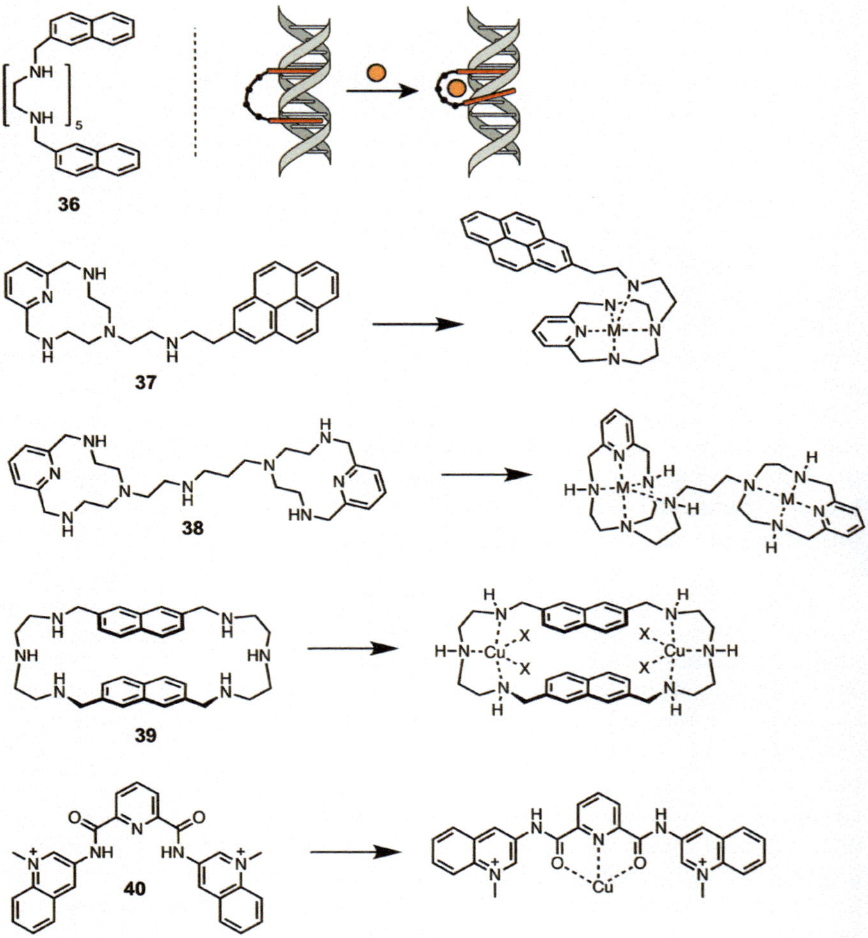

FIGURE 10 Selected examples where addition of small metal ions regulates the DNA-binding properties of small molecules.

in DNA-binding ability was reflected in the varying cytotoxicity of the open and metal-bound ligands, in which the open ligand was cytotoxic and could induce DNA damage response. In comparison, the Cu^{II} and Zn^{II} bound complexes were tolerated at much higher concentrations. The Zn^{II} complex could also be visualized in cells, showing that this lack of cytotoxicity was not due to differing uptake and that the Zn^{II} complex also did not induce any DNA damage response. A more detailed mechanistic study into the binding of the free and metal-complexed ligands to double and single-stranded DNA was also conducted [76].

Recent work was carried out by González-García and co-workers, in which they investigated ditopic scorpiand ligands (for example **38**) [77]. Upon the complexation of Zn^{II}, the number of available ammonium groups and the overall charge of the molecule decreases. This in turn affects how the molecule can interact with DNA and RNA. The free compounds were able to selectively interact with dsRNA compared to ct-DNA. After the coordination of either one or two Zn^{II} ions, the ability of the complexes to displace ethidium bromide or DAPI from RNA was decreased, along with its thermal stabilization. Finally, these results were reflected in biological assays, in which the free ligands showed high cytotoxicity whereas the Zn^{II} complexes did not.

An interesting approach has been taken by Granzhan and co-workers, in which they modulate the ability of a bis-naphthalene macrocycle (**39**) to stabilize homopyrimidine (T:T) DNA mismatches [78]. They first showed how these macrocycles can template the hybridization of two single-stranded DNA sequences containing T:T mismatches, acting as 'molecular glue'. The addition of Cu^{II} leads to the formation of a binuclear copper complex, in which the relative conformation of the two naphthalene units is locked in a displaced antiparallel conformation compared with the eclipsed parallel one found when the macrocycle is bound to a T:T mismatch. This leads to a denaturation of the heteroduplex structure. By designing a single-stranded sequence with a molecular beacon attached, they subsequently were able to modulate the fluorescence emission of their system by cycling the addition of Cu^{II} and EDTA.

Mergny and co-workers have used a metal-mediated conformational switch to control a ligand (**40**) which targets G-quadruplex DNA [79]. They took advantage of the fact that the well-studied G4 DNA ligand, 360A, includes a pyridocarboxamide motif. In its free form, the hydrogen atoms of the amide bond can hydrogen bond to the pyridine, leading to a compact 'V'-shaped molecule. However, this motif is also a tridentate metal chelator via the two carbonyl and pyridine units. This flips the orientation of the quinolinium unit and leads to decreased G4 DNA interactions. Interestingly, Cu^{II} also affects the ability of single-stranded DNA to form G4 structures. The authors were able to use both effects in tandem to efficiently cycle between a completely unfolded DNA state with a non-interacting ligand and a highly stable state in which a G4 unit was stabilized by 360A in its active conformation. The cycling was achieved via repeated addition of $CuSO_4$ to the system, followed by EDTA to remove the Cu^{II} ions.

3.3 Metal-Catalyzed Activation

All the previously discussed examples utilize compounds which contain metal-coordinating motifs and bind to DNA. In some cases, these are metallodrugs in which the metal center plays a role in the binding of the compound to DNA in its active state, and in others, the coordination of a metal ion can be used to assemble/disassemble separate units or lock compounds in favorable/unfavorable conformations. Both can be described via changes to the metal coordination, whether via ligand substitution or differing geometry.

The following set of compounds are examples of metal complexes that control the DNA-binding properties of a separate molecule via catalysis (Figure 11).

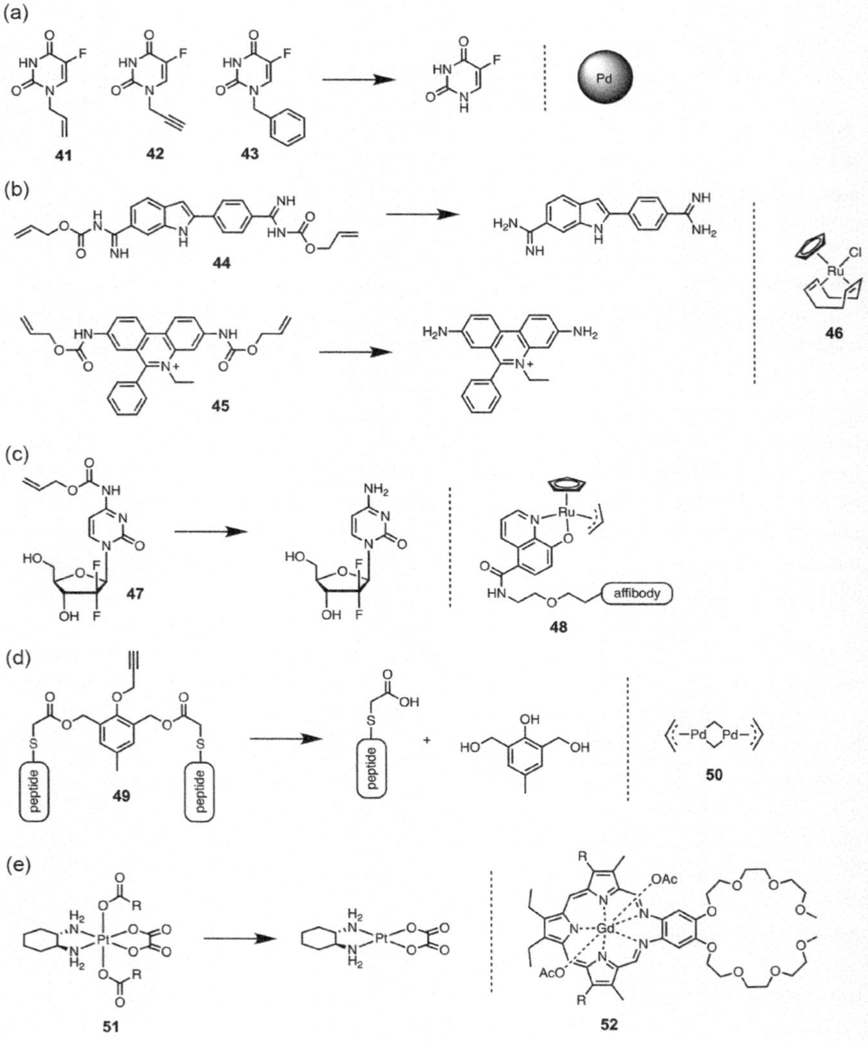

FIGURE 11 Selected examples where the activation of prodrugs takes place via metal-catalyzed processes.

The general mechanism of action in these systems is via the protection of essential functional groups in a DNA-binding molecule to form a prodrug. These protecting groups can then be selectively cleaved by metal complexes in a biological environment. Importantly, these types of reactions have no close biological equivalent, affording a high degree of spatiotemporal control. Many of the following examples have used doxorubicin, a currently used chemotherapy drug which targets DNA, as a proof of concept.

In 2014, Unciti-Broceta and co-workers demonstrated the first example of the release of a chemotherapeutic drug via metal-catalyzed de-caging [80]. They showed that a Pd^0-containing resin could be used to bioorthogonally activate 5-fluorouracil (5FU) protected with allyl (**41**), propargyl (**42**), or benzyl (**43**) moieties (5FU-pro). 5FU can be converted into active nucleotidic metabolites, which either can inhibit thymidylate synthase or be incorporated into DNA and RNA, disrupting their functions. The authors showed the combination of 5FU-pro and Pd^0-resin could be used to initiate a cytotoxic effect in cancer cells lines comparable to 5FU, and importantly that either component on its own had no effect.

Pioneering work was also carried out by Mascareñas and co-workers [81]. They demonstrated that the addition of allyl carbamate groups to both DNA groove binders (DAPI, **44**) and intercalators (EtBr, **45**) led to a 20–40-fold decrease in binding ability, ascribed to the loss of electrostatic and hydrogen bonding of the caged amidinium groups. In both cases, treatment with a combination of a Ru catalyst and thiophenol led to a near complete de-caging within 5 min and 1 h, respectively. In live cell experiments, the authors showed that treatment with their caged DAPI derivate led to an even cellular distribution of dye. However, upon the addition of thiophene and their Ru catalyst, a redistribution of the dye to the cell nucleus took place, as the uncaged DAPI became bound to nuclear DNA. A similar pattern was observed for their caged EtBr derivative. Finally, they also showed that a bis-benzamidine complex that had been similarly caged showed a 5–10-fold decrease in cytotoxicity when compared to the free analog.

The bioavailability and biocompatibility of the metal catalysts required for uncaging is a major limiting factor in their potential clinical use. Some steps to improve this have been taken already, through attachment of targeting molecules with enhanced permeability [82]. An alternative method is the use of antibody-drug conjugates. Here, Mao and co-workers have attached an affibody (proteins which function in a similar way to an antibody but are generally much smaller) directly to the metal catalyst rather than the drug [83]. They chose an affibody which targets the HER2 receptor, which is overexpressed in many tumors [84], hoping to achieve simultaneous tumor-targeting delivery of the metal catalyst and tumor growth inhibition via the blockade of the HER2 signaling pathway. The catalyst they used (**48**) was a hydroxyquinoline Ru(Cp) derivative with a maleimide for convenient bioconjugation. The resulting affibody conjugate was used in conjunction with an N-allyloxycarbonyl-caged gemcitabine prodrug (GPD, **47**). Gemcitabine is a nucleoside analog, which acts via its incorporation into native DNA strands in which it causes chain termination and DNA damage due to its recognition as a 'faulty' base. The authors showed that the catalytic activity of the Ru conjugate was retained and could completely convert the prodrug within 12 h. Next, the authors demonstrated that the combinational therapy of Ru-HER2 and GPD against a range of cell lines resulted in uncaging of GPD and a subsequent increase in cytotoxicity correlated with HER2 expression levels. They were able to quantify DNA damage levels using various biomarkers and showed a significant difference in HER2 positive and negative cell lines.

Finally, zebrafish xenograft experiments demonstrated that the Ru-HER2 and GBD combination was highly effective at limiting tumor growth *in vivo*.

Mascareñas and co-workers have used a metal-catalyzed cleavage reaction to deactivate a DNA binder [85]. As discussed above, GCN4 dimers based on the dimeric basic regions of bZIP transcription factors can bind to duplex DNA. Here, two cysteine-containing peptides (brC) based on the basic region of GCN4 were linked to a cleavable core containing a propargylic protecting group with two ortho arylether derivatives (**49**). Treatment with Pd catalyst **50** led to disappearance of the dimer within 3 h. The authors then used EMSA gel experiments and CD spectra to show that this cleavage process could disassemble the peptide/DNA complex.

An alternative method has been taken by Sessler and co-workers. As previously discussed, Pt^{IV} prodrugs can be activated via a redox process involving electron transfer to the Pt^{IV} center. However, in some cases, the complexes are too inert and cannot be reduced via biological reducing agents. One solution is to use photoactivation (Figure 7, compounds **28** and **29**), but this too suffers from various drawbacks. Motexafin gadolinium (MGd, **52**) is an imaging agent which has been found to accumulate preferentially in cancer cells. Interestingly, it can also act as a redox mediator, promoting electron transfer between reducing metabolites. Sessler and co-workers showed that Pt^{IV} complexes (e.g., **51**) could act as electron acceptors, leading to activation of the complex in the presence of MGd [86]. They showed that by using a hydrophilic Pt^{IV} complex they could block cellular uptake, keeping the complex in low ascorbate conditions. Then, via the tumor-selective local concentration of MGd, the complex could be reduced to the Pt^{II} form, and subsequently be taken up into cells to produce a cytotoxic effect.

A number of groups have used metal complexes to activate prodrugs of doxorubicin (Figure 12). Doxorubicin interacts with DNA via intercalation, inhibiting the progression of topoisomerase II during transcription. In 2014, Meggers and co-workers used a ruthenium catalyst to uncage allyl carbamate groups to form primary amines [87]. Building on their pioneering work using a [Cp*Ru(cod)Cl] catalyst [88], they screened various organo-ruthenium complexes using a fluorogenic reaction. They identified a quinoline complex (**54**) capable of deprotecting allyl carbamate groups under biologically relevant conditions such as in the presence of glutathione. They then applied this catalyst in live cells to de-cage a rhodamine dye and finally an allyl carbamate-protected Dox derivative (**53**), providing the first example of intracellular metal-catalyzed prodrug activation.

In 2017, Weissleder and co-workers loaded a [PdCl$_2$(TFP)$_2$] catalyst (**56**) in a PEG-based nanoparticle (Pd-NP) which could cleave alloc and allyl carbamate-protected Dox (**55**) [89]. Furthermore, they attempted to incorporate their Dox-prodrugs into nanoparticles for more efficient delivery. They were able to show that treatment of cancer cells with their proDox system and the Pd-NP counterpart led to a dramatic increase in cytotoxicity, and that the proDox molecule showed virtually no retention in live cells. There was also a prominent increase in DNA damage biomarkers. A subsequent follow-up study aimed to

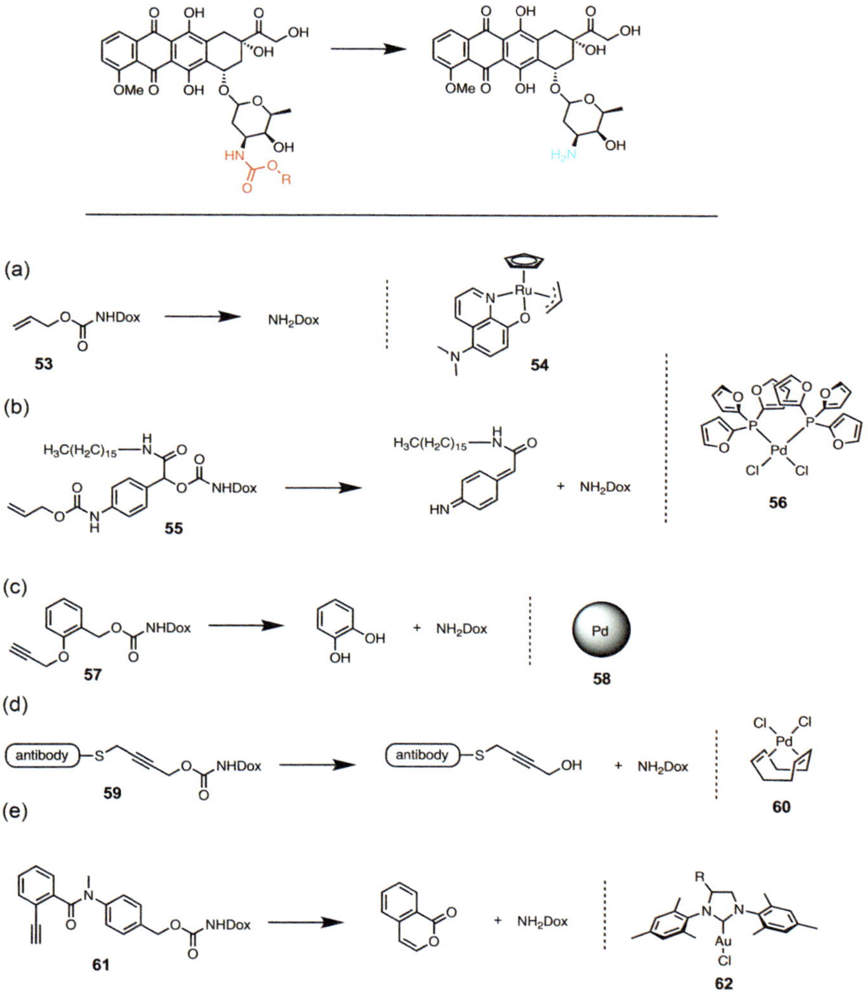

Stimuli-Responsive DNA-Binding Metal Complexes 181

FIGURE 12 Selected examples where the activation of prodrugs containing doxorubicin takes place via metal-catalyzed processes.

improve the nanoparticle loading of Dox [90]. In this case, they functionalized a self-immolative linker with three modular components: a biorthogonal metal-catalyzed trigger, a caged drug, and a 'nanoencapsulation anchor', in this case, a C_{18} chain in order the trap the entire system in a polymeric micelle. This led to enhanced permeability and retentions, and effective tumor growth suppression.

Unciti-Broceta and co-workers have investigated how it might be possible to use metal-containing implantable devices to control metal-catalyzed uncaging. They proposed that the surgical insertion of a Pd-containing species into a tumor could be used to activate multiple doses of a Pd-activatable prodrug [91]. In this work, they used propargyloxybenzylcarbonyl (PBC) protected Dox (**57**) along with some Pd-containing beads ranging from 10 to 110 μm in diameter (**58**). They demonstrated that the PBC-caged version of Dox did not induce lethality even at very high concentrations. Next, they injected mice tumors with Pd-containing beads and showed that they could catalytically release Dox for 21 days, in which the prodrug was only activated in the tumor, leading to DNA double-strand breaks (as shown by γH2AX foci).

Bernardes and co-workers synthesized a bifunctional cleavable linker in which Dox was conjugated to an antibody to form the drug conjugate **59** [92]. This concept built on work by Wood and co-workers, in which kinase inhibitors were conjugated to a HaloTag via an allyl carbamate linker. Developed for use in pull-down assays, the palladium-catalyzed cleavage of the linker could be used to more effectively identify captured drug targets [93]. In their work, Bernardes moved from cell lysates to cancer cells, aiming to selectively deliver and release a cytotoxic cancer drug in which their antibody could interact with HER2 receptors overexpressed in cancer cells. They first identified which palladium catalyst and functionalized propargyl carbamate pair could most effectively release a given payload, choosing a thioether functionalized linker which could be attached to any proteins containing a cysteine. Through a series of cell viability experiments, they showed that Dox attached to a PEG functionalized version of the linker was ten times less toxic than the parent drug, but when [Pd(cod)Cl$_2$] (**60**) was introduced, cell viability dropped significantly, showing the de-caging was working as expected. Finally, they conjugated Dox to a nanobody which targets the HER2 antigen and demonstrated that the ADC became twice as toxic upon treatment with [Pd(cod)Cl$_2$] against an HER2-positive cell line.

Tanaka and co-workers have aimed to increase the diversity of metal-based uncaging of biomolecules, as most examples so far utilized Ru or Pd [94]. Additionally, they wanted their protecting group to be able to be further derivatized, in order to ensure that it could sufficiently block a drug's mechanism of action. They set out to develop an appropriate Au-catalyzed unmasking of a 2-alkynylbenzamide (Ayba) protecting group, in which a secondary amide would be released [95]. Using a mixture of Ayba-protected endoxifen and proc or alloc-protected Dox (**61**), they demonstrated that either Au (e.g., **61**) or Ru/Pd could be used to orthogonally release their drug of choice. Next, in order to circumvent the requirement of the drug containing a secondary amine, they coupled the Ayba group to a methylamino-benzyloxycarbonyl (PMBC) spacer which would release a primary amine. After synthesizing a small library of Dox-PMBC-Ayba derivatives, they showed how treatment with a non-cytotoxic concentration of their Au catalyst led to a 16–36-fold increase in cytotoxicity. Finally, by increasing the hydrophilicity of their molecule via Ayba derivatization, they showed how they could block passive diffusion of the prodrug into cells, leading to a 2,000–6,500-fold increase in cytotoxicity upon metal-mediated uncaging.

A potential limitation of metal-catalyzed uncaging is that it is challenging to carry out cleavage reactions intracellularly. While extracellular cleavage can be achieved via the use of Pd-containing beads or resins, the poor uptake, poor solubility, and instability of many Pd catalytic systems can limit the effectiveness of their direct usage. Therefore, Bernardes and co-workers sought to develop a more biologically friendly approach [96]. Rather than directly introducing the Pd^0 source, they utilized the fact that the water-soluble Pd^{II} salt, Na_2PdCl_4, can be reduced to Pd^0 by sodium ascorbate. Using this mechanism, they were able to cleave allyl ethers and allyl carbamates in a cell culture medium. They then applied this concept in live cells, using the DNA minor-groove binder duocarmycin protected with an allyl ether and Dox protected with an allyl carbamate. They showed that pre-incubation of cells of the prodrug and Na_2PdCl_4, followed by incubation with NaAsc, led to a significant decrease in cell viability. Interestingly, pre-incubation with all three components did not lead to any significant change, demonstrating that the presence of intracellular biomolecules is necessary for the stabilization of the active Pd^0 species.

4 GENERAL CONCLUSIONS

The wide range of geometries, variable oxidation states, and unique properties (e.g., catalytic, photochemical, and structural) of metal complexes make them very attractive for the development of novel therapeutic approaches. However, to ensure that more metal complexes progress from preclinical studies to clinical applications, it is important to address some of their shortcomings such as poor bioavailability, unwanted toxicity, poor selectivity, and off-target effects. As has been discussed throughout this review, several strategies are being explored to control the activity of metal complexes that target DNA. By carefully selecting the triggers that regulate their activity, it has already been possible to improve significantly some of the shortcomings highlighted above. The systems herein discussed have already shown remarkable improvements in the activity of a broad range of DNA-targeting metallodrugs – *in vitro*, in cells and, in a few examples, *in vivo*. The field has reached a level of maturity that promises to deliver exciting new DNA-binding metal complexes that are more likely to progress to clinical studies in the near future.

ACKNOWLEDGMENTS

We acknowledge the funding support from "Laboratory for Synthetic Chemistry and Chemical Biology" under the Health@InnoHK Program launched by Innovation and Technology Commission, The Government of Hong Kong Special Administrative Region of the People's Republic of China.

ABBREVIATIONS

3MC   metal-centered triplet state
3MLCT   metal-to-ligand charge-transfer triplet state
5FU   5-fluorouracil

Ac	acetate
AIE	aggregation-induced emission
Asc	ascorbate
Ayba	2-alkynylbenzamide
Bpy	bipyridine
br	basic region
brC	cysteine-containing peptides
bZIP	basic leucine zippers
CD	circular dichroism
cod	cyclooctadiene
COX-2	cyclooxygenase-2
Cp	cyclopentadienyl
Cryo-SXT	cryosoft X-ray tomography
ct-DNA	calf thymus DNA
DAPI	4′, 6-diamidino-2-phenylindole
DNA	deoxyribonucleic acid
Dox	doxorubicin
dsDNA	double-stranded DNA
EDTA	ethylenediaminetetraacetic acid
EMSA	electrophoretic mobility shift assay
En	1,2-diaminoethane
EtBr	ethidium bromide
G4	guanine quadruplex
GPD	caged gemcitabine prodrug
HCM	hybrid coordination motifs
HDAC	histone deacetylase
HER2	human epidermal growth receptor 2
HPMA	hydroxypropylmethacrylamide
IDA	iminodiacetic acid
MGd	motexafin gadolinium
NIR	near infrared
NP	nanoparticle
PACT	photoactivated chemotherapy
PBC	propargyloxybenzylcarbonyl
PDT	photodynamic therapy
Phen	1,10-phenanthroline
PMBC	methylamino-benzyloxycarbonyl
Py	pyridine
RNA	ribonucleic acid
ROS	reactive oxygen species
TAT	transactivator of transcription
UV	ultraviolet
Vis	visible light
XANES	X-ray absorption near edge structure
XRF	X-ray fluorescence

REFERENCES

1. X. Wang, X. Wang, S. Jin, N. Muhammad, Z. Guo, *Chem. Rev.* **2019**, *119*, 1138–1192.
2. J. Rodriguez, J. Mosquera, S. Learte-Aymamí, M. E. Vázquez, J. L. Mascareñas, *Acc. Chem. Res.* **2020**, *53*, 2286–2298.
3. T. C. Johnstone, K. Suntharalingam, S. J. Lippard, *Chem. Rev.* **2016**, *116*, 3436–3486.
4. D. Gibson, *ChemMedChem* **2021**, *16*, 2188–2191.
5. Z. Wang, Z. Deng, G. Zhu, *Dalton Trans.* **2019**, *48*, 2536–2544.
6. V. Venkatesh, P. J. Sadler, in *Metallo-Drugs: Development and Action of Anticancer Agents*, Vol. 18 of *Metal Ions in Life Sciences*, Eds A. Sigel, H. Sigel, R. K. O. Sigel, De Gruyter, Berlin/Boston, **2018**, pp. 69–108.
7. M. Ravera, E. Gabano, M. J. McGlinchey, D. Osella, *Dalton Trans.* **2022**, *51*, 2121–2134.
8. M. D. Hall, H. R. Mellor, R. Callaghan, T. W. Hambley, *J. Med. Chem.* **2007**, *50*, 3403–3411.
9. S. Abramkin, S. M. Valiahdi, M. A. Jakupec, M. Galanski, N. Metzler-Nolte, B. K. Keppler, *Dalton Trans.* **2012**, *41*, 3001–3005.
10. C. M. Fadzen, J. M. Wolfe, W. Zhou, C.-F. Cho, N. von Spreckelsen, K. T. Hutchinson, Y.-C. Lee, E. A. Chiocca, S. E. Lawler, O. H. Yilmaz, S. J. Lippard, B. L. Pentelute, *J. Med. Chem.* **2020**, *63*, 6741–6747.
11. J. Ma, Q. Wang, Z. Huang, X. Yang, Q. Nie, W. Hao, P. G. Wang, X. Wang, *J. Med. Chem.* **2017**, *60*, 5736–5748.
12. W. H. Ang, I. Khalaila, C. S. Allardyce, L. Juillerat-Jeanneret, P. J. Dyson, *J. Am. Chem. Soc.* **2005**, *127*, 1382–1383.
13. L. Ma, R. Ma, Y. Wang, X. Zhu, J. Zhang, H. C. Chan, X. Chen, W. Zhang, S.-K. Chiu, G. Zhu, *Chem. Comm.* **2015**, *51*, 6301–6304.
14. S. Dhar, S. J. Lippard, *Proc. Natl. Acad. Sci. USA* **2009**, *106*, 22199–22204.
15. S. Jin, N. Muhammad, Y. Sun, Y. Tan, H. Yuan, D. Song, Z. Guo, X. Wang, *Angew. Chem. Int. Ed.* **2020**, *59*, 23313–23321.
16. R. Raveendran, J. P. Braude, E. Wexselblatt, V. Novohradsky, O. Stuchlikova, V. Brabec, V. Gandin, D. Gibson, *Chem. Sci.* **2016**, *7*, 2381–2391.
17. M. v. Babak, Y. Zhi, B. Czarny, T. B. Toh, L. Hooi, E. K. Chow, W. H. Ang, D. Gibson, G. Pastorin, *Angew. Chem. Int. Ed.* **2019**, *58*, 8109–8114.
18. D. Y. Q. Wong, C. H. F. Yeo, W. H. Ang, *Angew. Chem. Int. Ed.* **2014**, *53*, 6752–6756.
19. D. Gibson, *Dalton Trans.* **2016**, *45*, 12983–12991.
20. D. Gibson, *ChemMedChem* **2021**, *16*, 2188–2191.
21. K. M. Deo, J. Sakoff, J. Gilbert, Y. Zhang, J. R. Aldrich Wright, *Dalton Trans.* **2019**, *48*, 17217–17227.
22. H. Kostrhunova, J. Zajac, V. Novohradsky, J. Kasparkova, J. Malina, J. R. Aldrich-Wright, E. Petruzzella, R. Sirota, D. Gibson, V. Brabec, *J. Med. Chem.* **2019**, *62*, 5176–5190.
23. E. Petruzzella, J. P. Braude, J. R. Aldrich-Wright, V. Gandin, D. Gibson, *Angew. Chem. Int. Ed.* **2017**, *56*, 11539–11544.
24. S. Bandeira, J. Gonzalez-Garcia, E. Pensa, T. Albrecht, R. Vilar, *Angew. Chem. Int. Ed.* **2018**, *57*, 310–313.
25. M. J. Clarke, S. Bitler, D. Rennert, M. Buchbinder, A. D. Kelman, *J. Inorg. Biochem.* **1980**, *12*, 79–87.
26. L. Cardo, M. J. Hannon, in *Metallo-Drugs: Development and Action of Anticancer Agents*, Vol. 18 of *Metal Ions in Life Sciences*, Eds A. Sigel, H. Sigel, R. K. O. Sigel, De Gruyter, Berlin/Boston, **2018**, pp. 303–324.
27. E. Alessio, L. Messori, *Molecules* **2019**, *24*, 1995.

28. D. C. Ware, B. D. Palmer, W. R. Wilson, W. A. Denny, *J. Med. Chem.* **1993**, *36*, 1839–1846.
29. J. B. J. Milbank, R. J. Stevenson, D. C. Ware, J. Y. C. Chang, M. Tercel, G.-O. Ahn, W. R. Wilson, W. A. Denny, *J. Med. Chem.* **2009**, *52*, 6822–6834.
30. P. B. Cressey, A. Eskandari, P. M. Bruno, C. Lu, M. T. Hemann, K. Suntharalingam, *ChemBioChem* **2016**, *17*, 1713–1718.
31. G. Schilling, E. Amtmann, M. Zöller, H. Wesch, *Cancer Chemother. Pharmacol.* **2001**, *47*, 461–466.
32. M. Galanski, C. Baumgartner, V. Arion, B. K. Keppler, *Eur. J. Inorg. Chem.* **2003**, *2003*, 2619–2625.
33. S. M. Valiahdi, A. E. Egger, W. Miklos, U. Jungwirth, K. Meelich, P. Nock, W. Berger, C. G. Hartinger, M. Galanski, M. A. Jakupec, B. K. Keppler, *J. Biol. Inorg. Chem.* **2013**, *18*, 249–260.
34. J. R. Rice, J. L. Gerberich, D. P. Nowotnik, S. B. Howell, *Clin. Cancer Res.* **2006**, *12*, 2248–2254.
35. R. Walther, J. Rautio, A. N. Zelikin, *Adv. Drug Deliv. Rev.* **2017**, *118*, 65–77.
36. H. Liu, Y. Li, Z. Lyu, Y. Wan, X. Li, H. Chen, H. Chen, X. Li, *J. Mater. Chem. B* **2014**, *2*, 8303–8309.
37. S.-L. Li, Y. Hou, Y. Hu, J. Yu, W. Wei, H. Lu, *Biomat. Sci.* **2017**, *5*, 1558–1566.
38. J. M. Rademaker-Lakhai, C. Terret, S. B. Howell, C. M. Baud, R. F. de Boer, D. Pluim, J. H. Beijnen, J. H. M. Schellens, J.-P. Droz, *Clin. Cancer Res.* **2004**, *10*, 3386–3395.
39. C. Imberti, P. Zhang, H. Huang, P. J. Sadler, *Angew. Chem. Int. Ed.* **2020**, *59*, 61–73.
40. N. J. Farrer, L. Salassa, P. J. Sadler, *Dalton Trans.* **2009**, 10690–10701.
41. L. Gourdon, K. Cariou, G. Gasser, *Chem. Soc. Rev.* **2022**, *51*, 1167–1195.
42. S. Bonnet, *Dalton Trans.* **2018**, *47*, 10330–10343.
43. J. K. White, R. H. Schmehl, C. Turro, *Inorg. Chim. Acta* **2017**, *454*, 7–20.
44. R. E. Mahnken, M. A. Billadeau, E. P. Nikonowicz, H. Morrison, *J. Am. Chem. Soc.* **1992**, *114*, 9253–9265.
45. M. A. Billadeau, H. Morrison, *J. Inorg. Biochem.* **1995**, *57*, 249–270.
46. T. N. Singh, C. Turro, *Inorg. Chem.* **2004**, *43*, 7260–7262.
47. B. S. Howerton, D. K. Heidary, E. C. Glazer, *J. Am. Chem. Soc.* **2012**, *134*, 8324–8327.
48. N. A. Kratochwil, M. Zabel, K.-J. Range, P. J. Bednarski, *J. Med. Chem.* **1996**, *39*, 2499–2507.
49. N. A. Kratochwil, J. A. Parkinson, P. J. Bednarski, P. J. Sadler, *Angew. Chem. Int. Ed.* **1999**, *38*, 1460–1463.
50. F. S. Mackay, J. A. Woods, P. Heringová, J. Kašpárková, A. M. Pizarro, S. A. Moggach, S. Parsons, V. Brabec, P. J. Sadler, *Proc. Natl. Acad. Sci. USA* **2007**, *104*, 20743–20748.
51. N. J. Farrer, J. A. Woods, L. Salassa, Y. Zhao, K. S. Robinson, G. Clarkson, F. S. Mackay, P. J. Sadler, *Angew. Chem. Int. Ed.* **2010**, *49*, 8905–8908.
52. E. M. Bolitho, C. Sanchez-Cano, H. Shi, P. D. Quinn, M. Harkiolaki, C. Imberti, P. J. Sadler, *J. Am. Chem. Soc.* **2021**, *143*, 20224–20240.
53. G. Thiabaud, J. F. Arambula, Z. H. Siddik, J. L. Sessler, *Chem. Eur. J.* **2014**, *29*, 8942–8947.
54. Z. Deng, C. Li, S. Chen, Q. Zhou, Z. Xu, Z. Wang, H. Yao, H. Hirao, G. Zhu, *Chem. Sci.* **2021**, *12*, 6536–6542.
55. Z. Deng, N. Wang, Y. Liu, Z. Xu, Z. Wang, T.-C. Lau, G. Zhu, *J. Am. Chem. Soc.* **2020**, *142*, 7803–7812.

56. H. Shi, J. Kasparkova, C. Soulié, G. J. Clarkson, C. Imberti, O. Novakova, M. J. Paterson, V. Brabec, P. J. Sadler, *Chem. Eur. J.* **2021**, *27*, 10711–10716.
57. D. Wei, Y. Huang, B. Wang, L. Ma, J. Karges, H. Xiao, *Angew. Chem. Int. Ed.* **2022**, *61*, e202201486.
58. T. Kench, P. A. Summers, M. K. Kuimova, J. E. M. Lewis, R. Vilar, *Angew. Chem. Int. Ed.* **2021**, *60*, 10928–10934.
59. J. Mosquera, M. I. Sánchez, M. E. Vázquez, J. L. Mascareñas, *Chem. Commun.* **2014**, *50*, 10975–10978.
60. J. Rodriguez, J. Mosquera, S. Learte-Aymamí, M. E. Vázquez, J. L. Mascareñas, *Acc. Chem. Res.* **2020**, *53*, 2286–2298.
61. B. Cuenoud, A. Schepartz, *Science* **1993**, *259*, 510–513.
62. C. Park, J. L. Campbell, W. A. Goddard, *J. Am. Chem. Soc.* **1996**, *118*, 4235–4239.
63. M. Zhang, B. Wu, H. Zhao, J. W. Taylor, *J. Pept. Sci.* **2002**, *8*, 125–136.
64. X. Wang, W. Cao, A. Cao, L. Lai, *Biophys. J.* **2003**, *84*, 1867–1875.
65. E. Oheix, A. F. A. Peacock, *Chem. Eur. J.* **2014**, *20*, 2829–2839.
66. M. I. Sánchez, O. Vázquez, M. E. Vázquez, J. L. Mascareñas, *Chem. Eur. J.* **2013**, *19*, 9923–9929.
67. M. I. Sánchez, J. Mosquera, M. E. Vázquez, J. L. Mascareñas, *Angew. Chem. Int. Ed.* **2014**, *53*, 9917–9921.
68. J. Rodríguez, J. Mosquera, M. E. Vázquez, J. L. Mascareñas, *Chem. Eur. J.* **2016**, *22*, 13474–13477.
69. S. Learte-Aymamí, N. Curado, J. Rodríguez, M. E. Vázquez, J. L. Mascareñas, *J. Am. Chem. Soc.* **2017**, *139*, 16188–16193.
70. S. J. Smith, R. J. Radford, R. H. Subramanian, B. R. Barnett, J. S. Figueroa, F. A. Tezcan, *Chem. Sci.* **2016**, *7*, 5453–5461.
71. R. J. Radford, P. C. Nguyen, T. B. Ditri, J. S. Figueroa, F. A. Tezcan, *Inorg. Chem.* **2010**, *49*, 4362–4369.
72. Y. Azuma, M. Imanishi, T. Yoshimura, T. Kawabata, S. Futaki, *Angew. Chem. Int. Ed.* **2009**, *48*, 6853–6856.
73. N. Lomadze, E. Gogritchiani, H.-J. Schneider, M. T. Albelda, J. Aguilar, E. García-España, S. V. Luis, *Tetrahedron Lett.* **2002**, *43*, 7801–7803.
74. N. Lomadze, H.-J. Schneider, M. T. Albelda, E. García-España, B. Verdejo, *Org. Biomol. Chem.* **2006**, *4*, 1755–1759.
75. M. Inclán, M. T. Albelda, J. C. Frías, S. Blasco, B. Verdejo, C. Serena, C. Salat-Canela, M. L. Díaz, A. García-España, E. García-España, *J. Am. Chem. Soc.* **2012**, *134*, 9644–9656.
76. M. Inclán, L. Guijarro, I. Pont, J. C. Frías, C. Rotger, F. Orvay, A. Costa, E. García-España, M. T. Albelda, *Chem. Eur. J.* **2017**, *23*, 15966–15973.
77. L. Guijarro, Á. Martínez-Camarena, J. U. Chicote, A. García-España, E. García-España, M. Inclán, B. Verdejo, J. González-García, *Molecules* **2021**, *26*, 3957.
78. N. Kotera, R. Guillot, M.-P. Teulade-Fichou, A. Granzhan, *ChemBioChem* **2017**, *18*, 618–622.
79. D. Monchaud, P. Yang, L. Lacroix, M.-P. Teulade-Fichou, J.-L. Mergny, *Angew. Chem. Int. Ed.* **2008**, *47*, 4858–4861.
80. J. T. Weiss, J. C. Dawson, K. G. Macleod, W. Rybski, C. Fraser, C. Torres-Sánchez, E. E. Patton, M. Bradley, N. O. Carragher, A. Unciti-Broceta, *Nat. Commun.* **2014**, *5*, 3277.
81. M. I. Sánchez, C. Penas, M. E. Vázquez, J. L. Mascareñas, *Chem. Sci.* **2014**, *5*, 1901–1907.
82. J. Clavadetscher, E. Indrigo, S. v. Chankeshwara, A. Lilienkampf, M. Bradley, *Angew. Chem. Int. Ed.* **2017**, *56*, 6864–6868.

83. Z. Zhao, X. Tao, Y. Xie, Q. Lai, W. Lin, K. Lu, J. Wang, W. Xia, Z. Mao, *Angew. Chem. Int. Ed.* **2022**, *61*, e202202855.
84. S. Ménard, S. M. Pupa, M. Campiglio, E. Tagliabue, *Oncogene* **2003**, *22*, 6570–6578.
85. J. Rodríguez, C. Pérez-González, M. Martínez-Calvo, J. Mosquera, J. L. Mascareñas, *RSC Adv.* **2022**, *12*, 3500–3504.
86. G. Thiabaud, R. McCall, G. He, J. F. Arambula, Z. H. Siddik, J. L. Sessler, *Angew. Chem. Int. Ed.* **2016**, *55*, 12626–12631.
87. T. Völker, F. Dempwolff, P. L. Graumann, E. Meggers, *Angew. Chem. Int. Ed.* **2014**, *53*, 10536–10540.
88. C. Streu, E. Meggers, *Angew. Chem. Int. Ed.* **2006**, *45*, 5645–5648.
89. M. A. Miller, B. Askevold, H. Mikula, R. H. Kohler, D. Pirovich, R. Weissleder, *Nat. Commun.* **2017**, *8*, 15906.
90. M. A. Miller, H. Mikula, G. Luthria, R. Li, S. Kronister, M. Prytyskach, R. H. Kohler, T. Mitchison, R. Weissleder, *ACS Nano* **2018**, *12*, 12814–12826.
91. T. L. Bray, M. Salji, A. Brombin, A. M. Pérez-López, B. Rubio-Ruiz, L. C. A. Galbraith, E. E. Patton, H. Y. Leung, A. Unciti-Broceta, *Chem. Sci.* **2018**, *9*, 7354–7361.
92. B. J. Stenton, B. L. Oliveira, M. J. Matos, L. Sinatra, G. J. L. Bernardes, *Chem. Sci.* **2018**, *9*, 4185–4189.
93. R. Friedman Ohana, S. Levin, M. G. Wood, K. Zimmerman, M. L. Dart, M. K. Schwinn, T. A. Kirkland, R. Hurst, H. T. Uyeda, L. P. Encell, K. V. Wood, *ACS Chem. Biol.* **2016**, *11*, 2608–2617.
94. P. Destito, C. Vidal, F. López, J. L. Mascareñas, *Chem. Eur. J.* **2021**, *27*, 4789–4816.
95. K. Vong, T. Yamamoto, T. Chang, K. Tanaka, *Chem. Sci.* **2020**, *11*, 10928–10933.
96. J. Konč, V. Sabatino, E. Jiménez-Moreno, E. Latocheski, L. R. Pérez, J. Day, J. B. Domingos, G. J. L. Bernardes, *Angew. Chem. Int. Ed.* **2022**, *61*, e202113519.

8 How Do Cationic Pt(II) Complexes Modify the Higher-Order Structure of DNA?

Seiji Komeda and Masako Uemura
Faculty of Pharmaceutical Sciences, Suzuka University of Medical Science, Suzuka 513–8670, Japan
komedas@suzuka-u.ac.jp, masako-u@suzuka-u.ac.jp

Yuko Yoshikawa and Kenichi Yoshikawa
Faculty of Life and Medical Sciences, Doshisha University, Kyotanabe 610-0321, Japan
yoshi2989r@gmail.com, kyoshikawd@gmail.com

CONTENTS

1 Introduction 190
    1.1 Cationic Azolato-Bridged Dinuclear Platinum(II) Complexes 191
2 DNA Interactions 193
    2.1 Reactions with Nucleobases/Mononucleotides........................... 193
    2.2 Secondary DNA Structural Changes.. 195
    2.3 Higher-Order DNA Structural Changes 197
3 Comparison between Derivatives of 5-H-Y.. 199
    3.1 Derivatives with a Linear Alkyl Chain 199
        3.1.1 Secondary Structural Changes 199
        3.1.2 Higher-Order Structural Changes 201
    3.2 Derivatives with Other Substituents 201
        3.2.1 Secondary Structural Changes 202
        3.2.2 Higher-Order Structural Changes 205
4 General Conclusions 206
Acknowledgments.. 206
Abbreviations and Definitions 207
References.. 207

DOI 10.1201/9781003270201-8

Abstract

Cationic tetrazolato-bridged dinuclear Pt(II) complexes ([{cis-Pt(NH$_3$)$_2$}$_2$(μ-OH)(μ-5-R-tetrazolato)]$^{x+}$ where $x=1$ or 2; tetrazolato-bridged complexes) are promising candidates for development as next-generation platinum-based drugs because of their potent anticancer activities. However, they also bind to DNA in a unique manner and very efficiently induce DNA shrinkage/compaction by surface charge neutralization. In this chapter, we review our recent studies on the interactions of tetrazolato-bridged complexes with DNA. Reactions with nucleobases/mononucleotides and natural dsDNA (double-stranded DNA) were investigated using spectroscopic techniques such as circular dichroism. To gain insight into the higher-order structure of dsDNA, single-molecule observations were performed by means of fluorescence microscopy and transmission electron microscopy. In most cases, upon addition of the tetrazolato-bridged complexes to calf thymus DNA, the secondary structure of the DNA was changed from the B- to C-form. In addition, it was found that genome-sized DNA underwent a higher-order structural change and was efficiently shrunken/compacted by all of the tetrazolato-bridged complexes examined in the present study, as observed in a giant phage DNA (169 kbp). Our evaluations of a variety of tetrazolato-bridged complexes reveal how the DNA compaction efficiency of the complexes changes with respect to the substituent at the tetrazolate 5-position.

KEYWORDS

Azole; Cationic Platinum Complex; Circular Dichroism; DNA Shrinkage/Compaction; Fluorescence Microscopy; Single-Molecule Observation; Transmission Electron Microscopy

1 INTRODUCTION

Genomic DNA is a long, semiflexible nucleotide polymer that carries the complete genetic information of an organism. The nucleotides of genomic DNA are arranged with two chains by forming a double helix in what is known as the B-conformation. Under certain circumstances, genomic DNA can undergo conformation changes in its higher-order structure; for example, it can be folded into a compact state to reduce its size for storage within a cell, or it can be unfolded loosely to facilitate transcription and duplication. It is known that charge neutralization plays an essential role in causing the folding transition from an elongated coil to a tightly packed globule [1–4]. These changes in the second- and higher-order structure of DNA can be induced by the interaction of the DNA with inorganic [5] and organic [6] cations. For example, it is well-known that the conformation of double-stranded DNA (dsDNA) is regulated by divalent alkaline-earth metal ions [7, 8] such as Mg^{2+}, which can bind to DNA either directly or indirectly via hydrogen bonds between the coordinating water molecules surrounding the metal ion and the DNA [9]. In biological systems, intracellular Mg^{2+} is abundant, and it neutralizes the negative charge of the phosphate backbone of DNA to control the second- and higher-order DNA structure, modulating the folding or unfolding of chromatin [10]. Similarly, multivalent transition-metal ions such as Fe^{3+} are also known to induce conformational changes in DNA [11]. Cationic transition-metal complexes that non-covalently interact with DNA without disrupting the stability of the ligand(s) bound to the metal have also been reported, many of which bind to the minor groove [12] or the phosphate backbone [13–15] of dsDNA, or possibly act as DNA intercalators [16, 17]. Due to the unique geometry of these cationic transition-metal complexes, they attract negatively charged DNA to which they bind via interaction between the complex ligands and the DNA [18]. Thus, transition-metal complexes show potential for development as agents that can be used to precisely control the conformation both of the second-order and higher-order structures of DNA.

1.1 Cationic Azolato-Bridged Dinuclear Platinum(II) Complexes

Platinum (Pt) is not an essential metal for living organisms, and it is therefore excreted as a potentially toxic heavy metal. However, the covalent interaction between Pt and DNA has been successfully harnessed in the clinic for the treatment of cancer. Platinum-based antineoplastic drugs (platins) are a group of chemotherapeutics that are widely used for the treatment of a variety of cancers. The first, and most studied, of these drugs is the platinum(II) complex *cis*-diamminedichloridoplatinum(II) (cisplatin, Figure 1) [19], which has been shown to exert its anticancer effects by forming covalent Pt–DNA adducts [20,21], such as 1,2-intrastrand crosslinks [22,23] (see Figure 1a) and interstrand crosslinks [24,25]. Recently, Pt(II) complexes with distinctively different structures from those of the currently available platins have been synthesized as drug candidates that show high efficacy against chemotherapy-insensitive cancers and, possibly, cancers that have acquired resistance to the currently available Pt-based drugs [26]. Since the current platins are all electronically neutral mononuclear Pt(II) complexes, some cationic di- or trinuclear Pt(II) complexes have been developed and are considered good candidates [27]. During the development of these new Pt(II) complexes, several unique covalent and non-covalent Pt(II)–DNA interactions related to their anticancer effects have been described [28–32].

Some research groups have introduced a series of cationic dinuclear platinum(II) complexes ([{*cis*-Pt(NH$_3$)$_2$}$_2$(μ-OH)(μ-azolato)]$^{2+}$; hereafter, azolato-bridged complexes, Figure 1) bridged by OH$^-$ and an azolate such as pyrazolate (AMPZ) [33], 1,2,3-triazolate (AMTA) [34], or tetrazolate (5-H-X and 5-H-Y) [35]. These azolato-bridged complexes form 1,2-intrastrand crosslinks with minimal bending of DNA helix axis via substitution of a nitrogen atom of a nucleobase for the OH$^-$ bridge of the azolato-bridged complex (see Figures 1b, c, and 2) [33, 36, 37], whereas those formed by cisplatin are known to bend the axis significantly as illustrated in Figure 1a [22, 23]. Among these azolato-bridged complexes, we have found that the tetrazolato-bridged dinuclear Pt(II) complex 5-H-Y ([{*cis*-Pt(NH^3)^2}$_2$(μ-OH)(μ-tetrazolato-N2,N3)](ClO^4)^2) has potent anticancer activity and remarkably high antitumor efficacy in xenograft mouse models of human pancreatic cancer [35, 38], and the most studied azolato-bridged complexes as the drug candidates are derivatives of 5-H-Y. During our drug-discovery studies

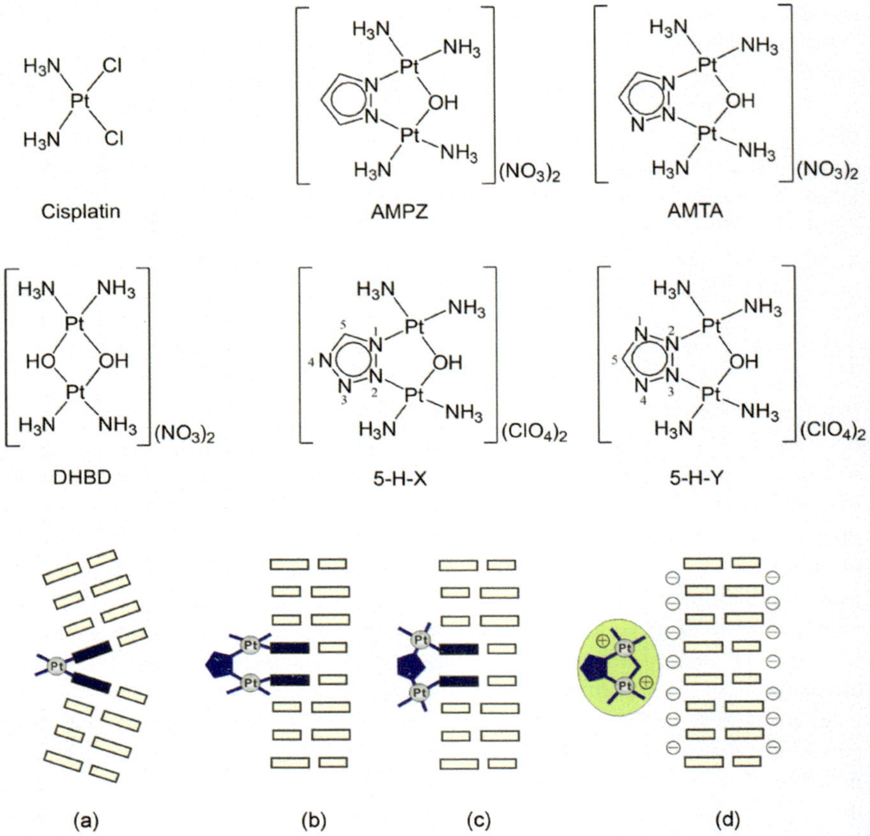

FIGURE 1 (Upper) Structures of cisplatin, pyrazolato-bridged complex (AMPZ), 1,2,3-triazolato-bridged complex (AMTA), dihydroxido-bridged dimer (DHBD), and tetrazolato-bridged complexes (5-H-X, 5-H-Y). (Lower) Schematics of major platinum-DNA adducts: (a) 1,2-intrastrand crosslink with severe DNA distortion (cisplatin analogues); (b) 1,2-intrastrand crosslink with minimal DNA distortion (AMPZ [b]; AMTA, 5-H-X, or 5-H-Y [c]); and (d) electrostatic association common for azolato-bridged complexes.

searching for a new anticancer agent, it was found that 5-H-Y and its derivatives induce dramatic conformational changes in the second- and higher-order structures of DNA via unique covalent and non-covalent DNA bindings (see Figure 1b–d), which have not been reported for the current platins. This suggests that these Pt(II) complexes may also be used as molecular tools to control the higher-order structure of DNA. In this chapter, based on circular dichroism (CD) measurements and single-molecule observations made by fluorescence microscopy (FM) and transmission electron microscopy (TEM), we review how 5-H-Y and its derivatives induce changes in the secondary and higher-order structures of DNA.

2 DNA INTERACTIONS

2.1 REACTIONS WITH NUCLEOBASES/MONONUCLEOTIDES

Our synthesis of 5-H-Y yielded not only 5-H-Y but also its linkage isomer 5-H-X ([{cis-Pt(NH$_3$)$_2$}$_2$(μ-OH)(μ-tetrazolato-*N1,N2*)] (ClO$_4$)$_2$, Figure 1) in a molar ratio of 6.5:3.5 (5-H-X:5-H-Y), and the two linkage isomers were separated and purified by reverse-phase liquid chromatography [35]. We then investigated the reactions of 5-H-X and 5-H-Y with the guanine derivatives 9-ethylguanine (9EtG) [39] and guanosine 5′-monophosphate (GMP) [40], and we characterized the final products by means of ^{1}H and ^{195}Pt nuclear magnetic resonance spectroscopy, since guanine is the most preferentially bound nucleobase by platins [41, 42]. Azolato-bridged complexes are known to bind two equivalents of guanine derivative at the N7 nitrogen atom of the guanine base [33, 34, 43], and Figure 2 shows the possible steps in the reactions of 5-H-X and 5-H-Y with 9EtG or GMP. Both 5-H-X and 5-H-Y yielded an identical final product ([{cis-Pt(NH$_3$)$_2$(9EtG-*N7*)}$_2$(μ-tetrazolato-*N1,N3*)]$^{3+}$ with 9EtG and [{cis-Pt(NH$_3$)$_2$(GMP-*N7*)}$_2$(μ-tetrazolato-*N1,N3*)]$^-$ with GMP), which is an asymmetric compound with N1,N3 platinum coordination resulting from a Pt(II) migration process on the tetrazolate ring [39, 40]. Thus, substitution of the N7 nitrogen atom of the guanine base for

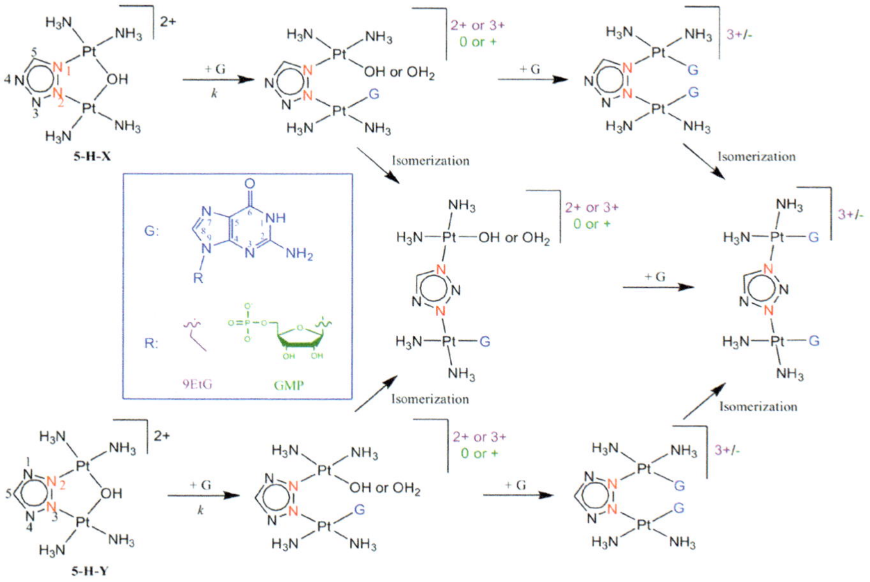

FIGURE 2 Proposed steps in the reaction of 5-H-X and 5-H-Y with two molar equivalents of 9-ethylguanine (9EtG) or guanosine 5′-monophosphate (GMP). *k* is the second-order reaction rate constant. The first step in both reaction pathways, the substitution of the OH$^-$ bridge for the N7 nitrogen atom in the guanine base of 9EtG or GMP, is the rate-determining step.

the μ-hydroxido bridge of the linkage isomer is the beginning of the reaction pathway, followed by a slightly different isomerization process.

The formation of 1,2-intrastrand DNA adducts (i.e., crosslinking with adjacent purine bases) by the pyrazolato-bridged complex AMPZ, which cannot be isomerized [33], is known to accompany no significant bend in the helix axis [44, 45], and the Watson–Crick base-pairing remains intact (see Figure 1b) [36]. Given that isomerization occurs during formation of the 1,2-intrastrand DNA adduct by 5-H-X and 5-H-Y, we predicted that the local DNA structure at the platinated site would be slightly distorted compared to that formed by AMPZ [36]. However, isomerization is not likely to increase the curvature of dsDNA, induce unwinding of the double helix, or induce compression of the major groove, as predicted by a simulation study for AMTA, which is isomerized (see Figure 1c) [37]. Accordingly, 5-H-X and 5-H-Y are likely to produce 1,2-intrastrand DNA adducts similar to those formed by AMTA, which is known to induce the second- and higher-order structural change of DNA [46].

The reactions of 5-H-X and 5-H-Y with 9EtG or GMP were kinetically analyzed in unbuffered D_2O or 0.1 M phosphate-buffered D_2O solution at 310 K. Based on our previous findings [33, 34, 47], the rate-determining step was considered to be the substitution of the N7 nitrogen atom in the guanine base of 9EtG or GMP for the OH$^-$ bridge; therefore, second-order kinetics were applied to the reactions of both linkage isomers. This is in contrast to the rate-determining step for cisplatin binding to DNA ($t_{1/2}$ approx. 2 h at 310 K) [48], which is a hydrolysis reaction and therefore can be analyzed by first-order kinetics. Table 1 shows the values determined for the second-order rate constant (k) for the rate-determining step and the half-lives ($t_{1/2}$) of the reactant. The reactions of 5-H-X and 5-H-Y with 9EtG in unbuffered D_2O proceeded at almost the same rate, and 5-H-X

TABLE 1
Results of a Kinetic Analysis of the Reaction of 5-H-X or 5-H-Y with Two Molar Equivalents of 9-Ethylguanine (9EtG) or Guanosine 5′-Monophosphate (GMP) at 310 K

| Complex | 9EtG | | GMP | | | |
| | In D_2O | | In D_2O | | In 0.1 M Phosphate-Buffered D_2O Solution (pD 6.9) | |
	k (M^{-1}s^{-1})	$t_{1/2}$ (h)	k (M^{-1}s^{-1})	$t_{1/2}$ (h)	k (M^{-1}s^{-1})	$t_{1/2}$ (h)
5-H-X	3.97×10^{-4}	87.4	N.D.[a]	N.D.[a]	5.62×10^{-4}	61.8
5-H-Y	3.87×10^{-4}	89.8	14.5×10^{-4}	23.8	4.75×10^{-4}	73.1

Source: Taken with permission from Refs. [39, 40].
k, second-order reaction rate constant; $t_{1/2}$, reactant half-life.
[a] Not determined because of precipitate formation.

reacted with GMP at slightly faster rate than 5-H-Y in 0.1 M phosphate-buffered D_2O solution. In the case of 5-H-Y, the reactions with GMP proceeded faster than those with 9EtG, and the reactivity with GMP dramatically increased in unbuffered D_2O solution, both of which are common tendencies among azolato-bridged complexes [34, 40, 43, 49]. This indicates the affinity of the OH^- bridge and/or ammine ligands of the platinum complexes for phosphate (i.e., the phosphate in the buffer competitively binds to the platinum complexes electrostatically and competes with the phosphate groups of GMP). Therefore, these complexes can be expected to have a high non-covalent (dipolar) affinity for the phosphate backbone of DNA, which might be important for non-covalent DNA interaction processes such as minor-groove binding.

2.2 Secondary DNA Structural Changes

The secondary structure of DNA can take one of several forms (A-, B-, or C-form for right-handed helixes; Z-form for left-handed helixes). A-form DNA has a tighter helical turn compared with that of the B-form. DNA transitions from the B- to A-form occur under low relative humidity (<75%). The form of a given sample of DNA can be identified by examination of its CD profile, which is strongly affected by stacking interactions [50]. For B-form DNA, the CD spectrum shows a positive peak at around 275 nm (positive Cotton effect) and a negative peak at around 240 nm (negative Cotton effect). For A-form DNA, the CD spectrum shows a blue shift of the positive peak, the negative peak at around 240 nm disappears, and a new negative peak emerges at around 210 nm. Another type of right-handed DNA is the C-form, which is also observed under conditions of low relative humidity [51] but in association with metal ions such as Li^+, Mg^{2+}, and Na^+ [52,53], which are densely charged and bind strongly to phosphate oxygen. C-form DNA is a slightly more wound form than the B-form [54] and is characterized by negative Cotton effects at around 235 and 278 nm. The left-handed helical turn in Z-DNA is the most elongated among the four forms, with a helical periodicity of around 12 bp per turn. Z-DNA shows an almost reversed spectrum compared to that of B-DNA, with a positive Cotton effect at around 260 nm and a negative Cotton effect at around 290 nm.

We examined the changes in the CD spectra of calf thymus (CT) DNA exposed to 5-H-X or 5-H-Y [55] (Figure 3) to investigate how these complexes alter the secondary structure of dsDNA. CT DNA is a dsDNA with an average size of 15–23 kbp and is often used to examine the relationship between the second-order structures and DNA-binding drugs [56]. First, we examined the changes immediately after exposure to different molar ratios of 5-H-X and 5-H-Y at 310 K (Figure 3a). The magnitude of both the positive and negative Cotton effects decreased with increasing molar ratio, with the change of the positive Cotton effect at around 278 nm being much greater than that of the negative Cotton effect at around 235 nm. This finding indicates that the CT DNA was transformed from B- to C-form. We then examined the changes in the CD spectra over time after exposure of 30 µM CT DNA to a fixed amount (10 µM) of 5-H-X or 5-H-Y at

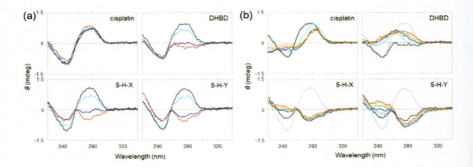

FIGURE 3 Circular dichroism spectra of 30 µM calf thymus (CT) DNA in the presence of cisplatin, dihydroxo-bridged dimer (DHBD), 5-H-X, or 5-H-Y. (a) Spectra obtained immediately after addition of the complexes at a molar ratio (Pt complex:phosphate) of 0 (black), 0.0333 (light blue), 0.167 (blue), or 0.333 (red). (b) Spectra obtained for the reaction between CT DNA and 10 µM azolato-bridged complex for 0 (black), 6 (light blue), 12 (blue), 24 (green), 48 (orange), and 72 h (red) at 310 K. The gray line shows the control (no platinum(II) complex added). (Reproduced by permission from Ref. [55]; copyright 2012 the Royal Society of Chemistry.)

310 K (Figure 3b). Characteristic spectral changes of platinated dsDNA were observed in the CD spectra at around 243 nm and the magnitude of these changes increased in a time-dependent manner. However, the spectral change at around 243 nm was not observed when the reactions were conducted at 277 K, even though 5-H-X and 5-H-Y still induced transformation of the CT DNA from B- to C-form. This indicated that the interaction of 5-H-X or 5-H-Y with CT DNA is a two-step process involving first non-covalent interactions that cause an immediate decrease in the positive Cotton effect at around 278 nm, and then covalent interactions that cause a later decrease in the negative Cotton effect at around 243 nm.

The first step of the interaction of 5-H-X and 5-H-Y with CT DNA likely occurs through non-covalent interactions with the DNA, as indicated by the rapid changes of the spectra even at the lower temperature. Cisplatin, an electronically neutral complex, induced only slight dose-dependent changes in the spectra (Figure 3a). However, a spectral change similar to those of 5-H-X and 5-H-Y was observed at around 275 nm in the case of cis-$[Pt(NH_3)_2(\mu\text{-}OH)]_2(NO_3)_2$ (dihydroxido-bridged dimer, DHBD, see Figure 1 for its structure), which has a 2+ positive charge, the same as 5-H-X and 5-H-Y. Therefore, it is likely that the positive charge of the compounds contributes to the pre-association of the complexes with negatively charged DNA. Both 5-H-X and 5-H-Y induced spectral changes at around 278 nm, even at much lower concentrations compared with bare metal cations such as Li^+ and Cs^+ [52, 53], which are also known to induce DNA transition from B- to C-form. This indicates that the non-covalent interactions include not only simple electrostatic associations but also other interactions such as hydrogen bonds.

2.3 HIGHER-ORDER DNA STRUCTURAL CHANGES

Unlike the helix-to-coil transition (melting transition) and the secondary structural transition, the fundamental characteristics of the higher-order structure of DNA become apparent only for long DNA molecules above several tens of kilobase pairs (kbp) in length. dsDNA in the B-form is physically characterized by a persistence length of around 50 nm (150 bp), indicating that short DNA behaves as a rigid rod (Figure 4a). In contrast, long DNA behaves as a semiflexible polymer (Figure 4b). This implies that individual short DNA molecules below the size of several hundreds of base pairs never exhibit transition from an elongated state to a compacted state. A long DNA molecule undergoes a marked change in its higher-order structure; for example, by adding a multivalent cation such as polyamine, long DNA undergoes a folding transition from elongated coil (coil, C) to compact globule (globule, G), accompanied by a volume decrease on the order of 10^{-4} to 10^{-5} [1–4] (Figure 4b–d). In this section, we describe the higher-order structural changes induced by Pt(II) complexes in long DNA molecules with lengths greater than 100 kbp.

Note that FM observation of single, long DNA molecules affords useful information on the higher-order structural changes that occur in solution (Figure 4c and d), regardless of the relatively low, sub-micrometer resolution of the approach compared with the higher resolution of TEM (Figure 4e) and atomic force microscopy (AFM). Therefore, TEM and AFM observations provide high-resolution images of DNA molecules adsorbed on a solid surface, that is, for the fixed state without Brownian motion, whereas FM provides images of individual DNA molecules under Brownian fluctuation by suppressing the artificial effect of surface adsorption.

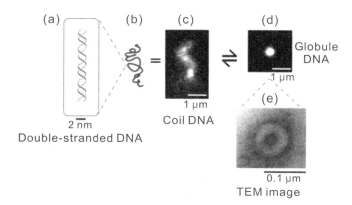

FIGURE 4 (a–e) Schematic representation of the higher-order structural transition of genome-sized long DNA, as observed by (c, d) fluorescence microscopy (FM) and (e) transmission electron microscopy (TEM). Transition between the elongated coil state and a compacted globule state induced by the addition of spermidine (3+) was observed by FM and TEM for a single duplex T4 phage DNA (166 kbp). (Reproduced by permission from Ref. [4]; Copyright 2002 CRC press, Boca Raton.)

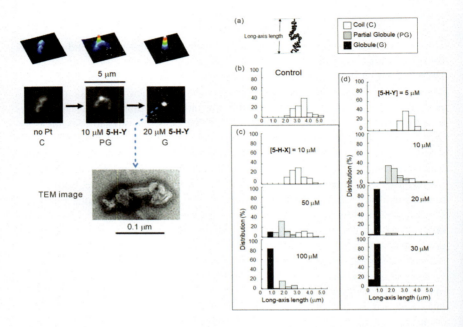

FIGURE 5 (Left) Schematic representation of a fluorescent image of T4 DNA and transmission electron miscroscopy image of compact T4 DNA particle in the presence of 5-H-Y. (Right) Size distributions for the long-axis length of T4 DNA in solution, together with the conformation type observed in images of the DNA. (a) In buffer solution. (b) In the presence of cisplatin. (c) In the presence of 5-H-X. (d) In the presence of 5-H-Y. (Reproduced by permission from Ref. [57]; copyright 2011 American Chemical Society.)

Figure 5 (left) shows representative FM images of single T4 DNA molecules in an aqueous solution at different concentrations of 5-H-Y (i.e., under Brownian motion with intramolecular and translational fluctuations) [57]. In the absence of 5-H-Y, the DNA existed in an elongated coil conformation. In the presence of 10 μM 5-H-Y, the DNA shrank by partial compaction along the molecular chain (i.e., by intramolecular phase separation or partial globule generation). When the concentration of 5-H-Y was increased to 20 μM, the DNA fully formed a globule. These partial and full globule states were stable, even at a high concentration (100 mM) of NaCl, indicating that the resultant platinated DNAs were also stable. TEM observation indicated that 5-H-X and 5-H-Y both induced collapse of the DNA into an irregularly packed structure [57]. This DNA compaction is markedly different from that induced by trivalent condensing agents such as spermidine and $[Co(NH_3)_6]^{3+}$, which shrink DNA into a well-ordered toroidal structure (Figure 4e) [58–60].

Figure 5 (right) shows the size distribution of the long-axis length of T4 DNA together with the conformation of the DNA (coil, partial globule, or globule). 5-H-Y induced partial globule and full globule formation at lower concentrations than did 5-H-X, and the potency of this compaction decreased in the order

5-H-Y > 5-H-X >> cisplatin. Cisplatin, even at 100 µM, had little effect on the conformation of the DNA molecules, indicating the strength of the effect of 5-H-Y on the higher-order structure of DNA.

3 COMPARISON BETWEEN DERIVATIVES OF 5-H-Y

3.1 Derivatives with a Linear Alkyl Chain

Derivatization of 5-H-Y has been carried out [61], and it would be very interesting to see how substitution at the C5 atom of the tetrazolate ring affects the DNA conformational changes induced by azolato-bridged complexes. In addition, lengthening the alkyl chain not only makes platinum(II) complexes more hydrophobic, but also affords them a surfactant-like property. Therefore, we synthesized nine derivatives of 5-H-Y with linear alkyl chains of various lengths ([{cis-Pt(NH$_3$)$_2$}$_2$(µ-OH)(µ-5-R-tetrazolato-$N2,N3$)](NO$_3$)$_2$ where R=(CH$_2$)$_n$CH$_3$, n=0–8, complexes **1–9**, Figure 6) and examined the efficiency by which they induce DNA conformational changes [62].

3.1.1 Secondary Structural Changes

To examine the secondary DNA structural changes induced by derivatives **1–9**, we conducted a CD study using CT DNA and various concentrations of the derivatives (Figure 7a) [62]. Upon addition of the derivatives to CT DNA, the spectral changes were comparable to those induced by 5-H-X and 5-H-Y, indicating that the derivatives each induced a B- to C-form transition in the structure of the CT DNA. These spectral changes were weakened in the presence of a high concentration of NaCl (200 mM), indicating that electrostatic attractions between the phosphate groups of the CT DNA and the positively charged Pt complexes contributed to the induced secondary structural changes.

To compare the ability of derivatives **1–9** to induce the secondary DNA structural changes, $\Delta\theta$, which is the difference between ellipticities at 278 nm observed

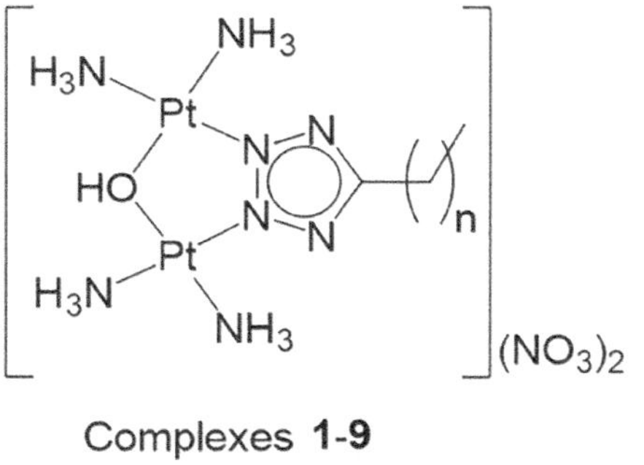

Complexes 1-9

1, n = 0
2, n = 1
3, n = 2
4, n = 3
5, n = 4
6, n = 5
7, n = 6
8, n = 7
9, n = 8

FIGURE 6 Structures of a series of 5-H-Y derivatives, 5-alkyl-tetrazolato-bridged dinuclear Pt(II) complexes (**1–9**), with the general formula [{cis-Pt(NH$_3$)$_2$}$_2$(µ-OH)(µ-5-R-tetrazolato-$N2,N3$)](NO$_3$)$_2$, where R=(CH$_2$)$_n$CH$_3$ (n=0–8).

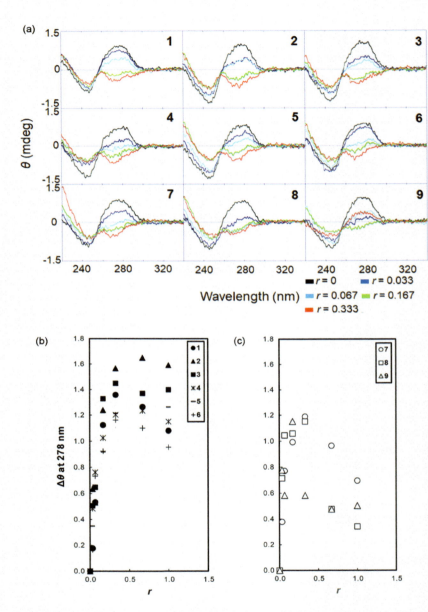

FIGURE 7 (a) Circular dichroism spectra of 30 μM calf thymus DNA obtained immediately after adding different concentrations of complexes **1–9**. *r* indicates the molar ratio used (Pt complex:phosphate). (Lower) Plots of $\Delta\theta$ at 278 nm *vs. r*. $\Delta\theta$ is the difference in ellipticity at 278 nm determined in the absence of platinum(II) complex (θ_0) and at the molar ratio *r* (θ_r). Plots are drawn by classifying them into 5-H-Y-type (b) and non-5-H-Y-type (c). (Reproduced by permission from Ref. [62]; copyright 2017 by American Chemical Society.)

in the absence of a platinum(II) complex (θ_0) and those obtained at the molar ratio of r (θ_r), is calculated by using the following equation:

$$\Delta\theta = \theta_0 - \theta_r$$

Plots of $\Delta\theta$ versus r for derivatives **1–9** are shown in Figure 7b and c. There are two plots: 5-H-Y-type (b) and non-5-H-Y-type (c). In both types, as the molar ratio increased, $\Delta\theta$ also increased. In the 5-H-Y-type plot, for **1–6**, the plots peak at around $r=0.333$ and further addition of complex results in a slight decrease in $\Delta\theta$. In the non-5-H-Y-type plot, for **7–9**, $\Delta\theta$ decreased with increasing molar ratio, indicating that the positive band in the CD spectra at around 278 nm increased in intensity until it was comparable with that for DNA that was predominantly in the B-form. This kind of spectral change has previously been reported for the cationic surfactant n-cetyltrimethylammonium bromide, for which the change was attributed to the compaction and decompaction of individual CT DNA molecules [63]. Derivatives **1–9** were all water-soluble cationic complexes with a 2+ charge. However, the alkyl chain substituted at C5 of the tetrazole ring was a hydrophobic moiety. Therefore, derivatives **7–9** with a relatively long linear alkyl chain were expected to have surfactant-like properties. Based on this assumption, the critical micelle concentrations (cmc) of **7–9** were determined by means of an electrical conductance method; no determinable cmc was obtained below saturating concentration of derivative **6** [62], and the results indicated that non-5-H-Y-type spectral changes are likely the result of the surfactant-like behavior of derivatives **7–9**.

3.1.2 Higher-Order Structural Changes

Figure 8 shows representative FM images of single T4 phage DNA molecules in the presence of derivative **2**, **5**, or **9**. These derivatives caused transition of the DNA conformation from the coil (C) state to the globule (G) state via the partial globule (PG) state. Figure 9 shows how the conformation of T4 phage DNA changes depending on the concentration of derivatives **1–9** and 5-H-Y. Single-molecule observations revealed that the probability of the DNA being in the fully compact state or in the globule state was more than 80% [62]. Here, a bimodal effect was observed with respect to the ability of the derivatives to cause folding of the DNA into the globule state. That is, as the length of the alkyl chain increased, the DNA compaction efficiency of 5-H-Y and **1–4** decreased, whereas that of **5–7** increased. DNA compaction efficiency plateaued with **7–9**, probably due to the surfactant-like properties of these complexes and their ability to form micelles. The different morphologies of the globule DNA in the presence of **2** or **8** were elucidated by TEM studies and representative images are shown in Figure 9 [62].

3.2 Derivatives with Other Substituents

In addition to the derivatives of a linear alkyl chain, we synthesized three derivatives of 5-H-Y with different substituents at the tetrazolate C5

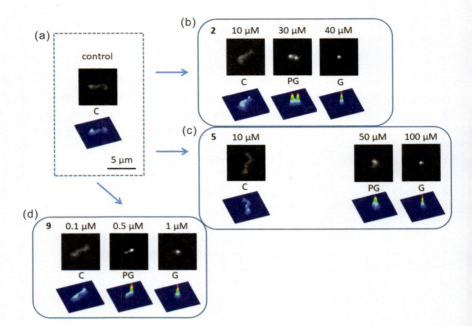

FIGURE 8 Representative fluorescence microscopy (FM) images of individual T4 phage DNA molecules moving freely in solution, and the corresponding quasi-three-dimensional profiles of fluorescence intensity. (a) Control: FM image of a single T4 phage DNA molecule exhibiting Brownian motion in a buffered solution. (b–d) Upon addition of **2**, **5**, or **9**, concentration-dependent conformational changes in the structure of the T4 phage DNA were observed. C, coil; PG, partial globule; G, globule. (Reproduced by permission from Ref. [62]; copyright 2017 American Chemical Society.)

([{cis-Pt(NH$_3$)}$_2$(μ-OH)(μ-5-R-tetrazolato-$N2,N3$)]$^{x+}$ where R=C$_6$H$_5$ (**10**), CH$_2$COOCH$_2$CH$_3$ (**11**), or CH$_2$COO$^-$ (**12**), $x=2$ for **10** and **11**, and 1 for **12**) (Figure 10) [38]. Derivative **10** has a phenyl ring attached at tetrazolate C5. **12** is a hydrolysis product of **11**, both of which possess different total positive charges of 2+ and 1+ for **11** and **12**, respectively. We then evaluated the changes these derivatives induced in the second- and higher-order DNA structures and compared them with the changes induced by 5-H-Y and **1**.

3.2.1 Secondary Structural Changes

Figure 11 shows CD spectra obtained from a study using CT DNA and different molar ratios of four derivatives of 5-H-Y: **1**, **10**, **11**, and **12** [64]. The most strikingly different spectra were obtained for **10**, which showed increased ellipticity at around 260 nm and decreased ellipticity at around 278 nm compared to the control spectrum shown in black. Further addition of **10** in molar ratios of 0.667 and 1.00 to CT DNA increased the intensity of the positive Cotton effect at around 260 nm and induced a small redshift. A similar increase in ellipticity at around

How Do Cationic Pt(II) Complexes Modify the Structure of DNA?

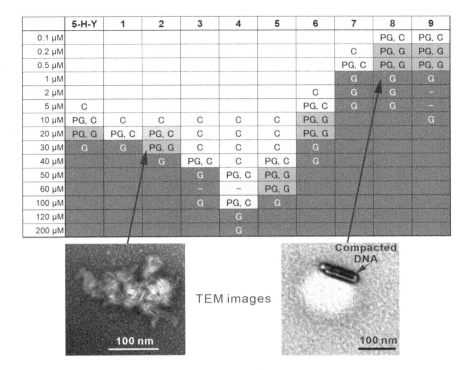

FIGURE 9 (Upper) Conformational states of T4 DNA in the presence of various concentrations of 5-H-Y [57], **1** [64], or **2–9** [62]. C, coil; PG, partial globule; G, globule. Cells marked with a label represent the results of our observation of 50–100 DNA molecules. (Lower) Representative transmission electron microscopy (TEM) images of compacted T4 DNA particles (0.1 μM) in the presence of 20 μM of **2** (left); rod-like compacted T4 DNA molecules on the surface of the spherical self-assembled structures formed by 1 μM **8** (right). (Reproduced by permission from Ref. [62]; copyright 2017 American Chemical Society.)

265 nm has been reported in CD measurements of a dsDNA with increasing molar ratio of phenyltetrazoles synthetically attached to consecutive nucleobases [65]. This implies that, after binding, **10** is arranged in a regular manner along the helix of the CT DNA.

Compared with 5-H-Y and **1**, **11** induced small dose-dependent changes at around 278 nm and almost no change at around 243 nm, and **12** induced almost no spectral changes at all. This suggests that **11** changes the secondary DNA structure from the B- to C-form but is less potent than 5-H-Y or **1**. Under physiological conditions, DNA is highly negatively charged due to the phosphate groups in the deoxyribose-phosphate backbone. Therefore, electrostatic attraction between the negatively charged DNA and the positively charged tetrazolato-bridged complexes is generated. As mentioned in Sections 2.2 and 3.1.1, electrostatic interactions are

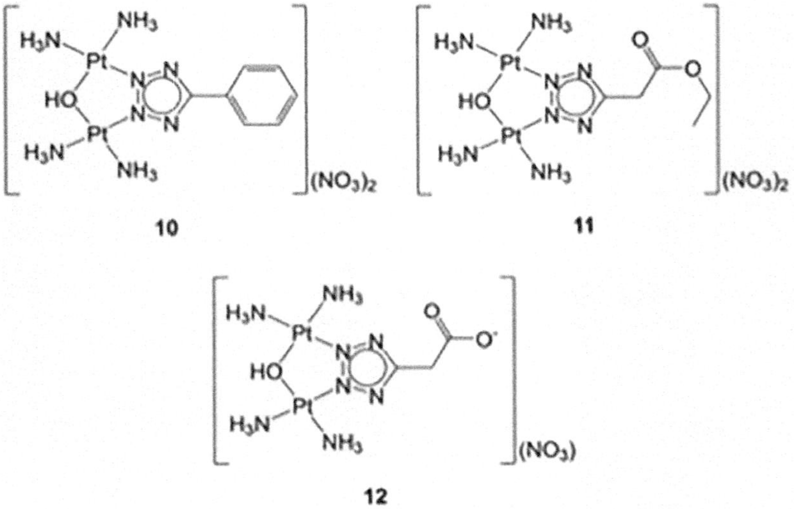

FIGURE 10 Structures of 5-H-Y derivatives with the general formula [{cis-Pt(NH$_3$)$_2$}$_2$(μ-OH)(μ-5-R′-tetrazolato-$N2,N3$)](NO$_3$)$_y$, where R′=C$_6$H$_5$ (**10**), CH$_2$COOC$_2$H$_5$ (**11**), or COO$^-$ (**12**); y=1 (**12**) or 2 (**10** and **11**).

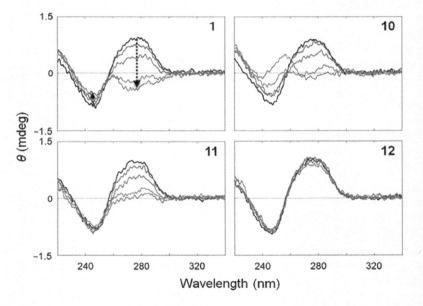

FIGURE 11 Circular dichroism spectra of 30 μM calf thymus DNA obtained immediately after adding different concentrations of complexes **1** and **10–12**. The molar ratios (Pt complex:phosphate) were 0, 0.033, 0.067, 0.167, and 0.333. (Reproduced by permission from Ref. [64]; copyright 2013 Elsevier.)

likely to be strongly involved in the observed dose-dependent spectral changes for three reasons: (1) the changes were elicited immediately after the derivatives were added; (2) the changes were observed even at 277 K, which is a temperature at which covalent bonds are not readily formed; and (3) the changes disappeared after the addition of NaCl. All three of these observations were made in the case of **11**. Thus, **11** can induce secondary structural changes of DNA from the B- to C-form by electrostatic attractions like other tetrazolato-bridged complexes with a 2+ charge. In contrast, **12** possesses an acetate group, the pK_a of which is 3.23, as determined by titration [64]. Thus, **12** primarily exists in an ionic form with a 1+ charge when in solution buffered at pH 7.4 (the proportion of ions to total molecules calculated using the Henderson-Hasselbalch equation is 99.993%). The extremely decreased spectral change induced by **12** indicates that the magnitude of the positive charge of tetrazolato-bridged complexes is positively correlated with the potency of the complexes to induce the B- to C-form transition of DNA.

3.2.2 Higher-Order Structural Changes

Figure 12 shows the change of the higher-order structure of T4 phage DNA by the addition of 5-H-Y, **1**, **10**, **11**, or **12**, as determined by single-molecule observations by FM. All of the derivatives caused the folding of the DNA from a coil into a globule via an intermediate partial globule state. Of the derivatives, **12** had the highest potency to induce compaction, and this potency was similar to that of 5-H-Y. However, it should be noted that **12** had a negligible effect on the secondary structure of DNA, indicating that the effects of a derivative on the secondary structure and on the higher-order structure show no correlation. Because **12** possesses a potential hydrogen bond acceptor in the form of an acetate group, it is likely that **12** binds strongly to the minor and major grooves of DNA by hydrogen bonding with the nucleobases.

	5-H-Y	1	10	11	12
1 µM					C
2 µM					PG, C
5 µM	C				–
10 µM	PG, G	C	C	C	PG, C
20 µM	G	PG, C	–	C	G
30 µM		G	–	PG, C	
100 µM			C	PG, C	
150 µM			PG, G	G	
200 µM			G		

FIGURE 12 Conformational states of T4 phage DNA in the presence of various concentrations of 5-H-Y [68], **1** [64], or **10–12** [64]. C, coil; PG, partial globule; G, globule. Cells marked with a label represent the results of our observation of 50–100 DNA molecules. (Reproduced by permission from Ref. [64]; copyright 2013 Elsevier.)

This investigation would ultimately provide useful information regarding the relationship between DNA structural changes and how substituents at the tetrazolate C5 atom and different molecular charges influence the ability of the derivatives to induce second- or higher-order DNA structural changes.

4 GENERAL CONCLUSIONS

The tetrazolato-bridged complexes are a series of promising candidates for development as the next generation of platinum-based drugs. Our DNA conformational study showed that the tetrazolato-bridged complexes can modulate the higher-order structure of DNA. It was found that DNA can be compacted very efficiently by covalent and non-covalent binding by these complexes. Also, it is known that 5-H-Y induces folding of chromatin, which is a complex of DNA and protein, much more efficiently than the Mg^{2+} ion does [66]. In addition, the advantage of these complexes (other than complex **11**) is that they are incorporated into cancer cells much more than cisplatin is [49, 61, 66], suggesting the possibility of using these complexes to affect changes in the structure of chromatin within cells. We have also found that the efficiency of DNA compaction can be controlled by changing the length of the alkyl chain of the substituent at the tetrazole C5 atom. There is no doubt that the positive charge of the tetrazolato-bridged complex is very important for DNA compaction; however, even if the total positive charge of the complex is low, the complex may induce DNA compaction, as indicated by our comparison between complexes **11** and **12**. These observations suggest that the induction of second- and higher-order DNA structural changes by these complexes is not necessarily related to one another. Indeed, it has been reported that spermidine and $[Co(NH_3)_6]^{3+}$ induce DNA compaction without inducing any changes in the CD spectrum using a T7 DNA (40 kbp) [60] or λ DNA (48 kbp) [67]. Furthermore, our findings show that the non-covalent interactions between the complexes and DNA can be divided into two distinctive types – one originating from ionic attraction and the other originating from hydrogen bonding and/or van der Waals interactions, both of which are followed by covalent interactions. Finally, although the rate of formation of covalent DNA adducts is slow, we confirmed that they eventually do form. However, this suggests that it may be possible to design a reagent that causes DNA shrinkage/compaction without the formation of covalent DNA adducts [68-71], enabling reversible DNA conformational changes to be induced. Thus, there are many avenues of research still open for exploration in this field and rationally designed derivatives with high DNA compaction efficiency are expected in the near future.

ACKNOWLEDGMENTS

We are grateful to Drs S. Harusawa and H. Yoneyama at Osaka Medical and Pharmaceutical University for providing the synthetic materials for the dinuclear Pt(II) complexes. This work was partially supported by JSPS KAKENHI Grant Number 20H01877 (K.Y.) and 19K07018 (S. K.).

ABBREVIATIONS AND DEFINITIONS

5-H-X and 5-H-Y	tetrazolato-bridged dinuclear Pt(II) complexes
θ	ellipticity
9EtG	9-ethylguanine
AFM	atomic force microscopy
AMPZ	pyrazolato-bridged dinuclear Pt(II) complex
AMTA	1,2,3-triazolato-bridged complex dinuclear Pt(II) complex
azolato-bridged complex	azolato-bridged dinuclear platinum(II) complex
CD	circular dichroism
cmc	critical micelle concentration
CT	calf thymus
DHBD	dihydroxido-bridged dimer
dsDNA	double-stranded deoxyribonucleic acid
FM	fluorescence microscopy
GMP	guanosine 5'-monophosphate
k	second-order rate constant
platin	platinum-based antineoplastic drug
$t_{1/2}$	half-life
TEM	transmission electron microscopy

REFERENCES

1. K. Yoshikawa, M. Takahashi, V. Vasilevskaya, A. Khokhlov, *Phys. Rev. Lett.* **1996**, *76*, 3029.
2. K. Yoshikawa, Y. Yoshikawa, T. Kanbe, *Chem. Phys. Lett.* **2002**, *354*, 354–359.
3. A. Estevez-Torres, D. Baigl, *Soft Matter* **2011**, *7*, 6746–6756.
4. K. Yoshikawa, Y. Yoshikawa, in *Pharmaceutical Perspectives of Nucleic Acid-Based Therapy*, Eds R. I. Mahato, S. W. Kim, CRC Press, Boca Raton, **2002**, pp. 123–147.
5. V. A. Bloomfield, *Biopolymers* **1997**, *44*, 269–282.
6. K. Hirano, M. Ichikawa, T. Ishido, M. Ishikawa, Y. Baba, K. Yoshikawa, *Nucleic Acids Res.* **2012**, *40*, 284–289.
7. C. Tongu, T. Kenmotsu, Y. Yoshikawa, A. Zinchenko, N. Chen, K. Yoshikawa, *J. Chem. Phys.* **2016**, *144*, 205101.
8. M. Osawa, A. Dace, K. I. Tong, A. Valiveti, M. Ikura, J. B. Ames, *J. Biol. Chem.* **2005**, *280*, 18008–18014.
9. J. Anastassopoulou, *J. Mol. Struct.* **2003**, *651*, 19–26.
10. P. J. Horn, C. L. Peterson, *Science* **2002**, *297*, 1824–1827.
11. Y. Yamasaki, K. Yoshikawa, *J. Am. Chem. Soc.* **1997**, *119*, 10573–10578.
12. M. R. Gill, J. A. Thomas, *Chem. Soc. Rev.* **2012**, *41*, 3179–3192.
13. S. Komeda, T. Moulaei, M. Chikuma, A. Odani, R. Kipping, N. P. Farrell, L. D. Williams, *Nucleic Acids Res.* **2011**, *39*, 325–336.
14. S. Komeda, T. Moulaei, K. K. Woods, M. Chikuma, N. P. Farrell, L. D. Williams, *J. Am. Chem. Soc.* **2006**, *128*, 16092–16103.
15. E. Kikuta, N. Katsube, E. Kimura, *J. Biol. Inorg. Chem.* **1999**, *4*, 431–440.
16. H.-K. Liu, P. J. Sadler, *Acc. Chem. Res.* **2011**, *44*, 349–359.

17. B. M. Zeglis, V. C. Pierre, J. K. Barton, *Chem. Comm.* **2007**, 4565–4579.
18. A. C. Komor, J. K. Barton, *Chem. Comm.* **2013**, *49*, 3617–3630.
19. B. Rosenberg, L. VanCamp, J. E. Trosko, V. H. Mansour, *Nature* **1969**, *222*, 385–386.
20. A. M. Fichtinger-Schepman, A. T. van Oosterom, P. H. Lohman, F. Berends, *Cancer Res.* **1987**, *47*, 3000–3004.
21. A. M. Fichtinger-Schepman, J. L. van der Veer, J. H. den Hartog, P. H. Lohman, J. Reedijk, *Biochemistry* **1985**, *24*, 707–713.
22. P. M. Takahara, A. C. Rosenzweig, C. A. Frederick, S. J. Lippard, *Nature* **1995**, *377*, 649–652.
23. A. Gelasco, S. J. Lippard, *Biochemistry* **1998**, *37*, 9230–9239.
24. H. Huang, L. Zhu, B. R. Reid, G. P. Drobny, P. B. Hopkins, *Science* **1995**, *270*, 1842–1845.
25. J.-M. Malinge, M. Leng, in *Cisplatin: Chemistry and Biochemistry of a Leading Anticancer Drug*, Ed B. Lippert, VHCA and Wiley-VCH, Zurich and Weinheim, **1999**, pp. 159–180.
26. S. Komeda, *Metallomics* **2011**, *3*, 650–655.
27. N. Farrell, *Met. Ions Biol. Syst.* **2004**, *42*, 251–296.
28. J. Suryadi, U. Bierbach, *Chem. Eur. J.* **2012**, *18*, 12926–12934.
29. S. M. Aris, N. P. Farrell, *Eur. J. Inorg. Chem.* **2009**, 1293–1302.
30. G. Y. Park, J. J. Wilson, Y. Song, S. J. Lippard, *Proc. Natl. Acad. Sci. U S A* **2012**, *109*, 11987–11992.
31. J. Malina, J. Kasparkova, N. P. Farrell, V. Brabec, *Nucleic Acids Res.* **2011**, *39*, 720–728.
32. T. C. Johnstone, G. Y. Park, S. J. Lippard, *Anticancer Res.* **2014**, *34*, 471–476.
33. S. Komeda, H. Ohishi, H. Yamane, M. Harikawa, K.-i. Sakaguchi, M. Chikuma, *J. Chem. Soc., Dalton Trans.* **1999**, 2959–2962.
34. S. Komeda, M. Lutz, A. L. Spek, Y. Yamanaka, T. Sato, M. Chikuma, J. Reedijk, *J. Am. Chem. Soc.* **2002**, *124*, 4738–4746.
35. S. Komeda, Y. L. Lin, M. Chikuma, *ChemMedChem* **2011**, *6*, 987–990.
36. S. Teletchea, S. Komeda, J.-M. Teuben, M.-A. Elizondo-Riojas, J. Reedijk, J. Kozelka, *Chem. Eur. J.* **2006**, *12*, 3741–3753.
37. A. Magistrato, P. Ruggerone, K. Spiegel, P. Carloni, J. Reedijk, *J. Phys. Chem. B* **2006**, *110*, 3604–3613.
38. S. Komeda, H. Takayama, T. Suzuki, A. Odani, T. Yamori, M. Chikuma, *Metallomics* **2013**, *5*, 461–468.
39. M. Uemura, T. Suzuki, K. Nishio, M. Chikuma, S. Komeda, *Metallomics* **2012**, *4*, 686–692.
40. M. Uemura, S. Komeda, *J. Inorg. Biochem.* **2017**, *177*, 359–367.
41. R. M. Wing, P. Pjura, H. R. Drew, R. E. Dickerson, *EMBO J.* **1984**, *3*, 1201–1206.
42. B. Lippert, *Coord. Chem. Rev.* **2000**, *200–202*, 487–516.
43. S. Komeda, H. Yamane, M. Chikuma, J. Reedijk, *Eur. J. Inorg. Chem.* **2004**, 4828–4835.
44. J. Mlcouskova, J. Kasparkova, T. Suchankova, S. Komeda, V. Brabec, *J. Inorg. Biochem.* **2012**, *114*, 15–23.
45. J. Mlcouskova, J. Malina, V. Novohradsky, J. Kasparkova, S. Komeda, V. Brabec, *Biochim. Biophys. Acta* **2012**, *1820*, 1502–1511.
46. N. Kida, Y. Katsuda, Y. Yoshikawa, S. Komeda, T. Sato, Y. Saito, M. Chikuma, M. Suzuki, T. Imanaka, K. Yoshikawa, *J. Biol. Inorg. Chem.* **2010**, *15*, 701–707.
47. S. Komeda, S. Bombard, S. Perrier, J. Reedijk, J. Kozelka, *J. Inorg. Biochem.* **2003**, *96*, 357–366.

48. D. P. Bancroft, C. A. Lepre, S. J. Lippard, *J. Am. Chem. Soc.* **1990**, *112*, 6860–6871.
49. M. Uemura, M. Hoshiyama, A. Furukawa, T. Sato, Y. Higuchi, S. Komeda, *Metallomics* **2015**, *7*, 1488–1496.
50. K. Nakamoto, M. Tsuboi, G. D. Strahan, Vol. 51 of *Drug-DNA Interactions: Structures and Spectra*, John Wiley & Sons, **2008**.
51. G. D. Fasman, *Circular Dichroism and the Conformational Analysis of Biomolecules*, Springer Science & Business Media, **2013**.
52. W. A. Baase, W. C. Johnson Jr, *Nucleic Acids Res.* **1979**, *6*, 797–814.
53. V. I. Ivanov, L. Minchenkova, A. Schyolkina, A. Poletayev, *Biopolymers* **1973**, *12*, 89–110.
54. L. van Dam, M. H. Levitt, *J. Mol. Biol.* **2000**, *304*, 541–561.
55. M. Uemura, Y. Yoshikawa, M. Chikuma, S. Komeda, *Metallomics* **2012**, *4*, 641–644.
56. S. U. Rehman, T. Sarwar, M. A. Husain, H. M. Ishqi, M. Tabish, *Arch. Biochem. Biophys.* **2015**, *576*, 49–60.
57. Y. Yoshikawa, S. Komeda, M. Uemura, T. Kanbe, M. Chikuma, K. Yoshikawa, T. Imanaka, *Inorg. Chem.* **2011**, *50*, 11729–11735.
58. N. V. Hud, I. D. Vilfan, *Annu. Rev. Biophys. Biomol. Struct.* **2005**, *34*, 295–318.
59. Y. Yoshikawa, K. Yoshikawa, T. Kanbe, *Langmuir* **1999**, *15*, 4085–4088.
60. L. C. Gosule, J. A. Schellman, *Nature* **1976**, *259*, 333–335.
61. S. Komeda, H. Yoneyama, M. Uemura, T. Tsuchiya, M. Hoshiyama, T. Sakazaki, K. Hiramoto, S. Harusawa, *Data in Brief* **2022**, *40*, 107697.
62. S. Komeda, H. Yoneyama, M. Uemura, A. Muramatsu, N. Okamoto, H. Konishi, H. Takahashi, A. Takagi, W. Fukuda, T. Imanaka, T. Kanbe, S. Harusawa, Y. Yoshikawa, K. Yoshikawa, *Inorg. Chem.* **2017**, *56*, 802–811.
63. E. Grueso, C. Cerrillos, J. Hidalgo, P. Lopez-Cornejo, *Langmuir* **2012**, *28*, 10968–10979.
64. M. Uemura, Y. Yoshikawa, K. Yoshikawa, T. Sato, Y. Mino, M. Chikuma, S. Komeda, *J. Inorg. Biochem.* **2013**, *127*, 169–174.
65. N. K. Andersen, N. Chandak, L. Brulíková, P. Kumar, M. D. Jensen, F. Jensen, P. K. Sharma, P. Nielsen, *Bioorg. & Med. Chem.* **2010**, *18*, 4702–4710.
66. R. Imai, S. Komeda, M. Shimura, S. Tamura, S. Matsuyama, K. Nishimura, R. Rogge, A. Matsunaga, I. Hiratani, H. Takata, M. Uemura, Y. Iida, Y. Yoshikawa, J. C. Hansen, K. Yamauchi, M. T. Kanemaki, K. Maeshima, *Sci. Rep.* **2016**, *6*, 24712.
67. J. Widom, R. L. Baldwin, *J. Mol. Biol.* **1980**, *144*, 431–453.
68. J. Malina, N. P. Farrell, V. Brabec, *Angew. Chem. Int. Ed.* **2014**, *126*, 13026–13030.
69. J. Malina, N. P. Farrell, V. Brabec, *Inorg. Chem.* **2014**, *53*, 1662–1671.
70. J. Malina, K. Čechová, N. P. Farrell, V. Brabec, *Inorg. Chem.* **2019**, *58*, 6804–6810.
71. S. Komeda, Y. Qu, J. B. Mangruma, A. Hegmans, L. D. Williams, N. P. Farrell, *Inorg. Chim. Acta* **2016**, *452*, 25–33.

9 Metals in Genotyping
From SNPs to Sequencing

Tuomas Lönnberg
Department of Chemistry, University of Turku,
Henrikinkatu 2, 20500 Turku, Finland
tuanlo@utu.fi

CONTENTS

1	Introduction		212
2	Metals in Identification of Single-Nucleotide Polymorphisms		213
	2.1	Metal-Mediated Base Pairing in Otherwise Conventional Hybridization Probes	213
		2.1.1 Linear Probes	213
		2.1.2 Molecular Beacons	217
	2.2	Metallated Probes with Base-Specific Reporter Complexes	218
3	Metals in Sequencing		219
	3.1	Electron Microscopy Sequencing	219
	3.2	Nanopore Sequencing	222
4	General Conclusions		224
Abbreviations and Definitions			224
References			224

Abstract

The base moieties of nucleic acids react with a wide range of transition metal ions through formation of either coordinate or organometallic bonds. In many cases, the reactions are sufficiently selective toward a given nucleobase to serve as a basis for elucidation of sequence information. Two fundamentally different approaches can be envisaged. Firstly, a metallated nucleobase can engage in metal-mediated base pairing with a natural nucleobase of the opposite strand and this interaction can be quite distinct from canonical Watson–Crick base pairing in terms of both affinity and selectivity. Secondly, a heavy metal ion can act as a contrast-enhancing label, altering the physicochemical properties of a nucleobase to make it detectable against a background of unmodified nucleobases. The first approach has found use in oligonucleotide hybridization probes for the detection of single-nucleotide polymorphisms (SNPs) and the second one in electron microscopy or nanopore sequencing. The potential of metals in genotyping has been studied for more than half a century but never very intensively. This chapter attempts to bring together the scattered reports in this field and to identify the most promising achievements as well as challenges that need to be met.

DOI: 10.1201/9781003270201-9

KEYWORDS

Genotyping; Sequencing; Single-Nucleotide Polymorphism; Base Paring; Hybridization; Probe; Metal Coordination

1 INTRODUCTION

Determining the primary structure of nucleic acids, whether at a single polymorphic site or over an entire genome, is of tremendous importance in various fields, such as medicine, anthropology, or forensics. The most visible example is undoubtedly the massive ongoing effort to screen for the SARS-CoV-2 virus in patients with symptoms of a respiratory infection. While the virus can be detected by fast and relatively inexpensive antibody tests, sequencing of the viral RNA by polymerase chain reaction (PCR) is still needed for reliable identification. A significant fraction of the national healthcare budgets worldwide is devoted to carrying out the latter task on an unprecedented scale. There is, hence, a clear demand for cheaper alternatives to the present methods, especially in less developed parts of the world.

Single-base extension [1] and PCR [2] are perhaps the most obvious approaches for the detection and identification of single-nucleotide polymorphisms (SNPs), relying on the high fidelity of polymerase enzymes. In addition, many enzyme-independent methods based on linear [3, 4], binary [5], and molecular beacon [6–8] oligonucleotide hybridization probes have been developed [9, 10]. The primary structure of longer tracts of nucleic acids, on the other hand, can be elucidated by Maxam–Gilbert [11], Sanger [12], pyro- [13], reversible dye terminator [14], ligation [15], single-molecule real-time (SMRT) [16] or nanopore [17] sequencing. With the notable exception of Maxam–Gilbert and nanopore sequencing, all of these methods rely on the same phenomenon as the transmission of genetic information in biological systems, i.e. Watson–Crick base pairing. While undeniably natural and elegant, such approaches also have inherent deficiencies. For example, while a canonical Watson–Crick base pair is usually much stronger than any of the mispairs, the latter tend to have rather similar stabilities so that several hybridization probes are typically needed for reliable identification of one SNP. Rare nucleobases present another obvious challenge, as they can be either incorrectly recognized as one of the canonical nucleobases or remain unidentified altogether.

Besides Watson–Crick base pairing, nucleobases can also engage in strong and often very selective interactions with soft transition metals. These interactions can take the form of a coordinate bond [18–20] to an endo- or exocyclic nitrogen atom or a metal–carbon bond [21, 22] formed through displacement of a C–H proton [23]. Formation of coordinate and organometallic metal–nucleobase complexes could both find use in genotyping and the first steps on this path have been taken recently. This chapter reviews these efforts and attempts to shed light on future prospects.

2 METALS IN IDENTIFICATION OF SINGLE-NUCLEOTIDE POLYMORPHISMS

The approaches that utilize metal ions in identification of SNPs fall into three distinct categories. Firstly, the metal ion may be involved in a metal-mediated base pair [21, 24–29] between the polymorphic base and an oligonucleotide probe, and genotyping is based on the hybridization affinity of the probe with the target sequence. Secondly, a metal complex within the probe sequence may produce a signal that is dependent on the identity of a proximal nucleobase within the target sequence. Thirdly, a metal complex may act as a passive label in a system where the recognition is based solely on Watson–Crick base pairing [30–33]. The third category falls outside the scope of this chapter.

2.1 METAL-MEDIATED BASE PAIRING IN OTHERWISE CONVENTIONAL HYBRIDIZATION PROBES

Metal-mediated base pairs are roughly coplanar assemblies of two canonical nucleobases or their artificial analogs linked to each other through coordination with a common metal ion. Cases, where inter-base hydrogen bonds (notably those between canonical nucleobases or their close analogs) are replaced or augmented by metal coordination, might be more correctly referred to as "metal-modified base pairs", reserving the term "metal-mediated" for pairs that only form in the presence of the appropriate metal ion [34]. However, the term "metal-mediated base pair" has become the convention in the field and it is also used throughout this chapter for simplicity. Metal-mediated base pairs between two natural, between one natural and one artificial, and between two artificial bases have all been reported, the first two cases being potentially useful for SNP genotyping [35]. Formal replacement of hydrogen bonds with coordinate ones can lead to substantial stabilization of the base pair, which in turn often translates into an elevated melting temperature of a corresponding double helix. Even more importantly from the point of view of identification of SNPs, in some cases, the melting temperatures of duplexes varying only in the natural component of the metal-mediated base pair are separated by a much wider margin than those of the respective unmodified duplexes.

2.1.1 Linear Probes

The melting temperatures of short double helices are sensitive to the presence of even a single mismatch within the sequence, providing a simple method for the detection of SNPs. As the four canonical Watson–Crick base pairs are all considerably more stable than any of the mispairs, hybridization with a single linear oligonucleotide probe is usually enough to establish whether a polymorphic site contains the expected nucleobase or one of the other three. Discrimination between the various mismatches, however, is much weaker and less predictable and as many as four probes are typically needed for reliable identification of an unknown polymorphic nucleotide.

Metal-mediated base-pairing preferences of a canonical nucleobase may be quite different from the Watson–Crick base-pairing preferences of the same nucleobase and in some cases more conducive to SNP genotyping. For example, in the middle of an 11-mer DNA duplex, thymine formed the expected strong Watson–Crick base pair with adenine and a weak mispair with cytosine and, in the presence of one equivalent of Hg(II), Hg(II)-mediated base pairs of intermediate strength with guanine and thymine [36]. The melting temperatures of all duplexes were separated by at least 5°C, a clear improvement compared to the same duplexes in the absence of transition metals (Figure 1a). Similar results were obtained on Ag(I)-mediated base pairing of cytosine by employing a probe featuring the α anomer of the 2′-deoxycytidine residue at the recognition site, in addition to its natural all-β counterpart (Figure 1b) [37].

Not surprisingly, artificial nucleobases specifically designed for metal-mediated base pairing can exhibit superior discriminatory power compared to their natural counterparts. For example, the melting temperatures of 13-mer DNA duplexes incorporating a central Ag(I)-mediated base pair between imidazophenanthroline glycol nucleic acid (GNA) and either cytosine or thymine differed by 13°C (Figure 2) [38]. Interestingly, both duplexes exhibited nearly identical melting temperatures in the absence of Ag(I) and addition of one equivalent of Ag(I) strongly stabilized the former and destabilized the latter.

Organometallic nucleobase analogs have been studied as a means to expand the scope of metal-mediated base pairing to biological systems [21, 29]. Arylmercury nucleobases, in particular, have also proven useful in SNP genotyping. The melting temperatures of 11-mer double-helical oligodeoxyribonucleotides featuring a

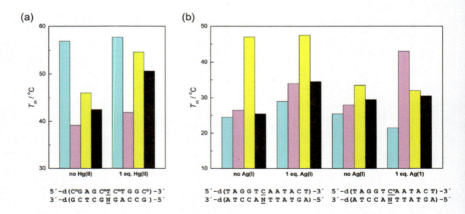

FIGURE 1 Comparison of melting temperatures of oligonucleotide duplexes featuring either a hydrogen-bonded or (a) [35] a Hg(II)- or (b) [36] a Ag(I)-mediated base pair between canonical nucleobases. In the sequences, C^m refers to 5-methyl-2′-deoxycytidine, C^α to the α-anomer of 2′-deoxycytidine and N to either adenine (cyan), cytosine (magenta), guanine (yellow) or thymine (black) and the residues involved in metal-mediated base pairing are underlined. For detailed experimental conditions, please refer to the original publications.

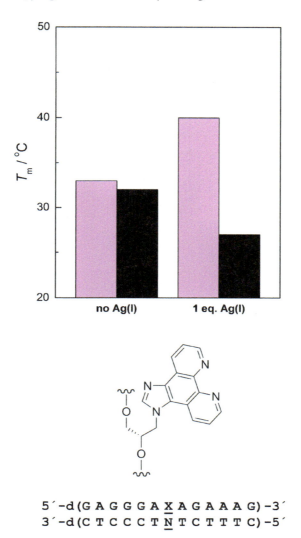

FIGURE 2 Comparison of melting temperatures of oligonucleotide duplexes featuring either a hydrogen-bonded or a Ag(I)-mediated base pair between imidazophenanthroline and canonical pyrimidine nucleobases [37]. In the sequences, X refers to imidazophenanthroline GNA nucleoside and N to either cytosine (magenta) or thymine (black) and the residues involved in metal-mediated base pairing are underlined. For detailed experimental conditions, please refer to the original publication.

central Hg(II)-mediated base pair between the organometallic nucleobase analog 3-fluoro-2-mercuri-6-methylaniline and each of the canonical nucleobase, for example, were all separated from each other by a margin of at least 7 °C (Figure 3) [39]. The most stable duplexes were obtained when either guanine or

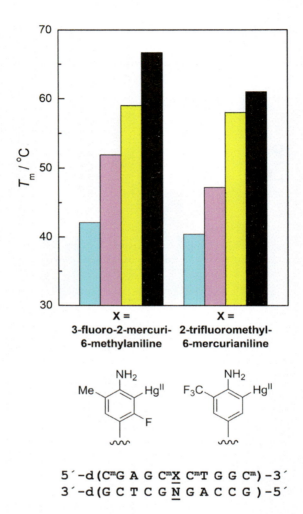

FIGURE 3 Comparison of melting temperatures of oligonucleotide duplexes featuring either a Hg(II)-mediated base pair between either 3-fluoro-2-mercuri-6-methylaniline or 2-trifluoromethyl-6-mercurianiline and one of the canonical nucleobases. In the sequences, C^m refers to 5-methyl-2′-deoxycytidine, X to either 3-fluoro-2-mercuri-6-methylaniline or 2-trifluoromethyl-6-mercurianiline and N to either adenine (cyan), cytosine (magenta), guanine (yellow) or thymine (black) and the residues involved in metal-mediated base pairing are underlined. For detailed experimental conditions, please refer to the original publications.

thymine was placed opposite to the organometallic base, in line with the known tendency of Hg(II) to coordinate to N1 and N3 of these nucleobases by displacement of the relatively acidic proton [18, 40]. Discrimination by 2-trifluoromethyl-6-mercurianiline, lacking the fluoro substituent on the Watson–Crick face, was otherwise similar but the melting temperatures of duplexes pairing this organometallic base with guanine or thymine differed by only 3°C (Figure 3) [41].

2.1.2 Molecular Beacons

A linear hybridization probe can be converted into a molecular beacon by incorporating it into the loop region of a hairpin oligonucleotide, the termini of which are functionalized with a suitable reporting group. The most commonly employed reporting group is a Förster resonance energy transfer (FRET) pair, consisting of a fluorophore at one terminus and a quencher at the other terminus. Hybridization of the loop with the target sequence leads to unwinding of the double-helical stem, greatly increasing the distance between the fluorophore and the quencher and thus rendering the molecular beacon emissive (Figure 4). In other words, while SNP detection by a molecular beacon also relies on different stabilities of matched and mismatched duplexes, the readout is faster than with linear probes as no time-consuming heating and cooling ramps are needed.

The first molecular beacon-type hybridization probe featuring a metal-mediated base pair with the polymorphic base was created by incorporating the aforementioned imidazophenanthroline GNA nucleoside in the middle of the loop region and 6-carboxyfluorescein (FAM) and 4-{[4-(dimethylamino)phenyl]azo}benzoic acid (dabcyl) at the 3'- and 5'-termini, respectively [38]. In line with the UV melting temperatures of duplexes formed by the respective linear probe, a two-fold increase of fluorescence emission was observed only with the target placing cytosine opposite to the imidazophenanthroline base and only in the presence of Ag(I). Despite being limited to discrimination between the two pyrimidine bases, molecular beacons based on Ag(I)-mediated base pairing of imidazophenanthroline could nonetheless find use in diagnostics as medicinally relevant examples of both C→T and T→C transitions exist [42–45].

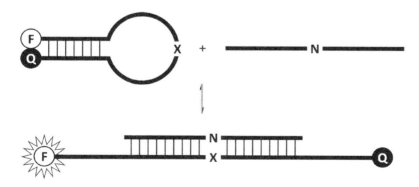

FIGURE 4 General working principle of a FRET-based molecular beacon-type hybridization probe. Hybridization of the loop region with a complementary target sequence forces opening of the double-helical stem and turns on fluorescence. X and N refer to the nucleobases (natural or artificial) involved in SNP detection, F to a fluorophore and Q to a quencher.

The organometallic nucleobase surrogate 3-fluoro-2-mercuri-6-methylaniline discussed above has also been incorporated in a molecular beacon-type hybridization probe [46]. The same fluorophore (FAM) and quencher (dabcyl) were used as in the imidazophenanthroline-based probe discussed above, but owing to their sensitivity to the mercuration conditions these groups had to be conjugated to the mercurated oligonucleotide post-synthetically by strain-promoted azide–alkyne cycloaddition (SPAAC) or peptide coupling, respectively. The additional synthetic effort proved worthwhile, as the organometallic molecular beacon was able to discriminate between all of the canonical nucleobases. At 55°C, the fluorescence emission of the probe increased 3-, 8-, 17- and 31-fold on addition of a target sequence pairing the organometallic nucleobase analog with adenine, cytosine, guanine, and thymine, respectively.

2.2 Metallated Probes with Base-Specific Reporter Complexes

In addition to having base-pairing preferences different from those of the canonical nucleobases, artificial nucleobase analogs and surrogates can have unique properties that facilitate SNP detection. Well-known examples include fluorophores and spin labels, both of which have been employed successfully in conjunction with metal-mediated base pairing. Electrochemical labeling is an attractive alternative and the label most widely used with nucleic acids, namely ferrocene, has shown potential in discriminating between proximal nucleobases. Ideally, a nucleobase analog would form base pairs with canonical nucleobases in a predictable manner and each of the base pairs would give out a unique signal.

Pyrrolo- and imidazolocytosines are fluorescent nucleobase analogs that retain the Watson–Crick base-pairing properties of cytosine [47]. These nucleobases are useful in monitoring oligonucleotide hybridization as base stacking quenches their fluorescence emission. In addition to the hydrogen-bonded Watson–Crick base pair with guanine, pyrrolo- and imidazolocytosines also form stable mononuclear Ag(I)-mediated base pairs with cytosine and extremely stable dinuclear Ag(I)-mediated homo base pairs with themselves [48–51]. One might expect the fluorescence spectra of these base pairs to be sufficiently characteristic to allow identification of SNPs but this hypothesis remains to be tested in practice. In this regard, it is also interesting to note that the molar absorptivities of oligonucleotide duplexes incorporating a central Pd(II)-mediated base pair between a phenylpyridine palladacycle and each of the canonical nucleobases were systematically higher than those of the corresponding unmodified duplexes and apparently dependent on the identity of the canonical base-pairing partner [52]. While this phenomenon as such would probably not be useful with longer nucleic acids having higher background absorptivity, it nonetheless suggests that SNP detection based on different absorption (and perhaps also emission) spectra of metal-mediated base pairs with different canonical nucleobases might be feasible.

^{19}F NMR spectrometry has been studied extensively as a means to monitor changes in nucleic acid secondary structure [53, 54]. The fluorine atoms of the aforementioned 2-trifluoromethyl-6-mercurianiline [41] and, especially, 3-fluoro-2-mercuri-6-methylaniline [39], lie close to the opposite nucleobase and their chemical shifts could, hence, be expected to reflect changes not only in the secondary structure of the oligonucleotide but also in the Hg(II)-mediated base pairing itself. This was indeed found to be the case and the base-pairing partner of both of these organometallic nucleobase analogs could be identified reliably based on the ^{19}F NMR spectrum of the respective double-helical oligonucleotide. Separation of the chemical shifts was greater with 3-fluoro-2-mercuri-6-methylaniline than with 2-trifluoromethyl-6-mercurianiline, consistent with the location of the fluoro substituent on the Watson–Crick face. Interestingly, pairing of 3-fluoro-2-mercuri-6-methylaniline with either adenine or guanine gave rise to two ^{19}F NMR signals, whereas only one was observed when pairing with cytosine or thymine. N1/N7 dichotomy is a known phenomenon in the coordination of arylmercury compounds to purine nucleosides [40] and it is tempting to speculate that the two signals correspond to two Hg(II)-mediated base pairs, one formed through N1 and the other one through N7 coordination.

While examples discussed above are all based on inner-sphere coordination of the polymorphic nucleobase to a metal ion of the reporter group, such coordination is not an absolute requirement. Indeed, interesting results have been obtained on hybridization probes placing a ferrocene moiety opposite to the polymorphic base [55]. Square wave voltammetry (SWV) current changes of 15-mer DNA duplexes incorporating the ferrocene residue in various positions of the sequence showed a clear dependence on the "base-pairing partner" but even more so on the neighboring bases. The strongest SNP discrimination was observed when the ferrocene residue was flanked by a purine base on both sides. Interaction of ferrocene with the neighboring bases probably involves stacking but interaction with the opposite base remains enigmatic. The complex dependence of the SWV current change on the environment of the ferrocene moiety makes an interpretation of the results challenging but electrochemical labels nonetheless appear to be a promising alternative to fluorophores and spin labels also in the context of SNP genotyping.

3 METALS IN SEQUENCING

The natural pyrimidine nucleobases react with certain heavy metal ions and complexes under conditions where the other bases are inert [56–58]. Alternatively, the bases can be first modified chemoselectively to generate the desired metal binding sites. In either case, the resulting coordination or organometallic complexes are clearly distinct from any of the natural nucleobases in terms of molecular weight as well as steric and electronic properties. These differences could be exploited for example in electron microscopy or nanopore sequencing. Initial studies on both methods have yielded encouraging results.

3.1 Electron Microscopy Sequencing

Direct visualization of DNA by electron microscopy [59–61] offers the promise of improved read lengths, compared with the state-of-the-art next-generation sequencing methods [62–68]. The similar size and elemental composition of the four canonical nucleobases make unmodified DNA hardly suitable for this approach but base-specific introduction of even a single heavy metal atom provides a sufficient contrast. Non-specific staining with heavy metal salts had been used for electron microscopic visualization of DNA already in the early 1960s [69]. The first attempts at rendering such staining base-specific involved chemoselective introduction of anionic ligands to cytosine [70] or guanine residues [71–73], followed by soaking in an aqueous uranyl acetate solution. In these studies, selectivity toward a given base was inferred from comparison of reactivities of nucleotides or their homopolymers and the chemical structure of the products remained somewhat obscure. The electron micrographs of the labeled DNAs showed rows of dots assigned as the heavy atom markers but did not allow unambiguous determination of the sequence.

In addition to anionic ligands, carbon–carbon double bonds of furan and imidazole rings have been studied as reactive sites for introduction of heavy metals. Selective labeling of cytosine bases with furan moieties has been achieved by sodium bisulfite-promoted treatment with O-furfurylhydroxylamine (Figure 5a) [74]. Treatment with chloroacetaldehyde, on the other hand, selectively converts both adenine and cytosine bases to the corresponding etheno derivatives, extending the heteroaromatic ring system with an additional fused imidazole (Figure 5b) [75]. In this case, differentiation between adenine and cytosine residues could be achieved by acid-catalyzed depurination of the former. Both furan and imidazole labels have been shown to react with both osmium tetroxide and mercury acetate, through formation of osmate esters [74, 76, 77] or organomercury derivatives [74, 75], respectively. None of these studies, however, have been followed up by actual electron microscopy experiments.

By the early 2010s, technological advances had finally brought sequencing by electron microscopy within the realms of possibility. Mercury was again used as the contrast-enhancing heavy atom label, but in contrast to the earlier studies, it was incorporated by enzymatic polymerization rather than by chemical treatment of natural DNA [78]. Specifically, thymidine-5'-triphosphate was completely replaced by 2'-deoxy-5-methylmercurythiouridine-5'-triphosphate in the polymerization mixture, yielding a product in which each thymine/uracil residue bore a methylmercury label (Figure 6). The test sequences prepared in this way were thousands of nucleotides in length. In principle, a similar approach could be used for labeling of any of the four canonical nucleobases.

The methylmercury-labeled DNAs were separated and linearized on an amorphous carbon film and visualized by annular dark field scanning transmission electron microscopy (ADF-STEM) [78]. Individual heavy atoms could be detected with fair confidence and spatial separation of the signals was consistent with the pattern predicted based on the sequence and helical parameters under the experimental conditions [79]. For labels that were relatively far apart (>1 nm), variability of the observed distance was too high for unambiguous determination of the number of intervening residues. A higher labeling density, i.e. labeling

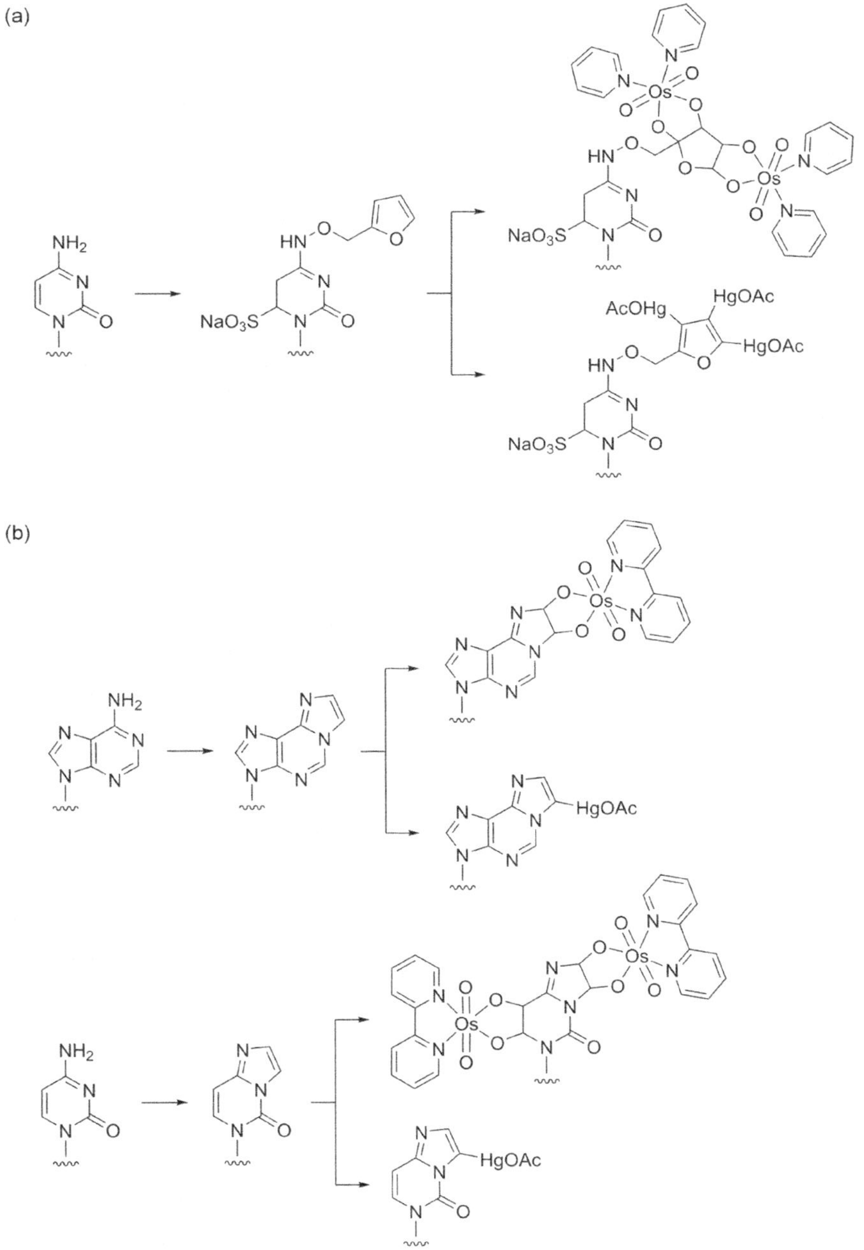

FIGURE 5 Chemoselective introduction of a reactive "handle" to adenine and cytosine residues ((a) sodium bisulfite-promoted treatment with O-furfurylhydroxylamine, (b) treatment with chloroacetaldehyde), followed by reaction with heavy metals.

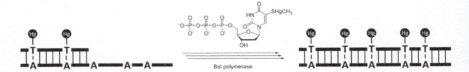

FIGURE 6 Heavy atom labeling of DNA through enzymatic polymerization, using 2′-deoxy-5-methylmercurythiouridine-5′-triphosphate instead of thymidine-5′-triphosphate.

of more than one type of nucleobase with the same sequence, was suggested to address this issue but no such report is yet forthcoming. Nevertheless, electron microscopy employing heavy metal contrast-enhancing labels has the potential to become a viable sequencing method once the remaining technical problems are solved.

3.2 Nanopore Sequencing

Nanopore sequencing is based on nucleobase-specific perturbations in ionic current as a single strand of DNA passes through a nanopore set in an electrical field (Figure 7) [17]. Unlike sequencing by electron microscopy, nanopore sequencing is a proven method in regular use. However, while it can be carried out on unmodified DNA, nanopore sequencing would also benefit from more pronounced differences between the nucleobases in terms of steric and electronic properties. It is therefore not surprising that the same solution as with electron microscopy

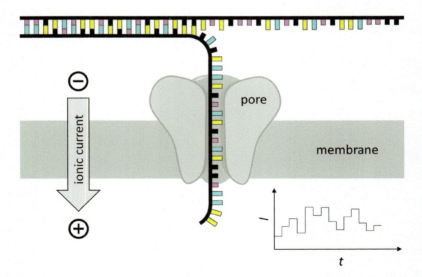

FIGURE 7 General working principle of nanopore sequencing. The pore can be either natural, such as an alpha-hemolysin (α-HL) or *Mycobacterium smegmatis* porin A (MspA) protein or an artificial solid-state pore.

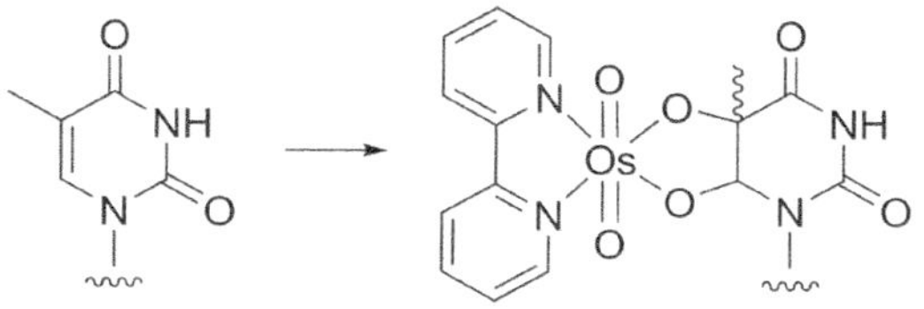

FIGURE 8 Labeling of thymine residues by treatment with osmium tetroxide 2,2'-bipyridine.

sequencing, namely base-specific labeling by heavy metal ions, has been proposed also to improve the reliability of nanopore sequencing [80].

Unpaired thymine residues of DNA can be selectively labeled by treatment with 3.15 mM osmium tetroxide 2,2'-bipyridine for 60 min at room temperature (Figure 8), greatly increasing their steric bulk [81, 82]. Under harsher conditions (14.2 mM osmium tetroxide 2,2'-bipyridine for 11 h at room temperature), also cytosine residues are being similarly labeled, while the purine residues remain unreactive. These results could be generalized to apply also to respective labeling of RNA [83]. Passage of any of the osmylated residues through a nanopore gives rise to a signal clearly distinct from those of any of the unlabeled residues [84]. Selective labeling of either thymine or all pyrimidine residues on both of the constituent single strands of double-helical DNA, followed by nanopore discrimination of labeled *vs.* unlabeled residues on all of the resulting four strands, should, hence, allow complete elucidation of the sequence, with greater confidence than what would be achievable with unlabeled DNA.

In addition to the similar size and electronic properties of the four canonical nucleobases, early approaches at nanopore sequencing suffered from too fast translocation of the DNA substrate through the nanopore, making detection of current changes associated to passage of an individual base impossible [85]. Incorporation of a phi29 DNA polymerase enzyme on the upstream side of the pore solves this problem [86–88] but may actually slow down the translocation too much from the point of view of sequencing whole genomes [85, 89]. Treatment of pyrimidine bases with osmium tetroxide 2,2'-bipyridine, on the other hand, increased their dwell times to detectable levels even in the absence of an additional processing enzyme [90]. Curiously, dwell times of osmylated cytosine and thymine within an alpha-hemolysin (α-HL) pore were quite different from each other and showed no clear correlation with the current modulation.

While artificial nanopores can, in principle, be engineered to a desired length, protein nanopores have a given length that is not necessarily optimal for sequencing purposes. The *Mycobacterium smegmatis* porin A (MspA) pore, for example, accommodates a sequence of four nucleotides and the α-HL pore is even longer [87]. In other words, the observed signal corresponds to a short nucleic acid sequence, rather than a single nucleotide, making interpretation of the data challenging. Osmium tetroxide bipyridine labeling of pyrimidine residues appears to improve this resolution – for example, the commercially available

MinION device, employing a CsgG lipoprotein pore, was reported to sense a two-nucleotide sequence within an osmylated substrate as opposed to a five-nucleotide sequence within a native substrate [83].

4 GENERAL CONCLUSIONS

Metals show great promise in genotyping, through alteration of either the base-pairing properties of oligonucleotide hybridization probes or the size of certain nucleobases within a longer nucleic acid sequence. Both approaches represent a step away from the paradigm of Watson–Crick base pairing as the basis of sequence recognition and could, hence, prove useful especially with target sequences featuring non-canonical nucleobases. No applications have yet reached widespread use and one cannot escape the feeling that this is at least in part due to biosciences and inorganic chemistry being two different worlds, with few people able to appreciate both. Hopefully, this chapter will, for its part, serve to bring these two worlds closer to each other.

ABBREVIATIONS AND DEFINITIONS

α-HL	alpha-hemolysin
ADF	annular dark field
Dabcyl	4-{[4-(dimethylamino)phenyl]azo}benzoic acid
DNA	deoxyribonucleic acid
FAM	6-carboxyfluorescein
FRET	Förster resonance energy transfer
GNA	glycol nucleic acid
MspA	*Mycobacterium smegmatis* porin A
NMR	nuclear magnetic resonance
PCR	polymerase chain reaction
RNA	ribonucleic acid
SARS-CoV-2	severe acute respiratory syndrome coronavirus
SMRT	single-molecule real-time
SNP	single-nucleotide polymorphism
SPAAC	strain-promoted azide–alkyne cycloaddition
STEM	scanning transmission electron microscopy
SWV	square wave voltammetry

REFERENCES

1. A.-C. Syvänen, *Hum. Mutat.* **1999**, *13*, 1–10.
2. M. V Myakishev, Y. Khripin, S. Hu, D. H. Hamer, *Genome Res.* **2001**, *11*, 163–169.
3. H. Frickmann, A. E. Zautner, A. Moter, J. Kikhney, R. M. Hagen, H. Stender, S. Poppert, *Crit. Rev. Microbiol.* **2017**, *43*, 263–293.
4. N. M. Guimarães, N. F. Azevedo, C. Almeida, *Methods Mol. Biol.* **2021**, *2246*, 17–33.
5. D. M. Kolpashchikov, *Chem. Rev.* **2010**, *110*, 4709–4723.

6. N. Bidar, M. Amini, F. Oroojalian, B. Baradaran, S. S. Hosseini, M. A. Shahbazi, M. Hashemzaei, A. Mokhtarzadeh, M. R. Hamblin, M. de la Guardia, *TrAC Trends Anal. Chem.* **2021**, *134*, 116143.
7. S. Mao, Y. Ying, R. Wu, A. K. Chen, *iScience* **2020**, *23*, 101801.
8. J. Huang, J. Wu, Z. Li, *Rev. Anal. Chem.* **2015**, *34*, 1–27.
9. D. M. Kolpashchikov, *Acc. Chem. Res.* **2019**, *52*, 1949–1956.
10. J. X. Chen, C. Shi, X. Y. Kang, X. T. Shen, X. Z. Lao, H. Zheng, *Anal. Methods* **2020**, *12*, 884–893.
11. A. M. Maxam, W. Gilbert, *Biochemistry* **1977**, *74*, 560–564.
12. F. Sanger, S. Nicklen, A. R. Coulson, *Proc. Natl. Acad. Sci. U.S.A.* **1977**, *74*, 5463–5467.
13. P. Nyrén, B. Pettersson, M. Uhlén, *Anal. Biochem.* **1993**, *208*, 171–175.
14. B. Canard, R. S. Sarfati, *Gene* **1994**, *148*, 1–6.
15. F. Barany, *Proc. Natl. Acad. Sci. U.S.A.* **1991**, *88*, 189–193.
16. J. Eid, A. Fehr, J. Gray, K. Luong, J. Lyle, G. Otto, P. Peluso, D. Rank, P. Baybayan, B. Bettman, A. Bibillo, K. Bjornson, B. Chaudhuri, F. Christians, R. Cicero, S. Clark, R. Dalal, A. DeWinter, J. Dixon, M. Foquet, A. Gaertner, P. Hardenbol, C. Heiner, K. Hester, D. Holden, G. Kearns, X. Kong, R. Kuse, Y. Lacroix, S. Lin, P. Lundquist, C. Ma, P. Marks, M. Maxham, D. Murphy, I. Park, T. Pham, M. Phillips, J. Roy, R. Sebra, G. Shen, J. Sorenson, A. Tomaney, K. Travers, M. Trulson, J. Vieceli, J. Wegener, D. Wu, A. Yang, D. Zaccarin, P. Zhao, F. Zhong, J. Korlach, S. Turner, *Science* **2009**, *323*, 133–138.
17. J. J. Kasianowicz, E. Brandin, D. Branton, D. W. Deamer, *Proc. Natl. Acad. Sci. U.S.A.* **1996**, *93*, 13770–13773.
18. R. B. Martin, *Acc. Chem. Res.* **1985**, *18*, 32–38.
19. H. Sigel, *Chem. Soc. Rev.* **1993**, *22*, 255–267.
20. P. Zhou, R. Shi, J. feng Yao, C. fang Sheng, H. Li, *Coord. Chem. Rev.* **2015**, *292*, 107–143.
21. D. Ukale, T. Lönnberg, *ChemBioChem* **2021**, *22*, 1733–1739.
22. K. Kowalski, *Coord. Chem. Rev.* **2021**, *432*, 213705.
23. B. Lippert, *Coord. Chem. Rev.* **2000**, *200–202*, 487–516.
24. S. Naskar, R. Guha, J. Müller, *Angew. Chem. Int. Ed.* **2020**, *59*, 1397–1406.
25. B. Jash, J. Müller, *Chem. Eur. J.* **2017**, *23*, 17166–17178.
26. Y. Takezawa, J. Müller, M. Shionoya, *Chem. Lett.* **2017**, *46*, 622–633.
27. Y. Takezawa, M. Shionoya, *Acc. Chem. Res.* **2012**, *45*, 2066–2076.
28. G. H. Clever, M. Shionoya, *Coord. Chem. Rev.* **2010**, *254*, 2391–2402.
29. D. Ukale, S. Maity, M. Hande, T. Lönnberg, *Synlett* **2019**, *30*, 1733–1737.
30. E. Paleček, M. Bartošík, *Chem. Rev.* **2012**, *112*, 3427–3481.
31. E. Paleček, *Electroanalysis* **2009**, *21*, 239–251.
32. K. Matsumoto, *Handb. Phys. Chem. Rare Earths* **2020**, *57*, 119–191.
33. K. Hashino, M. Ito, K. Ikawa, C. Hosoya, T. Nishioka, K. Matsumoto, *Anal. Biochem.* **2006**, *355*, 278–284.
34. B. Lippert, *J. Biol. Inorg. Chem.* **2022**, *27*, 215–219.
35. S. Taherpour, O. Golubev, T. Lönnberg, *Inorg. Chim. Acta* **2016**, *452*, 43–49.
36. D. Ukale, V. S. Shinde, T. Lönnberg, *Chem. Eur. J.* **2016**, *22*, 7917–7923.
37. X. Guo, F. Seela, *Chem. Eur.J* **2017**, *23*, 11776–11779.
38. B. Jash, P. Scharf, N. Sandmann, C. Fonseca Guerra, D. A. Megger, J. Müller, *Chem. Sci.* **2017**, *8*, 1337–1343.
39. A. Aro-Heinilä, T. Lönnberg, P. Virta, *Bioconjugate Chem.* **2019**, *30*, 2183–2190.
40. R. B. Simpson, *J. Am. Chem. Soc.* **1964**, *86*, 2059–2065.

41. A. Aro-Heinilä, A. Lepistö, A. Äärelä, T. A. Lönnberg, P. Virta, *J. Org. Chem.* **2022**, *87*, 137–146.
42. B. Jash, J. Müller, *Eur. J. Inorg. Chem.* **2017**, *2017*, 3857–3861.
43. M. Yokota, S. Ichihara, T. L. Lin, N. Nakashima, Y. Yamada, *Circulation* **2000**, *101*, 2783–2787.
44. E. Ziv, J. Cauley, P. A. Morin, R. Saiz, W. S. Browner, *JAMA J. Am. Med. Assoc.* **2001**, *285*, 2859–2863.
45. E. Martinez, F. Silvy, F. Fina, M. Bartoli, M. Krahn, F. Barlesi, D. Figarella-Branger, J. Iovanna, R. Laugier, M. Ouaissi, D. Lombardo, E. Mas, E. Martinez, F. Silvy, F. Fina, M. Bartoli, M. Krahn, F. Barlesi, D. Figarella-Branger, J. Iovanna, R. Laugier, M. Ouaissi, D. Lombardo, E. Mas, *Oncotarget* **2015**, *6*, 39855–39864.
46. A. Aro-Heinilä, T. Lönnberg, P. M. Virta, *ChemBioChem* **2020**, *22*, 354–358.
47. M. Bood, S. Sarangamath, M. S. Wranne, M. Grøtli, L. M. Wilhelmsson, *Beilstein J. Org. Chem.* **2018**, *14*, 114–129.
48. H. Mei, S. A. Ingale, F. Seela, *Chem. Eur. J.* **2014**, *20*, 16248–16257.
49. H. Yang, H. Mei, F. Seela, *Chem. Eur. J.* **2015**, *21*, 10207–10219.
50. H. Mei, I. Röhl, F. Seela, *J. Org. Chem.* **2013**, *78*, 9457–9463.
51. S. K. Jana, X. Guo, H. Mei, F. Seela, *Chem. Commun.* **2015**, *51*, 17301–17304.
52. S. K. Maity, T. Lönnberg, *Chem. Eur. J.* **2018**, *24*, 1274–1277.
53. D. Gimenez, A. Phelan, C. D. Murphy, S. L. Cobb, *Beilstein J. Org. Chem.* **2021**, *17*, 293–318.
54. H. Chen, S. Viel, F. Ziarelli, L. Peng, *Chem. Soc. Rev.* **2013**, *42*, 7971–7982.
55. R. Abdullah, S. Xie, R. Wang, C. Jin, Y. Du, T. Fu, J. Li, J. Tan, L. Zhang, W. Tan, *Anal. Chem.* **2019**, *91*, 2074–2078.
56. R. M. K. Dale, D. C. Livingston, D. C. Ward, *Proc. Natl. Acad. Sci. U.S.A.* **1973**, *70*, 2238–2242.
57. R. M. K. Dale, E. Martin, D. C. Livingston, D. C. Ward, *Biochemistry* **1975**, *14*, 2447–2457.
58. M. Beer, S. Stern, D. Carmalt, K. H. Mohlhenrich, *Biochemistry* **1966**, *5*, 2283–2288.
59. R. P. Feynman, *J. Microelectromechanical Syst.* **1992**, *1*, 60–66.
60. M. Beer, E. N. Moudrianakis, *Proc. Natl. Acad. Sci. U.S.A.* **1962**, *48*, 409–416.
61. F. P. Ottensmeyer, *Ann. Rev. Biophys. Bioeng.* **1979**, *8*, 129–144.
62. S. C. Schuster, *Nat. Methods* **2008**, *5*, 16–18.
63. R. Xue, R. Li, F. Bai, *Sci. Bull.* **2015**, *60*, 33–42.
64. W. W. Soon, M. Hariharan, M. P. Snyder, *Mol. Syst. Biol.* **2013**, *9*, 640.
65. S. Moorthie, C. J. Mattocks, C. F. Wright, *Hugo J.* **2011**, *5*, 1–12.
66. M. Kircher, J. Kelso, *BioEssays* **2010**, *32*, 524–536.
67. X. Teng, H. Xiao, *Sci. China Ser. C Life Sci.* **2009**, *52*, 7–16.
68. S. El-Metwally, O. M. Ouda, M. Helmy, *New Horizons in Next-Generation Sequencing*, Springer, New York, **2014**.
69. W. Stoeckenius, *J. Biophys. Biochem. Cytol.* **1961**, *11*, 297–310.
70. L. Gal-Or, J. E. Mellema, E. N. Moudrianakis, M. Beer, *Biochemistry* **1967**, *6*, 1909–1915.
71. E. N. Moudrianakis, M. Beer, *Proc. Natl. Acad. Sci. U.S.A.* **1965**, *53*, 564–571.
72. E. N. Moudrianakis, M. Beer, *Nature* **1964**, *204*, 685–686.
73. E. N. Moudrianakis, M. Beer, *BBA Nucleic Acids Protein Synth.* **1965**, *95*, 23–39.
74. S. D. Rose, M. Beer, *Bioinorg. Chem.* **1978**, *9*, 231–243.
75. S. D. Rose, *BBA Nucleic Acids Protein Synth.* **1974**, *361*, 231–235.
76. L. G. Marzilli, B. F. Hanson, L. Kapili, S. D. Rose, M. Beer, *Bioinorg. Chem.* **1978**, *8*, 531–534.

77. R. F. Hartman, S. D. Rose, M. D. Cole, S. D. Rose, J. W. Wiggins, M. Beer, A. A. Waldrop, L. G. Marzilli, *J. Org. Chem.* **1981**, *46*, 4340–4345.
78. D. C. Bell, W. K. Thomas, K. M. Murtagh, C. A. Dionne, A. C. Graham, J. E. Anderson, W. R. Glove, *Microsc. Microanal.* **2012**, *18*, 1049–1053.
79. D. Bensimon, A. J. Simon, V. Croquette, A. Bensimon, *Phys. Rev. Lett.* **1995**, *74*, 4754.
80. A. Kanavarioti, *Nanotechnology* **2015**, *26*, 134003.
81. A. Kanavarioti, K. L. Greenman, M. Hamalainen, A. Jain, A. M. Johns, C. R. Melville, K. Kemmish, W. Andregg, *Electrophoresis* **2012**, *33*, 3529.
82. A. Kanavarioti, *Beilstein J. Nanotechnol.* **2016**, *7*, 1434–1446.
83. M. Sultan, A. Kanavarioti, *Sci. Rep.* **2019**, *9*, 14180.
84. R. Y. Henley, A. G. Vazquez-Pagan, M. Johnson, A. Kanavarioti, M. Wanunu, *PLoS One* **2015**, *10*, e0142155.
85. G. Maglia, A. J. Heron, D. Stoddart, D. Japrung, H. Bayley, *Methods Enzymol.* **2010**, *475*, 591–623.
86. J. Chu, M. González-López, S. L. Cockroft, M. Amorin, M. R. Ghadiri, *Angew. Chem. Int. Ed.* **2010**, *49*, 10106–10109.
87. E. A. Manrao, I. M. Derrington, A. H. Laszlo, K. W. Langford, M. K. Hopper, N. Gillgren, M. Pavlenok, M. Niederweis, J. H. Gundlach, *Nat. Biotechnol.* **2012**, *30*, 349–353.
88. K. R. Lieberman, G. M. Cherf, M. J. Doody, F. Olasagasti, Y. Kolodji, M. Akeson, *J. Am. Chem. Soc.* **2010**, *132*, 17961–17972.
89. F. Haque, J. Li, H. C. Wu, X. J. Liang, P. Guo, *Nano Today* **2013**, *8*, 56–74.
90. Y. Ding, A. Kanavarioti, *Beilstein J. Nanotechnol.* **2016**, *7*, 91–101.

10 Nucleic Acids for the Preparation and Control of Continuous Hybrid Metallic Assemblies

Miguel A. Galindo
Departamento Química Inorgánica,
Universidad de Granada, Spain
magalindo@ugr.es

Fátima Linares
Centro de Instrumentación Científica
(CIC), Universidad de Granada, Spain
flinaor@ugr.es

*Alicia Domínguez-Martín and
Antonio Pérez-Romero*
Departamento Química Inorgánica,
Universidad de Granada, Spain
adominguez@ugr.es, antperrom@ugr.es

CONTENTS

1 Introduction 230
2 Toward Continuous Metallized DNA Systems 232
3 Metal-DNA Systems Using 7-Deazaadenine and 7-Deazaguanine 239
4 Metal Complexes Complementary to Single-Stranded DNA
  Sequences 244
5 General Conclusions 249
Abbreviations and Definitions 250
References 251

Abstract

New nanomaterials' development depends on the correct organization and positioning of matter at the nanometric scale, giving rise to new physicochemical properties that can be exploited in emerging technologies. In this respect, nucleic acids play an important role. DNA is a well-known water-soluble biopolymer relatively easy to synthesize and whose structure can be programmed to form almost any assembly at the nanometric scale (1D, 2D, or 3D). If these DNA assemblies could have properties of technological interest, such as conductive, photoluminescent or catalytic properties, superior nanomaterials could be prepared on demand. In particular, metals can provide these properties if arranged correctly, and DNA can serve as a template or scaffold to guide the formation of customized nanoscale metal assemblies precisely.

This chapter will describe the methodologies and strategies used to create continuous metal-DNA hybrid systems, where DNA molecules are transformed into corresponding metal assemblies. Despite the significant progress made in this regard, this goal is not as simple as it seems. For this reason, the chapter will present main advances in this matter, the unresolved challenges, and new strategies to overcome them.

KEYWORDS

Bioinorganic Chemistry; Nucleic Acids; DNA Metallization; Metal-Mediated Base Pair; Supramolecular Chemistry

1 INTRODUCTION

The proposal of the helical structure of DNA by Watson and Crick in 1953 certainly revolutionized science [1]. This research work was published under the title "Molecular Structure of Nucleic Acids: A Structure for Deoxyribose Nucleic Acid". It is worth mentioning that the contributions of other scientists made this achievement possible, among which we highlight here Phoebus Levene, Erwin Chargaff, Rosalind Franklin, and Maurice Wilkins. Even though the Watson–Crick double-helical structure, so-called B-DNA, is still considered the most representative structure of DNA in the human genome, it is only one of the various molecular structures currently described for DNA, a biopolymer which turned out to be more flexible and versatile than ever imagined, and which marked the beginning of genetics and molecular biology studies.

The folding of the different DNA conformations, and additional DNA interactions with other biomolecules, are driven by the formation of distinct non-covalent interactions, i.e., hydrogen bonding, π-π-stacking, and electrostatic interactions. The nature and strength of such interactions are determined by the identity and the relative position of each nucleobase forming the DNA strands. Therefore, it is evident that the DNA structure strongly depends on the base sequence. Indeed, one of the most remarkable properties of nucleic acids is their ability to base-pair recognition [2–4]. Interestingly, the exquisite specificity of such interactions allows for predicting DNA self-assembly into secondary and tertiary structures and their approximate thermodynamic stability, just based on the DNA sequence. Furthermore, folding stability *in vivo* is also conditioned by the cellular environment, including metal ion concentration, hydration, or crowding conditions [5].

In the past decades, the continuous development of high-resolution techniques, mainly X-ray crystallography and nuclear magnetic resonance, has transformed the structural DNA landscape, allowing to confirm the atomic details not only of the B-DNA helical structure but also describing two other types of DNA helices, i.e., A-DNA or the left-handed Z-DNA [6–9], and additional non-canonical structures such as triplexes [10], three-way (3WJ) and four-way (4WJ) junction structures [11–13], G-quadruplexes (G4) [14, 15] and i-motifs [16]. Non-canonical structures should not be considered artifacts. On the contrary, their existence has been related to numerous processes concerning gene regulation [17–20].

Understanding the structural diversity of DNA, including the rationale for the non-covalent interactions on which it is based, has been of paramount importance in developing and programming novel self-assembled synthetic DNA-based nanomaterials [21–25]. In this context, DNA origami technology has proved to be an exceptionally robust and successful strategy for the bottom-up design of accurate DNA architectures thanks to the involvement of powerful bioinformatic tools [22, 26, 27]. Nonetheless, further work still needs to be done to fully understand the thermodynamics and kinetics of scaffolded assembly within DNA nanotechnology.

DNA nanotechnology research not only seeks efficient control of the engineering process for the design and construction of DNA nanostructures but also fosters the development of new DNA-based nanomaterials with potential nanotechnological applications [28–30]. The optical and electronic properties of DNA itself are limited [31, 32]. Therefore, functionalization is required to make DNA-based nanomaterials more interesting for the industry [30, 33, 34].

If DNA nanomaterials are to be considered for industrial applications, we first must achieve simple and inexpensive synthetic methods. The development of modified DNA sequences is mainly based on the solid-phase methodology, which has significantly improved the synthetic process, allowing the introduction of a variety of specific modifications, and providing pure and high-yield DNA products in a short time at a moderately low cost [35]. Nevertheless, enzymatic DNA synthesis seems to be gaining interest again [36]. The modifications can be introduced at different locations, i.e., terminal 3′- and 5′-ends, 2′- and 4′-sites at the ribose ring, and various positions within the four aromatic nucleobases [37]. A more aggressive synthetic approach would consider the deletion of natural nucleobases/nucleosides and their substitution by artificial nucleobases/nucleosides or other related ligands. An additional functionalization strategy that successfully introduces new physicochemical properties into synthetic DNA nanomaterials, such as enhanced luminescent, magnetic, or electronic properties in such novel nanomaterials [38–41], is the introduction of metal ions or small metal complexes, i.e., the so-called "metal-mediated" and "metal-modified" base-pair approach [42, 43]. DNA structures with one or a few metallo-base pairs have been shown to maintain their integrity. The slighter the changes, the more preserved the non-covalent interactions present in the natural sequence, thus staying closer to the native structure. However, keeping the DNA conformation closer to nature is not always the goal. For instance, different research groups in the field thoroughly study extraordinary metallo-base pairs systems that involve mismatches and artificial ligands [44–47]. The metallization of the DNA molecules throughout the whole structure is more challenging and has been classically done by the deposition of metal ions all over the structure. However, this can be also achieved by using metallo-base pairs. In particular, DNA molecules containing 7-deazaadenine and 7-deazaguanine nucleobases that substitute adenine and guanine, respectively, can be applied. This strategy can convert DNA assemblies into the corresponding metallized DNA, yet with the metals being stacked throughout the interior of the double strands [48–50]. This strategy, discussed below, offers alternatives to resolve some of the challenges associated with the metallization of complete DNA assemblies, mainly related to the lack of control in; (1) uniform, homogeneous and selective metallization of the whole structure, (2) stoichiometry of the metallization, (3) maintaining the hybridization ability of DNA, aiming to metallize DNA assemblies without loss of their original shape and geometry (junctions, networks), and (4) dynamic instability, necessary to afford dynamic applications such as nanorobots for drug delivery systems [51, 52]. Therefore, if these factors can be controlled, it is possible to think that well-defined DNA assemblies can be metallized in a regular, homogeneous, and controlled manner, giving rise to a metallized assembly with the preconceived structure. In addition, if metal ions are well-positioned all over the structure, they can be reduced to produce well-organized continuous nanometallic entities throughout the structure, serving as nucleation/catalytic sites for further metal growth. This achievement would open the door to preparing an infinity of possible metallic structures at the nanometric scale, with potential conductive, photoluminescent, catalytic, and/or cytotoxic properties, giving rise to new applications of industrial and biomedical interest.

In this chapter, we want to put into perspective the advances made in the complete and continuous metallization of DNA structures to evaluate the possibility of converting highly organized DNA assemblies (for example, DNA origami) into their corresponding metallized versions, to obtain personalized metallic nanostructures.

2 TOWARD CONTINUOUS METALLIZED DNA SYSTEMS

Metal ions are commonly associated with biological systems owing to their essential role in living cells, protein structure, and physiological functions. In other cases, the interaction of metal ions with biological systems is related to toxicity problems and harmful effects on health. However, from a scientific and technological point of view, the association of metal ions with DNA molecules can also give rise to metal-DNA assemblies with remarkable properties and potential applications. The properties and structure of metal-DNA systems will depend on many factors, including the type of metal used, its oxidation state, mode of interaction, the amount of metal, and its arrangement within the structure. From a general perspective, nucleic acids offer three prominent locations for metal binding: phosphate oxygen atoms, sugar oxygen atoms, and/or nucleobase donor atoms. The interaction possibilities between metals and DNA and the following structural consequences are enormous, which is reflected in the extensive published literature on the subject [53–58]. In general, the alkali and alkaline earth metals, lanthanoides and actinoides preferentially bind to phosphate groups. In contrast, transition metals can bind to phosphate and nucleobase sites with different affinities, which also depends on the metal concentration as well as hard-soft properties of metals and donor atoms [57, 59]. It is worth mentioning that the mode of interaction of metal ions with nucleobases may be different in free nucleobases, including ss-DNA, compared to when the bases are paired in ds-DNA.

Although almost all nucleobase atoms can be subject to metallization (Figure 1), the N7(G) and N7(A) purine atoms, facing the DNA major groove, are the most frequent metal-binding sites. Binding at minor groove positions, such as purine-N3 and pyrimidine-O2 atoms, is also possible, but considerably less relevant [60–63]. In ds-DNA, atoms participating in Watson–Crick hydrogen bonds may need nucleobases to undergo conformational changes that facilitate their exposure to metals, such as a *syn-anti* conformational change [64]. On the other hand, atoms like N3(T), N1(G), and exocyclic amino groups may also require more specific conditions to favor deprotonation prior to metal binding or alterations of their preferred tautomer state, therefore being generally slightly less favored for metallization.

Among the metals that favorably interact with different donor atoms of nucleobases, some stand out, such as Pt^{II}, Pd^{II}, Rh^{III}, Ru^{III}, Ag^{I}, Zn^{II}, Hg^{II}, and Cu^{II}. However, some metal ions preferentially bind to a specific position. In particular, Hg^{II} and Ag^{I} have shown a specific high affinity for N3(T) and N3(C), forming

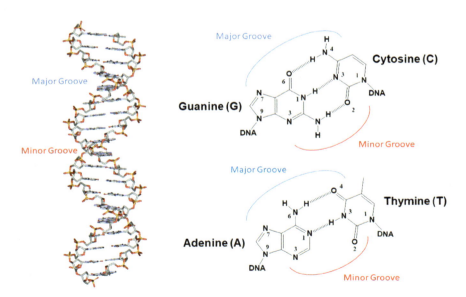

FIGURE 1 Nucleobase pairs in ds-DNA and atom numbering scheme. Location of the nucleobase atoms relative to their position in the major or minor groove of the double helix.

well-established T–Hg^{II}–T and C–Ag^{I}–C metallo-base pairs, respectively, inside ds-DNA molecules [65–67].

Classically, and in particular, since the discovery of the antitumor activity of cisplatin, the interaction of metal ions and metal complexes with DNA has attracted the attention of scientists in the field of bioinorganic and medical chemistry [68]. However, during the last two decades, the interaction of transition metal ions with DNA molecules has also been seen from a nanotechnological viewpoint. For instance, the binding of free metal ions to nucleobases has been exploited to develop DNA-based metal sensors [69]. Notably, the pioneering work of Braun and colleagues [70] evoked new interest in creating conductive metallic materials at the nanometric scale using DNA molecules that serve as templates or scaffolds to organize the metallic material. In addition, Dickson and colleagues also showed that photoluminescent metal nanoclusters can be prepared by exploiting the affinity of Ag^{I} for DNA sequences, acting as a capping agent that stabilizes such metallic entities [71]. Since then, interest in developing conducting and photoluminescent metallic DNA-based assemblies has grown exponentially [56, 72, 73]. These relatively new research areas are only two examples demonstrating the usefulness of metal-DNA systems in opening up new frontiers to generate functional nanomaterials.

In particular, creating conducting and/or photoluminescence nanowires using DNA molecules is very attractive for the nanoelectronics industry. However, despite some controversy, DNA seems to behave as an insulated wire at low bias and across long sections [74]. In this context, scientists are looking for ways to improve the conducting properties of nucleic acids, and metals are excellent candidates since the metallization of DNA has proven to afford metal-DNA nanowires with enhanced conductivity [56, 70, 75–77].

The metallization of entire DNA molecules is usually achieved by using the following general approach (Figure 2). First, a prearranged DNA structure is designed, prepared, and placed on a surface, acting as a template or scaffold for metallation (the DNA structure could also carry chemical modification that facilitates specific metal ion interactions). Secondly, metal cations are bound to

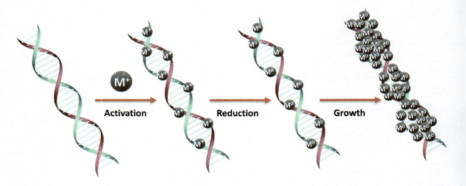

FIGURE 2 Scheme showing a general pathway to metallize complete DNA molecules.

the anionic nucleic acids by electrostatic interactions or by exploiting their affinity toward phosphate groups, nucleobases, or chemical modifications introduced (activation step). This process can also be done in solution by mixing DNA molecules and the desired metal ions, but this methodology often leads to unforeseen metal-DNA networks. Finally, chemical agents are used for reducing excess metal ions bound to the DNA to create continuous metal entities on the surface of the DNA (reduction step). These metallic entities will act as catalyst nuclei to promote further metallic growth (growth step). It is worth mentioning that reducing agents can also lead to secondary side reactions, denature, or destroy the DNA assembly. Therefore, chemical-free approaches such as photoreduction [78] and electrochemical deposition [79] have also been investigated.

There is enough experimental evidence demonstrating that metal deposition on DNA molecules (for instance, Ag, Au, Pt, Pd, Cu, Rh) results in higher electron transfer throughout the structure than through bare DNA. Thus, these metal-DNA systems can be envisioned as conductive nanowires. Nevertheless, comparing conductivity values for different metal-DNA wires can be misleading due to the various conducting measurement techniques used, the measurement conditions, and the nature of the metal-DNA structure obtained [80, 81]. Furthermore, the physicochemical mechanism that explains their conductive performances is not yet fully established, but studies point toward a charge transport process through nanometal granules on the surface of metallized DNA [82–84].

The above-described templated methodology has been and continues to be widely used because it is simple, direct, and cheap. However, it does not offer control over the interaction process of metals with DNA in terms of stoichiometry and location. These limitations often lead to metal-DNA systems with unevenly metallized sections compromising the continuity of the metallic array and affecting their conductive properties. Furthermore, nonspecific metallic structures often contaminate the surroundings of the system. The metal deposition on DNA molecules can also be achieved using already-formed metallic assemblies. For instance, silver-gold nanoparticles have been demonstrated to preferentially bind to poly(dG)-poly(dC) duplexes, leading to more uniform metal-DNA [85]. Still, none of the strategies described above combines the programmable assembly ability of DNA molecules with the metallization process. To obtain metallo-DNA-based networks, the original DNA assemblies are usually first immobilized on a surface; otherwise, if done in solution, nonspecific metal interactions could destabilize, collapse, or destroy the native design. However, ideally, the metallization and the DNA network assembly process should be compatible, without limiting one another.

An alternative approach is the selective metallization of the interior of the DNA strands by forming metallo-base pairs, where a metal ion bridges two bases (natural or artificial), creating a coordination bond with each one. Metallo-base-pair formation provides unprecedented control over metal-binding position and stoichiometry in ds-DNA. Despite the earlier suggestion of the existence of T–Hg^{II}–T metal-mediated base pairs [65, 86], it has not been until the last two decades that scientists focused their attention on creating customized metallo-base pairs inside DNA molecules, using canonical bases and substitutes [87]. This approach offers new possibilities for preparing metal-DNA systems whose structures and applications are under continuous study [40, 41, 43, 88]. At this point, it is worth mentioning that the terminology to define metallo-base pairs can be misleading. In this regard, Lippert offers helpful interpretations that can help clarify this issue [42].

In theory, almost any metallo-base pair could be introduced into DNA and placed at desired positions, which means that specific metals can be wisely positioned inside the double helix. To do this, ds-DNA molecules are prepared using complementary sequences that incorporate ligand-like nucleobases at a specific position to allow them to face each other when the oligonucleotides anneal to form the double strand. Subsequent addition of a metal ion results in metal-mediated base-pair formation at that precise position. It is important to mention that correct ligand design is crucial to promoting metallo-base pairing over other undesired metal-DNA interactions. The concept was initially proposed by Shionoya [87], and the first artificial metal-mediated base pair incorporated in DNA was Dipic–Cu^{II}–P (Dipic=pyridine-2,6-dicarboxylate, P=pyridine), which significantly increased the thermal stability of the duplex, consistent with the formation of a coordination bond between the strands [89, 90]. Since then, numerous DNAs containing metal-mediated base pairs have been prepared, often using metals that provide linear (Ag^{I}, Hg^{II}) and square-planar (Cu^{II} and Pd^{II}) coordination geometries facilitating a coplanar arrangement consistent with natural base pairs. However, other metal ions have been also used, such as Mn^{III}, Zn^{II}, Ni^{II}, or Gd^{III} [40]. The correct ligand design can permit more sophisticated metal-binding modes. For example, some ligands form dinuclear and trinuclear metal-mediated base pairs holding more than one metal ion, on the same side of the molecule [91–94] or at different sides [95]. Ligands such as 5-hydroxyuracil act as bifacial nucleobase analogs, allowing either metal- or hydrogen-bonded base-pair formation, depending on the absence or presence of metal ions and which side of the molecule is involved [96]. Besides, the artificial base 5-carboxyuracil forms several base pairs with variable nucleobases depending on the metal ions present [97]. Thiolated nucleobases also provide an alternative to introducing metal ions into DNA [98–100]. These examples show the incredible versatility of this approach in creating metal-DNA systems. More comprehensive reviews on this matter are available in the literature [40, 41, 43, 88].

However, while the arrangement of one or a few metallo-base pairs is typical, creating DNA with continuous metallo-base pairs is more challenging. It stimulates great interest in developing DNA-based metal nanowires. The problem of preparing DNA containing many metallo-base pairs arises from using the correct ligands. Replacing all canonical bases with artificial ligands to form continuous metallo-base pairs would be a significant synthetic challenge. But overall, the resulting molecule would not be an actual DNA molecule. Therefore, another approach must be sought to prepare DNA molecules comprising consecutive metal base pairs. Ideally, the strategy should be based on canonical nucleobases or close analogs to maintain the nature and unique properties of DNA. Gwinn and collaborators demonstrated that poly(dC) and poly(dG) strands form metal-DNA duplexes structures comprising contiguous silver-metallated C–Ag^I–C and G–Ag^I–G base pairs, respectively [101–103]. Müller and collaborators used 1-deazaadenine (D) as a nucleobase analog to achieve similar results [104]. This base is analogous to adenine but with the N1 position replaced by a CH group. Therefore, D pairs with T by forming Hoogsteen-type hydrogen bonds, and this D-T base pair hybridizes in double-stranded structures [105]. This study revealed that adding Ag^I gives rise to the formation of silver-modified D–Ag^I–T base pairs across the entire duplex, with silver-coordination bonds replacing hydrogen bonds at each base pair. Also, the 1,3-dideazaadenine base analog was employed to form sequential dinuclear silver-modified base pairs in DNA [106]. DNA homopolymers containing continuous metallo-base pairs are an excellent template for creating long straight nanowires. However, the use of homopolymers could not be applied to generate more complicated customizable arrays, including connections or programmable lattices, as base-pair recognition cannot be exploited. It is also possible to create contiguous metallo-base pairs using canonical bases only. Kondo and collaborators showed that adding Ag^I to DNA sequences containing all four canonical bases can lead to a silver-DNA molecule comprising continuous metallo-base pairs. The structure was characterized by high-resolution X-ray crystallography revealing the formation of three metal-mediated T–Ag^I–T, C–Ag^I–C and G–Ag^I–G homobase pairs and one metal-modified G–Ag^I–C heterobase pair. These metallo-base pairs alternately form an endless silver chain along the DNA helical axis [107], but adenine does not participate in any of the metallo-base pairs but rather dangles from the duplex. In the metallo-homobase pairs the Ag^I coordinates to N3(C), N7(G) and N3(T) atoms. However, a different guanine-binding mode occurs in the unprecedented metal-modified G–Ag^I–C heterobase pair. In this case, the Ag^I bridges the two bases through deprotonated N1(G) and N3(C) atoms, forming the second reported silver-modified Watson–Crick base pair to date. An earlier gold-modified G–Au^{III}–C base pair was described in which G and C act as bidentate ligands via their Watson–Crick faces [108]. These results are remarkable because they demonstrate that, under the right conditions, Watson–Crick base pairs can be metallated while maintaining their natural arrangement. Importantly, this Ag-DNA structure unequivocally confirms that it is possible to create an unbroken chain of ions running throughout the DNA helix axis while retaining a classical B-form. Yet, despite the outstanding achievement, the silver-DNA structure obtained does not obey the initial hydrogen-bonded DNA design that should have contained hydrogen-bonded A-T, G-C base pairs, and two C-C mismatches. These latter mismatches seem to be the metallation target to create two C–Ag^I–C pairs in the duplex, as previously accomplished in the corresponding RNA molecule [109]. Instead, the DNA strands underwent a strand displacement to form the observed silver-DNA system, whose structure appears to be a favorable thermodynamic arrangement. Another example of a silver-DNA structure has been accomplished using sequences containing G, C, and ^{Br}U (bromouracil). In this case, an uninterrupted silver chain is derived from the formation of well-established C–Ag^I–C and G–Ag^I–G homobase pairs and new G–Ag^I–^{Br}U heterobase pairs, with the Ag^I coordinating the N3(C), N7(G) and deprotonated N1(^{Br}U) atoms [110]. Yet again, this structure does not contain Watson–Crick base pairs. All these extraordinary X-ray structures clearly demonstrated that DNA is an ideal structure for forming continuous Ag^I chains containing silver-silver interactions.

Inspired by the research mentioned above and, in an effort, to overcome the challenge of creating predictable metal-DNA systems containing contiguous Watson–Crick metallo-base pairs, we explored the use of DNA molecules containing 7-deazaadenine/thymine and 7-deazaguanine/cytosine base pairs to create DNA assemblies with continuous silver-modified base pairs [48, 49]. This methodology will be discussed in more detail in the next section due to the exclusive peculiarities of these nucleobase analogs.

DNA molecules containing metallo-base pairs can be used for different applications [41]. However, the study of their conductive properties has been the focus of many studies due to the potential to serve as DNA-based nanowires. For this purpose, the charge transfer capabilities of different DNA molecules containing different metallo-base pairs have been investigated using different approaches. Again, as with the conductive properties of DNA-based nanowires prepared by metal deposition (*vide supra*), the conclusions drawn from these studies will depend on several factors, including the nature and number of metallo-base pairs, the DNA sequence, experimental conditions, and the technique used for the measurement. The majority of the conducting studies have shown increased conducting properties in DNA-containing metallo-base pairs, including T–Hg^{II}–T [84, 111, 112], H–Cu^{II}–H (H=hydroxypyridone) [113], and C–Ag^I–C [83, 84]. Notably, two of these studies were performed on single molecules [83, 113]. However, other studies indicate the contrary, the charge transfer resistance increases in DNA-containing Im–Ag^I–Im [114] and C–Ag^I–C [115] base pairs. The conducting properties of molecules comprising continuous C–Ag^I–C base pairs have been more extensively studied, probably due to their stability and easier preparation. Long strands of poly(dC) can be converted into strands containing continuous C–Ag^I–C base pairs, and this system also showed increased conducting properties [116]. The stacking of individual C–Ag^I–C base pairs outside the DNA context can lead to supramolecular assemblies comparable to those formed in DNA [39, 117–120], although these assemblies behave as insulators [39, 118, 119]. However, the conducting and photoluminescence properties of these structures were enhanced by reducing the Ag^I to metallic silver using photoreduction and cold hydrogen plasma methodologies. The results suggest that continuous metallo-base pairs can be transformed into a continuum of metallic silver units inside DNA molecules. This is further supported by other studies demonstrating that metallic silver chains can be accommodated inside DNA duplexes upon reducing bound Ag^I ions [121, 122], although forming continuous silver clusters capped by the DNA strands is also feasible [123, 124].

Overall, enough experimental evidence suggests that the correct organization of metal ions along the central DNA axis can increase conductivity. Furthermore, metal ions exclusively bound inside duplexes can also be reduced to form well-organized metallic entities that could further improve these properties, including also photoluminescence.

Despite all this significant progress, the scientific development to build devices for nanoelectronics or nanophotonics using DNA-containing metallo-base pairs is arguably still in its infancy. Although metallo-base pairing is an excellent strategy for controlling the positioning and stoichiometry of metal ions inside DNA, some challenges are still to be overcome. For example, in a more straightforward and controlled manner, new approaches should be investigated to form long metal-DNA wires comprising continuous metallo-base pairs using different metals, bases, and ligands. Also, there is the challenge of developing complex assemblies (interconnections, joints, 3D structures) that contain continuous metallo-base pairs and are not limited to wire forms.

To this end, and inspired by the approach of the metallo-base pair, new approaches were investigated to prepare metal-DNA systems containing continuous metallo-base pairs. These approaches are presented in the following sections. The first method is based on the metallization of DNA molecules derived from 7-deazaadenine/thymine and 7-deazaguanine/cytosine base pairs. The other strategy utilizes a self-assembly reaction between particular metal complexes and ss-DNA to create highly customizable continuous metal-DNA systems.

3 METAL-DNA SYSTEMS USING 7-DEAZAADENINE AND 7-DEAZAGUANINE

Since Seeman proposed using DNA molecules to form customized DNA shapes, extraordinary assemblies and materials have been made based on this approach [25, 30, 125]. If the same principles could be exploited in combination with metal ions, a plethora of new DNA-based functional materials could evolve. In this context, many researchers investigated novel strategies to introduce consecutively transition metal ions into the ds-DNA core, while respecting the original base-pairing composition. Ideally, canonical base pairs should be transformed into metal-modified base pairs A–M^{n+}–T and G–M^{n+}–C (M^{n+} = metal ion) while maintaining their original Watson–Crick arrangement. However, the formation of these metallo-base pairs is mainly hindered by the preferential binding of metal ions toward the purine-N7 position, which generally occurs in silver-DNA systems [107, 110, 126]. Only two examples demonstrate that N1(G) can be deprotonated inside DNA to form metallo-Watson–Crick base pairs, although these were not anticipated [107, 108]. Considering these facts, we envisaged that removing the N7(G, A) atoms in DNA molecules would not alter the canonical self-assembly capabilities. Still, it can promote metal ion interactions with N1(G) and N1(A) atoms (Figure 3) [48, 49, 127]. In this regard, 7-deazaadenine (X) and 7-deazaguanine (Y) base analogs can serve this purpose, as a CH group replaces their N7 atoms. This very subtle modification maintains the ability of the bases to form 7-deazaDNA molecules (^{7C}DNA). Moreover, they are commercially available and can be employed in standardized synthesizers and enzymatic DNA synthesis [128, 129]. Other 7-deazapurine derivatives could also form metal base pairs, but substituting N7 with chemical groups more complex than CH would substantially affect the chemical properties of the purine

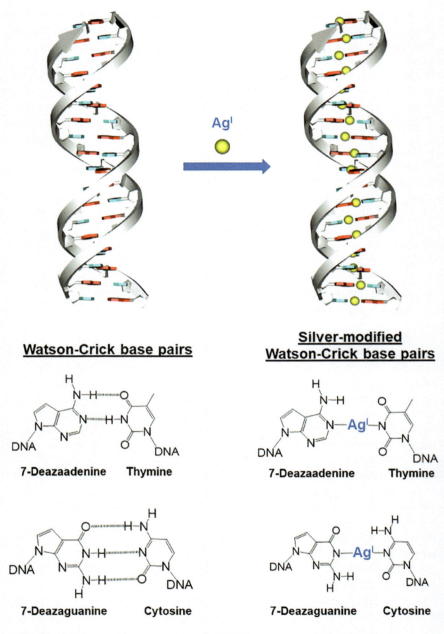

FIGURE 3 Schematic representation of DNA comprising Watson–Crick hydrogen-bonded 7-deazaadenine/thymine and 7-deazaguanine/cytosine and its transformation to silver-DNA metal-containing silver-modified base pairs.

nucleobases. The nucleosides 5-aza-7-deazapurine and 8-aza-7-deazapurine are also good alternatives to 7-deazapurine as they shift the N7 atom to a new N5 or N8 position, respectively [127, 130]. However, the purine-N8 atom could also participate in metal-binding [131] and the 5-aza-7-deazaguanine nucleoside loses its ability to form the established three hydrogen bonds with cytosine.

Therefore, the use of X and Y nucleosides provides exceptional control over the positioning and stoichiometry for DNA metallization and, at the same time, respects the natural ability of nucleic acids to self-assemble. Furthermore, in principle, ^{7C}DNA-based nanostructures could be rationally designed and prepared following the established base-pairing rules, as proposed by Seeman [25]. Subsequently, the interior of these double helixes could be lined with metal ions to form coordination bonds that substitute Watson–Crick hydrogen bonds. The resulting metal-^{7C}DNA structure would contain metal-modified Watson–Crick base pairs and, in principle, could resemble the original design as base-pair recognition can remain unaltered.

To demonstrate this hypothesis, ^{7C}DNA sequences were prepared to replace canonical purine A and G bases with 7-deazaadenine (X) and 7-deazaguanine (Y) base analogs, respectively.

Metals ions such as Ag^I and Hg^{II} ions provide linear coordination geometry that mimics hydrogen bonds and, therefore, are good candidates to serve this purpose. However, the initial studies focused on using Ag^I ions to yield stable linear coordination bonds between the bases due to their borderline Lewis acidity and lower toxicity.

The first work toward this aim focused on studying the metallation of the X-T base pair using self-complementary oligonucleotide sequence ODN1 with alternating X and T bases (X = 7-deazaadenine, T = thymine) (Table 1).

In the absence of Ag^I ions, the octadecamer ODN1 forms duplex **I** comprising consecutive X-T base pairs. This duplex shows a typical sigmoidal two-state denaturing curve. In the presence of Ag^I ions, the melting curves shift to higher temperatures and suggest stabilization upon adding one equivalent per base pair. Unfortunately, the final plateau of the melting curve could not be determined due to the high thermal stability of the **I**+Ag species. Still, the DNA melting studies indicate that the presence of Ag^I stabilizes duplex **I**, in agreement with the formation of coordination bonds to generate metal-modified X–Ag^I–T base pairs that replace the original Watson–Crick base pairs. CD spectroscopy also demonstrates the interaction of Ag^I with duplex **I**. In the absence of Ag^I ions, the CD spectrum displays a characteristic profile for a duplex B-DNA conformation, closely related to $d(AT)_n$ and $d(IC)_n$ duplexes [132]. Upon the addition of Ag^I, the CD spectrum undergoes significant changes until one equivalent of the metal ion (per base pair) is present in the solution, after which no significant additional changes are observed. These data also prove the interaction between Ag^I and duplex **I** and reveal a 1:1 stoichiometry per Ag:base pair. Control experiments were recorded for canonical duplex **Ic**, prepared using ODN1c comprising A-T

TABLE 1
Sequences of DNA Strands Used to Study the Formation of Continuous Metal-Modified Base Pairs Using X=7-Deazaadenine and Y=7-Deazaguanine Base Analogs

DNA Duplexes	Sequences	Sequences Code
I	5'- d(TXTXTXTXTXTXTXTXTX)-3' 3'- d(XTXTXTXTXTXTXTXTXT)-5'	ODN1
Ic	5'- d(TATATATATATATATATA) -3' 3'- d(ATATATATATATATATAT) -5'	ODN1c
II	5'- d(YYC YCC) -3' 3'- d(CCY CYY) - 5'	ODN2
IIc	5'- d(GGC GCC) -3' 3'- d(CCG CGG) -5'	ODN2c
III	5'- d(YC YC YC YC YC YC YC) -3' 3'- d(CY CY CY CY CY CY CY) -5'	ODN3
IIIc	5'- d(CG CG CG CG CG CG CG) -3' 3'- d(GC GC GC GC GC GC GC) -5'	ODN3c
IV	3'- d(CYT XCY TXC YTX CYT XCY) -5' 5'- d(YCX TYC XTY CXT YCX TYC) -3'	ODN4
IVc	3'- d(CGT ACG TAC GTA CGT ACG) -5' 5'- d(GCA TGC ATG CAT GCA TGC) -3'	ODN4c

instead of X-T base pairs. The interaction studies performed for **Ic** and Ag^I gave entirely different results. The CD curve experiences an inversion between 250 and 300 nm upon adding Ag^I, proving that the presence of the adenine-N7 affects the mode of interaction between Ag^I and the duplex structure.

Subsequently, the next step was to investigate the transformation of Y-C base pairs into metallated Y–Ag^I–C analogs using duplexes **II** and **III**, derived from hybridizing sequences with six (ODN2) or fourteen (ODN3) bases, respectively. Duplex **II** is a hexamer designed to have lower thermal stability, thus allowing to determine complete melting curves in the presence of Ag^I. Indeed, a significant increase in T_m could be observed for both duplexes **II** and **III** upon adding two equivalents of Ag^I per base pair. Thus, the presence of Ag^I stabilizes the duplexes comprising Y-T pairs and suggests the formation of silver-coordination bonds between them. The CD titration experiments also reached the same conclusions. Duplex **II** and **III** have CD profiles that resemble the B-form conformation described for poly(CG) molecules [133, 134]. Nevertheless, in the presence of Ag^I, their profile experiences notable changes during the addition of two equivalents of Ag^I, with no significant differences thereafter. Once again, there is an ellipticity decrease in the 240–300 nm region while the curve retains its profile. However, the experiments led to different CD results when using canonical duplexes **IIc** and **IIIc** comprising G-C base pairs. In these cases, the presence of Ag^I provokes an inversion of the curve in the 240–300 nm region and a general ellipticity decrease at all wavelengths. This trend resembles those published for the interaction of Ag^I with oligonucleotides containing canonical C and G bases [101, 102], indicating that the silver-binding mode is different when N7(G) is present, most likely to form N7(G)–Ag^I–N7(G) or N7(G)–Ag^I–C base pairs. Interestingly, the metal-binding stoichiometry is different for the X–Ag^I–T and Y–$(Ag^I)_2$–C modified base pairs, which has been further corroborated by other authors reporting the same findings for Y-C pairs [127]. DFT calculations performed on $[Y–(Ag^I)_2–C]_2$ dinucleotides indicate that the first silver is inserted into the Y-C base-pair binding the N1(Y) and N3(C) atoms (as described for the canonical G–Ag^I–C base-pair) [107]. Notably, the second silver is found at interplanar positions binding the keto and/or amino groups of two successive Y-C base pairs. However, these findings could also be sequence-dependent and additional studies need to confirm it.

Finally, to demonstrate the full potential of this approach, the interaction of Ag^I was studied in duplex **III**, which contains both X-T and Y-C base pairs. Sequence ODN3 hybridizes to form duplex **III**, similar to its canonical homolog ODN3c forming **IIIc**. Both duplexes display similar melting behavior, but **III** has a lower T_m due to the weaker Watson–Crick hydrogen bonds formed by X and Y bases. The addition of Ag^I to a solution of **III** shifts the melting curves toward higher temperatures, increasing the thermal stability of the system and suggesting the formation of silver-modified base pairs. The CD titration experiment confirms the interaction of Ag^I with duplex **III**, showing changes in the ellipticity curves up to the addition of 1.5–2 equivalents of metal ions. This stoichiometry can be related to the binding of more than one Ag^I ion at each base pair, as seen for **II**. However, the need for excess ions to fully form the mono-metallated Ag^I-mediated base pairs cannot be ruled out due to the weak-to-medium strength and thermodynamic character of silver-coordination bonds. Notably, the CD curves undergo intensity changes while retaining their sinusoidal profile, as observed above for **I** and **II**, indicating that the structure of **III**+Ag is closely related to that of free **III**. When investigating canonical **IIIc**, these experiments show different results, and the CD spectra resemble those reported for the interaction between canonical sequences and Ag^I.

In general, these results highlight that the purine-N7 atoms participate in the formation of Ag-DNA systems when canonical G and A are employed, and the use of X and Y bases leads to different silver-binding patterns that can only occur at the interior positions of the double helix. It is worth mentioning that silver-binding at G-N7 and A-N7 atoms (Hoogsteen face) can also take place in the center of a double helix if the bases adopt a non-canonical *syn* conformation around the glycosidic bond [107, 110, 126]. The strategy using X and Y bases can be applied to form consecutive and predictable Watson–Crick metal-modified X–Ag^I–T and Y–Ag^I–C base pairs in a DNA molecule. Notably, the metallization of the interior of the double helix respects the initial hybridization pattern, allowing the preconceived structure to be maintained (with some deviations due to the insertion of metal ions in the central axis of the double helix).

Maintaining the initial hybridization pattern between the bases is essential for designing preconceived structures where the DNA molecules are fully metallized exclusively inside. DNA molecules comprising X-T and Y-C pairs offer unprecedented control to achieve this goal. Moreover, it is worth mentioning that we have recorded high-resolution NMR measurements on these Ag-DNA systems, and the results further confirm that it is possible to metallize the X-T and Y-C base pairs while respecting the original hybridization pattern [135]. Ultimately, creating metal-DNA systems capable of following the base-pairing rules to prepare preconceived DNA networks may be possible by following this strategy. Further studies should be done in this direction.

4 METAL COMPLEXES COMPLEMENTARY TO SINGLE-STRANDED DNA SEQUENCES

ss-DNA molecules hold a unique molecular organization and association capacity via base-pair recognition. They constitute a precise template for ordering molecules that can selectively interact with the nucleobases. The correct association of single molecules, such as chromophores, can lead to well-organized supramolecular assemblies with properties otherwise absent. In this context, many researchers have equipped individual molecules with functionalities that allow them to interact with the nucleobases so that they can be recognized and organized by ss-DNA sequences [136]. The interactions between these molecules and ss-DNA often rely on hydrogen-bonding interactions, as they offer base recognition capabilities and self-correction, thus preventing products obtained by kinetic control and favoring thermodynamic products. But self-assembly reactions between metal ions and suitable organic ligands can also lead to thermodynamically stable complex molecular architectures with self-correction interactions [137]. These characteristics could be also used to organize metallo-base pairs along ss-DNA sequences using a self-assembly reaction. It has been shown that metal complexes can be customized to exhibit higher affinity and selectivity between nucleobases [138–140]. This concept can be exploited to prepare a custom continuum of nucleobase-metal-ligand arrays where metal complexes target particular bases in a self-assembly reaction. Furthermore, if different metal complexes were designed to recognize other nucleobases selectively, more ambitious metal-DNA arrays could be designed to contain different metal complexes in specific sections. We have explored this bottom-up strategy to prepare DNA systems comprising continuous metallo-base pairs [50]. For this, we used metal complexes capable of forming cooperative hydrogen and coordination bonds at the Watson–Crick face of the nucleobase and stacking interactions with neighboring units. Following this strategy, it will be possible to rationally create DNA hybrids containing an endless array of metal ions and functional ligands. The sequence will regulate the number of metal complexes and their positioning. In addition, coordination bonds will give the nucleobase-complex assemblies significant stability, making it possible to work over a higher temperature range than with recognition events between ligands and nucleobases based solely on hydrogen bonds. Finally, the formation of complementary hydrogen bonds with the nucleobases could help to promote base recognition and obtain a coplanar arrangement of the metallo-base pair. This alignment will favor stacking interactions and increase stability for the overall supramolecular assembly.

Thus, this new approach can create well-organized DNA-metal-ligand hybrid systems at room temperature using self-assembly reactions between ss-DNA sequences and complementary coordination compounds. The resultant assembly will emulate the organization of ds-DNA molecules containing one strand of DNA, a second strand formed by stacked ligands, and an endless metal array running through the double helix axis.

To prove this concept, highly organized Pd-DNA double helices were prepared by using a self-assembly reaction between single-stranded dA_{15} and dX_{15} homopolymers and the complex [Pd(Cheld)(CH$_3$CN)], which was obtained by the reaction of Pd^{II} and chelidamic acid (Cheld) (Figure 4) [50]. Initially, the interaction of [Pd(Cheld)(CH$_3$CN)] with the individual bases 9-ethyladenine (EtA) and 9-propyl-7-deazaadenine (PrX) was studied to gain knowledge of the complex-base binding patterns. The PrX base serves as a reference to evaluate exclusive binding at the N1 atom because a CH group replaces the N7 atom.

NMR spectroscopy was used to follow the reaction between the Pd complex and the alkylated nucleobases. The ^{1}H NMR spectra revealed the co-existence of [Pd(Cheld)(*N1*-EtA)] and [Pd(Cheld)(*N7*-EtA)] isomers in solution, but an excess of [Pd(Cheld)(CH$_3$CN)] did not lead to bispalladium *N1,N7* species. As expected, in the case of PrX only signals for [Pd(Cheld)(*N1*- PrX)] were observed. In both cases, ESI mass spectrometry confirmed the formation of monopalladium species.

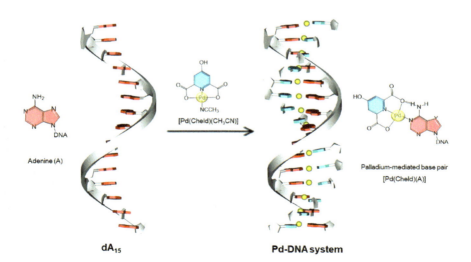

FIGURE 4 Example of the bottom-up strategy employed to prepare metal-DNA systems comprising continuous metal-mediated base pairs. This self-assembly reaction involves dA_{15} and the complex [Pd(Cheld)(CH$_3$CN)]. (Adapted from Ref. [50].)

Crystallization from a solution containing both isomers of the EtA complexes only yielded crystals of the N1-isomer. Single-crystal X-ray diffraction revealed the molecular structure of [Pd(Cheld)(*N1*-EtA)], and powder X-ray diffraction confirmed that this was the only isomer in the bulk polycrystalline sample. The molecular structure of [Pd(Cheld)(*N1*-EtA)] showed Pd(II) adopting a square-planar geometry to bind the Cheld ligand and the EtA base. Cheld acts as a tridentate ligand through both carboxylic groups and the endocyclic N-atom, and EtA acts as a monodentate ligand through the purine-N1 atom. Significantly, intramolecular hydrogen bonds form between the NH_2(EtA) group and a CO(Cheld) group, leading to a coplanar arrangement between the units and facilitating stacking interactions between contiguous complexes. Unsurprisingly, the molecular structure of [Pd(Cheld)(*N1*-PrX)] shows comparable organization. These structural features are ideal for organizing [Pd(Cheld)] units all over ss-DNA molecules to form a supramolecular stack of palladium-mediated base pairs. With this aim, Pd-dA_{15} and Pd-dX_{15} molecules were prepared using a self-assembly reaction between [Pd(Cheld)(CH_3CN)] and the corresponding homopolymer dA_{15} and dX_{15}, respectively. The reactions were studied by CD spectroscopy titrations. In both cases, the spectra showed new induced CD bands, indicating the binding of the metal complex to the oligonucleotides. Moreover, the presence of isodichroic points revealed the expected transition between the two-states population that can be related to free ss-DNA and metallized ss-DNA. Finally, the spectroscopic variations stabilized upon adding one equivalent of complex per base, confirming a 1:1 stoichiometry (base:complex). The close similarities observed between the spectra of Pd-dA_{15} and Pd-dX_{15} suggest the formation of identical B-form conformations. This indicates that the interaction of [Pd(Cheld)] with the homopolymers occurs through the N1(A) and N1(X) atoms, respectively, as seen in the crystallographic studies. ESI-MS further confirmed the existence of the Pd-DNA hybrids, and deconvoluted spectra showed peaks for each homopolymer with 15 [Pd(Cheld)] units, even in the presence of an excess of the complex. In addition, the fluorescence of ethidium bromide (EB) increases when Pd-dA_{15} is formed in solution compared to free dA_{15}, suggesting better intercalation of EB due to improved stacking interactions between coplanar metallized base pairs. Small-angle X-ray scattering (SAXS) recorded for Pd-dA_{15} demonstrates the existence of a monodisperse sample. The simulated scattering data obtained from a right-handed B-DNA-like model matches the experimental results, further supporting the formation of the proposed Pd-dA_{15}.

The experimental data obtained for the single [Pd(Cheld)(*N1*-EtA)] complex and the supramolecular Pd-dA_{15} assembly provided complete information to build a theoretical model. Consequently, a Pd-dA_{12} structure was modeled, composed of 12 palladium-mediated base pairs completing a helical turn. In addition, sodium ions were included as counterions to the phosphate groups, and water molecules were placed close to all acceptor and donor atoms. This Pd-dA_{12} structure was optimized using ab-initio calculations. The result showed a double helix conformation resembling ds-DNA with one strand being replaced by a supramolecular stack of Pd^{II} complexes (Figure 5). The structure contains an

Nucleic Acids for Continuous Hybrid Metallic Assemblies 247

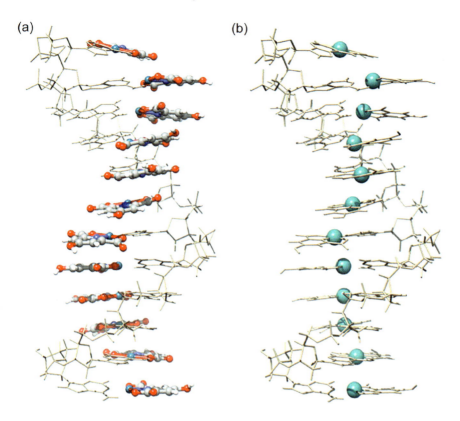

FIGURE 5 Two different representations of the optimized geometry structure of Pd-dA$_{12}$ show the organization of [Pd(Cheld)] lengthwise the system (a) and the formation of a continuous 1D array of Pd^{II} ions (b). Sodium cations and water molecules have been omitted for clarity. Atom color code: carbon, gray; hydrogen, white; nitrogen, light blue; oxygen, red; palladium, cyan; dA$_{12}$, tan (in (a) and (b)); Cheld, tan (in (b)). (Copyright 2021 Angew. Chem. Int. Ed. [50].)

uninterrupted one-dimensional Pd^{II} array running through the center of the helix with Pd···Pd distances in the range of 3.447–3.765 Å.

This remarkable result demonstrates that it is possible to use a bottom-up approach to create continuous palladium-mediated base pairs through poly(deoxyadenylic acid), controlling the stoichiometry, the organization, and the binding pattern. Notably, this strategy allows metal complexes to be modified to carry additional functionalities (i.e., chromophores or monomeric precursors of conducting polymers), opening the gate to create customized metal-DNA conjugates with superior properties. Moreover, this methodology can be further exploited to develop different metal-mediated base pairs with other nucleobases. If complexes are correctly designed, they could interact with specific bases in a sequence, as demonstrated by the recognition of thymine by Zn^{II}-cyclen complexes [139, 140], giving rise to more sophisticated supramolecular assemblies.

The properties of the resulting system would be highly modelable and would undoubtedly be very interesting, especially if several metals and ligands could be rationally introduced in the same structure.

In this regard, we have prepared a different palladium complex to recognize cytosine. The following results have not yet been published in a peer-reviewed journal and will be soon, but it is worth briefly exposing some results to highlight the potential of this methodology [141]. The reaction between the ligand 8-amino-4-hydroxyquinoline-2-carboxylic acid (Hq) and Pd^{II} affords the complex [Pd(Hq)(H$_2$O)] (Figure 6). This palladium complex has one amino and one carboxyl group capable of forming two complementary hydrogen bonds with cytosine. The reaction of [Pd(Hq)(H$_2$O)] and N1-methylcytosine (mC) led to the complex [Pd(Hq)(mC)], as confirmed by ^{1}H NMR and ESI-MS. The self-assembly reaction between [Pd(Hq)(H$_2$O)] and the homooligomer dC$_{15}$ also led to the formation of the supramolecular Pd-dC$_{15}$ assembly, which was confirmed utilizing CD spectroscopy and ESI-MS. Interestingly, although a 1:1 complex-base stoichiometry can be controlled in this assembly, an excess of palladium complex

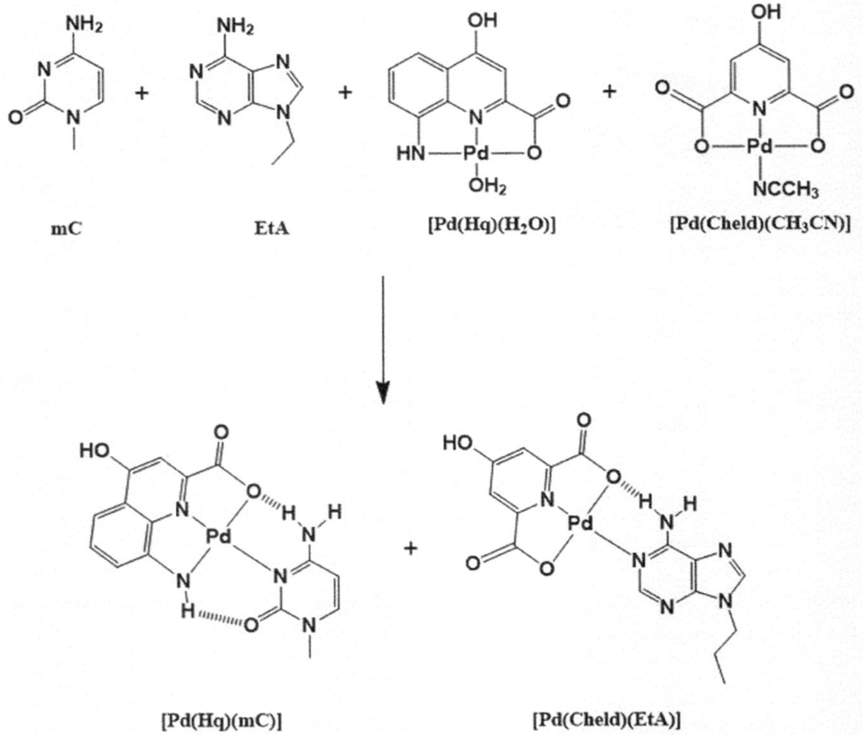

FIGURE 6 Reaction scheme showing the binding preference of [Pd(Hq)(H$_2$O)] and [Pd(Cheld)(CH$_3$CN)] for nucleobases 1-methylcytosine (mC) and 9-ethyladenine (EtA), respectively, forming metal-mediated [Pd(Hq)(mC)] and [Pd(Cheld)(EtA)] base pairs.

gave rise to structures with higher metal content. This could be due to the binding of a second Pd[II] complex to the O2(C) or N4(C) position after a first metal-binding interaction with the preferential N3(C) atom. Although more studies will be necessary to evaluate these possibilities, they cannot be ruled out since other similar examples have been described in the literature [142, 143]. Thus, Pd-dC$_{15}$ supramolecular assemblies can also be prepared using a self-assembly reaction between poly(deoxycytidylic acid) and cytosine-complementary complexes, as previously demonstrated for Pd-dA$_{15}$.

The next and most ambitious step requires testing whether [Pd(Cheld)(CH$_3$CN)] and [Pd(Hq)(H$_2$O)] complexes can preferentially bind to the nucleobases A and C, respectively. In this regard, competitive binding assays followed by ^{1}H NMR spectroscopy using the complexes [Pd(Hq)(H$_2$O)] and [Pd(Cheld)(CH$_3$CN)] and the bases mC and EtA showed that the most prevalent species formed were [Pd(Hq)(mC)] and [Pd(Cheld)(EtA)] (Figure 6). This result is in agreement with the formation of two hydrogen bonds in [Pd(Hq)(mC)] and only one hydrogen bond in [Pd(Cheld)(EtA)], which may facilitate the formation of these species (Figure 6). Moreover, complex [Pd(Cheld)(mC)] would be less favorable due to repulsion between the cytosine- and Cheld-keto groups.

It was also observed that if complex [Pd(Hq)(EtA)] is formed first, the addition of mC displaces EtA, leading to [Pd(Hq)(mC)]. However, other species were also found in solution due to ligand exchange processes, although in considerably less quantity. DFT calculations performed on [Pd(Hq)(mC)] and [Pd(Cheld)(EtA)] indicate that the binding energy between the precursor complexes and the nucleobases may not be large enough to yield two exclusive complexes, despite the formation of two hydrogen bonds in [Pd(Hq)(mC)] relative to one, or none, formed in other combinations. However, we can foresee that the correct design of the metal complexes could lead to a specific and more favorable interaction with the target nucleobases. Hence, the creation of metal-DNA systems can be extended to systems containing metallo-base pairs of different nature and organized according to a specific base sequence. The properties of such an assembly will depend on the metal, the ligand employed, and their organization. Therefore, this bottom-up strategy using ss-DNA molecules and custom metal complexes offers numerous possibilities for obtaining novel functional DNA-based nanomaterials, but could also find application in antisense and antigenic strategies based on custom metal complexes [144, 145] and in analytical applications.

5 GENERAL CONCLUSIONS

The development of nanotechnology based on DNA molecules makes it possible to design and create nanometric structures with high precision. The metallization of these assemblies gives rise to metal-DNA hybrid systems whose physicochemical properties are improved by the presence of metallic entities. However, the correct positioning of metal species in DNA assemblies remains a subject of research. Converting a DNA assembly into a corresponding metallic DNA assembly that maintains the initial design and structure remains a challenge for scientists. Continuous metallization of DNA systems throughout their structure has been successfully achieved. However, control over metal-DNA stoichiometry and homogeneous positioning of metals throughout the design still needs to be improved. The development of metallo-base pairs offers new advances in this area. This strategy allows the introduction of metal ions inside the DNA chains in a specific and controlled way. Still, the formation of DNA structures where all base pairs are metallized is a complex task that requires demanding synthetic processes. And above all, the way to metallize the interior of DNA while maintaining its initial structure is still being investigated.

One recent strategy offers alternatives to meet these challenges. It is based on the use of DNA molecules with 7-deazaadenine/thymine and 7-deazaguanine/cytosine base pairs. These base pairs allow a rational design of DNA assemblies based on canonical base pairs and promote the interaction of metal ions inside the double helix, maintaining the conceived base-pair arrangement. That is, it simplifies the conversion of Watson–Crick-type base pairs to their metallized counterparts, metal-modified Watson–Crick base pairs. Following this methodology, DNA duplexes with metal ions inside have been prepared, and the results indicate that the metal-DNA structure remains very close to the initial conformation. However, more research using different base sequences and more complex DNA assemblies is needed to assess the potential of this methodology to form metal-DNA structures on demand and to anticipate whether undesired mismatches could occur.

The use of metallo-base pairs can also be exploited using a bottom-up strategy. Correctly designed metal complexes and ss-DNA sequences can react in a self-assembly reaction leading to supramolecular metal-DNA systems comprising consecutive metal-mediated base pairs. This metal-DNA assembly contains highly organized metal ions running through the center of the helix and stacked organic ligands throughout the structure. The versatility of this methodology allows the design of different coordination compounds that could recognize different nucleobases so that the metal-DNA can be prepared to contain several metal ions and ligands in distinct sections of customized ss-DNA sequences.

ABBREVIATIONS AND DEFINITIONS

3WJ	three-way junction
4WJ	four-way junction
CD	circular dichroism
D	1-deazaadenine
Dipic	pyridine-2,6-dicarboxylate
ds-DNA	double-stranded DNA
EB	ethidium bromide
ESI-MS	electrospray ionization mass spectrometry
EtA	9-ethyladenine
H	hydroxypyridone

Hq	8-amino-4-hydroxyquinoline-2-carboxylic acid
mC	1-methylcytosine
NMR	nuclear magnetic resonance
ODN	oligodeoxyribonucleotide
P	pyridine
PrX	9-propyl-7-deazaadenine
SAXS	small-angle X-ray scattering
ss-DNA	single-stranded DNA
T_m	melting temperature
X	7-deazaadenine
Y	7-deazaguanine

REFERENCES

1. J. D. Watson, F. H. C. Crick, *Nature* **1953**, *171*, 737–738.
2. F. A. Hays, A. Teegarden, Z. J. R. Jones, M. Harms, D. Raup, J. Watson, E. Cavaliere, P. S. Ho, *Proc. Natl. Acad. Sci. USA* **2005**, *102*, 7157–7162.
3. K. J. Breslauer, R. Frank, H. Blöcker, L. A. Marky, *Proc. Natl. Acad. Sci. USA* **1986**, *83*, 3746–3750.
4. R. E. Dickerson, A. Klug, *J. Mol. Biol.* **1983**, *166*, 419–441.
5. R. J. Ellis, A. P. Minton, *Nature* **2003**, *425*, 27–28.
6. R. E. Franklin, X. R. G. Goslino, *Acta Cryst* **1953**, *6*, 673.
7. A. H. J. Wang, G. J. Quigley, F. J. Kolpak, J. L. Crawford, J. H. van Boom, G. van der Marel, A. Rich, *Nature* **1979**, *282*, 680–686.
8. R. Wing, H. Drew, T. Takano, C. Broka, S. Tanaka, K. Itakura, R. E. Dickerson, *Nature* **1980**, *287*, 755–758.
9. R. E. Dickerson, H. R. Drew, B. N. Conner, R. M. Wing, A. V. Fratini, M. L. Kopka, *Science* **1982**, *216*, 475–485.
10. G. Felsenfeld, D. R. Davies, A. Rich, *J. Am. Chem. Soc.* **2002**, *79*, 2023–2024.
11. D. R. Duckett, A. I. H. Murchie, S. Diekmann, E. von Kitzing, B. Kemper, D. M. J. Lilley, *Cell* **1988**, *55*, 79–89.
12. D. M. J. Lilley, *Quart. Rev. Biophys.* **2000**, *33*, 109–159.
13. C. Altona, J. A. Pikkemaat, F. J. J. Overmars, *Curr. Op. Struct. Biol.* **1996**, *6*, 305–316.
14. M. Gellert, M. N. Lipsett, D. R. Davies, *Proc. Natl. Acad. Sci. USA* **1962**, *48*, 2013–2018.
15. D. Sen, W. Gilbert, *Nature* **1988**, *334*, 364–366.
16. K. Gehring, J. L. Leroy, M. Guéron, *Nature* **1993**, *363*, 561–565.
17. X. Du, D. Wojtowicz, A. A. Bowers, D. Levens, C. J. Benham, T. M. Przytycka, *Nucleic Acids Res.* **2013**, *41*, 5965–5977.
18. R. Hänsel-Hertsch, D. Beraldi, S. V. Lensing, G. Marsico, K. Zyner, A. Parry, M. Di Antonio, J. Pike, H. Kimura, M. Narita, D. Tannahill, S. Balasubramanian, *Nat. Genet.* **2016**, *48*, 1267–1272.
19. S. Pandey, A. M. Ogloblina, B. P. Belotserkovskii, N. G. Dolinnaya, M. G. Yakubovskaya, S. M. Mirkin, P. C. Hanawalt, *Nucleic Acids Res.* **2015**, *43*, 6994–7004.
20. S. Kendrick, H. J. Kang, M. P. Alam, M. M. Madathil, P. Agrawal, V. Gokhale, D. Yang, S. M. Hecht, L. H. Hurley, *J. Am. Chem. Soc.* **2014**, *136*, 4161–4171.
21. G. M. Whitesides, J. P. Mathias, C. T. Seto, *Science* **1991**, *254*, 1312–1319.

22. P. W. K. Rothemund, *Nature* **2006**, *440*, 297–302.
23. Z. G. Wang, B. Ding, *Acc. Chem. Res.* **2014**, *47*, 1654–1662.
24. N. C. Seeman, *Ann. Rev. Biochem.* **2010**, *79*, 65–87.
25. N. C. Seeman, *J. Theor. Biol.* **1982**, *99*, 237–247.
26. F. Hong, F. Zhang, Y. Liu, H. Yan, *Chem. Rev.* **2017**, *117*, 12584–12640.
27. N. C. Seeman, *J. Biomol. Struct. Dyn.* **1990**, *8*, 573–581.
28. A. V. Pinheiro, D. Han, W. M. Shih, H. Yan, *Nat. Nanotechnol.* **2011**, *6*, 763–772.
29. F. Zhang, J. Nangreave, Y. Liu, H. Yan, *J. Am. Chem. Soc.* **2014**, *136*, 11198–11211.
30. N. C. Seeman, H. F. Sleiman, *Nat. Rev. Mat.* **2017**, *3*, 1–23.
31. Y. W. Kwon, D. H. Choi, J. I. Jin, *Polymer J.* **2012**, *44*, 1191–1208.
32. H. W. Fink, C. Schönenberger, *Nature* **1999**, *398*, 407–410.
33. M. Madsen, K. V. Gothelf, *Chem. Rev.* **2019**, *119*, 6384–6458.
34. E. Stulz, in *Molecular Architectonics and Nanoarchitectonics*, Eds T. Govindaraju, K. Ariga, Springer Nature, Switzerland AG, **2022**.
35. S. L. Beaucage, M. H. Caruthers, *Tetrahedron Lett.* **1981**, *22*, 1859–1862.
36. M. Eisenstein, *Nat. Biotechnol.* **2020**, *38*, 1113–1115.
37. T. J. Bandy, A. Brewer, J. R. Burns, G. Marth, T. N. Nguyen, E. Stulz, *Chem. Soc. Rev.* **2010**, *40*, 138–148.
38. K. Tanaka, A. Tengeiji, T. Kato, N. Toyama, M. Shionoya, *Science* **2003**, *299*, 1212–1213.
39. F. Linares, E. García-Fernández, F. J. López-Garzón, M. Domingo-García, A. Orte, A. Rodríguez-Diéguez, M. A. Galindo, *Chem. Sci.* **2019**, *10*, 1126–1137.
40. Y. Takezawa, J. Müller, M. Shionoya, *Chem. Lett.* **2017**, *46*, 622–633.
41. B. Jash, J. Müller, *Chem. Eur. J.* **2017**, *23*, 17166–17178.
42. B. Lippert, *J. Biol. Inorg. Chem.* **2022**, *27*, 215–219.
43. J. Müller, *Coord. Chem. Rev.* **2019**, *393*, 37–47.
44. A. Ono, H. Kanazawa, H. Ito, M. Goto, K. Nakamura, H. Saneyoshi, J. Kondo, *Angew. Chem. Int. Ed.* **2019**, *58*, 16835–16838.
45. Y. Takezawa, S. Sakakibara, M. Shionoya, *Chem. Eur. J.* **2021**, *27*, 16626–16633.
46. I. Schönrath, V. B. Tsvetkov, M. Barceló-Oliver, M. Hebenbrock, T. S. Zatsepin, A. V. Aralov, J. Müller, *J. Inorg. Biochem.* **2021**, *219*, 111369.
47. A. Zhang, S. Budow-Busse, P. Leonard, F. Seela, *Chem. Eur. J.* **2021**, *27*, 10574–10577.
48. J. M. Méndez-Arriaga, C. R. Maldonado, J. A. Dobado, M. A. Galindo, *Chem. Eur. J.* **2018**, *24*, 4583–4589.
49. N. Santamaría-Díaz, J. M. Méndez-Arriaga, J. M. Salas, M. A. Galindo, *Angew. Chem. Int. Ed.* **2016**, *55*, 6170–6174.
50. A. Pérez-Romero, A. Domínguez-Martín, S. Galli, N. Santamaría-Díaz, O. Palacios, J. A. Dobado, M. Nyman, M. A. Galindo, *Angew. Chem. Int. Ed.* **2021**, *60*, 10089–10094.
51. S. M. Douglas, I. Bachelet, G. M. Church, *Science* **2012**, *335*, 831–834.
52. Q. Hu, H. Li, L. Wang, H. Gu, C. Fan, *Chem. Rev.* **2018**, *119*, 6459–6506.
53. Ed N. V. Hud, *Nucleic Acid-Metal Ion Interactions*, Royal Society of Chemistry, Cambridge, **2008**.
54. Eds N. Hadjiliadis, E. Sletten, *Metal Complex-DNA Interactions*, John Wiley & Sons Ltd, Chichester, **2009**.
55. H. Sigel, *Chem. Soc. Rev.* **1993**, *22*, 255–267.
56. Z. Chen, C. Liu, F. Cao, J. Ren, X. Qu, *Chem. Soc. Rev.* **2018**, *47*, 4017–4072.
57. B. Lippert, *Coord. Chem. Rev.* **2000**, *200–202*, 487–516.
58. B. Lippert, P. J. Sanz Miguel, *Acc. Chem. Res.* **2016**, *49*, 1537–1545.

59. S. A. Kazakov, S. M. Hecht, Nucleic Acid–Metal Ion Interactions. *Encyclopedia of Inorganic Chemistry*, John Wiley & Sons Ltd, **2006**, pp. 1–34.
60. Y. Liu, J. Vinje, C. Pacifico, G. Natile, E. Sletten, *J. Am. Chem. Soc.* **2002**, *124*, 12854–12862.
61. M. A. Galindo, A. Houlton, *Inorg. Chim. Acta* **2009**, *362*, 625–633.
62. M. A. Galindo, D. Amantia, A. M. Martinez, W. Clegg, R. W. Harrington, V. M. Martinez, A. Houlton, *Inorg. Chem.* **2009**, *48*, 10295–10303.
63. M. A. Galindo, D. Amantia, A. Martinez-Martinez, W. Clegg, R. W. Harrington, V. M. Martinez, A. Houlton, *Inorg. Chem.* **2009**, *48*, 11085–11091.
64. Eds G. M. Blackburn, M. J. Gait, D. Loakes, D. M. Williams, *Nucleic Acids in Chemistry and Biology*, Royal Society of Chemistry, Cambridge, **2007**.
65. S. Katz, *Nature* **1962**, *195*, 997–998.
66. A. Ono, S. Cao, H. Togashi, M. Tashiro, T. Fujimoto, T. Machinami, S. Oda, Y. Miyake, I. Okamoto, Y. Tanaka, *Chem. Comm.* **2008**, 4825–4827.
67. Y. Miyake, H. Togashi, M. Tashiro, H. Yamaguchi, S. Oda, M. Kudo, Y. Tanaka, Y. Kondo, R. Sawa, T. Fujimoto, T. Machinami, A. Ono, *J. Am. Chem. Soc.* **2006**, *128*, 2172–2173.
68. Ed B. Lippert, *Cisplatin: Chemistry and Biochemistry of a Leading Anticancer Drug*, VHCA Zürich and Wiley-VCH, **1999**.
69. W. Zhou, R. Saran, J. Liu, *Chem. Rev.* **2017**, *117*, 8272–8325.
70. E. Braun, Y. Eichen, U. Sivan, G. Ben-Yoseph, *Nature* **1998**, *391*, 775–778.
71. J. T. Petty, J. Zheng, N. V. Hud, R. M. Dickson, *J. Am. Chem. Soc.* **2004**, *126*, 5207–5212.
72. A. Gonzàlez-Rosell, C. Cerretani, P. Mastracco, T. Vosch, S. M. Copp, *Nanoscale Adv.* **2021**, *3*, 1230–1260.
73. R. Guha, S. M. Copp, *Chapter 12 of this book*.
74. P. J. de Pablo, F. Moreno-Herrero, J. Colchero, J. Gómez Herrero, P. Herrero, A. M. Baró, P. Ordejón, J. M. Soler, E. Artacho, *Phys. Rev. Lett.* **2000**, *85*, 4992–4995.
75. A. Houlton, S. M. D. Watson, *Ann. Rep. Prog. Chem. Sect. A* **2011**, *107*, 21–42.
76. H. D. A. Mohamed, S. M. D. Watson, B. R. Horrocks, A. Houlton, *J. Mat. Chem. C* **2015**, *3*, 438–446.
77. M. Al-Hinai, R. Hassanien, S. M. D. Watson, N. G. Wright, A. Houlton, B. R. Horrocks, *Nanotech.* **2016**, *27*, 095704.
78. L. Berti, A. Alessandrini, P. Facci, *J. Am. Chem. Soc.* **2005**, *127*, 11216–11217.
79. S. M. D. Watson, H. D. A. Mohamed, B. R. Horrocks, A. Houlton, *Nanoscale* **2013**, *5*, 5349–5359.
80. T. Bayrak, N. S. Jagtap, A. Erbe, *Int. J. Mol. Sci.* **2018**, *19*, 3019.
81. S. M. D. Watson, A. R. Pike, J. Pate, A. Houlton, B. R. Horrocks, *Nanoscale* **2014**, *6*, 4027–4037.
82. D. Porath, N. Lapidot, J. Gomez-Herrero, *Lect. Note Phys.* **2006**, *680*, 411–444.
83. E. Toomey, J. Xu, S. Vecchioni, L. Rothschild, S. Wind, G. E. Fernandes, *J. Phys. Chem. C* **2016**, *120*, 7804–7809.
84. Z. Lin, X. Li, H.-B. Kraatz, *Anal. Chem.* **2011**, *83*, 6896–6901.
85. G. Eidelshtein, N. Fardian-Melamed, V. Gutkin, D. Basmanov, D. Klinov, D. Rotem, Y. Levi-Kalisman, D. Porath, A. Kotlyar, *Adv. Mat.* **2016**, *28*, 4839–4844.
86. S. Katz, *Biochim. Biophys. Acta* **1963**, *68*, 240–253.
87. K. Tanaka, M. Shionoya, *J. Org. Chem.* **1999**, *64*, 5002–5003.
88. M. Hebenbrock, J. Müller, in *Comprehensive Inorganic Chemistry III*, Eds J. Reedijk, K. Poeppelmeier, Elsevier, in press (doi: 10.1016/B978-0-12-823144-9.00033-9).

89. E. Meggers, P. L. Holland, W. B. Tolman, F. E. Romesberg, P. G. Schultz, *J. Am. Chem. Soc.* **2000**, *122*, 10714–10715.
90. S. Atwell, E. Meggers, G. Spraggon, P. G. Schultz, *J. Am. Chem. Soc.* **2001**, *123*, 12364–12367.
91. S. K. Jana, X. Guo, H. Mei, F. Seela, *Chem. Comm.* **2015**, *51*, 17301–17304.
92. S. Mandal, A. Hepp, J. Müller, *Dalton Trans.* **2015**, *44*, 3540–3543.
93. I. Okamoto, K. Iwamoto, Y. Watanabe, Y. Miyake, A. Ono, *Angew. Chem. Int. Ed.* **2009**, *48*, 1648–1651.
94. A. Fujii, O. Nakagawa, Y. Kishimoto, T. Okuda, Y. Nakatsuji, N. Nozaki, Y. Kasahara, S. Obika, *Chem. Eur. J.* **2019**, *25*, 7443–7448.
95. D. U. Ukale, T. Lönnberg, *Angew. Chem. Int. Ed.* **2018**, *57*, 16171–16175.
96. Y. Takezawa, K. Nishiyama, T. Mashima, M. Katahira, M. Shionoya, *Chem. Eur. J.* **2015**, *21*, 14713–14716.
97. Y. Takezawa, A. Suzuki, M. Nakaya, K. Nishiyama, M. Shionoya, *J. Am. Chem. Soc.* **2020**, *142*, 21640–21644.
98. J. Kondo, T. Sugawara, H. Saneyoshi, A. Ono, *Chem. Comm.* **2017**, *53*, 11747–11750.
99. I. Okamoto, T. Ono, R. Sameshima, A. Ono, *Chem. Comm.* **2012**, *48*, 4347–4349.
100. L. L. G. Al-Mahamad, O. El-Zubir, D. G. Smith, B. R. Horrocks, A. Houlton, *Nat. Comm.* **2017**, *8*, 1–7.
101. S. M. Swasey, E. G. Gwinn, *New J. Phys.* **2016**, *18*, 045008.
102. S. M. Swasey, L. E. Leal, O. Lopez-Acevedo, J. Pavlovich, E. G. Gwinn, *Sci. Rep.* **2015**, *5*, 10163.
103. S. M. Swasey, F. Rosu, S. M. Copp, V. Gabelica, E. G. Gwinn, *J. Phys. Chem. Lett.* **2018**, *9*, 6605–6610.
104. F.-A. Polonius, J. Müller, *Angew. Chem. Int. Ed.* **2007**, *46*, 5602–5604.
105. F. Seela, T. Wenzel, *Helv. Chim. Acta* **1994**, *77*, 1485–1499.
106. D. A. Megger, C. Fonseca Guerra, J. Hoffmann, B. Brutschy, F. M. Bickelhaupt, J. Müller, *Chem. Eur. J.* **2011**, *17*, 6533–6544.
107. J. Kondo, Y. Tada, T. Dairaku, Y. Hattori, H. Saneyoshi, A. Ono, Y. Tanaka, *Nat. Chem.* **2017**, *9*, 956–960.
108. E. Ennifar, P. Walter, P. Dumas, *Nucleic Acids Res.* **2003**, *31*, 2671–2682.
109. J. Kondo, Y. Tada, T. Dairaku, H. Saneyoshi, I. Okamoto, Y. Tanaka, A. Ono, *Angew. Chem. Int. Ed.* **2015**, *54*, 13323–13326.
110. T. Atsugi, A. Ono, M. Tasaka, N. Eguchi, S. Fujiwara, J. Kondo, *Angew. Chem. Int. Ed.* **2022**, *61*, e202204798.
111. H. Isobe, N. Yamazaki, A. Asano, T. Fujino, W. Nakanishi, S. Seki, *Chem. Lett.* **2011**, *40*, 318–319.
112. E. Xu, Y. Lv, J. Liu, X. Gu, S. Zhang, *RSC Adv.* **2015**, *5*, 49819–49823.
113. S. Liu, G. H. Clever, Y. Takezawa, M. Kaneko, K. Tanaka, X. Guo, M. Shionoya, *Angew. Chem. Int. Ed.* **2011**, *50*, 8886–8890.
114. J. C. Léon, Z. She, A. Kamal, M. H. Shamsi, J. Müller, H.-B. Kraatz, *Angew. Chem. Int. Ed.* **2017**, *56*, 6098–6102.
115. H. Gong, X. Li, *Analyst* **2011**, *136*, 2242–2246.
116. N. Fardian-Melamed, L. Katrivas, G. Eidelshtein, D. Rotem, A. Kotlyar, D. Porath, *Nano Lett.* **2020**, *20*, 4505–4511.
117. R. M. Smith, I. Colliard, M. Amiri, M. A. Galindo, M. Nyman, *Cryst. Growth Des.* **2022**, *22*, 2294–2306.
118. L. Mistry, O. El-Zubir, G. Dura, W. Clegg, P. G. Waddell, T. Pope, W. A. Hofer, N. G. Wright, B. R. Horrocks, A. Houlton, *Chem. Sci.* **2019**, *10*, 3186–3195.
119. L. Mistry, O. El-Zubir, T. Pope, P. G. Waddell, N. Wright, W. A. Hofer, B. R. Horrocks, A. Houlton, *Cryst. Growth Des.* **2021**, *21*, 4398–4405.

120. A. Terrón, B. Moreno-Vachiano, A. Bauzá, A. García-Raso, J. J. Fiol, M. Barceló-Oliver, E. Molins, A. Frontera, *Chem. Eur. J.* **2017**, *23*, 2103–2108.
121. D. J. E. Huard, A. Demissie, D. Kim, D. Lewis, R. M. Dickson, J. T. Petty, R. L. Lieberman, *J. Am. Chem. Soc.* **2019**, *141*, 11465–11470.
122. D. Schultz, K. Gardner, S. S. R. Oemrawsingh, N. Markešević, K. Olsson, M. Debord, D. Bouwmeester, E. Gwinn, *Adv. Mat.* **2013**, *25*, 2797–2803.
123. C. Cerretani, H. Kanazawa, T. Vosch, J. Kondo, *Angew. Chem. Int. Ed.* **2019**, *58*, 17153–17157.
124. S. M. Copp, D. Schultz, S. Swasey, J. Pavlovich, M. Debord, A. Chiu, K. Olsson, E. Gwinn, *J. Phys Chem. Lett.* **2014**, *5*, 959–963.
125. N. C. Seeman, N. R. Kallenbach, *Biophys. J.* **1983**, *44*, 201–209.
126. H. Liu, F. Shen, P. Haruehanroengra, Q. Yao, Y. Cheng, Y. Chen, C. Yang, J. Zhang, B. Wu, Q. Luo, R. Cui, J. Li, J. Ma, J. Sheng, J. Gan, *Angew. Chem. Int. Ed.* **2017**, *56*, 9430–9434.
127. X. Guo, P. Leonard, S. A. Ingale, J. Liu, H. Mei, M. Sieg, F. Seela, *Chem. Eur. J.* **2018**, *24*, 8883–8892.
128. E. Eremeeva, M. Abramov, L. Margamuljana, P. Herdewijn, *Chem. Eur. J.* **2017**, *23*, 9560–9576.
129. F. Seela, H. Thomas, *Helv. Chim. Acta* **1995**, *78*, 94–108.
130. H. Zhao, P. Leonard, X. Guo, H. Yang, F. Seela, *Chem. Eur. J.* **2017**, *23*, 5529–5540.
131. A. Domínguez-Martín, D. Choquesillo-Lazarte, J. A. Dobado, H. Martínez-García, L. Lezama, J. M. González-Pérez, A. Castiñeiras, J. Niclós-Gutiérrez, *Inorg. Chem.* **2013**, *52*, 1916–1925.
132. J. Kypr, I. Kejnovská, D. Renčiuk, M. Vorlíčková, *Nucleic Acids Res.* **2009**, *37*, 1713–1725.
133. A. Parkinson, M. Hawken, M. Hall, K. J. Sanders, A. Rodger, *Phys. Chem. Chem. Phys.* **2000**, *2*, 5469–5478.
134. S. I. Nakano, L. Wu, H. Oka, H. T. Karimata, T. Kirihata, Y. Sato, S. Fujii, H. Sakai, M. Kuwahara, H. Sawai, N. Sugimoto, *Mol. BioSyst.* **2008**, *4*, 579–588.
135. M. A. Galindo, J. Plavec, U. Javornik, M. Nyman, M. Bera, O. Palacios, unpublished results.
136. M. Surin, S. Ulrich, *Chem. Open* **2020**, *9*, 480–498.
137. S. Pullen, J. Tessarolo, G. H. Clever, *Chem. Sci.* **2021**, *12*, 7269–7293.
138. A. Aro-Heinilä, T. Lönnberg, *Chem. Eur. J.* **2017**, *23*, 1028–1031.
139. E. Kimura, M. Shionoya, *Met. Ions Biol. Syst.* **1996**, *33*, 29–52.
140. E. Kimura, H. Kitamura, K. Ohtani, T. Koike, *J. Am. Chem. Soc.* **2000**, *122*, 4668–4677.
141. M. A. Galindo, A. Pérez-Romero, O. Palacios, C. López-Chamorro, unpublished results.
142. S. Coşar, M. B. L. Janik, M. Flock, E. Freisinger, E. Farkas, B. Lippert, *J. Chem. Soc., Dalton Trans.* **1999**, 2329–2336.
143. L. Yin, P. J. Sanz Miguel, W. Hiller, B. Lippert, *Inorg. Chem.* **2012**, *51*, 6784–6793.
144. J. Müller, M. Drumm, M. Boudvillain, M. Leng, E. Sletten, B. Lippert, *J. Biol. Inorg. Chem.* **2000**, *5*, 603–611.
145. M. B. L. Janik, B. Lippert, *J. Biol. Inorg. Chem.* **1999**, *4*, 645–653.

11 Recent Advances in the Development of Metal-Responsive Functional DNAs Based on Metal-Mediated Artificial Base Pairing

Yusuke Takezawa and Mitsuhiko Shionoya**
Department of Chemistry, Graduate School of
Science, The University of Tokyo, Tokyo, Japan
takezawa@chem.s.u-tokyo.ac.jp,
shionoya@chem.s.u-tokyo.ac.jp

CONTENTS

1	Introduction	258
2	Stabilization of DNA Duplexes by Metal-Mediated Base Pairing	260
	2.1 Metal-Mediated Base Pairing with Natural Nucleobases	260
	2.2 Cu^{II}-Mediated Hydroxypyridone Base Pair	263
	2.3 Metal-Mediated Base Pairs with Carboxyimidazole and Its Analogs	266
3	Metal-Responsive Functional DNAs with Metal-Mediated Base Pairs Consisting of Natural Nucleobases	268
	3.1 Metal-Responsive RNA-Cleaving DNAzymes	268
	3.2 Metal-Responsive Peroxidase-Mimicking DNAzymes	270
	3.3 Metal-Responsive DNA Aptamers	272
4	Metal-Responsive Functional DNAs with Metal-Mediated Base Pairs Consisting of Artificial Nucleobases	273
	4.1 Metal-Responsive Split DNAzymes	273
	4.2 Metal-Responsive Single-Stranded DNAzymes	275
	4.3 Metal-Responsive DNA Aptamers	277

---

* Corresponding authors

DOI: 10.1201/9781003270201-11

4.4 AND-Logic Gate DNAzyme Responsive to Two Different
Metal Ions 278
5 Development of Metal-Responsive Bifacial Nucleobases for
Future Applications 279
5.1 Design Concept of Metal-Responsive Bifacial Nucleobases 279
5.2 Bifacial Base-Pairing Behavior of 5-Hydroxyuracil Bases 281
5.3 Hydrogen-Bonded and Metal-Mediated Base Pairing of
5-Carboxyuracil Bases 282
5.4 Applications of the Bifacial Nucleobases 283
6 Concluding Remarks 285
Abbreviations 286
References 287

Abstract

Metal ions have a large impact on the structure and stability of DNA. The most studied metal-DNA interaction is the formation of interstrand metal complexes between opposing nucleobases and a bridging metal ion. These 2:1 metal complexes are called metal-mediated base pairs because they function as alternative base pairs for DNA duplexes. Natural pyrimidine nucleobases, T and C, are known to form such metallo-base pairs with Hg[II] and Ag[I] ions, respectively. In addition, a variety of unnatural nucleobases that can form metal-mediated base pairs have been synthesized to date. In most cases, the metal-mediated base pairing allows for metal-dependent stabilization of DNA duplexes. Recently, the metal-mediated base pairing has been applied to the development of metal-responsive functional DNAs and recognized as versatile building blocks in DNA supramolecular chemistry and DNA nanotechnology. For example, metal-mediated base pairs have been incorporated into previously obtained DNAzymes (catalytic DNA) and DNA aptamers. Their catalytic activity and binding ability can be regulated in response to metal ions that induce the formation of metal-mediated base pairs in functionally active structures. Furthermore, ligand-type nucleobases that form both metal-mediated base pairs and hydrogen-bonded base pairs were newly devised as metal-responsive building units. Thus, the development and application of metal-mediated artificial base pairing have become an active research area in DNA chemistry. This chapter reviews recent progress in the study of metal-mediated artificial base pairing, focusing primarily on the development of metal-responsive functional DNAs.

KEYWORDS

Artificial Base Pair; Metal-Mediated Base Pairing; DNAzyme; DNA Nanotechnology; Coordination Chemistry; Molecular Switching

1 INTRODUCTION

DNA molecules carry the genetic information of living organisms, which is encoded as a sequence of nucleotide monomers, A, T, G, and C. Natural DNA molecules normally form right-handed anti-parallel duplexes, with complementary hydrogen bonds forming Watson-Crick base pairs (i.e., A–T and G–C). In a typical B-DNA duplex, nucleobase pairs are regularly stacked, with an inter-base-pair distance of about 3.3–3.4 Å. DNA has excellent molecular recognition capabilities based on base pairing, allowing for sequence-specific hybridization. Metal ions have a significant impact on the structure and stability of DNA [1]. The stability of DNA duplexes is greatly affected by the concentration of metal cations such as Na^I and Mg^{II}, which reduce the electron repulsion between negatively charged phosphate groups. It is also well known that G-quadruplex structures consisting of G-rich sequences are stabilized by K^I ions [2]. The K^I ions are located between two stacked G-quartet planes and coordinated by the eight O6 carbonyl groups of the G bases. In addition to phosphate groups and carbonyl oxygen atoms, endocyclic nitrogen atoms such as N3 of pyrimidine bases and N7 of purine bases are also good metal-binding sites. For example, the well-known metallodrug cisplatin (*cis*-[PtCl$_2$(NH$_3$)$_2$]) binds primarily to the N7 positions of two adjacent G bases [3].

The most studied metal-DNA interaction is the formation of interstrand metal complexes between opposing nucleobases and a bridging metal ion. These 2:1 metal complexes are called metal-mediated base pairs [4–7] or metal-modified base pairs [8] because they function as alternative base pairs for DNA duplexes (Figure 1). In most cases, metal-mediated base pairing results in metal-dependent stabilization of DNA duplexes, which is easily confirmed by duplex melting analysis. The natural pyrimidine nucleobases, T and C, are known to form such metallo-base pairs with Hg^{II} and Ag^I ions, respectively [9]. There are also a great number of excellent reports on metal crosslinks between natural nucleobases with other metal ions such as the binding of transplatin [10]. A variety of

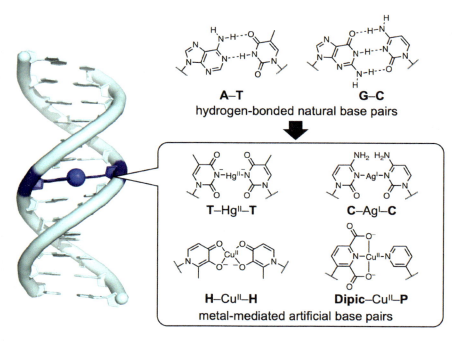

FIGURE 1 Schematic diagram of a DNA duplex containing a metal-mediated artificial base pair. Examples of metal-mediated base pairs are those consisting of natural nucleobases (T–Hg^{II}–T and C–Ag^I–C) and synthetic nucleobases (**H**–Cu^{II}–**H** and **Dipic**–Cu^{II}–**P**).

unnatural nucleobases that can form metal-mediated base pairs have been synthesized. The first example of a fully artificial metal-mediated base pair, developed by Tanaka and Shionoya in 1999, consists of a synthetic nucleoside bearing an *o*-phenylenediamine ligand as the nucleobase [11]. This nucleoside was reported to form a Pd^{II}-mediated base pair at the monomeric level, but was not successfully introduced into oligonucleotides for synthetic reasons. Subsequently, in 2000, Schultz et al. demonstrated Cu^{II}-mediated base pairing within a DNA duplex using an artificial nucleoside with pyridine-2,6-dicarboxylic acid (**Dipic**) and pyridine ligands (**P**) [12]. In metal-metal-mediated base pairing, metal ions that prefer linear coordination (such as Hg^{II} and Ag^{I}) or square-planar coordination (such as Cu^{II} and Ni^{II}) are used as bridging metal ions, because the resulting complexes can adopt a planar structure suitable for base-pair stacking within DNA duplexes. Artificial ligand-type nucleosides are generally synthesized by coupling reactions between a deoxyribose derivative and a metal ligand as the nucleobase moiety. After the reactive functional group of the ligand moiety is protected if necessary, the nucleoside can be incorporated into the desired position of the DNA oligomer by using an automated DNA synthesizer. DNA duplexes containing ligand-bearing nucleotide pairs form complexes with appropriate metal ions to form metal-mediated base pairs. The metal-mediated base pairing can be characterized by duplex melting experiments, UV-vis absorption spectroscopy, NMR spectroscopy, EPR spectroscopy, mass spectrometry, and single-crystal X-ray diffraction analysis.

Metal-mediated base pairs have recently been applied to the development of metal-responsive functional DNAs and recognized as versatile building blocks in DNA supramolecular chemistry and DNA nanotechnology. For example, metal-mediated base pairs have been incorporated into known DNAzymes (catalytic DNA) and DNA aptamers. Their catalytic activity and molecular recognition ability can be controlled in a manner responsive to metal ions that induce the formation of metal-mediated base pairs in the functionally active structures. In addition, novel ligand-type nucleobases that form both metal-mediated and hydrogen-bonded base pairs have been devised as metal-responsive building units. Thus, the development and application of metal-mediated artificial base pairing have become an active research area in DNA chemistry. This chapter reviews recent studies on the metal-mediated artificial base pairing, with a particular focus on the development of metal-responsive functional DNAs.

2 STABILIZATION OF DNA DUPLEXES BY METAL-MEDIATED BASE PAIRING

2.1 Metal-Mediated Base Pairing with Natural Nucleobases

The metal-mediated base pairing was first proposed for the interaction of Hg^{II} ions with natural thymine (T) bases in the early 1960s [13–15]. Hg^{II}-mediated T–Hg^{II}–T base pairing was characterized and came into the limelight in the late 2000s [16, 17]. In the T–Hg^{II}–T base pair, the T bases, from which the two imine protons dissociate, coordinate linearly to the Hg^{II} ion. T–Hg^{II}–T base pairs can be easily constructed inside DNA duplexes composed exclusively of natural nucleotides, which allows for a wide range of applications [9]. One of the typical features of metal-mediated base pairing is the metal-dependent stabilization of DNA duplexes. DNA duplexes containing one T–T mismatch are stabilized by the addition of Hg^{II} ions (ΔT_m=+10 °C under certain conditions) by the formation of the T–Hg^{II}–T base pair [16, 18]. The addition of other metal ions does not result in the stabilization of the duplex, clearly indicating metal specificity. Isothermal titration calorimetry (ITC) revealed that the association constant (K_a) of 1:1 binding of Hg^{II} to a DNA duplex containing a T–T mismatch pair to form a T–Hg^{II}–T base pair is in the order of 5×10^5 M^{-1} [18]. The structure of the T–Hg^{II}–T base pair in DNA duplexes was first clarified by NMR spectroscopy [17]. The addition of Hg^{II} caused the imino proton signal to disappear and the ^{15}N resonance at the N3 positions to shift significantly downfield (about +30 ppm), suggesting that the Hg^{II} ion is bound to the deprotonated N3 atom of the T bases. The N3–Hg^{II}–N3 linkage was also confirmed by the two-bond ^{15}N–^{15}N coupling across the metal ion ($^2J_{N,N}$=2.4 Hz) observed in a duplex with ^{15}N-labeled T bases. The T–Hg^{II}–T base pair was also characterized by single-crystal X-ray diffraction analysis [19]. The crystal structure of a DNA duplex with two consecutive T–Hg^{II}–T base pairs revealed that the Hg^{II} ions are located between the opposing T residues. The C1′–C1′ distance was 9.5–9.6 Å, shorter than that of natural Watson-Crick base pairs (10.7 Å), but the T–Hg^{II}–T base pairing did not distort the right-handed B-DNA helix. Binding modes of Hg^{II} ions to thymine bases in DNA duplexes are still being actively studied [20]. It is also noteworthy that structurally related uracil (U) nucleobases have been found to form similar U–Hg^{II}–U base pairs in RNA duplexes [21].

Cytosine (C) nucleobases form an Ag^{I}-mediated C–Ag^{I}–C base pair, with the Ag^{I} ion coordinating linearly to the N3 atoms [22]. A DNA duplex containing a C–C mismatch pair is significantly stabilized by the addition of Ag^{I} ions (ΔT_m = +8 °C), confirming the formation of a C–Ag^{I}–C base pair in the duplex. Other metal ions exhibit no significant stabilizing effect, indicating that Ag^{I} binds to the C–C mismatch in a highly specific manner. The association constant (K_a) of C–Ag^{I}–C within a DNA duplex has been estimated to be 4×10^5 M^{-1} [23]. In terms of thermodynamic parameters, the T–Hg^{II}–T and the C–Ag^{I}–C base pairs were found to have comparable stability. Single-crystal X-ray analysis revealed that the C–Ag^{I}–C base pair has an A-type duplex structure in the RNA duplex [24]. The C1′–C1′ distance was 9.1–9.6 Å, shorter than that of Watson-Crick base pairs. The propeller twist angle (−29° to −27°) of the C–Ag^{I}–C base pairs was significantly greater than those of natural base pairs inside RNA duplexes (−12°). This deviation was due to the repulsion between the amino groups of the C bases. The structure of the C–Ag^{I}–C base pair in the DNA duplex was further determined by NMR spectroscopy in solution [25]. The N3–Ag^{I}–N3 bonding was directly confirmed by the ^{15}N–^{109}Ag coupling ($^1J_{Ag,N}$=83–84 Hz). The exocyclic N4 atoms exhibited triplet resonances, indicating that the 4-NH$_2$ group did not tautomerize or metal-coordinate. The structure determined by NOEs showed that the C–Ag^{I}–C base pairs have a propeller twist of −18°, but do not distort the B-form duplex structure.

Metal-mediated base-pairing structures found in the crystal structures of DNA have received increasing attention recently; in addition to T–Hg^{II}–T and C–Ag^{I}–C base pairs, metal-mediated base pairs of natural nucleobases have been observed in the crystal state. For example, Kondo et al. reported that the DNA dodecamer 5′-d(GGA CT[BrC]C GAC TCC)-3′ ([BrC]: 5-bromo-2′-deoxycytidine) forms a nonstandard duplex structure consisting only of Ag^I-mediated base pairs in the crystal (Figure 2a) [26]. Not only C–Ag^I–C base pairs, but also T–Ag^I–T, G–Ag^I–C, and G–Ag^I–G base pairs were formed by the coordination of endocyclic nitrogen atoms. The T–Ag^I–T pair has a very similar structure to the T–Hg^{II}–T base pair, with deprotonated T bases binding to the central metal ion. The G–Ag^I–C pair is similar to the canonical Watson-Crick G–C base pair because the Ag^I ion formally replaces the central proton of the G–C base pair. The G–Ag^I–G base pair consists of two G residues with a *syn* conformation that coordinate to the Ag^I ion via the N7 position. The metallo-duplexes were linked to each other by the formation of intermolecular G–Ag^I–G base pairs, forming an uninterrupted, one-dimensional Ag^I array along the DNA helix axis. Hydrogen bonds between base pairs were formed in the major groove and, as a result, the entire metal-DNA duplex structure is stabilized.

A short DNA oligomer 5′-d(GCA CGC GC)-3′ was found to form a double-stranded structure containing C–Ag^I–C and G–Ag^I–G base pairs in the crystal state [27]. While the glycosidic bonds in the C–Ag^I–C base pair normally have a cisoid arrangement in the B-form duplex, the C–Ag^I–C pairs found in the crystal have a transoid form. The G–Ag^I–G base pairs are formed by the coordination of the N7 atoms of the two G bases. The G residue adopts a reversed Hoogsteen orientation, which is different from the structure described above. Very recently, a rod-shaped DNA

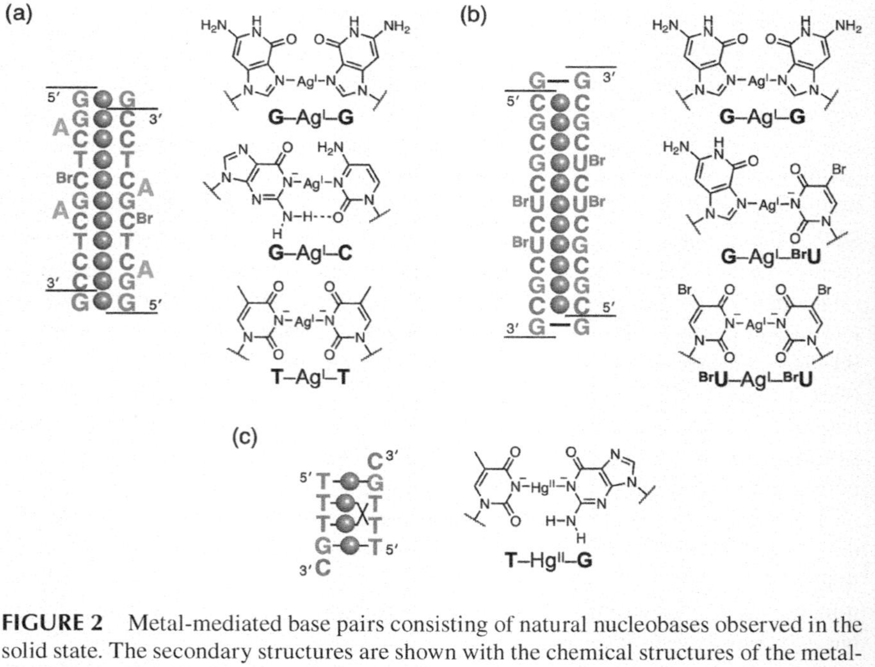

FIGURE 2 Metal-mediated base pairs consisting of natural nucleobases observed in the solid state. The secondary structures are shown with the chemical structures of the metal-mediated base pairs. The structures of the classic T–Hg^{II}–T and C–Ag^I–C base pairs are not shown.

structure containing 11 Ag^I ions was constructed using the oligonucleotide 5'-d(CGC GC^{Br}U C^{Br}UC GCG)-3' (^{Br}U: 5-bromo-2'-deoxyuridine) [28]. Crystallographic analysis showed that the oligomer formed a double-helical structure consisting of C–Ag^I–C, G–Ag^I–G, G–Ag^I–^{Br}U, and ^{Br}U–Ag^I–^{Br}U base pairs (Figure 2b). In the new G–Ag^I–^{Br}U base pair, the G residue adopted a *syn* conformation and the Ag^I was linearly coordinated by the N7 of the G base and the N3 of the deprotonated ^{Br}U base. The structure of the ^{Br}U–Ag^I–^{Br}U base pair was identical to that of the T–Ag^I–T base pair. Spectroscopic titration studies as well as mass spectrometry suggested the formation of a similar rod-shaped metallo-DNA duplex in solution.

The crystal structure of a short oligonucleotide 5'-d(TTT GC)-3' with Hg^{II} ions revealed a new base pair mediated by Hg^{II} (Figure 2c) [29]. The oligomer formed a double-stranded structure containing two T–Hg^{II}–T base pairs and two T–Hg^{II}–G base pairs. The T–Hg^{II}–G base pair was formed by the coordination of the N3 of the T base and the N1 of the G base. Hg^{II}–N distances (2.2–2.4 Å) confirmed that both nucleobases were deprotonated. Circular dichroism (CD) spectroscopy and mass spectrometry showed that the Hg^{II}-DNA complex is also present in the solution.

Metal-mediated base pairing consisting of natural nucleobases can be easily incorporated into the molecular architecture of DNA and is widely used in the field of DNA nanotechnology. In addition to DNA-based molecular sensors that detect Hg^{II} [30] and Ag^I ions [22], various metal-responsive DNA systems have been developed that utilize T–Hg^{II}–T and C–Ag^I–C base pairing. As evidenced by the examples of metallo-base pairs found in the crystal structures, Hg^{II} and Ag^I can also bind to other nucleobases. Thus, metal-mediated base pairing with unnatural ligand-type nucleobases and other metal ions is becoming increasingly important in terms of advanced DNA system design. The use of various metal ions also expands the functional diversity of the resulting metallo-DNA complexes. The following is an overview of typical examples of metal-mediated base pairing with synthetic nucleobases.

2.2 Cu^{II}-Mediated Hydroxypyridone Base Pair

The most studied metal-mediated artificial base pair is the 3-hydroxy-4-pyridone ligand-type nucleobase (**H**) reported by Tanaka and Shionoya (Figure 3) [31]. Hydroxypyridone is known as a bidentate ligand that forms 2:1 square-planar complexes with metal ions such as Cu^{II}. **H**-bearing nucleoside was synthesized by coupling reaction of the ligand moiety and the deoxyribose, and incorporated into the DNA strand using a standard automated DNA synthesizer. The **H** nucleosides were found to form a stable Cu^{II}-mediated base pair (**H**–Cu^{II}–**H**) within the DNA duplexes, as confirmed by melting analysis, UV, and electron paramagnetic resonance (EPR) spectroscopy. In the UV spectra of a duplex containing an **H**–**H** pair, a new absorption band appeared around 314 nm after the addition of Cu^{II} ions. This spectral change indicated metal complexation of the **H** ligands with deprotonation of the hydroxy group. The EPR spectra showed that the Cu^{II} ion was present in the square-planar ligand field, which also confirmed the formation of the **H**–Cu^{II}–**H** complex. A crystal structure of the **H**–Cu^{II}–**H** pair within

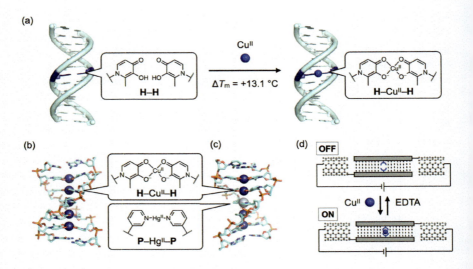

FIGURE 3 Cu^{II}-mediated base pairing of artificial hydroxypyridone-bearing nucleotides (**H**). (a) Stabilization of a duplex by **H**–Cu^{II}–**H** base pairing. (b) Assembly of homologous metals by DNA templates based on five **H**–Cu^{II}–**H** base pairs. (c) Heterologous metal assembly by a DNA template based on four **H**–Cu^{II}–**H** and one **P**–Hg^{II}–**P** base pairs. (d) Cu^{II}-dependent regulation of the conductivity of metallo-DNA devices filling gaps in carbon nanotubes.

the DNA duplex has not been reported, but the crystal structure within a simplified DNA analog (glycol nucleic acid) was elucidated by Meggers et al. [32]. The **H**–Cu^{II}–**H** base pair had a square-planar geometry in the *cis* configuration as expected. The C1′–C1′ distance of the **H**–Cu^{II}–**H** base pair was found to be 10.7 Å, slightly shorter than that of Watson-Crick base pairs (about 12.7 Å). The **H**–Cu^{II}–**H** base pair is thought to have almost the same structure inside the DNA duplexes. Importantly, CD spectroscopy suggested that the **H**–Cu^{II}–**H** base pairing hardly distorts the standard B-type duplex structure.

The formation of the **H**–Cu^{II}–**H** base pair increased the thermal stability of the entire duplex (Figure 3a) [31]. Replacing a natural A–T base pair with an **H**–**H** pair greatly destabilized the duplex ($\Delta T_m = -7.2°C$), indicating that **H**–**H** behaves as a mismatch pair. In the presence of one equivalent of Cu^{II} ions, the duplex with an **H**–**H** pair was significantly stabilized ($\Delta T_m = +13.1°C$). In contrast, the addition of Cu^{II} ions to the natural DNA duplex did not stabilize it. These results indicate that the DNA duplex was stabilized by the formation of an **H**–Cu^{II}–**H** base pair. Such a duplex stabilization was not observed with other transition metal ions such as Mn^{II}, Co^{II}, Ni^{II}, Zn^{II}, Pd^{II}, and Pt^{II} [33]. In addition, Hg^{II} and Ag^{I}, which can form metal-mediated base pairs with natural nucleobases, did not improve the stability of the duplex with an **H**–**H** pair. This metal specificity plays an important role in the application of **H**–Cu^{II}–**H** base pairing as discussed below.

This stable **H**–Cu^{II}–**H** base pairing was first applied to the construction of discrete metal arrays (Figure 3b) [34]. Oligonucleotides, 5′-d(G**H**$_n$C)-3′ ($n = 1$–5), consisting of consecutive **H** nucleotides and terminal natural-type nucleotides were used as the template ligands for metal assembly. Complexation with Cu^{II} ions led to the formation of the multinuclear complexes, Cu$^{II}{}_n$·(5'-d(GH$_n$C)-3')$_2$ (n = 1–5), which contain consecutive **H**–Cu^{II}–**H** base pairs. As a result, arrays of one to five Cu^{II} ions could be constructed inside the DNA duplexes. Interestingly, EPR measurements revealed that the Cu^{II} ions were ferromagnetically coupled. The distances between Cu^{II} ions were estimated to be about 3.7 Å, suggesting that this is comparable to the distance between stacked natural base pairs. Furthermore, the assembly of two different metal ions, Cu^{II} and Hg^{II}, in combination with a pyridine-based Hg^{II}-mediated base pair (**P**–Hg^{II}–**P**), using DNA as a template was demonstrated (Figure 3c) [35]. Oligonucleotides containing both **H** and **P** nucleotides (e.g., 5'-d(**GHPHC**)-3') were found to form double-stranded heteronuclear complexes (e.g., Cu$^{II}{}_2$·Hg^{II}·(5'-d(**GHPHC**)-3')$_2$) as characterized by UV and CD titration analyses and mass spectrometry. These results indicated that arrays of heterologous metal ions (e.g. Cu^{II}–Hg^{II}–Cu^{II}) were constructed inside the DNA duplexes. The sequence of metal ions can be determined specifically by the sequence of the ligand-type nucleobases on the DNA strands.

Recently, **H**–Cu^{II}–**H** base pairing has been applied to modulate the electrical conductivity of DNA duplexes (Figure 3d) [36]. Direct conductance measurements were performed using a carbon nanotube device covalently bridged with DNA duplexes containing **H**–Cu^{II}–**H** base pairs. The analysis showed that the conductance of the metallo-DNA duplexes was greater than that without Cu^{II} ions. It was also demonstrated that alternating addition of Cu^{II} and the chelating agent ethylenediamine-N,N,N',N'-tetraacetate (EDTA) causes periodic on–off switching of conductivity. These results indicate that **H**–Cu^{II}–**H** base pairs are a versatile building block for constructing metal-dependent switching devices composed of DNA.

The incorporation of unnatural ligand-type nucleotides, such as **H** nucleotides, into DNA strands is generally done by conventional solid-phase synthesis. Recent studies have demonstrated that **H** nucleotides can be incorporated using standard enzymes, providing a new synthetic method (Figure 4) [33]. A Klenow fragment of DNA polymerase I lacking proofreading activity (KF exo$^-$) was found to incorporate **H** nucleotide triphosphate (dHTP) into a DNA primer when the opposite base on the template is A or T. Further elongation after **H**–A/T mismatch pair was not observed with KF exo$^-$. However, the subsequent addition of natural nucleotides (dNTPs) and a lesion-bypass polymerase (Dpo IV) further promoted the extension reactions to yield the full-length product. As a result, DNA oligomers containing one **H** nucleotide in the middle were enzymatically synthesized by a two-step primer extension reaction using two DNA polymerases (i.e., KF exo$^-$ and Dpo IV) and a natural DNA template (Figure 4a). Polymerase incorporation of dHTP and subsequent enzymatic ligation reactions made it possible to introduce two or more **H** nucleotides at distant positions (Figure 4b) [37]. Furthermore, the lesion-bypass Dpo IV polymerase was used to consecutively incorporate **H** nucleotides at a predetermined position under optimized conditions [38]. This enzymatic synthesis was further applied to the development of metal-responsive functional DNAs as described below (see Section 4).

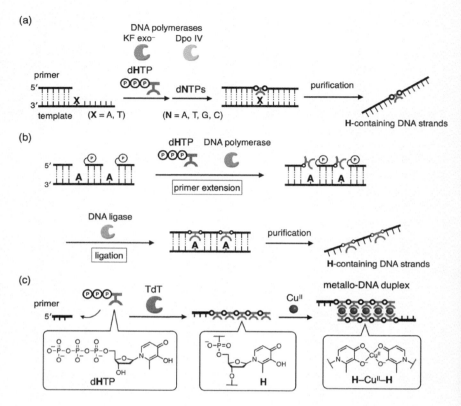

FIGURE 4 Enzymatic synthesis of artificial DNA strands containing ligand-type hydroxypyridone (**H**) nucleotides (a) with two DNA polymerase (KF exo⁻ and Dpo IV), (b) with DNA polymerase and ligase, and (c) with template-independent DNA polymerase (TdT).

The reaction with terminal deoxynucleotidyl transferase (TdT), a template-independent polymerase, produced DNA oligomers with several **H** nucleotides attached at the 3′-terminus (Figure 4c) [39]. In particular, DNA duplexes with a 3′-protruding end were tailed site-specifically with an average of 5.5 **H** nucleotides. The resulting **H**-tailed duplex formed a dimeric structure by the formation of **H**–Cu^{II}–**H** base pairs, which was confirmed by native polyacrylamide gel electrophoresis (PAGE) analysis. Template-independent polymerase reactions could be used for post-synthetic modification of DNA structures and would be a novel tool for building metal-responsive DNA-based supermolecules.

2.3 Metal-Mediated Base Pairs with Carboxyimidazole and Its Analogs

4-Carboxyimidazole (**Im^C**) nucleosides form one of the most stabilizing metal-mediated base pairs with Cu^{II} ions (Figure 5); the **Im^C**–Cu^{II}–**Im^C** base pair was

Metal-Responsive Functional DNAs Based on Artificial Base Pairing 267

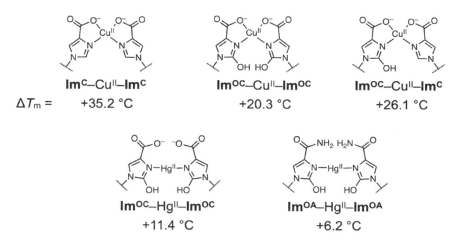

FIGURE 5 Metal-mediated base pairs consisting of nucleotides with carboxyimidazole and its analogs. ΔT_m represents the difference in melting temperature (T_m) of a duplex containing a metal-mediated base pair relative to that of the corresponding metal-free duplex.

first reported by Müller et al. in 2019 [40]. In the first report, Cu^{II}-mediated base pairing was studied in a pH 9.0 buffer; the addition of Cu^{II} ions increased the melting temperatures (T_m) of duplexes containing an **Im^C–Im^C** pair by about +20°C, suggesting the formation of an **Im^C–Cu^{II}–Im^C** base pair. The **Im^C** nucleobases of both strands bind the Cu^{II} ion as bidentate ligands to form a square-planar complex. In 2020, a metal-responsive DNAzyme (see Section 4.1) was reported by Takezawa and Shionoya et al. using the same metallo-base pair [41]. In the course of this study, the **Im^C–Cu^{II}–Im^C** base pairing was found to greatly stabilize the duplex under neutral conditions, and the DNAzyme reactions were examined under the same conditions. A 15-mer duplex with an **Im^C–Im^C** mismatch in the middle was used for duplex melting analysis at pH 7.0. In the absence of Cu^{II} ions, the T_m value was estimated to be 22.5°C, significantly lower than that of the natural duplex $(T_m = 44.2°C)$. Notably, the duplex containing an **Im^C–Im^C** pair is less stable than the duplex containing an **H–H** pair (37.0°C). The large destabilization of the duplex was interpreted to be the result of electric repulsion between the two negatively charged **Im^C** bases. The addition of one equivalent of Cu^{II} ions markedly improved the duplex stability $(T_m = 57.7°C, \Delta T_m = +35.2°C)$ due to the formation of an **Im^C–Cu^{II}–Im^C** base pair. The **Im^C–Cu^{II}–Im^C** base pair is arguably one of the most stabilizing metal-mediated base pairs reported to date.

In addition to Cu^{II} ions, other divalent transition metal ions were found to stabilize the duplexes containing an **Im^C–Im^C** pair [41]. For instance, the addition of Co^{II} $(\Delta T_m = +11.3°C)$, Ni^{II} (+14.0°C), and Zn^{II} ions (+15.9°C) improved the duplex stability. However, their stabilization effect (ΔT_m) is significantly smaller than that of Cu^{II}. Interestingly, the metal-dependent stabilization trend follows the Irving-Williams series $(Co^{II} < Ni^{II} < Cu^{II} > Zn^{II})$, which is known to explain the typical binding affinity of the first-row transition metal ions. Furthermore, the **Im^C** base was found to form Ag^I- and Hg^{II}-mediated base pairs presumably by N–Ag^I/Hg^{II}–N monodentate coordination. Under neutral conditions, a duplex with an **Im^C–Im^C** pair was stabilized by the addition of Ag^I and Hg^{II} ions (ΔT_m=+17.7 °C and +12.6 °C, respectively). However, **Im^C–Ag^I–Im^C** and **Im^C–Hg^{II}–Im^C** base pairs are less stabilizing than the **Im^C–Cu^{II}–Im^C** base pair.

More recently, structurally related base pairs were developed by Takezawa and Shionoya et al. (Figure 5) [42]. The metal-mediated base-pairing properties of a novel 2-oxo-imidazole-4-carboxylate (**Im^{OC}**) nucleobase and the previously reported 2-oxo-imidazole-4-carboxamide (**Im^{OA}**) nucleobase [43] were studied under neutral conditions. Both nucleobases have an NH group and a carboxylate/carboxamide as coordinating sites as well as an additional carbonyl group. The corresponding nucleosides can be easily derived from commercially available 5-bromo-2'-deoxyuridine by a ring contraction reaction. Duplex melting analysis and mass spectrometric measurements revealed that the **Im^{OC}** base forms a stable Cu^{II}-mediated base pair (**Im^{OC}–Cu^{II}–Im^{OC}**), in contrast to **Im^{OA}**. The duplex containing the **Im^{OC}–Im^{OC}** pair was stabilized by +20.3 °C by the formation of the **Im^{OC}–Cu^{II}–Im^{OC}** base pair, in which both the carboxy group and the deprotonated N3 atoms are thought to coordinate to the Cu^{II} center. The effects of other divalent metal ions (Mn^{II} to Zn^{II}, Pd^{II}, and Pt^{II}) were examined, and it was found that only Cu^{II} ions substantially stabilize the duplex. In other words, **Im^{OC}** showed superior metal selectivity compared to the previous **Im^C** nucleobase. The **Im^{OC}** base also combined with **Im^C** to form an unsymmetric metallo-base pair (**Im^{OC}–Cu^{II}–Im^C**). Interestingly, the ΔT_m of the **Im^{OC}–Cu^{II}–Im^C** base pair (+26.1°C) is intermediate between those of the two symmetric base pairs, **Im^{OC}–Cu^{II}–Im^{OC}** (+35.2°C) and **Im^C–Cu^{II}–Im^C** (+20.3°C). Like the **Im^C** base, **Im^{OC}** and **Im^{OA}** also formed Hg^{II}-mediated base pairs, **Im^{OC}–Hg^{II}–Im^{OC}** and **Im^{OA}–Hg^{II}–Im^{OA}**, showing Hg^{II}-dependent duplex stabilization (ΔT_m=+11.4 °C and +6.2 °C, respectively). However, the addition Ag^I ions did not change the duplex stability. Thus, the **Im^{OC}** and **Im^{OA}** bases have improved metal selectivity compared to the **Im^C** base, presumably due to the need to remove imino protons for metal complexation.

3 METAL-RESPONSIVE FUNCTIONAL DNAS WITH METAL-MEDIATED BASE PAIRS CONSISTING OF NATURAL NUCLEOBASES

3.1 METAL-RESPONSIVE RNA-CLEAVING DNAZYMES

DNAzymes, also called deoxyribozymes, are short DNA oligomers that catalyze chemical reactions similar to protein enzymes [44, 45]. Since the discovery of a DNAzyme catalyzing RNA cleavage in 1994 [46], a number of DNAzymes catalyzing various reactions such as ligation, peptide linkage, and oxidation have been reported to date. DNAzymes are generally obtained by a method called Systematic Evolution of Ligands by EXponential Enrichment (SELEX) or *in vitro* selection.

DNA oligomers with catalytic activity (i.e., DNAzymes) are selected from a large library of random DNA sequences. Most DNAzymes require metal ions (or metal complexes) such as Mg^{II} for their catalytic function. DNAzymes are widely used as components of molecular sensors, molecular devices, and molecular machines because of the ease of chemical modification and sequence-dependent hybridization of oligonucleotides. For such applications, the development of stimuli-responsive DNAzymes has attracted increasing attention. In particular, metal-dependent DNAzymes can be rationally designed by using metal-mediated base pairs.

Hg^{II}-mediated T–Hg^{II}–T base pairing was first applied by Lu et al. to the design of metal-responsive DNAzymes (Figure 6a) [47]. The Hg^{II}-responsive DNAzyme was designed based on the sequence of a UO_2^{2+}-dependent RNA-cleaving DNAzyme obtained by *in vitro* selection [48]. The UO_2^{2+}-dependent DNAzyme is composed of a catalytic domain, a substrate-binding domain, and a

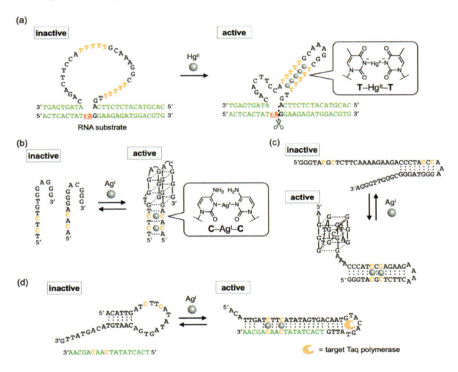

FIGURE 6 Metal-responsive functional DNAs with metal-mediated base pairs consisting of natural nucleobases. The base sequence is shown in both inactive and active secondary structures. (a) Design of a Hg^{II}-responsive RNA-cleaving DNAzyme based on T–Hg^{II}–T base pairing. The "rA" in the substrate represents the cleavage site, adenine ribonucleotide. (b, c) Design of Ag^{I}-responsive horseradish peroxidase (HRP)-mimicking DNAzymes based on C–Ag^{I}–C base pairing. The induced G-quadruplex structures exhibit peroxidase activity in the presence of the cofactor hemin. (d) Design of an Ag^{I}-responsive DNA aptamer based on C–Ag^{I}–C base pairing. The aptamer binds to Taq DNA polymerase in the presence of Ag^{I} ions.

variable stem loop. One-to-six T–T mismatch pairs were inserted into the stem region to allow the modified DNAzymes to form the catalytically active structure through the formation of T–Hg^{II}–T base pairs. All DNAzymes with T–T mispairs showed higher RNA-cleaving activity in the presence of Hg^{II} ions than in the absence of Hg^{II}. For example, the activity of the DNAzyme with five T–T pairs was increased 153-fold by the addition of Hg^{II} ions. These results suggest that the DNAzyme activity was restored because the catalytically active structure was stabilized by the formation of T–Hg^{II}–T base pairs. The resulting Hg^{II}-dependent DNAzyme was converted into a catalytic beacon for Hg^{II} detection by labeling the substrate with a fluorescent dye and a quencher. Addition of Hg^{II} ions activated the DNAzyme and increased fluorescence. This DNAzyme sensor showed high selectivity for Hg^{II} ions and the detection limit was determined to be 2.4 nM.

Willner et al. developed metal-responsive DNAzymes [49] based on a different RNA-cleaving DNAzyme named E6 [50]. The E6 DNAzyme was fragmented into two subunits and T–T mismatches were introduced into the stem duplex. The two fragments dissociated in the absence of Hg^{II} ions because the stem duplex was too short. As a result, DNAzyme activity was significantly reduced. The RNA-cleavage activity increased with increasing concentrations of Hg^{II} ions. This is because the T–Hg^{II}–T base pairing helped to hybridize the two split strands and to reassemble the structure of the active DNAzyme. The addition of other metal ions resulted in less activity, and as a result, the metal selectivity was found to be good. Removal of Hg^{II} ions with dihydrolipoic acid-functionalized magnetic particles also switched off DNAzyme activity. Cycles of activation and inactivation were repeated by alternating treatment of the DNAzyme with Hg^{II} ions and the modified magnetic beads. Similarly, an Ag^{I}-responsive split DNAzyme based on the Ag^{I}-mediated C–Ag^{I}–C base pairing was developed [49]. The DNAzyme activity increased when more Ag^{I} ions were added, indicating a good response to Ag^{I} ions. The selectivity for Ag^{I} ions was also confirmed. When Ag^{I} ions were removed by dithiol-functionalized magnetic beads, the catalytic function of the DNAzyme was inactivated, and when Ag^{I} ions were re-added, the DNAzyme activity was restored. Thus, it was confirmed that the addition and removal of Ag^{I} ions can switch the activation and inactivation of the DNAzyme.

These Hg^{II}- and Ag^{I}-responsive DNAzymes were developed by modification of *in vitro*-selected DNAzymes with T–T and C–C mismatch pairs, which form T–Hg^{II}–T and C–Ag^{I}–C base pairs in the presence of the corresponding metal ions. Molecular sensors have also been constructed using these metal-responsive DNAzymes to detect Hg^{II} or Ag^{I} ions. Because DNA oligomers composed entirely of natural nucleotides are readily prepared, Hg^{II}- and Ag^{I}-responsive DNAzymes have a wide range of applications.

3.2 Metal-Responsive Peroxidase-Mimicking DNAzymes

DNAzymes that mimic horseradish peroxidase (HRP) belong to another class of DNAzymes that have been well studied [51]. The HRP-mimicking DNAzyme consists of a G-quadruplex structure and a hemin cofactor and catalyzes oxidation reactions in the presence of H_2O_2, like catalase. DNAzyme-catalyzed oxidation reactions can be easily monitored by the color change of ABTS (2,2′-azino-bis(3-ethylbenzothiazoline-6-sulfonic acid)) and by luminol chemiluminescence. Thus, the G-quadruplex–hemin DNAzymes have been widely used to create DNA-based molecular sensors. Similar to RNA-cleaving DNAzymes, Hg^{II}- and Ag^{I}-responsive HRP-mimicking DNAzymes have been developed based on metal-mediated base pairing.

The earliest example is the Ag^{I}-responsive split DNAzyme reported by Dong et al. (Figure 6b) [52]. They designed an intermolecular G-quadruplex consisting of two G-rich DNA strands and introduced two C–C mismatch pairs in its appended duplex region. In the absence of Ag^{I} ions, the DNAzyme showed very low activity, mainly due to the inherent catalytic activity of hemin itself. This result indicates that the DNAzyme loses its catalytic activity due to the low stability of the G-quadruplex structure. In the presence of Ag^{I} ions, oxidation of the substrate (ABTS) was clearly observed by the color change. The formation of the C–Ag^{I}–C pairs facilitated the assembly of the G-quadruplex and the binding of the hemin cofactor, resulting in the Ag^{I}-mediated activation of the DNAzyme. The DNAzyme activity was enhanced at higher Ag^{I} concentrations. Therefore, quantitative detection of Ag^{I} ions by the colorimetric method was performed using this system, and the detection limit was determined to be 2.5 nM. Importantly, the DNAzyme showed higher selectivity for Ag^{I} than for other metal ions. Note that Hg^{II} ions slightly inhibited the DNAzyme activity. This is presumably because Hg^{II} ions bind to the T residues in the structure and prevent the G-quadruplex from folding. The addition of cysteine, which can remove Ag^{I} ions from the DNAzyme, reduced the DNAzyme activity. The same design principle was adopted by Kong et al. who developed an Hg^{II}-responsive split HRP-mimicking DNAzyme containing three T–T mismatch pairs [53]. This DNAzyme was activated by the formation of T–Hg^{II}–T base pairs and applied to detect Hg^{II} ions in water. Competition experiments showed that the DNAzyme is highly selective for Hg^{II} ions.

Another Ag^{I}-responsive DNAzyme was also developed based on a different strategy [54]. This DNAzyme consists of only a single strand comprising a catalytic G-quadruplex sequence and an appended domain containing a duplex-forming sequence (Figure 6c). In the absence of Ag^{I} ions, the oligonucleotide folded into an intramolecular duplex by hybridization of the G-rich and appended domains. Therefore, it was not possible to form a catalytically active G-quadruplex. In the presence of Ag^{I} ions, the appended domain formed an intramolecular duplex containing C–Ag^{I}–C base pairs, and the remaining G-rich domain folded into a G-quadruplex. The results showed that the DNAzyme efficiently catalyzes H_2O_2-mediated oxidation reactions in the presence of hemin cofactors. This mechanism was verified by CD and UV-vis spectroscopy. A similar Ag^{I}-responsive DNAzyme was developed by using two strands of different length [55]. In the absence of Ag^{I} ions, the blocker strand binds to the quadruplex-forming domain of the DNAzyme strand and inhibits its catalytic activity. The addition of Ag^{I} ions caused a portion of the DNAzyme strand to fold into an intramolecular duplex via the formation of multiple C–Ag^{I}–C base pairs, and the blocker strand to dissociate. As a result, the

DNAzyme strand formed a G-quadruplex structure. Thus, the HRP-mimicking DNAzyme was activated in response to the addition of Ag^I ions.

3.3 Metal-Responsive DNA Aptamers

DNA aptamers are DNA oligomers that recognize and bind to target molecules including proteins. The metal-mediated base pairing was also applied to control the functions of DNA aptamers [56]. Park et al. reported metal-dependent reversible switching of DNA aptamer functions. The function of DNA aptamers binding to Taq DNA polymerases could be regulated by the formation of $T-Hg^{II}-T$ and $C-Ag^I-C$ base pairs. The results showed that the DNA polymerases were activated and inactivated in response to Hg^{II} and Ag^I ions. The Hg^{II}-responsive DNA aptamer (designated TQ21D) was derived from the known DNA aptamer TQ21 [57]. The TQ21D aptamer has many thymine (T) bases in the loop region, which are considered essential for binding to the target. In the absence of Hg^{II} ions, the aptamer bound to the target, resulting in complete inhibition of the DNA polymerases. When a large excess of Hg^{II} ions was added, the DNA polymerase regained activity. This suggests that the DNA aptamer lost its binding ability. This is because the structure of the TQ21D aptamer has been distorted by the binding of Hg^{II} ions to the T bases. The DNA aptamer was further activated by the addition of cysteine, which binds strongly to Hg^{II} ions. Alternate addition of Hg^{II} and cysteine reversibly switched the binding ability of the DNA aptamer. The TQ21D aptamer was found to have high specificity to Hg^{II} ions.

In addition, an Ag^I-responsive DNA aptamer (TQ30D) based on the $C-Ag^I-C$ base pairing was developed (Figure 6d) [56]. The TQ30D aptamer was designed by modifying the sequence of another DNA aptamer (TQ30) that can inhibit Taq polymerase [57]. The system consists of two strands, an extended DNA aptamer that forms a hairpin structure and a blocker DNA. These strands were complementary to each other except for two C–C mismatch pairs. In the absence of Ag^I ions, the two strands were separated and the aptamer formed an inactive hairpin structure. Thus, the DNA aptamer did not inhibit the DNA polymerase. When Ag^I ions were added, the DNA aptamer recovered its binding affinity to the DNA polymerase and inhibited the polymerization reaction. The Ag^I-mediated activation of the aptamer was explained by the binding of the blocker DNA to the aptamer via $C-Ag^I-C$ base pairing, inducing the formation of an active structure that can inhibit the polymerase. Other metal ions did not activate the TQ30D aptamer, indicating high specificity for Ag^I ions. Furthermore, reversible ON–OFF switching of the aptamer function was demonstrated by the addition of Ag^I ions and cysteine, which removes Ag^I from the aptamer.

In both cases, the metal-mediated base pairing alters the structure of the known aptamers, resulting in metal-dependent regulation of the aptamer function. A number of DNA aptamers have been discovered that bind to various molecules and inhibit target enzymes. Therefore, incorporation of $T-Hg^{II}-T$ and $C-Ag^I-C$ base pairs into their sequences would be a promising approach to regulate biological functions, such as enzyme activity, using metal ions as stimuli.

4 METAL-RESPONSIVE FUNCTIONAL DNAs WITH METAL-MEDIATED BASE PAIRS CONSISTING OF ARTIFICIAL NUCLEOBASES

4.1 Metal-Responsive Split DNAzymes

By incorporating metal-mediated base pairs into DNA strands, we can construct metal-responsive functional DNAs. However, the metal ions used as stimuli are limited to Hg^{II} and Ag^{I} ions when only natural nucleotides are used. Because Hg^{II} and Ag^{I} bind strongly to natural T and C bases, the development of Hg^{II}- and Ag^{I}-responsive DNA systems often involves the binding of metal ions at unexpected positions. Artificial metal-mediated base pairing consisting of unnatural ligand-type nucleobases has been employed to solve this problem.

In 2019, Takezawa and Shionoya et al. reported the first metal-responsive DNAzymes using Cu^{II}-mediated artificial base pairing [33]. Compared to Hg^{II} and Ag^{I} ions, Cu^{II} ions interfere little with natural nucleobases, making sequence design simpler. A Cu^{II}-responsive DNAzyme was developed by introducing a Cu^{II}-mediated hydroxypyridone base pair (**H**–Cu^{II}–**H**) [31] into a known RNA-cleaving DNAzyme (E5 DNAzyme [50]) (Figure 7a). E5 DNAzyme was split into

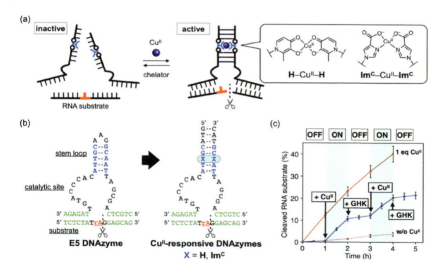

FIGURE 7 Development of metal-responsive split DNAzymes using metal-mediated base pairs consisting of artificial nucleobases. (a) Schematic diagram of Cu^{II}-responsive RNA-cleaving DNAzymes based on **H**–Cu^{II}–**H** or **Im^C**–Cu^{II}–**Im^C** base pairs. (b) Base sequences of the original RNA-cleaving E5 DNAzyme and Cu^{II}-responsive split DNAzymes. The "rA" in the substrate represents the cleavage site, adenine ribonucleotide. (c) Repetitive switching of the activity of **Im^C**-modified DNAzyme by the addition and removal of Cu^{II} ions. Cu^{II} (1 equiv.), GHK (2 equiv.), Cu^{II} (2 equiv.), and GHK (4 equiv.) were sequentially added. [DNAzyme] = 1.0 μM, [substrate] = 10 μM, 25 °C, $N = 3$. The activity in the presence (red solid lines) and absence of Cu^{II} ions (red dotted lines) is also shown.

two fragments, with one set of **H** nucleotides incorporated into the variable stem duplex. Although the split DNAzyme lost its catalytic activity, it was expected to regain its catalytically active structure by forming **H**–Cu^{II}–**H** base pairs in the presence of Cu^{II} ions. Therefore, the length of the stem region and the position of the **H**–**H** pair were varied to find the optimal sequence. As a result, a DNAzyme with an 8-bp stem duplex containing an **H**–**H** pair at the third position from the catalytic core showed a good response to Cu^{II} ions (Figure 7b).

Next, the RNA-cleaving activity of the modified DNAzyme was evaluated in the presence of ten equivalents of substrate and the apparent first-order rate constants (k_{obs}) were compared. In the absence of Cu^{II} ions, the k_{obs} for the modified DNAzyme was 0.029 h^{-1}, significantly lower than that of the original E5 DNAzyme (0.23 h^{-1}). The results clearly showed that the introduction of an **H**–**H** mismatch pair efficiently suppressed the DNAzyme activity. The addition of one equivalent of Cu^{II} ions improved the k_{obs} to 0.16 h^{-1} and the ON–OFF ratio was found to be about 5.5. In contrast, the RNA-cleaving activity of E5 DNAzyme was not increased by the addition of Cu^{II}. Accordingly, it was concluded that the addition of Cu^{II} ions enhanced the catalytic activity of the modified **H**-DNAzyme. Titration of Cu^{II} ions showed that equimolar amounts of Cu^{II} ions were sufficient to activate the modified DNAzyme. These results suggest that the quantitative formation of an **H**–Cu^{II}–**H** base pair induced the hybridization of the split strands and reconstructed the catalytically active DNAzyme structure. The activity of the **H**-modified DNAzyme can be reversibly regulated by the addition and removal of Cu^{II} ions. The addition of Cu^{II} ions caused a rapid increase in the DNAzyme activity. Next, the DNA enzyme was found to be efficiently inactivated by the addition of a Cu^{II}-binding peptide (GHK) [58], which can trap Cu^{II} ions. Equimolar amounts of Cu^{II} and GHK were added alternately to repeatedly switch DNAzyme activity. Furthermore, the DNAzyme activity can be regulated according to the oxidation state of the Cu ions. When sodium ascorbate was added to a mixture of **H**-modified DNAzyme and Cu^{II} ions, the DNAzyme activity was markedly reduced to the level comparable to that observed without Cu^{II}. The results showed that the **H**-modified DNAzyme was inactivated by reducing Cu^{II} ions. Conversely, the addition of an oxidant restored DNAzyme activity.

The switching efficiency of the metal-responsive split DNAzyme was improved by using another Cu^{II}-mediated base pair, **Im^C**–Cu^{II}–**Im^C** (Figure 7a) [41]. As described in Section 2.3, the **Im^C**–Cu^{II}–**Im^C** base pairing leads to higher duplex stabilization (ΔT_m=+35.2°C) than the **H**–Cu^{II}–**H** base pairing (+13.1°C) under neutral conditions. The parent E5 DNAzyme strand [50] was then split in two and a pair of **Im^C** nucleotides was incorporated at the same position as in the **H**-modified split DNAzyme (Figure 7b). In the absence of Cu^{II} ions, the activity of the **Im^C**-modified DNAzyme was significantly suppressed. This may be due to the electric repulsion between the negatively charged **Im^C** bases in the stem region, which greatly destabilized the structure of the active DNAzyme. In the presence of one equivalent of Cu^{II} ions, the catalytic activity of the DNAzyme increased 12-fold. The Cu^{II}-mediated activation was attributed to the reconstruction of the active DNA enzyme structure by the formation of **Im^C**–Cu^{II}–**Im^C** base pairs. The ON–OFF ratio (12) was found to be higher than that of the **H**-modified DNAzyme (5.5). The DNAzyme activity was reversibly regulated by the addition, removal, and reduction of Cu^{II} ions. The sequential addition of Cu^{II} and GHK also demonstrated repetitive switching of the DNAzyme activity (Figure 7c).

Both **H**- and **Im^C**-modified DNAzymes showed high specificity for Cu^{II} ions [33, 41]. The addition of other transition metal ions such as Fe^{II}, Co^{II}, Ni^{II}, Zn^{II}, Pd^{II}, and Pt^{II} did not improve the DNAzyme activity at all. This metal selectivity is in good agreement with the case of metal-mediated stabilization of DNA duplexes containing an **H–H** or an **Im^C–Im^C** base pair. Importantly, the modified DNAzymes were not activated by the addition of Hg^{II} or Ag^{I} ions, which form the well-studied T–Hg^{II}–T or C–Ag^{I}–C base pairs. This high metal selectivity was used to demonstrate metal-dependent orthogonal regulation of the Cu^{II}- and Hg^{II}-responsive DNAzymes [33, 41]. A Cu^{II}-dependent split DNAzyme (**H**- or **Im^C**-modified DNAzyme) was mixed with a Hg^{II}-responsive DNAzyme that is activated by the formation of T–Hg^{II}–T base pairs. The two DNAzymes were designed to cleave different substrates. The addition of Cu^{II} ions to the mixture of the two DNAzymes selectively promoted cleavage of the substrate by the Cu^{II}-responsive DNAzyme. The addition of Hg^{II} ions enhanced the cleavage reaction catalyzed by the Hg^{II}-responsive DNAzyme. These results confirm that the two DNAzymes are activated orthogonally in a metal-dependent manner. Both DNAzymes were activated in the presence of both Cu^{II} and Hg^{II} ions.

It is worth noting that metal-responsive DNAzymes were developed by incorporating one metal-mediated base pair (**H–Cu^{II}–H** or **Im^C–Cu^{II}–Im^C**). In other words, a pair of unnatural ligand-type nucleotides (**H** or **Im^C**) was used as metal-recognition site. The design strategy of the split DNAzymes is advantageous for devising other metal-responsive functional DNAs because it requires minimal chemical modification.

4.2 Metal-Responsive Single-Stranded DNAzymes

It is also possible to develop metal-responsive DNAzymes without splitting the parent DNAzyme strands. Shionoya et al. reported a rational method for designing Cu^{II}-responsive single-stranded DNAzymes whose activity can be regulated by intrastrand structural changes through metal-mediated base pairing (Figure 8) [37]. A pair of **H** nucleotides was incorporated into the stem of known DNAzymes in a manner similar to the split DNAzymes described above. To reduce the DNAzyme activity without Cu^{II} ions, the loop sequence was modified to form a stable catalytically inactive secondary structure. For example, a sequence complementary to a part of the catalytic domain was inserted into the loop region. The formation of **H–Cu^{II}–H** base pairing was predicted to cause an intrastrand conversion from an inactive to a catalytically active structure, allowing allosteric regulation of the DNAzyme activity in response to Cu^{II} ions.

Based on the sequence of the RNA-cleaving E5 DNAzyme [50], the first example of a Cu^{II}-responsive non-split DNAzyme was developed (Figure 8a). The apparent rate constant (k_{obs}) of the **H**-modified non-split DNAzyme was

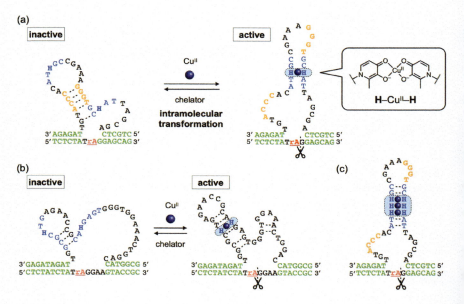

FIGURE 8 Development of metal-responsive single-stranded DNAzymes using H–Cu^{II}–H base pairing. (a) Design of a Cu^{II}-responsive DNAzyme based on the RNA-cleaving E5 DNAzyme. Both inactive and active secondary structures are shown. (b) Design of a Cu^{II}-responsive DNAzyme based on the RNA-cleaving NaA43 DNAzyme. (c) Cu^{II}-responsive DNAzyme containing multiple H–Cu^{II}–H base pairs. Only the active secondary structure is shown. The "rA" in the substrate represents the cleavage site, adenine ribonucleotide.

0.011 h^{-1} in the absence of Cu^{II} ions, but was increased to 0.073 h^{-1} in the presence of one equivalent of Cu^{II} ions. The addition of Cu^{II} increased the DNAzyme activity by 6.8-fold, indicating better performance compared to the H-modified split DNAzyme. The addition of excess Cu^{II} ions did not further increase the DNAzyme activity, indicating that equimolar Cu^{II} ions are sufficient for the DNAzyme activation. The Cu^{II}-mediated structural change was confirmed by a fluorescence assay using a DNAzyme strand containing a fluorescent pyrrolocytosine base. The DNAzyme activity was reversibly controlled by the addition and removal of Cu^{II} ions under isothermal conditions. The addition of Cu^{II} ions rapidly increased the DNAzyme activity, although an intrastrand structural conversion was required. Stepwise addition of Cu^{II} ions and a Cu^{II}-binding peptide, GHK, resulted in a sequential switching in the DNAzyme activity.

An RNA-cleaving DNAzyme called NaA43 [59] was also modified to develop another Cu^{II}-responsive DNAzyme (Figure 8b) [37]. A pair of H nucleotides was incorporated into the stem region of the parent DNAzyme to shorten the stem duplex, allowing it to form a catalytically inactive structure in the absence of Cu^{II} ions. The DNAzyme activity in the presence of one equivalent of Cu^{II} ions (k_{obs}=0.28 h^{-1}) was 5.9 times greater than in the absence of Cu^{II} ions (0.047 h^{-1}). The results indicate that the activity of the H-modified DNAzyme is allosterically regulated in response to Cu^II ions. As a result, it was concluded that metal-responsive DNAzyme can be designed by introducing metal-mediated artificial base pairs to various known DNAzymes.

A Cu^II-responsive DNAzyme containing multiple metal-mediated base pairs was also reported by Takezawa and Shionoya et al. (Figure 8c) [38]. The E5 DNAzyme [50] was modified by incorporating three consecutive **H–Cu^II–H** base pairs into the stem region. Furthermore, the loop sequence was modified to stabilize the catalytically inactive structure in the absence of Cu^II ions. The RNA-cleaving activity of the **H**-modified DNAzyme was 2.2-fold higher in the presence of three equivalents of Cu^II ions ($k_{obs} = 0.032\,h^{-1}$) than in the absence of Cu^II ions ($0.014\,h^{-1}$). This result indicates that the DNAzyme was activated by the addition of Cu^II ions. However, the ON–OFF efficiency was lower than that of the homologous DNAzyme containing only a single **H–Cu^II–H** pair. Sequence optimization would be necessary to achieve more efficient switching of the DNAzyme.

As overviewed, metal-responsive single-stranded DNAzymes have been developed by introducing **H–Cu^II–H** base pairs into previously reported DNAzymes and rationally designing base sequences. Rapid metal complexation of the **H–Cu^II–H** base pairs enabled rapid intramolecular structure conversion between the catalytically active and inactive states. The results showed that the activity of DNAzymes is allosterically regulated in response to Cu^II ions. By using metal ions which rarely interfere with natural nucleobases, it is possible to design metal-responsive DNAzymes in a simple and rational way. The design principle of metal-responsive single-stranded DNAzymes is expected to be applicable to allosteric regulation of various functional DNAs other than DNAzymes.

4.3 Metal-Responsive DNA Aptamers

Metal-mediated base pairing with unnatural nucleobases has also been applied to the creation of metal-responsive DNA aptamers. Müller et al. reported metal-responsive adenosine triphosphate (ATP) aptamers that can switch binding affinity through metal-mediated base pairing (Figure 9) [60]. A pair of imidazole-bearing nucleotides (**Im**) forming stable Ag^I-mediated base pairs (**Im–Ag^I–Im**) [61] was

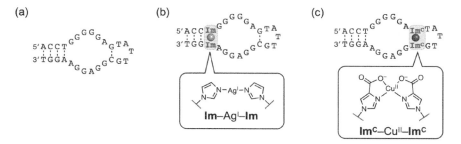

FIGURE 9 Development of metal-responsive DNA aptamers. (a) Base sequence of the original ATP-binding DNA aptamer. (b) Ag^I-responsive ATP aptamer based on **Im–Ag^I–Im** base pairing. (c) Cu^II-responsive ATP aptamer based on **Im^C–Cu^II–Im^C** base pairing.

incorporated into the stem duplex of a known ATP-binding DNA aptamer [62] with flexible bulges that bind to two ATP molecules (Figure 9b). The position of the **Im–Im** base pair was varied and the DNA sequence was optimized. Melting experiments showed that the **Im**-modified aptamers are stabilized by the addition of Ag^I ions (ΔT_m=+5 to +12°C). This is presumably due to the formation of the **Im–Ag^I–Im** base pair. The binding affinity of the aptamers was first evaluated by fluorescence assay and further analyzed using an ATP-loaded agarose gel. The results showed that incorporating the **Im–Im** mismatch pair near the ATP-binding domain efficiently reduced the binding affinity of the aptamer. When Ag^I ions were added, the binding affinity was restored. In some cases, the addition of excess Ag^I ions reduced the binding affinity. This may be due to the weak interactions between Ag^I ions and natural nucleobases. These results indicate that the aptamer regulates its function by forming an artificial **Im–Ag^I–Im** base pair.

The same group has recently developed Cu^{II}-responsive DNA aptamers by incorporating a Cu^{II}-mediated artificial base pair (Figure 9c) [63]. A Cu^{II}-mediated imidazole-4-carboxylate base pair (**Im^C–Cu^{II}–Im^C**) [40] allowed for regulating the function of the aptamer. An **Im^C–Im^C** mismatch pair was incorporated into the ATP aptamer [62]. The incorporation of the **Im^C–Im^C** pair significantly reduced the melting temperature of the aptamers. The thermal stability of the **Im^C**-modified aptamers was greatly enhanced by the addition of Cu^{II} ions, indicating the formation of the **Im^C–Cu^{II}–Im^C** base pair. The binding affinity for ATP was reduced in the absence of Cu^{II} ions, but the aptamer function was restored in the presence of Cu^{II} ions. Although the binding constants have not yet been determined, the binding affinity of the **Im^C**-modified aptamers was shown to be regulated in response to the addition of Cu^{II} ions. Similarly, a Cu^{II}-responsive arginine aptamer was also developed based on the **Im^C–Cu^{II}–Im^C** base pairing.

Although detailed analysis of aptamer function and sequence optimization are needed, these results suggest that the incorporation of metal-mediated base pairs consisting of unnatural nucleobases is a versatile method for developing metal-dependent functional DNAs. Since DNA aptamers are widely used in DNA nanotechnology and chemical biology, metal-responsive aptamers based on metal-mediated base pairing are expected to have a wide range of applications.

4.4 AND-Logic Gate DNAzyme Responsive to Two Different Metal Ions

The rational design strategy for metal-responsive functional DNA was applied to the development of an AND-logic gating system that responds to two types of metal ions. Based on the high metal selectivity of the **H–Cu^{II}–H** base pairing [31], a DNAzyme which exhibited an AND-logic gate response for Cu^{II} and Ag^I ions was developed by Takezawa and Shionoya et al. (Figure 10) [37]. An Ag^I-dependent RNA-cleaving DNAzyme Ag10c obtained by *in vitro* selection [64] was modified to show catalytic activity in the presence of Cu^{II} ions (Figure 10a). By introducing an **H–H** mismatch pair in the stem region and modifying the loop sequence, a catalytically inactive structure was stably formed under Cu^{II}-free conditions.

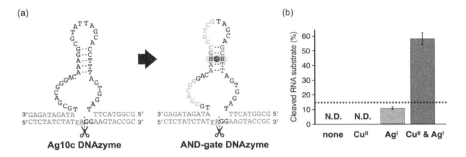

FIGURE 10 Development of an AND-gate DNAzyme responsive to Cu^{II} and Ag^{I} ions. (a) Base sequences of the original Ag^{I}-dependent DNAzyme (Ag10c) and of the AND-gate DNAzyme. Only the active structures are shown. The "rA" in the substrate represents the cleavage site, adenine ribonucleotide. (b) RNA-cleaving activity of the AND-gate DNAzyme upon the addition of Cu^{II} and/or Ag^{I} ions. [DNAzyme] = 1.0 µM, [substrate] = 10 µM, [$CuSO_4$] = 0 or 1.0 µM, [$AgNO_3$] = 0 or 10 µM in 10 mM HEPES buffer (pH 7.5), 200 mM $NaNO_3$, 25 °C, 1 h, $N=3$.

The RNA-cleaving activity of the modified DNAzyme was examined using Cu^{II} ions (1 equiv.) and Ag^{I} ions (10 equiv.) as input signals (i_1 and i_2, respectively) (Figure 10b). In the absence of Ag^{I} ions ((i_1, i_2) = (0, 0) or (1, 0)), the DNAzyme shows no catalytic activity at all and the output signal is "0". When only Ag^{I} was added but Cu^{II} was not present ((i_1, i_2) = (0, 1)), the DNAzyme showed only very low activity. This suggests that the modified DNAzyme becomes inactive in the absence of Cu^{II} ions as designed. This result corresponds to an output signal of "0". When both Cu^{II} and Ag^{I} ions are present ((i_1, i_2) = (1, 1)), the DNAzyme shows sufficient RNA-cleaving activity, indicating an output signal of "1". These results indicate that the **H**-modified DNAzyme functions as an AND-logic gate system responsive to Cu^{II} and Ag^{I} ions.

It is important to note that the metal-responsive AND-gate DNAzyme is composed of a single oligonucleotide with minimal chemical modification. It has been difficult to obtain functional DNAs that act as logic gates using conventional *in vitro* selection methods. Therefore, combining rational design strategies with metal-mediated base pair incorporation is a powerful way to develop highly functional DNAs.

5 DEVELOPMENT OF METAL-RESPONSIVE BIFACIAL NUCLEOBASES FOR FUTURE APPLICATIONS

5.1 Design Concept of Metal-Responsive Bifacial Nucleobases

Metal-mediated base pairing is an excellent tool for developing metal-responsive DNA supramolecules and nanostructures as described above. Metal-responsive bifacial nucleobases that form both hydrogen-bonded and metal-mediated base pairs were developed for more efficient switching of DNA structures in

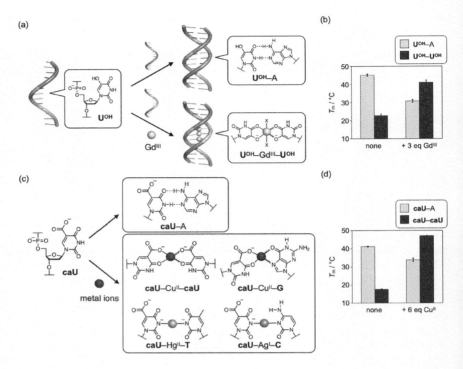

FIGURE 11 Hydrogen-bonded and metal-mediated base pairing of bifacial 5-modified pyrimidine nucleobases. (a) 5-Hydroxyuracil (U^{OH}) nucleobase. X represents additional coordinating ligands such as water molecules and adjacent nucleobases. (b) Melting temperatures (T_m) of 15-mer DNA duplexes containing three U^{OH}–A or U^{OH}–U^{OH} base pairs in the absence and presence of Gd^{III} ions. [duplex] = 2.0 μM, [Gd^{III}]/[duplex] = 0 or 3 in 10 mM HEPES buffer (pH 8.0), 100 mM NaCl. (c) 5-Carboxyuracil (**caU**) nucleobases. (d) T_m values of 15-mer DNA duplexes containing three **caU**–A or **caU**–**caU** base pairs in the absence and presence of Cu^{II} ions. [duplex] = 2.0 μM, [Cu^{II}]/[duplex] = 0 or 6 in 10 mM HEPES buffer (pH 7.0), 100 mM NaCl.

response to metal complexation (Figure 11). The prototype of bifacial nucleobases was reported by Lehn et al. [65], and several bifacial nucleobases have been synthesized. Conventional artificial bifacial nucleobases have two hydrogen-bonding faces to form two different hydrogen-bonded base pairs, similar to the purine bases that form Watson-Crick and Hoogsteen base pairs on the other sides. Metal-responsive bifacial nucleobases were designed to have a hydrogen-bonding face and a metal coordination site in one molecule. The first example was 5-hydroxyuracil (U^{OH}), where the 4-carbonyl group and an additional 5-hydroxy group act as a bidentate ligand to form a metal-mediated base pair (Figure 11a) [66]. The U^{OH} base, like natural thymine (T) and uracil (U) bases, retains the Watson-Crick face and can form a hydrogen-bonded base pair with natural adenine (A) bases. Subsequently, 5-carboxyuracil (**caU**) base was employed as a bifacial base

(Figure 11c) [67]. The 4-carbonyl and the 5-carboxy groups provide a bidentate metal-binding site for metal-mediated base pairing. The introduction of a coordinating group at the 5-position of pyrimidine-type nucleobases is expected to induce novel bifacial ligand-type nucleobases. The base-pairing properties of the U^{OH} and caU bases are described in the following sections.

5.2 Bifacial Base-Pairing Behavior of 5-Hydroxyuracil Bases

Hydroxyuracil (U^{OH}) is known to be naturally produced by oxidative degradation of cytosine (C) bases. Although U^{OH} was known to form a hydrogen-bonded U^{OH}–A base pair, its properties as a ligand had not been investigated. In 2015, Shionoya et al. reported that U^{OH} bases form metal-mediated homo base pairs (U^{OH}–M–U^{OH}) in the presence of most lanthanoide ions (Figure 11a) [66]. The metal-mediated base pairing was confirmed by DNA duplex melting analysis, UV titration experiments, and mass spectrometry. A DNA duplex containing three U^{OH}–U^{OH} pairs, (5′-d(CAC ATT U^{OH}U^{OH}U^{OH} GTT GTA)-3′)·(3′-d(GTG TAA U^{OH}U^{OH}U^{OH} CAA CAT)-5′), was used for the analysis. Melting experiments showed that the addition of three equivalents of Gd^{III} ions significantly increased the stability of the duplex (ΔT_m=+18.3°C). In contrast, duplexes in which the U^{OH}–U^{OH} pairs were replaced with U^{OH}–T or T–T were not stabilized by the addition of Gd^{III} ions. UV spectroscopy showed the appearance of a new absorption band around 310 nm, suggesting metal complexation of the U^{OH} bases. UV titration experiments, Job's plot analysis, and mass spectrometric measurements confirmed that three Gd^{III} ions were bound to the duplex. These results suggest that the three U^{OH}–Gd^{III}–U^{OH} base pairs are formed inside the duplex. Since lanthanoide ions generally have high coordination numbers, such as 8 or 9, it is possible that the Gd^{III} ions are coordinated not only by the two U^{OH} nucleobases but also by additional ligands such as water molecules and adjacent nucleobases. Note that a DNA duplex containing one U^{OH}–U^{OH} base pair was not stabilized at all by the addition of Gd^{III} ions. This may be because the structure of the U^{OH}–Gd^{III}–U^{OH} base pair did not fit well into the B-DNA duplex structure, as supported by CD spectroscopy.

The hydrogen-bonded U^{OH}–A base pair also exhibits metal-dependent behavior. The melting temperature of a DNA duplex containing three U^{OH}–A pairs, (5′-d(CAC ATT U^{OH}U^{OH}U^{OH} GTT GTA)-3′)·(3′-d(GTG TAA AAA CAA CAT)-5′), decreased when three equivalents of Gd^{III} ions were added (ΔT_m=−14.3°C). The binding of Gd^{III} ions to the U^{OH} bases affected the pK_a of the N3 atom and weakened the hydrogen-bonded base pairing. As summarized in Figure 11b, the thermal stability of the duplexes containing U^{OH}–U^{OH} and U^{OH}–A pairs was inversed by the addition of Gd^{III} ions. Under Gd^{III}-free conditions, the duplex with U^{OH}–A pairs (T_m=45.2°C) was more stable than the duplex with U^{OH}–U^{OH} pairs (22.8°C). In the presence of Gd^{III} ions (3 equiv.), the duplex containing U^{OH}–Gd^{III}–U^{OH} pairs (41.1°C) became more stable than the duplex with U^{OH}–A pairs (30.9°C). These results indicate that the hybridization preference of the U^{OH}-containing strand can change in response to Gd^{III} ions.

A similar behavior was observed for Zn^{II} ions [68]. The addition of Zn^{II} ions (3 equiv.) at pH 8 stabilized the duplex with U^{OH}–U^{OH} pairs (ΔT_m=+13.0°C) and destabilized the duplex with U^{OH}–A pairs (ΔT_m=–2.9°C). At pH 7.0, the addition of Zn^{II} hardly changed the melting temperatures, while the addition of Gd^{III} ions stabilized or destabilized the duplex. In other words, the stability of the U^{OH}-containing duplexes in the presence of Zn^{II} ions is highly dependent on the pH of the solution. These results can be explained by a pH-dependent complexation of the U^{OH} bases with Zn^{II} ions accompanied by the deprotonation of the 5-OH group of U^{OH} (pK_a=7.7).

Thus, U^{OH} bases form both hydrogen-bonded U^{OH}–A base pairs and metal-mediated U^{OH}–M–U^{OH} base pairs (M = Gd^{III}, Zn^{II}, etc.). Because the base-pairing partners of U^{OH} bases can be switched in response to the presence or absence and type of metal ions, the bifacial U^{OH} base is a promising building block for the construction of metal-responsive functional DNA systems.

5.3 Hydrogen-Bonded and Metal-Mediated Base Pairing of 5-Carboxyuracil Bases

5-Carboxyuracil (**caU**) is another example of a metal-responsive bifacial nucleobase (Figure 11c). The **caU** nucleobase has a carboxyl group at the 5-position and, like U^{OH}, functions as a bidentate metal ligand. In 2020, Shionoya et al. reported that successive incorporation of **caU**–**caU** mismatch pairs can lead to Cu^{II}-mediated **caU**–Cu^{II}–**caU** base pairing inside the DNA duplexes [67]. UV melting analysis revealed that a DNA duplex containing three **caU**–**caU** pairs, (5'-d(CAC ATT **caUcaUcaU** GTT GTA)-3')·(3'-d(GTG TAA **caUcaUcaU** CAA CAT)-5') was greatly stabilized by the addition of 3 equiv. of Cu^{II} ions (ΔT_m=+30.7 °C). The Cu^{II}-mediated stabilization of the duplex may be due to the formation of three **caU**–Cu^{II}–**caU** base pairs, which additionally cross-link the two strands. Note that the **caU**–Cu^{II}–**caU** base pairing showed a higher degree of duplex stabilization than the U^{OH}–Gd^{III}–U^{OH} base pairing. Furthermore, the quantitative formation of the **caU**–Cu^{II}–**caU** pairs was confirmed by mass spectrometry and titration experiments based on CD spectroscopy. In the putative structure of the **caU**–Cu^{II}–**caU** pair, the two glycosidic bonds (C1'–N1) are parallel to each other. Therefore, the B-DNA helix structure may be distorted by the **caU**–Cu^{II}–**caU** base pairing, as observed in the CD spectrum.

The degree of the Cu^{II}-dependent stabilization of the duplex was found to increase as the number of **caU**–Cu^{II}–**caU** pairs increased. Melting analysis was performed with DNA duplexes containing one to five **caU**–**caU** pairs, (5'-d(CAC ATT (**caU**)$_n$ GTT GTA)-3')·(3'-d(GTG TAA (**caU**)$_n$ CAA CAT)-5') (n=1–5), in the presence of equimolar Cu^{II} ions ([Cu^{II}]/[**caU**–**caU**] = 1.0). The duplex with a single **caU**–**caU** pair was not stabilized by the addition of Cu^{II} ions, while the duplex with two consecutive **caU**–**caU** pairs was stabilized by +14.2°C. The stability of the duplexes with three, four, and five **caU**–**caU** pairs was enhanced by +30.7°C, +37.9°C, and +39.8°C, respectively, upon the addition of Cu^{II} ions.

The **caU** base also forms a **caU**–A pair by hydrogen bonding at the Watson-Crick face. As is the case for the U^{OH}–A base pair, the **caU**–A pair was destabilized by the addition of Cu^{II} ions. For example, the melting temperature of a DNA duplex containing three **caU**–A pairs, (5′-d(CAC ATT **caUcaUcaU** GTT GTA)-3′)·(3′-d(GTG TAA AAA CAA CAT)-5′), was reduced by −7.3°C with excess Cu^{II} ions (6 equiv.). In the absence of Cu^{II} ions, the duplex with three **caU**–A pairs (T_m=41.2°C) was more stable than the duplex containing three **caU**–**caU** mispairs (17.7°C). The addition of Cu^{II} ions (6 equiv.) made the duplex with **caU**–**caU** (47.0°C) more stable than the duplex with **caU**–A (33.9°C). As a result, the addition of Cu^{II} ions reversed the order of the stability of the duplex (Figure 11d). These results suggest that the **caU** bases can be used as a molecular switch in response to Cu^{II} ions.

Notably, the **caU** base forms a metal-mediated base pair with other natural nucleobases, T, C, and G (Figure 11c). A duplex containing a **caU**–T pair was stabilized by +10.6°C in the presence of equimolar Hg^{II} ions. This is thought to be due to the formation of the **caU**–Hg^{II}–T base pair by N3 coordination as in the T–Hg^{II}–T pair. It is interesting to note that the duplex stabilization by the **caU**–Hg^{II}–T base pairing is greater than that observed with T–Hg^{II}–T. The **caU** base also forms an Ag^{I}-mediated base pair (**caU**–Ag^{I}–C) with the natural C base, similar to the C–Ag^{I}–C base pair. A duplex containing a **caU**–C mismatch was stabilized by +15.5°C by the addition of one equivalent of Ag^{I} ions. This degree of stabilization is higher than that observed for C–Ag^{I}–C base pairing (ΔT_m=+10.2°C for the same sequence). Finally, the **caU** bases were found to pair with the G bases in the presence of Cu^{II} ions. A DNA duplex containing three consecutive **caU**–G base pairs was stabilized by the addition of 3 equiv. of Cu^{II} ions (ΔT_m=+8.3°C), suggesting the formation of three **caU**–Cu^{II}–G base pairs. Since a duplex containing **caU**–7-deazaguanine base pairs was only slightly stabilized by the addition of Cu^{II} ions (ΔT_m=+3.1°C), the **caU**–Cu^{II}–G base pairs are considered to have an *N,O,O,O*-coordination geometry.

Taken altogether, it was revealed that the **caU** base forms base pairs with four types of natural nucleobases (**caU**–A, **caU**–Hg^{II}–T, **caU**–Ag^{I}–C, and **caU**–Cu^{II}–G) and with itself (**caU**–Cu^{II}–**caU**), depending on the coexisting metal ions. This suggests that the use of metal ions as an external stimulus can alter the hybridization partner of the **caU**-containing strands. Thus, the metal-dependent base-pairing behavior of **caU** has potential application in the development of metal-responsive DNA molecules.

5.4 Applications of the Bifacial Nucleobases

The metal responsiveness of the 5-modified pyrimidine bases allows for metal-dependent control of DNA hybridization as described above. Thus, the bifacial nucleobases could be applied to the fabrication of metal-responsive DNA materials. Recently, the 5-hydroxyuracil (**U^{OH}**) base was used to modulate the binding affinity of triplex-forming oligonucleotides (TFOs) (Figure 12) [69]. TFOs are oligonucleotides that bind to a target DNA duplex via Hoogsteen base pairing and have potential applications in gene regulation and the control of DNA assembly in DNA nanotechnology. TFOs containing **U^{OH}** bases were found to bind to target

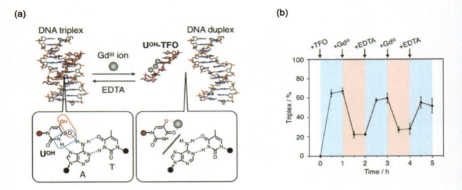

FIGURE 12 (a) Schematic diagram of metal-responsive reversible binding of triplex-forming oligonucleotides with 5-hydroxyuracil (U^{OH}) nucleobases. The structure of a U^{OH}·A–T base triad is shown. (b) Gd^{III}-responsive reversible binding of the U^{OH}-modified TFO to the target DNA duplex under isothermal conditions. [DNA duplex] = 1.5 μM in 10 mM HEPES buffer (pH 7.0), 140 mM NaCl, 10 mM $MgCl_2$. After the addition of U^{OH}-modified TFO (2.0 μM), $GdCl_3$ (6 equiv.), and EDTA (6 equiv.) were alternately added at 20°C. (Reprinted from Ref. [69]; copyright 2021 Royal Society of Chemistry.)

duplexes by forming U^{OH}·A–T base triads, similar to T·A–T base triads consisting of natural T bases. For example, the melting temperature corresponding to the dissociation of a TFO containing three U^{OH} bases, (5'-d(TC^{m}C^m TTU^{OH} TC^{m}T U^{OH}TC^m TU^{OH}T TTC^m C^{m}TT)-3'; C^m = 5-methylcytosine), from the target DNA duplex was determined as 45.2°C. This is only slightly lower than a TFO containing natural T bases instead of U^{OH} (T_m = 48.3°C).

The binding affinity of a U^{OH}-modified TFO was found to decrease with addition of Gd^{III} ions. The addition of six equiv. of Gd^{III} ions lowered the melting point to 29.7°C (ΔT_m = −15.6°C), but did not change the stability of the target DNA duplex. The dissociation temperature of the unmodified TFO was not affected by the addition of Gd^{III} ions. Thus, it was concluded that site-selective metal complexation of the U^{OH} bases disrupts the Hoogsteen U^{OH}·A base pair and reduces the binding affinity of the U^{OH}-modified TFO (Figure 12a).

The binding affinity of the U^{OH}-modified TFOs was reversibly regulated by the sequential addition and removal of Gd^{III} ions under isothermal conditions (Figure 12b). The addition of Gd^{III} ions (6 equiv.) released the TFO from the duplex. Subsequent addition of EDTA (6 equiv.), which removes Gd^{III} ions, reassociated the TFO. The Gd^{III}-dependent binding of U^{OH}-modified TFO was repeated at least twice, albeit with gradually decreasing efficiency.

As illustrated in the above example, it was shown that the DNA hybridization can be controlled in a metal-responsive manner by using bifacial nucleobases as metal-recognition sites. This strategy could be applied to DNA triplexes as well as other higher-order DNA nanostructures. Thus, the metal-induced switching of the base-pairing mode of 5-modified pyrimidine nucleobases is expected to be used to develop a variety of metal-responsive DNA materials and DNA molecular machines.

6 CONCLUDING REMARKS

Artificial metal-mediated DNA base pairing is becoming increasingly important not only in the field of bioinorganic chemistry, but also in the broader field of DNA chemistry. Metal-mediated base pairs are formed with natural nucleobases and an Ag^I or Hg^{II} ion, or with synthetic ligand-type nucleobases and a certain metal ion such as a Cu^{II} ion. In many cases, metal-mediated base pairing enhances the thermal stability of DNA duplexes in a metal-dependent manner. One excellent example is the recently reported Cu^{II}-mediated base pairing with a 4-carboxyimidazole (**Im^C**) nucleobase. The model duplex containing an **Im^C**–**Im^C** pair was greatly stabilized by the formation of an **Im^C**–Cu^{II}–**Im^C** base pair. The melting temperature (T_m) of the duplex increased by 35 °C with the addition of Cu^{II} ions. One of the latest and the most prominent applications of metal-mediated base pairing is the development of metal-responsive functional DNAs. This chapter reviews recent developments in this area. Metal-responsive DNA aptamers and DNAzymes (catalytic DNA) have been developed by introducing metal-mediated base pairs to pre-identified DNA sequences. Split DNAzymes, for example, were designed so that metal-mediated base pairing reorganizes the structure of the catalytic DNAzyme. The modified DNAzymes lost their catalytic activity in the absence of metal ions, and the addition of metal restored the activity of the DNAzyme. Furthermore, single-stranded metal-responsive DNAzymes were constructed through a more thoughtful sequence design. In addition to incorporation of metal-mediated base pairs, strategic changes were made to the base sequences. In the absence of metal ions, the resulting DNAzyme formed an inactive structure with a deformed catalytic domain. Once metal-mediated base pairs were formed, the DNAzymes changed to a catalytically active structure. As a result, the DNAzyme activity was regulated in response to metal ions. It is worth mentioning that based on this strategy, an AND-gate DNAzyme was developed that is active only when both Ag^I and Cu^{II} ions are present.

Metal-mediated base pairs consisting of natural nucleobases, namely T–Hg^{II}–T and C–Ag^I–C, have been widely used to construct metal-responsive functional DNAs. In addition, there are a variety of Hg^{II}/Ag^I-responsive DNA molecular devices and machines, such as DNA tweezers. However, if Hg^{II} or Ag^I ions happen to bind to natural nucleobases, functional DNA performance is compromised. Therefore, the use of other metal-mediated base pairs consisting of synthetic ligand-type nucleobases and metal ions other than Hg^{II} or Ag^I is expected. As described in this chapter, a variety of Cu^{II}-responsive DNAzymes and DNA aptamers have been devised using the **H**–Cu^{II}–**H** and **Im^C**–Cu^{II}–**Im^C** base pairs. The regulation of their activity via reduction/oxidation of copper ions was also demonstrated. Redox-based regulation of functional DNAs would be a promising application of metal-mediated base pairing.

Ligand-type bifacial nucleobases were newly designed as metal-responsive building blocks. Bifacial nucleobases such as 5-hydroxyuracil (**U^{OH}**) and 5-carboxyuracil (**caU**) have a bidentate metal-binding site in addition to the Watson-Crick hydrogen-bonding face. Thus, both hydrogen-bonded base pairs (such as caU–A) and metal-mediated base pairs (such as **caU**–Cu^{II}–**caU**) can be formed. Metal-mediated base pairing stabilizes DNA duplexes, but the addition of metal ions was found to destabilize duplexes containing hydrogen-bonded pairs composed of bifacial nucleobases. Because of this metal-dependent behavior, the bifacial ligand-type nucleobases are expected to be a promising tool for the construction of metal-responsive DNA materials.

The types of metal species applicable for metal-mediated base pairing will be expanded for future applications. The specific complexation between ligand-type nucleobases and metal ions would enable metal-dependent orthogonal responses and is expected to be applied to the construction of more advanced systems such as logic gates. Functional DNAs that respond to biologically relevant metal ions can be developed through novel metal-mediated base pairing, which will have new applications in life sciences. New synthetic methods, such as enzymatic incorporation of metal-mediated base pairs, will also be of interest. The development of metal-mediated base pairing has contributed to a wide range of areas of DNA chemistry, particularly the rapid progress of DNA nanotechnology.

ABBREVIATIONS

A	adenine
ABTS	2,2′-azino-bis(3-ethylbenzothiazoline-6-sulfonic acid)
ATP	adenosine triphosphate
bp	base pair(s)
^{Br}C	5-bromo-2′-deoxycytidine
^{Br}U	5-bromo-2′-deoxyuridine
C	cytosine
caU	5-carboxyuracil
CD	circular dichroism
C^m	5-methylcytosine
Dipic	pyridine-2,6-dicarboxylic acid
DNAzyme	deoxyribozyme (catalytic DNA)
dNTP	2′-deoxyribonucleoside 5′-triphosphate
Dpo IV	*Sulfolobus solfataricus* DNA polymerase IV
EDTA	ethylenediamine-*N*,*N*,*N*′,*N*′-tetraacetate
EPR	electron paramagnetic resonance
ESI	electron spray ionization
G	guanine
GHK	glycyl-L-histidyl-L-lysine (Cu^{II}-binding peptide)
H	3-hydroxy-4-pyridone
HRP	horseradish peroxidase
Im^C	4-carboxyimidazole
Im^{OA}	2-oxo-imidazole-4-carboxamide
Im^{OC}	2-oxo-imidazole-4-carboxylate
ITC	isothermal titration calorimetry

KF exo⁻	Klenow fragment lacking exonuclease activity
k_{obs}	apparent first-order rate constant
NOE	nuclear Overhauser effect
P	pyridine
PAGE	polyacrylamide gel electrophoresis
rA	adenine ribonucleotide
SELEX	systematic evolution of ligands by exponential enrichment
TdT	terminal deoxynucleotidyl transferase
TFO	triplex-forming oligonucleotide
T	thymine
T_m	melting temperature
U	uracil
U^{OH}	5-hydroxyuracil
UV	ultraviolet

REFERENCES

1. *Interplay between Metal Ions and Nucleic Acids*, Vol. 10 of *Metal Ions in Life Sciences*, Eds A. Sigel, H. Sigel, R. K. O. Sigel, Springer, Dordrecht, The Netherlands, **2012**, pp. 1–353.
2. N. H. Campbell, S. Neidle, in *Interplay between Metal Ions and Nucleic Acids*, Vol. 10 of *Metal Ions in Life Sciences*, Eds A. Sigel, H. Sigel, R. K. O. Sigel, Springer, Dordrecht, The Netherlands, **2012**, pp. 119–134.
3. S. E. Sherman, S. J. Lippard, *Chem. Rev.* **1987**, *87*, 1153–1181.
4. Y. Takezawa, M. Shionoya, *Acc. Chem. Res.* **2012**, *45*, 2066–2076.
5. Y. Takezawa, J. Müller, M. Shionoya, *Chem. Lett.* **2017**, *46*, 622–633.
6. Y. Takezawa, M. Shionoya, J. Müller, Vol. 4 of *Comprehensive Supramolecular Chemistry II*, Ed J. L. Atwood, Elsevier, Oxford, **2017**, pp. 259–293.
7. S. Naskar, R. Guha, J. Müller, *Angew. Chem. Int. Ed.* **2020**, *59*, 1397–1406.
8. B. Lippert, *J. Biol. Inorg. Chem.* **2022**, *27*, 215–219.
9. Y. Tanaka, J. Kondo, V. Sychrovský, J. Šebera, T. Dairaku, H. Saneyoshi, H. Urata, H. Torigoe, A. Ono, *Chem. Commun.* **2015**, *51*, 17343–17360.
10. F. Paquet, M. Boudvillain, G. Lancelot, M. Leng, *Nucleic Acid Res.* **1999**, *21*, 4261–4268.
11. K. Tanaka, M. Shionoya, *J. Org. Chem.* **1999**, *64*, 5002–5003.
12. E. Meggers, P. L. Holland, W. B. Tolman, F. E. Romesberg, P. G. Schultz, *J. Am. Chem. Soc.* **2000**, *122*, 10714–10715.
13. S. Katz, *Nature* **1962**, *194*, 569.
14. S. Katz, *Nature* **1962**, *195*, 997–998.
15. S. Katz, *Biochim. Biophys. Acta* **1963**, *68*, 240–253.
16. Y. Miyake, H. Togashi, M. Tashiro, H. Yamaguchi, S. Oda, M. Kudo, Y. Tanaka, Y. Kondo, R. Sawa, T. Fujimoto, T. Machinami, A. Ono, *J. Am. Chem. Soc.* **2006**, *128*, 2172–2173.
17. Y. Tanaka, S. Oda, H. Yamaguchi, Y. Kondo, C. Kojima, A. Ono, *J. Am. Chem. Soc.* **2007**, *129*, 244–245.
18. H. Torigoe, A. Ono, T. Kozasa, *Chem. Eur. J.* **2010**, *16*, 13218–13225.
19. J. Kondo, T. Yamada, C. Hirose, I. Okamoto, Y. Tanaka, A. Ono, *Angew. Chem. Int. Ed.* **2014**, *53*, 2385–2388.

20. S. Nehzati, A. O. Summers, N. V. Dolgova, J. Zhu, D. Sokaras, T. Kroll, I. J. Pickering, G. N. George, *Inorg. Chem.* **2021**, *60*, 7442–7452.
21. S. Johannsen, S. Paulus, N. Düpre, J. Müller, R. K. O. Sigel, *J. Inorg. Biochem.* **2008**, *102*, 1141–1151.
22. A. Ono, S. Cao, H. Togashi, M. Tashiro, T. Fujimoto, T. Machinami, S. Oda, Y. Miyake, I. Okamoto, Y. Tanaka, *Chem. Commun.* **2008**, *44*, 4825–4827.
23. H. Torigoe, I. Okamoto, T. Dairaku, Y. Tanaka, A. Ono, T. Kozasa, *Biochimie* **2012**, *94*, 2431–2440.
24. J. Kondo, Y. Tada, T. Dairaku, H. Saneyoshi, I. Okamoto, Y. Tanaka, A. Ono, *Angew. Chem. Int. Ed.* **2015**, *54*, 13323–13326.
25. T. Dairaku, K. Furuita, H. Sato, J. Šebera, K. Nakashima, J. Kondo, D. Yamanaka, Y. Kondo, I. Okamoto, A. Ono, V. Sychrovský, C. Kojima, Y. Tanaka, *Chem. Eur. J.* **2016**, *22*, 13028–13031.
26. J. Kondo, Y. Tada, T. Dairaku, Y. Hattori, H. Saneyoshi, A. Ono, Y. Tanaka, *Nat. Chem.* **2017**, *9*, 956–960.
27. H. Liu, F. Shen, P. Haruehanroengra, Q. Yao, Y. Cheng, Y. Chen, C. Yang, J. Zhang, B. Wu, Q. Luo, R. Cui, J. Li, J. Ma, J. Sheng, *Angew. Chem. Int. Ed.* **2017**, *56*, 9430–9434.
28. T. Atsugi, A. Ono, M. Tasaka, N. Eguchi, S. Fujiwara, J. Kondo, *Angew. Chem. Int. Ed.* **2022**, *61*, e202204798.
29. A. Ono, H. Kanazawa, H. Ito, M. Goto, K. Nakamura, H. Saneyoshi, J. Kondo, *Angew. Chem. Int. Ed.* **2019**, *58*, 16835–16838.
30. A. Ono, H. Togashi, *Angew. Chem. Int. Ed.* **2004**, *43*, 4300–4303.
31. K. Tanaka, A. Tengeiji, T. Kato, N. Toyama, M. Shiro, M. Shionoya, *J. Am. Chem. Soc.* **2002**, *124*, 12494–12498.
32. M. K. Schlegel, L.-O. Essen, E. Meggers, *J. Am. Chem. Soc.* **2008**, *130*, 8158–8159.
33. Y. Takezawa, T. Nakama, M. Shionoya, *J. Am. Chem. Soc.* **2019**, *141*, 19342–19350.
34. K. Tanaka, A. Tengeiji, T. Kato, N. Toyama, M. Shionoya, *Science* **2003**, *299*, 1212–1213.
35. K. Tanaka, G. H. Clever, Y. Takezawa, Y. Yamada, C. Kaul, M. Shionoya, T. Carell, *Nat. Nanotechnol.* **2006**, *1*, 190–194.
36. S. Liu, G. H. Clever, Y. Takezawa, M. Kaneko, K. Tanaka, X. Guo, M. Shionoya, *Angew. Chem. Int. Ed.* **2011**, *50*, 8886–8890.
37. T. Nakama, Y. Takezawa, D. Sasaki, M. Shionoya, *J. Am. Chem. Soc.* **2020**, *142*, 10153–10162.
38. T. Nakama, Y. Takezawa, M. Shionoya, *Chem. Commun.* **2021**, *57*, 1392–1395.
39. T. Kobayashi, Y. Takezawa, A. Sakamoto, M. Shionoya, *Chem. Commun.* **2016**, *52*, 3762–3765.
40. N. Sandmann, D. Defayay, A. Hepp, J. Müller, *J. Inorg. Biochem.* **2019**, *191*, 85–93.
41. Y. Takezawa, L. Hu, T. Nakama, M. Shionoya, *Angew. Chem. Int. Ed.* **2020**, *59*, 21488–21492.
42. L. Hu, Y. Takezawa, M. Shionoya, *Chem. Sci.* **2022**, *13*, 3977–3983.
43. C. Cadena-Amaro, S. Pochet, *Tetrahedron* **2005**, *61*, 5081–5087.
44. T. Lan, Y. Lu, in *Interplay between Metal Ions and Nucleic Acids*, Vol. 10 of *Metal Ions in Life Sciences*, Eds A. Sigel, H. Sigel, R. K. O. Sigel, Springer, Dordrecht, The Netherlands, **2012**, pp. 217–248.
45. L. Ma, J. Liu, *iScience* **2020**, *23*, 100815.
46. R. R. Breaker, G. F. Joyce, *Chem. Biol.* **1994**, *1*, 223–229.
47. J. Liu, Y. Lu, *Angew. Chem. Int. Ed.* **2007**, *46*, 7587–7590.
48. J. Liu, A. K. Brown, X. Meng, D. M. Cropek, J. D. Istok, D. B. Watson, Y. Lu, *Proc. Natl. Acad. Sci. USA* **2007**, *104*, 2056–2061.

49. S. Shimron, J. Elbaz, A. Henning, I. Willner, *Chem. Commun.* **2010**, *46*, 3250–3252.
50. R. R. Breaker, G. F. Joyce, *Chem. Biol.* **1995**, *2*, 655–660.
51. Y. Li, D. Sen, *Biochemistry* **1997**, *36*, 5589–5599.
52. T. Li, L. Shi, E. Wang, S. Dong, *Chem. Eur. J.* **2009**, *15*, 3347–3350.
53. D.-M. Kong, N. Wang, X.-X. Guo, H.-X. Shen, *Analyst* **2010**, *135*, 545–549.
54. X. H. Zhou, D. M. Kong, H. X. Shen, *Anal. Chim. Acta* **2010**, *678*, 124–127.
55. D.-M. Kong, L.-L. Cai, H.-X. Shen, *Analyst* **2010**, *135*, 1253–1258.
56. K. S. Park, C. Y. Lee, H. G. Park, *Chem. Commun.* **2016**, *52*, 4868–4871.
57. C. Dang, S. D. Jayasena, *J. Mol. Biol.* **1996**, *264*, 268–278.
58. L. Pickart, J. H. Freedman, W. J. Loker, J. Peisach, C. M. Perkins, R. E. Stenkamp, B. Weinstein, *Nature* **1980**, *288*, 715–717.
59. S.-F. Torabi, P. Wu, C. E. McGhee, L. Chen, K. Hwang, N. Zheng, J. Cheng, Y. Lu, *Proc. Natl. Acad. Sci. USA* **2015**, *112*, 5903–5908.
60. M. H. Heddinga, J. Müller, *Beilstein J. Org. Chem.* **2020**, *16*, 2870–2879.
61. S. Johannsen, N. Megger, D. Böhme, R. K. O. Sigel, J. Müller, *Nat. Chem.* **2010**, *2*, 229–234.
62. D. E. Huizenga, J. W. Szostak, *Biochemistry* **1995**, *34*, 656–665.
63. M. H. Heddinga, J. Müller, *Org. Biomol. Chem.* **2022**, *20*, 4787–4793.
64. R. Saran, J. Liu, *Anal. Chem.* **2016**, *88*, 4014–4020.
65. N. Branda, G. Kurz, J. M. Lehn, *Chem. Commun.* **1996**, *32*, 2443–2444.
66. Y. Takezawa, K. Nishiyama, T. Mashima, M. Katahira, M. Shionoya, *Chem. Eur. J.* **2015**, *21*, 14713–14716.
67. Y. Takezawa, A. Suzuki, M. Nakaya, K. Nishiyama, M. Shionoya, *J. Am. Chem. Soc.* **2020**, *142*, 21640–21644.
68. K. Nishiyama, Y. Takezawa, M. Shionoya, *Inorg. Chim. Acta* **2016**, *452*, 176–180.
69. K. Nishiyama, K. Mori, Y. Takezawa, M. Shionoya, *Chem. Commun.* **2021**, *57*, 2487–2490.

12 Nucleic Acid-Templated Metal Nanoclusters

Rweetuparna Guha
Department of Materials Science and Engineering, University of California, Irvine, California 92697-2585, USA
rweetupg@uci.edu

Stacy M. Copp[*]
Department of Materials Science and Engineering, University of California, Irvine, California 92697-2585, USA
Department of Physics and Astronomy, University of California, Irvine, California 92697-4575, USA
Department of Chemical and Biomolecular Engineering, University of California, Irvine, California 92697-4575, USA
stacy.copp@uci.edu

CONTENTS

1	Introduction	293
2	Synthesis, Purification, and Mass Characterization	296
	2.1 Synthesis	296
	2.1.1 High-Throughput Ag_N-DNA Synthesis	298
	2.2 Purification by HPLC	299
	2.3 Determination of Composition by Mass Spectrometry	300
3	Structure-Property Relationships of DNA-Stabilized Silver Nanoclusters	301
	3.1 Ag_N-DNA Structure Determination	301
	3.1.1 The Jellium Model for Metal Nanoclusters	302
	3.1.2 Evidence for Rod-Like Structure	302
	3.1.3 Magic Colors Are Correlated to Magic Numbers	303
	3.1.4 X-ray Spectroscopy	304
	3.1.5 Infrared Spectroscopy	305

---

[*] Corresponding author

　　　　　3.1.6　Circular Dichroism Spectroscopy Provides a
　　　　　　　　Bridge between Theory and Experiment.................. 306
　　　　　3.1.7　Crystal Structures... 307
　　3.2　Ag⁺-DNA Interaction – A Prerequisite for Ag$_N$-DNA
　　　　　Formation 310
4　Photophysical Properties 313
　　4.1　Anatomy of the Ag$_N$-DNA Fluorescence Spectrum 314
　　4.2　Time-Resolved Studies of Ag$_N$-DNA Excited State Dynamics ...315
　　4.3　Dark Excited State Behavior 317
　　4.4　Evidence for Initial Collective Electronic Excitation..................317
　　4.5　Alignment of Excitation and Emission Transition Dipole
　　　　　Moments..318
　　4.6　Large-Scale Studies of Ag$_N$-DNA Stokes Shift 318
　　4.7　Two-Photon Excitation 320
　　4.8　Environmental and Stimulus Effects on Emission Properties 320
　　4.9　DNA Ligand Effects on Emission Properties 321
5　Machine Learning-Guided Studies of Ag$_N$-DNAs.................................. 322
6　Applications and Future Opportunities 326
　　6.1　Sensing 327
　　6.2　Bioimaging 328
　　6.3　New NIR-Emitting Ag$_N$-DNAs... 329
　　6.4　DNA-Directed Nanocluster Architectures 329
　　6.5　Catalysis 331
　　6.6　Future Opportunities and Outlook 332
　　6.7　Structural Details 332
　　6.8　Ag$_N$-DNA Photophysics 332
　　6.9　Improved Chemical and Photostability..................................... 333
　　6.10　Purity... 333
　　6.11　Artificial Nucleic Acids.. 334
　　6.12　Beyond Silver 334
　　6.13　Cellular Uptake and Cytotoxicity 334
7　Concluding Remarks 334
Acknowledgments... 335
Abbreviations and Definitions 335
References... 336

Abstract

Nucleic acid-metal interactions can be exploited to form metal nanoclusters templated by DNA and RNA. These metal nanoclusters have unique properties that are conferred by their polydentate nucleic acid ligands and are promising for a range of functional applications. Silver nanoclusters templated by single-stranded DNA oligomers (Ag$_N$-DNA) are the most well-understood species of nucleic acid-stabilized nanoclusters and exhibit an especially diverse array of exciting optical properties that depend on oligomer sequence. Ag$_N$-DNAs exhibit bright, narrow-band fluorescence, displaying a wide palette of sequence-selected emission colors that range from visible to near-infrared (NIR) wavelengths and high quantum yields in select cases. These nanoclusters have demonstrated promise for bioimaging, chemical and biomolecular sensing,

Nucleic Acid-Templated Metal Nanoclusters

and nanophotonics and provide new opportunities to merge atomically precise nanochemistry with programmable DNA nanotechnology. Recent years have witnessed a significant leap in the fundamental understanding of the structure-property relationships of Ag_N-DNAs, facilitated by simultaneous breakthroughs in advanced purification methods to achieve atomically precise Ag_N-DNAs, spectroscopic and mass characterization of purified samples, crystallographic structure determination, and machine learning-driven high-throughput experiments. This chapter places nucleic acid-templated metal nanoclusters in the context of the field of nucleic acid-metal chemistry, presents the current fundamental understanding of Ag_N-DNA structure and optical properties in the context of recent advances, and describes future opportunities and challenges to realize the potential of these nanoclusters for applications.

KEYWORDS

DNA; Metal Nanoclusters; Templated Synthesis; Atomic Precision; Fluorescence; Photophysics; Machine Learning for Chemical Design; Biosensing

1 INTRODUCTION

Metal clusters, often termed "nanoclusters", are tiny nanoparticles of countably few metal atoms bonded together. Nanoclusters typically consist of $N=2-10^2$ atoms and provide a window into the transition from molecules to bulk metals [1]. Molecules exhibit discrete electronic structures and single-electron transitions, while bulk metals contain a sea of delocalized electrons in a conduction band that exhibits collective behavior such as plasmonic excitations. As one shrinks a metal particle to below 1 µm in size, new properties emerge from confinement of the electron gas, which produces the localized surface plasmon resonance. Reducing size further to the few nanometers scale, approaching the Fermi wavelength of the conduction electrons, leads to the emergence of discrete energy levels, quantized atomic sizes, and behaviors such as size-dependent photoluminescence. Detailed studies of these nanocluster properties have been carried out for decades in ultrahigh vacuum environments for bare metal clusters [1], which are highly reactive and easily undergo aggregation and oxidation to reduce surface energy. Stabilizing nanoclusters at ambient conditions requires protecting atomic or molecular ligands or supporting substrates or matrices. This approach has brought noble metal nanoclusters out of the vacuum and into the "real world", significantly expanding their potential applications [2]. Ligand-stabilized nanoclusters have structures and properties that are strongly affected by the choice of the protecting ligand, providing a route to tailor nanoclusters for specific functions. While many noble metal nanoclusters have been stabilized by small molecule ligands, forming the so-called monolayer-protected nanoclusters [3], macromolecules such as peptides, polymers, and oligonucleotides also serve as versatile templates for nanocluster synthesis [4, 5]. Because these macromolecules can be multidentate metal ligands, macromolecule-stabilized nanoclusters may allow chemists to further expand the structure-property relations and technological uses of nanoclusters.

This chapter focuses on metal nanoclusters stabilized by nucleic acids. In particular, we focus primarily on DNA-templated silver nanoclusters (Ag_N-DNAs), which are by far the most well-understood class of nucleic acid-protected nanoclusters and have attracted attention for their remarkable and tunable optical properties. Ag_N-DNAs were first reported by Petty, Dickson, and coworkers, who used a cytosine-rich 12-base oligomer to template the synthesis of Ag_N-DNAs by chemical reduction, yielding a product with fluorescence emission peaks between 400 and 600 nm [6]. Soon after, Vosch et al. reported an Ag_N-DNA that exhibited near-infrared (NIR) fluorescence, unusually high photostability, and excited dark-state behavior [7]. Early work by Gwinn et al. found that Ag_N-DNAs prefer single-stranded (ss) over double-stranded (ds) DNA hosts and that the Ag_N-DNA fluorescence spectrum depends sensitively on the nucleobase sequence of the stabilizing DNA oligomer, supporting that silver-nucleobase interactions are key to the stabilization of Ag_N-DNAs [8]. These early fundamental studies were quickly followed by reports of the sensitivity of Ag_N-DNA fluorescence properties to various chemical and biomolecular analytes [9–11]. These reports established the promise of Ag_N-DNAs as uniquely programmable fluorophores and biomolecular and chemical sensors [12–16].

Ag_N-DNAs are exceptional for their highly tunable photophysical properties (Figure 1). The structural and photophysical properties of the Ag_N-DNA are tuned by tailoring the DNA oligomer sequence, which determines the size and shape of the encapsulated silver cluster core that forms during chemical reduction. Because of this sequence tunability, Ag_N-DNAs exhibit a wide palette of emission colors ranging from 450 to 1,000 nm [17–21]. Certain Ag_N-DNAs have been reported with high chemical stabilities and photostabilities [7], high fluorescence quantum yields [22, 23], and high Stokes shifts [19]. Due to these properties, Ag_N-DNAs are emerging in applications including bioimaging; strand exchange on-off switches [24]; sensitive specific sensors for aptamers, nucleic acids sequences [9, 25, 26], proteins, enzymatic activity, and metal ions [27]; background-free fluorescence microscopy [28, 29]; and nanophotonics [30, 31]. Because Ag_N-DNAs can be highly fluorescent and are smaller in size than colloidal quantum dots and other luminescent nanoparticles [32], it is promising to pursue Ag_N-DNAs as biocompatible alternatives to organic dyes and quantum dots for *in-vivo* fluorescence imaging. Many organic dyes suffer from low photostability [33] and oxygen sensitivity, whereas quantum dots are toxic, larger in size and exhibit strong nonmolecular power-law fluorescence intermittency [34–38]. In contrast, Ag_N-DNAs display high emission rates, excellent photostability, strong antibunching, and non-blinking traits [7].

The literature contains a plethora of publications that present proof-of-principle applications of Ag_N-DNAs in diverse fields [12]. In order to further advance these and other yet-discovered technological applications of Ag_N-DNAs and other nucleic acid-stabilized metal nanoclusters, it is essential to understand the underlying fundamental principles that govern their formation, stability, structure, and optical and chemical properties. Numerous fascinating scientific challenges pertaining to Ag_N-DNAs remain to be fully addressed. While a few crystal structures of Ag_N-DNAs have emerged [39–42], the vast majority of structures remain unsolved. Also, the photophysical mechanisms governing Ag_N-DNA luminescence remain only partially understood. Although Ag_N-DNA synthesis is facile, purification is nearly always required to obtain compositionally pure Ag_N-DNA solutions. Because this

Nucleic Acid-Templated Metal Nanoclusters

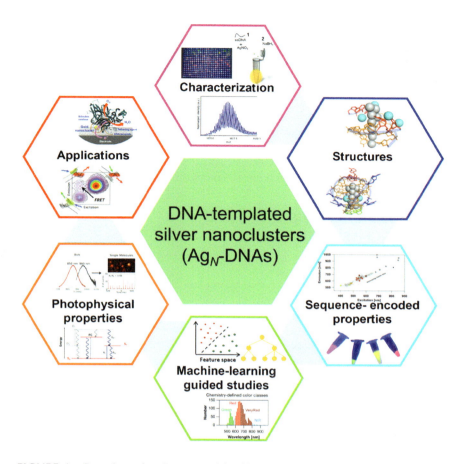

FIGURE 1 Overview of topics covered in this chapter, spanning fundamental understanding of Ag_N-DNA structures and properties, approaches to Ag_N-DNA design, and emerging applications. Images of crystal structures are created from PDB ID: 6NIZ, 6JR4 with PyMOL. (Figures are adapted from Swasey et al. [18], Chakraborty et al. [50] (adapted with permission from the American Chemical Society. Copyright 2015), Copp et al. [61] (adapted with permission from the American Chemical Society. Copyright 2018), Schultz et al. [65, 183] (Figure from Ref. [183] is adapted with permission from the American Chemical Society. Copyright 2013), and Liisberg et al. [175] (adapted with permission from the American Chemical Society. Copyright 2021).)

challenging step has often been skipped, the scientific literature on structure-property relations of Ag_N-DNAs contains inconsistencies as the field has evolved. Finally, the rules governing how DNA sequences encode Ag_N-DNA properties, including the fluorescence color, extinction coefficient, quantum yield, chemical, and photostability, are complex and challenging to discern by conventional methods. For nucleic acid-stabilized metal nanoclusters beyond Ag_N-DNAs, very little is known about their fundamental properties.

In this chapter, we present the state-of-art for synthesis and purification procedures to obtain and characterize compositionally pure Ag$_N$-DNA, which are critically needed to determine the structure-property relations of these nanoclusters (Figure 1). Next, we discuss what is currently known about the structures and photophysical properties of Ag$_N$-DNA, including indirect structure-property inferences from studies of purified Ag$_N$-DNAs and the first reported crystal structures for several Ag$_N$-DNA species. We describe how high-throughput experiments and machine learning (ML) classifiers are decoding how nucleobase sequence controls Ag$_N$-DNA properties. Finally, we discuss emerging applications of Ag$_N$-DNAs, as well as challenges and opportunities for future research in the field of nucleic acid-stabilized metal nanoclusters.

2 SYNTHESIS, PURIFICATION, AND MASS CHARACTERIZATION

2.1 Synthesis

Ag$_N$-DNA synthesis is a simple two-step process, carried out by mixing an aqueous solution of silver salt and oligonucleotides, followed by NaBH$_4$ reduction (Figure 2a). Typically, silver nitrate is used as the source of silver cations, and the synthesis is carried out in neutral pH solutions of ammonium acetate, phosphate [43], citrate [21, 44], or sodium cacodylate buffer [39], although other solution conditions have also been reported. Fluorescent products typically require cytosine-rich and/or guanine-rich DNA oligomers. In addition to the DNA sequence, the stoichiometry of silver ion to DNA strand and post-reduction incubation time can affect the product formation. The sequence dependence of Ag$_N$-DNAs likely results in part from the sequence dependence of the Ag$^+$–DNA complexes that are the precursors of these nanoclusters [45–47]. It is also possible to stabilize Ag$_N$-DNA with oligomers containing artificial nucleobases [48].

Early work found that fluorescent Ag$_N$-DNAs were not synthesized using WC-paired dsDNA, leading to the false assumption that only ssDNA can act as a template for Ag$_N$-DNA and that Ag$_N$-DNAs can be confined solely to single-stranded regions of DNA WC-paired complexes during chemical synthesis. However, as discussed in Section 3, Ag$^+$-nucleobase interactions can significantly reorganize DNA secondary structure, particularly for C-rich or G-rich DNA [46, 47]. Thus, it is not appropriate to assume that DNA will preserve its natural WC secondary structure after addition of silver ions. Well-controlled Ag$^+$–DNA complexes can, however, be used to control Ag$_N$-DNA formation, as shown by Léon et al. [25].

It is important to note that Ag$_N$-DNA synthesis by chemical reduction yields a heterogeneous mixture of products of fluorescent and dark (nonfluorescent) DNA-templated nanoclusters, Ag$^+$–DNA complexes, and larger colloidal silver nanoparticles. In many cases, the as-synthesized solution may contain multiple fluorescent Ag$_N$-DNAs containing varying numbers of silver atoms (N) and number of DNA strands (n_s), evolving with time. This heterogeneity challenges

Nucleic Acid-Templated Metal Nanoclusters

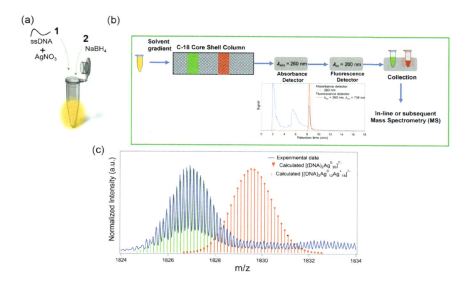

FIGURE 2 (a) Ag_N-DNA synthesis involves reduction of an aqueous of silver salt and DNA strands using $NaBH_4$. (b) Schematic of tandem HPLC-MS with in-line UV/Vis and fluorescence detectors to purify and characterize Ag_N-DNAs. (c) Experimental mass spectrum of the Ag_{30}-DNA product at the 7− charge state dimeric product (blue), with the calculated mass distribution (green bars) for a product with two DNA strands, $N_0 = 12\ Ag^0$, and $N_+ = 18\ Ag^+$ [18]. The calculated distribution for a product with no charged silvers (two DNA strands and 30 Ag^0, red bars), illustrates how the shift between the experimental and calculated isotopic finger distribution (green bars) can be used to accurately determine the numbers of Ag^0 and Ag^+ in an Ag_N-DNA product.

studies of Ag_N-DNA composition. Literature reports of the atomic composition of Ag_N-DNAs that have not been purified often contain errors for this reason. Hence, it is of utmost importance to obtain compositionally pure solution of a single Ag_N-DNA species prior to any further structural and spectral characterization. In Sections 2 and 3 of this book chapter, we primarily focus on Ag_N-DNAs that have undergone purification prior to characterization.

RNA has also been shown to template fluorescent nanoclusters using the same chemical reduction process as for Ag_N-DNAs. RNA and DNA oligomers of equal length and nucleobase sequence produce fluorescent products with different spectral properties, suggesting distinct cluster sizes/structures [49]. These distinctions may be caused by differences in the conformations that RNA and DNA can adopt around a tiny Ag_N. Variations in the backbone chemistry of nucleic acids may provide a way to expand the space of possible nucleic acid-stabilized metal nanoclusters.

Nanoclusters of metals other than silver have been stabilized using DNA ligands, although their fundamental properties remain much less characterized. Chakraborty et al. reported much smaller gold nanoclusters to form on a 30-mer DNA strand by reducing an Au^+–DNA mixture with dimethylamine borane [50].

Resulting products had sub-nanometer sizes as observed by transmission electron microscopy (TEM), and X-ray photoelectron spectroscopy (XPS) showed the presence of both Au(I) and Au(0) in the reduced mixture. The nanocluster displayed weak phosphorescence characterized by a μs-scale lifetime and high Stokes shift, which has been characteristic of other ligand-stabilized gold nanoclusters [51, 52]. Fluorescent copper nanoclusters have also been reported to form on DNA using ascorbic acid reduction, with A-T-rich duplex DNA appearing most suitable for stabilizing fluorescent products [53, 54]. However, so far reported DNA-stabilized copper nanoclusters are preferentially stabilized by thymine-rich sequences. These fluorescent copper nanoclusters have been utilized for detection of rutin and other analytes [55–58].

2.1.1 High-Throughput Ag$_N$-DNA Synthesis

The dependence of Ag$_N$-DNA properties on nucleobase sequence motivates the development of experimental methods for high-throughput synthesis and fluorescence characterization of Ag$_N$-DNAs. These approaches provide important insights because the chemical space of DNA ligands for silver nanoclusters is immense, with 4^L unique sequences of length L for the four canonical nucleobases. Typical DNA ligands for Ag$_N$-DNAs are $L=10–30$ nucleobases. Well-controlled experiments on $10^2–10^4$ DNA ligands can enable fundamental studies of the "sequence-structure-property relations" of Ag$_N$-DNAs and dramatically expedite the discovery of new Ag$_N$-DNAs. The scientific literature contains a range of Ag$_N$-DNA synthesis conditions, including stoichiometries, buffer conditions, and protocols, making it difficult to gather large datasets that connect Ag$_N$-DNA sequences to fluorescence properties directly from the published literature. Thus, it is critical to perform high-throughput Ag$_N$-DNA synthesis at uniform conditions to directly compare how DNA ligands of different sequences stabilize Ag$_N$-DNAs.

Richards et al. were the first to report the parallel synthesis of 384 Ag$_N$-DNAs on distinct DNA templates in a DNA microarray. These studies were confined to sequences of only cytosine, adenine, and thymine. Only five of the DNA sequences and associated Ag$_N$-DNA products were reported [43], which prohibited interrogation of Ag$_N$-DNA sequence-to-color relations.

Copp et al. developed an approach to synthesize and characterize Ag$_N$-DNAs in 384 microwell plates using robotic liquid handling followed by rapid parallel fluorimetry in well plate readers. Experiments proceed as follows. (1) Combine DNA oligomers suspended in ultrapure water with a solution of AgNO$_3$ and NH$_4$OAc, followed by mixing by pipetting. (2) Reduce DNA-AgNO$_3$-NH$_4$OAc mixtures with a freshly prepared aqueous solution of NaBH$_4$ about 18 min after the first step, followed by mixing by pipetting. (3) Centrifuge microwell plates at slow speed for a short time to remove any bubbles that may inhibit fluorimetry in well plates. (4) Store well plates at 4°C until measurement. (5) Using a well plate fluorimeter, measure fluorescence emission spectra of all fluorescent Ag$_N$-DNA products using universal excitation at 260 nm. The resulting distributions of peak fluorescence emission wavelength were initially reported for various stoichiometries and time points after synthesis [59].

Later reports have focused on Ag_N-DNAs that persist for 1 week after reduction, synthesized at stoichiometries of 20 μM DNA, 100 or 140 μM $AgNO_3$, $[NaBH_4]/[AgNO_3]=0.5$, and 10 mM NH_4OAc [60]. Each experiment includes several wells filled with a DNA control strand that forms brightly fluorescent Ag_N-DNAs, 5′-d(TTCCCACCCACCCCGGCCCGTT)-3′, which allows fluorescence intensities to be normalized across all high-throughput experiments performed over a decade on multiple instruments. This method has generated a data library of more than 3,000 distinct DNA ligand sequences correlated with the fluorescence spectral properties of the Ag_N-DNA products they stabilize [18, 60–62]. Unlike microarray-based high-throughput Ag_N-DNA synthesis, this method also avoids constraining DNA templates to a surface, which may affect formation of Ag_N-DNA products.

Recently, the Yeh group has significantly increased the throughput of Ag_N-DNA experimental screening using next-generation sequencing (NGS) chips to screen 10^4 Ag_N-DNAs [63]. This method specifically focuses on a class of Ag_N-DNA complexes with sensing functionality, called NanoCluster Beacons (NCBs) [63, 64]. These are composed of a nonfluorescent Ag_N-DNA and an "activator" DNA strand, which "lights up" the Ag_N-DNA upon binding. Because the mechanisms of these important Ag_N-DNA sensors are complex and not well understood, NGS approaches to experimental screening can dramatically increase the success rate of designing activator sequences that result in a dramatic increase in Ag_N-DNA fluorescence. It is important to note that the higher throughput capability of NGS chips comes with a trade-off in lower quality fluorescence emission data; NGS platforms use fluorescence microscopy for detection, meaning that an image at a specific excitation and emission wavelength is collected rather than a full fluorescence emission spectrum [63].

2.2 Purification by HPLC

Purification of Ag_N-DNAs can be performed by ion-pair reversed-phase high-performance liquid chromatography (RP-HPLC) containing core-shell C-18 columns. TEAA at pH 7.4 is commonly used as the ion-pairing agent, mixed with the mobile phase (methanol/water mixture) for improved separation. Under optimized conditions (which include a solvent gradient of mobile phase, ion-pairing agent, *etc.*), the Ag_N-DNA desorbs from the stationary phase depending on its composition and secondary structure. Aliquots then pass through an absorbance detector at 260 nm to monitor all species containing DNA and through a fluorescence detector to monitor fluorescent species (Figure 2b) [65]. It is advantageous to use 260-nm excitation because Ag_N-DNAs are universally excited through the nucleobases, in addition to size/shape-specific excitation peaks in the visible to NIR spectrum [22, 59]. Using this method, it is possible to separate DNA products that bear the fluorescent Ag_N-DNA of interest from the many other products formed during synthesis. The reader should note that not all fluorescent Ag_N-DNA will be sufficiently stable under HPLC conditions, which include high pressures and nonaqueous solvent conditions.

2.3 Determination of Composition by Mass Spectrometry

Electrospray ionization mass spectrometry (ESI-MS) is a versatile and valuable tool to characterize noncovalent nucleic acid complexes [66]. Because the negatively charged phosphate backbone of DNA is deprotonated at neutral pH, negative ion-mode ESI-MS is an ideal approach for native mass spectrometry of Ag$_N$-DNAs. Koszinowski and Ballweg first reported the composition of a nonfluorescent and partially oxidized (Ag$_6^{4+}$)-DNA, using high-resolution mass spectrometry (HRMS) by negative ion-mode ESI to resolve the total mass and charge of the product [67]. Gwinn and coworkers later used tandem HPLC-MS to correlate Ag$_N$-DNA optical properties with composition for many compositionally pure Ag$_N$-DNAs [22, 59, 65], providing valuable insights into how metal cluster size, charge and geometry are correlated with the photophysical properties of Ag$_N$-DNA. Here, we describe experimental methods for HRMS of purified Ag$_N$-DNAs and how these experiments can be used to fully determine mass and oxidation state of Ag$_N$-DNAs.

HRMS can be performed either by direct injection of purified Ag$_N$-DNAs or by tandem HPLC-MS [68]. For direct injection, solvents of aliquots collected from RP-HPLC are exchanged to ammonium acetate prior to injection. Ammonium acetate is a commonly used salt to enhance the resolution of native ESI-MS, as its volatility is ideal for desolvation and allows the use of soft ionization techniques to avoid fragmentation of DNA complexes [69]. Ammonium ions protonate the negatively charged phosphate backbone, forming volatile ammonia under ionization conditions and thus do not interfere with the ESI process. The use of organic solvents such as MeOH (≈20%) during an injection can further improve ESI yield. By these methods, it is possible to perform HRMS for Ag$_N$-DNAs and to resolve the isotopic abundance pattern of the silver atoms within the Ag$_N$-DNA product.

Analysis of the isotopic distribution of the Ag$_N$-DNA allows determination of the total number of silver atoms N as well as the oxidation state of the nanocluster. The oxidation state can be described in terms of the effective cationic (N_+) and neutral (N_0) silver content. (Note that for a few-atom nanocluster, individual metal atoms may not be strictly neutral or cationic; rather, this terminology presents a helpful way to describe the number of effective valence electrons within the nanocluster core.) Firstly, the z^- charge of the m/z peak is determined from the spacing between adjacent isotopic peaks (separated by $1/z$). The total charge of the complex corresponding to this m/z peak, $-ez$, is equal to the charge of the Ag$_N$, eN_+, minus the charge of the number of protons removed from the DNA, n_{pr}, to reach the total charge of $-ez$.

$$-z = N_+ - n_{pr} \qquad (1)$$

Now, since n_{pr} protons must be removed from an unionized DNA oligomer to reach the $z-$ charge state, the total mass m_{total} of the Ag$_N$-DNA is calculated as:

$$m_{total} = m_{DNA} n_s + m_{Ag}(N_+ + N_0) - n_{pr} \qquad (2)$$

where m_{DNA} is the mass of the unionized DNA oligomer and n_s is the number of DNA strands templating the nanocluster. (Note that during negative ion-mode ESI, protons are added to, not physically removed from, the already deprotonated DNA at neutral pH [66]. Rather, Equation 2 simply allows one to relate m_{total} to the mass of the unionized DNA strand m_{DNA}.) N_0 and N_+ can be precisely determined from the measured isotope distribution pattern by determining the value of N_+ that best fits the m/z isotope pattern (Figure 2c). These advancements to isolate and characterize compositionally pure Ag_N-DNAs have enabled researchers to correlate the atomically precise sizes of Ag_N-DNAs to their optical properties, providing key insights into structure-property relations of these nanoclusters, which we discuss in Section 3.

Inductively coupled plasma-atomic emission spectroscopy (ICP-AES) has been employed by Petty et al. to determine the relative stoichiometry of silver to DNA for a solution of Ag_N-DNAs [70]. Because this is a bulk solution method, ICP-AES can underestimate the size of the Ag_N-DNA for n_s greater than 1. It is, thus, necessary to determine n_s by other means in order to use ICP-AES for accurate determination of total silver composition N.

Purification and size determination methods have primarily been developed for Ag_N-DNAs, while methods for other DNA-stabilized nanoclusters remain to be reported. It is likely that many of the purification and size determination methods for Ag_N-DNAs would also be well-suited for other metals and charged nucleic acids. Because compositionally pure solutions are critical for building a fundamental understanding of structure-property relationships, it will be important to extend methods to prepare atomically precise DNA-stabilized nanoclusters beyond just Ag_N-DNAs.

3 STRUCTURE-PROPERTY RELATIONSHIPS OF DNA-STABILIZED SILVER NANOCLUSTERS

This section describes the current understanding of the structures and properties of Ag_N-DNAs, including how DNA sculpts silver nanocluster structure, what is known about the silver-DNA interaction, relation to Ag^+–nucleobase interactions, and photophysical properties. We focus primarily on studies for compositionally pure Ag_N-DNA solutions, as it is possible to correlate properties to a given atomic size and structure in such cases.

3.1 Ag_N-DNA Structure Determination

Prior to recent breakthrough X-ray crystallographic studies [39–42], Ag_N-DNA structural features were primarily inferred by experimentally observed correlations of Ag_N-DNA composition with optical spectra, in the general context of what is known about structure-to-optical property relationships for metal nanoclusters. X-ray spectroscopy and infrared spectroscopy provide important complementary information about the coordination environment of silver atoms within the Ag_N-DNAs.

3.1.1 The Jellium Model for Metal Nanoclusters

For readers primarily in the field of nucleic acids, we briefly introduce the electronic properties of simple metal clusters. These can be described by the spherical jellium model. The jellium model assumes that valence electrons in a metal cluster delocalize over the entire nanocluster, forming a jellium, i.e., a uniform electron gas distributed over a uniform positively charged background. A neutral nanocluster that contains N atoms of valency z will contain zN effective free electrons, and these electrons form 'superatomic' orbitals whose electronic shell structure is analogous to the shell structure of atomic nuclei. Experimental and computational studies show that neutral nanoclusters with closed shell configurations contain $zN = 2, 8, \ldots$ effective free electrons, often termed "magic numbers" in analogy to nuclear physics, and exhibit much greater stabilities and enhanced abundances than other nanocluster sizes [1, 71]. This model was first developed for naked gas-phase clusters and later extended to ligand-stabilized coinage metal nanoclusters, which also prefer to adopt compositions that correspond to spherical superatom magic numbers. The effective number of valence electrons in the cluster core for ligand-protected nanoclusters is given by $zN–M–Z$, where M is the number of electron-withdrawing ligands and Z is the total charge of the complex [2, 72]. Numerous ligand-stabilized nanoclusters with ultrahigh chemical stability are found to possess these spherical magic number properties, and these superatoms have significant utility for practical applications [3, 71].

3.1.2 Evidence for Rod-Like Structure

The jellium model can also be applied to Ag_N-DNAs when effective valence electron count is experimentally determined. Equation 2 in Section 2 describes how HRMS enables the resolution of the effective valence electron count for Ag_N-DNAs, N_0 [22, 59]. (Effective electron count is N_0 because silver has valency $z = 1$.) The correlation of N_0 with Ag_N-DNA peak absorption wavelengths then yields insights into Ag_N-DNA structure. Schultz et al. compared the peak absorbance energies of compositionally pure Ag_N-DNAs to those for bare Ag clusters with equal N_0, finding the first evidence that Ag_N-DNAs adopt anisotropic, rod-like shapes [22]. Bare Ag clusters with $N_0 = 2–20$ exhibit absorption spectra with multiple UV transitions between 3 and 5 eV, and these clusters adopt globular structures for Ag_7 and large sizes [73]. In contrast, compositionally pure Ag_N-DNAs were found to exhibit much simpler absorption spectra, featuring a single dominant peak in the visible to NIR range below 3 eV and an additional UV absorption band at 4.7 eV that corresponds almost exactly to the absorption spectrum of the DNA template strand. Peak visible to NIR absorption energies of Ag_N-DNAs shift to lower energies with increasing N_0. The dependence of Ag_N-DNA absorption energy on N_0 was found to correspond well with the findings of quantum chemical calculations for linear atomic chains of silver by Guidez and Aikens [74]. These calculations find that linear silver chains exhibit high amplitude low energy absorption peaks corresponding to collective electronic oscillations along the longitudinal axis of the linear chain, and these longitudinal peaks red-shift as chain length increases. A second weak, higher excitation peak (5–6 eV) arises from charge oscillations perpendicular to the chain axis and is independent of the chain length. This peak would be obscured for Ag$_N$-DNAs due to the strong absorption of DNA bases above 4 eV. The correlation between peak absorbance energy and N_0 of Ag$_N$-DNA agrees well with calculations on Ag atomic chains with one-atom cross section (gray line, Figure 3a). Deviations likely arise from variation of the longitudinal mode energy, which increases with the increase in aspect ratio (length *vs.* diameter) of the cluster [75]. This comparison provided early evidence that Ag$_N$-DNAs adopt rod-like structures, in contrast to the vast majority of similarly sized noble metal nanoclusters with globular shapes [3]. Shortly thereafter, density functional theory (DFT) calculations by Ramazanov and Kononov supported an elongated, "threadlike" shape for Ag$_N$-DNAs [76].

3.1.3 Magic Colors Are Correlated to Magic Numbers

Our large-scale study of Ag$_N$-DNAs stabilized by 10-base oligomers with randomly assigned sequences provided additional evidence that the silver cluster core within Ag$_N$-DNAs has anisotropic shape [59]. High-throughput experimental synthesis and fluorescence emission characterization found enhanced abundances of Ag$_N$-DNAs with emission wavelengths at about 540 nm, "Green", and 630 nm, "Red". An analysis of literature-reported emission wavelengths also shows the same enhanced abundances of these "magic colors." Enhanced abundances of certain sizes of metal nanoclusters typically point to magic number properties [1]. HPLC with tandem HRMS showed that "magic colored" Green and Red Ag$_N$-DNAs contain even numbers of effective valence electrons, $N_0 = 4$

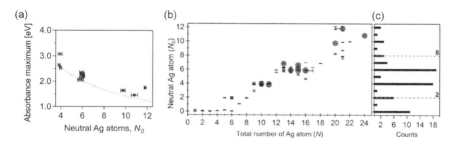

FIGURE 3 (a) Peak absorbance energies for purified Ag$_N$-DNAs characterized by HRMS as a function of the number of effective free electrons in the cluster, equal to N_0. Experimental data are well-described by simulations of silver nanorods with one-atom cross sections (gray line) [22]. (b) The number of neutral Ag atoms, N_0, as determined by HRMS for HPLC-purified Ag$_N$-DNAs, including brightly fluorescent Ag$_N$-DNAs (gray-filled circles) and Ag$_N$-DNAs without measurable fluorescence (black markers). (c) Histogram of N_0 values shows abundances of clusters with even N_0 as compared to magic numbers 2 and 8 predicted by the spherical 'superatom' model. ((b and c) Adapted from Copp et al. [59], with permission from the American Chemical Society. Copyright 2014.)

and 6, respectively (Figures 3b and c). Because spherical "superatom" silver nanoclusters exhibit magic numbers of $N_0=2$, 8, etc., the preferred values of N_0 for Ag$_N$-DNAs are consistent with a rod-like silver cluster core. The ellipsoidal shell model for nanoclusters predicts even magic numbers of N_0 for nanoclusters with sufficiently broken spherical symmetry.

DNA is a multidentate ligand for Ag$^+$, with individual nucleobases confined to the phosphate backbone. This spatial constraint of silver-nucleobase interactions may prefer rod-like nanoclusters, with energetically favored sizes of $N_0=4, 6, 10, 12, \ldots$, i.e., even numbers of effective free electrons that do *not* correspond to spherical superatoms (aspherical cluster cores will be energetically disfavored for closed spherical shell configurations due to the Jahn–Teller effect). Different values of N_0 will correspond to different nanocluster rod lengths, tuning fluorescence excitation and emission. Finer variations in fluorescence properties for Ag$_N$-DNAs with the same magic number could arise from variations in N_+ and the arrangement of these silver cations in the Ag$_N$-DNA complexes. Our molecular dynamics (MD) simulations of toy model Ag$_N$-DNA structures suggest that variations in Ag$^+$–nucleobase interactions can tune the shape of the Ag$_N$-DNA. Furthermore, large-scale studies of 500 Ag$_N$-DNA excitation spectra suggest variations in silver cluster core geometry, as reflected by a diversity of different excitation spectral features [77]. Thus, it is likely that nucleic acid ligands stabilize a rich space of Ag$_N$-DNAs with highly diverse structures and optical properties.

3.1.4 X-ray Spectroscopy

X-ray spectroscopy has also yielded important insights into the oxidation states and ligand coordination environment of silvers in Ag$_N$-DNAs. Petty et al. studied a dimly emissive violet Ag$_N$-DNA with an absorbance maximum at 400 nm, hosted by a 20-base ssDNA [78]. This violet species evolves into a strongly fluorescent NIR-emitting species upon DNA strand perturbation [21, 79]. The violet species was probed by HRMS, X-ray absorption near edge structure (XANES), and extended X-ray absorption fine structure (EXAFS) to interrogate the Ag:DNA stoichiometry, oxidation state, ligand coordination environment, and structure of this Ag$_N$-DNA [78]. MS and Ag L$_3$ edge XANES spectra established the presence of an Ag$_{10}^{6+}$ species in native aqueous environment. Ag K-edge EXAFS spectra elucidated the structure and coordination environment of the cluster. The experimental EXAFS spectrum was fitted with three calculated individual scattering paths (Figure 4a) that correspond to Ag$^+$–nucleobase interaction and two types of silver environment in the cluster core, where neutral silver atoms reside in the metal-like cluster core and Ag$^+$ dwell outside the cluster core to interact with the DNA template (or metal-like Ag$\cdots$Ag and long-distance Ag$\cdots$Ag interactions). Based on this, the authors proposed an octahedral geometry of the Ag$_{10}^{6+}$ nanocluster that contains Ag$^+$-mediated base pairings and in which not all the nucleobases interact with the Ag$_N$-DNA (Figure 4b).

Volkov et al. used X-ray photon spectroscopy (XPS) to compare an HPLC-purified Ag$_N$-DNA solution to the DNA template strand alone, the unreduced DNA–Ag$^+$ mixture, and larger silver nanoparticles [80]. The similarity in the

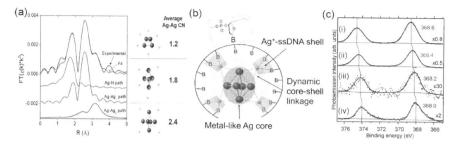

FIGURE 4 (a) Ag K-edge EXAFS (extended X-ray absorption fine structure) trace of the solution state Ag$_N$-DNAs. The experimental data (black) was fitted (gray) with three individual scattering paths displayed separately. (b) Proposed octahedral structure of Ag$_{10}^{6+}$ nanocluster core after combining all information from HRMS and EXAFS measurements. (Adapted from Petty et al. [78], with permission from the American Chemical Society. Copyright 2016.) (c) Ag 3d peak doublet for (i) Ag$^+$–DNA complexes, (ii) AgNO$_3$ salt, (iii) HPLC-purified fluorescent Ag$_N$-DNAs containing both neutral and cationic silver and (iv) metallic Ag nanoparticles [80]. (Adapted from Volkov et al. [80], with permission from the American Chemical Society. Copyright 2017.)

oxygen spectra of the bare DNA strand and the DNA–Ag$^+$ mixture supports that Ag$^+$ ions prefer to bind to nitrogen rather than oxygen atoms. Spectra obtained for the Ag$_N$-DNA (i.e., after reduction) showed evidence for binding of silver to oxygen, which agrees with crystal structures of Ag$_{16}$-DNAs (discussed below) in which Ag atoms were found to interact with oxygen that belongs to phosphodiester bonds [40–42]. In addition to this, the comparative analysis of Ag 3d core-level spectra for the HPLC-purified Ag$_N$-DNA species and larger silver nanoparticles showed that 3d$_{5/2}$ Ag peaks have lower binding energies for Ag^0-containing nanoparticles and Ag$_N$-DNA than for Ag$^+$–DNA complexes and AgNO$_3$, as expected for the difference between Ag^0 and Ag$^+$ (Figure 4c). These XPS studies support that Ag$_N$-DNAs consist of both neutral and cationic Ag species, consistent with HRMS studies [18, 59, 78].

3.1.5 Infrared Spectroscopy

Petty and Kohler and coauthors employed ultrafast time-resolved infrared (TRIR) spectroscopy to study the coordination environment of two Ag$_N$-DNAs hosted by 18-base oligonucleotides, 5′-d(CCCCACCCCTCCCXTTTT)-3′, where X=guanosine and its analog inosine, which lacks exocyclic C2-NH$_2$ [81]. HRMS and identical absorption/emission spectra prove the formation of Ag$_{10}^{6+}$ species on both oligonucleotides. TRIR spectra provide insights into the bonding interactions that control the electronic properties of Ag$_N$-DNA, showing that vibrational modes of cytidines, guanosines, and inosines bleach upon nanocluster formation, while spectral signatures corresponding to thymidine are absent. The lower affinity of Ag$^+$ ions for thymine at neutral pH has been well documented [46]. The decay of vibrational signatures and electronic relaxation of the nanocluster occur synchronously, pointing to strong interaction of specific nucleobases with the cluster core. Furthermore, the absence of ligation through deprotonated N1 of guanosine and inosine was observed.

3.1.6 Circular Dichroism Spectroscopy Provides a Bridge between Theory and Experiment

Electronic circular dichroism (CD) spectroscopy is a valuable and sensitive tool to study and characterize nucleic acid structures. Because CD spectra can be calculated by first-principles methods, the structure-sensitive chiroptical activity of Ag_N-DNAs allows comparison between experimental and computational studies. Swasey et al. compared CD spectra of four purified Ag_N-DNAs to their bare DNA and Ag^+–DNA precursors [82]. The similarity of the UV CD spectra of Ag_N-DNAs to spectra for unreduced Ag^+–DNA precursors indicates that the reduced Ag_N-DNA solution sustains much of the DNA structure that is imposed by interaction between the nucleobases and Ag^+ prior to reduction (Figure 5a). The visible to NIR features of Ag_N-DNA CD spectra are dependent on cluster size and structure, exhibiting dichroic peak(s) that align with the lowest energy absorbance peak, in addition to higher energy peaks that may arise from both nucleobase and nanocluster transitions (Figure 5b). These experimentally measured CD signatures of Ag_N-DNAs agree with quantum chemical calculations of CD spectra of bare neutral Ag clusters with helical, filamentary structures of the

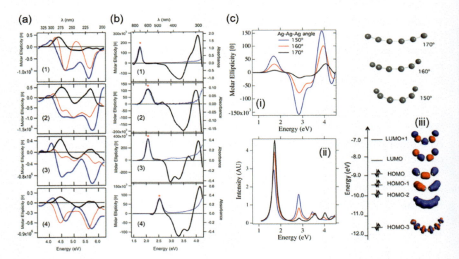

FIGURE 5 (a) UV CD spectra of different DNA templates used to form fluorescent Ag_N-DNAs. (The numbers (1)–(4) in (a) and (b) represent four different Ag_N-DNA species) Black curves are bare DNA templates in aqueous solution, red curves are Ag^+–DNA complexes, and blue curves are HPLC-purified fluorescent Ag_N-DNAs. (b) CD (black) and absorbance (blue) spectra of HPLC-purified Ag_N-DNAs. The CD peaks that overlie with the lowest energy absorbance peaks are marked in red stars. (c) Calculated CD (i) and absorbance (ii) spectra, and Kohn–Sham orbitals and energies (iii) for differently oriented neutral, filamentary Ag_6 clusters shown at top right [82]. (Adapted from Swasey et al. [82], with permission from the American Chemical Society. Copyright 2014.)

same chiral twist as DNA (Figure 5c) [82]. Chen et al. recently found evidence that silver-to-DNA transitions contribute to the chiroptical properties of Ag_N-DNAs in the visible CD region (below 3.0 eV), based on quantum mechanics/molecular mechanics (QM/MM) calculations [83]. These studies suggest that the nucleobase-metal interaction plays a critical role in the photophysical properties of Ag_N-DNAs. This intimate connection has also been supported by excited state dynamics of Ag_N-DNAs, as vibrational modes of the nucleobases have been found to be excited by visible excitation of the nanocluster, and these modes decay synchronously with the visible luminescence [81].

3.1.7 Crystal Structures

The first X-ray crystal structures for Ag_N-DNAs have provided key structural insights into Ag_N-DNAs and the DNA-silver interactions involved in stabilizing these nanoclusters. In 2019, Huard et al. reported the first crystal structure of an Ag_N-DNA with green fluorescence, which was reduced during or after crystallization [39]. (It should be noted that this Ag_N-DNA cannot be formed in solution because it likely requires the architecture of the crystal for stabilization.) Encapsulated by two copies of a 6-base strand, 5′-d(AACCCC)-3′, eight Ag atoms in this Ag_N-DNA arrange in a "Big Dipper"-like planar geometry. The handle of the Dipper is a zipper region of three C–Ag^+–C metallo-base pairs that form a stem-like duplex with parallel DNA strand orientation, in agreement with findings for C–Ag^+–C duplexes [47]. The zipper region is connected to an adenine-rich hairpin-like pocket that encapsulates a trapezoid-shaped planar Ag_5 cluster core. Ag⋯Ag distances within this trapezoid are ≈2.9 Å, comparable to bond distances in metallic silver [84] and reduced silver nanoclusters.

The Ag_5 cluster core interacts with four adenines (*via* endocyclic N1 and exocyclic N6) and two cytosines (*via* endocyclic N3 and exocyclic N4) (Figures 6b and c). The exocyclic N's of cytosine and adenines are believed to be deprotonated. In the three C–Ag^+–C metallo-base pairs, each Ag^+ interacts with endocyclic N3 of cytosine, forming a near linear geometry of these three Ag^+ (Figure 6a and b). Four additional Ag^+ are present near or at the interface of two symmetry-related adjacent Ag_N-DNAs and are assumed to contribute to the crystal packing (Figure 6a, cyan-colored silver atoms). Two of these Ag^+ are also found to interact with adenines of the Ag_N-DNA, and the remaining two Ag^+ ions were noted to be crystallographic artifacts due to their low occupancies. Interestingly, large-scale studies of 10^3 Ag_N-DNAs have found that adenine-rich nucleobase motifs are associated with green-fluorescent Ag_N-DNAs [60, 77] meaning that while the Big Dipper Ag_N-DNA cannot be chemically synthesized in solution, the silver-nucleobase interactions observed in the crystal structure, especially regarding the Ag_5-nucleobase interactions, have important relevance for solution-synthesized Ag_N-DNAs with green fluorescence.

Cerretani et al. reported the first X-ray crystal structure of a HPLC-purified Ag_N-DNA (Figure 6d and e) [42]. This NIR-emissive species is stabilized by a 10-base DNA ligand, 5′-d(CACCTAGCGA)-3′, discovered by Copp et al. [60], and exhibits an unusually large Stokes shift [19]. Because the Ag_N-DNA was

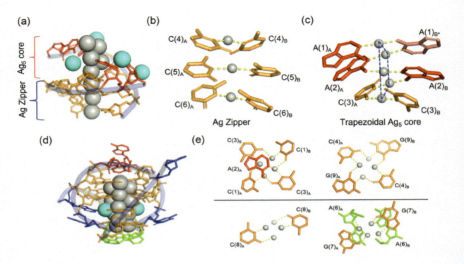

FIGURE 6 (a) Asymmetric unit of "Big Dipper"-shaped Ag$_8$-DNA reported by Huard et al. (Adenines and cytosines are shown in red and orange, respectively. Cyan-colored silver atoms are involved in crystal packing and two of them have low occupancies). (b) Nucleobase–silver interactions in the Ag-zipper section of the Ag$_8$-DNA nanocluster. (c) Nucleobase–silver interactions in the Ag$_5$ nanocluster core section of the Ag$_8$-DNA nanocluster. Adenine from adjacent unit cell is shown in light red [39]. (d) Asymmetric unit of Ag$_{16}$-DNA reported by Cerretani et al. [42] (Nucleobases that are not interacting with the nanocluster core are shown in blue, adenine residues at position 2 (A2) and position 6 (A6) are shown in red and green, respectively. Silver atoms with occupancy 1 are shown in gray spheres, whereas silver atoms with 0.3 occupancy are shown in cyan.) (e) Nucleobase–silver interactions shown from top view of the Ag$_{16}$-DNA. Images are created from PDB ID 6NIZ (a–c) and 6JR4 (d and e) with PyMOL. (The size of silver atoms is shown smaller in (b), (c), and (e) as compared to in (a) and (d) to highlight the interactions with nucleobases.)

synthesized in solution and HPLC-purified prior to crystallization, and its spectral properties are retained after crystallization, the X-ray crystal structure is highly relevant to the solution-phase structure. The structure shows a rod-shaped silver nanocluster core composed of 16 silvers with occupancy one (shown as gray spheres, Figure 6d) and two silvers with occupancy ~0.3 (shown as cyan spheres, Figure 6d). These lower occupancy silvers were hypothesized to be present in only some Ag$_N$-DNA repeating units of the crystal, motivating the assignment of the species as Ag$_{16}$-DNA. No WC-type base pairs are present in the crystal structure. Instead, two DNA strands are linked by silver-nucleobase and H-bonding interactions, forming "horseshoe-like" turns around the Ag$_{16}$. Analogous to the crystal structure reported by Huard et al. [39], Ag atoms form coordinate bonds with the N3 of cytosine and adenines *via* N1. Additional interacting sites are discovered for cytosine (O2) and N7 of adenine. In the case of guanines, interaction *via* N7, N1 and, O6 position are detected (Figure 6e). Interestingly, the terminal adenine, A10, is engaged in formation of A10–Ag$^+$–A10 base pairing with the neighboring asymmetric unit. Removal of this A10 from the 3′-end of the DNA strand has no considerable impact on the photophysical properties of Ag$_{16}$-DNA or its crystal structure [40]. Thymine at position 5 (T5) and adenine at position 10 (A10) (shown in blue, Figure 6d) do not participate in any interaction with the Ag$_{16}$ but rather ensure DNA strand flexibility and engage in π-stacking interactions that promote crystal packing. However, the similarity in asymmetric units for the crystal structure obtained upon deletion of the A10 rules out the impact of A10 on crystal packing.

Ag–N distances are 2.2–2.5 Å, whereas Ag–O bond lengths are 2.4–2.4 Å. The shorter bond length between N1 of G9 and Ag$^+$ (2.3–2.4 Å) suggests a deprotonated N1 guanine. The distances between two silver atoms in the Ag$_{16}$ nanocluster core are between 2.7 and 2.9 Å, well below the van der Waals radii (3.44 Å) [85] and similar to or shorter than their metallic radii (2.8 Å) [86].

A deeper insight into key interactions driving the properties of Ag$_N$-DNA was revealed by crystal engineering on the Ag$_{16}$-DNA. The nucleobase at position 5 of the DNA sequence, originally a thymine (T5), was mutated to X5 (abasic site), C5 (cytosine), A5 (adenine), and G5 (guanine) (5′-d(CACCRAGCGA)-3′, where R=X, A, C, G) [41]. Mutations still produced the NIR-emitting Ag$_{16}$ cluster core, as evidenced by minimal or no changes in structural and photophysical features. The mutation G5 also produced another G5-red emitter which could be removed by HPLC purification prior to crystallization. By comparing crystal structures of the Ag$_{16}$-DNA stabilized by six different DNA templates, one observes that a minimal pattern of 5′-d(CACC/AGCG/)-3′ is necessary to produce Ag$_{16}$-DNA. Mutations at non-interacting 5 and 10 nucleobase positions (shown in blue in Figure 6d) preserve the Ag$_N$ structure but can promote or alter crystal packing. This demonstrates that select nucleobase patterns in an oligonucleotide are more relevant than the sequential arrangement of all nucleobases, consistent with our ML-enabled findings of certain nucleobase 'motifs' involved in Ag$_N$-DNA stabilization (see Section 5) [62].

The HRMS spectrum of the reported Ag$_8$-DNA and Ag$_{16}$-DNA has not yet been reported. Determination of N_0 and N_+ for these species would enable accurate first-principles calculations of the electronic structure of Ag$_N$-DNAs for the first time. The Ag$_8$-DNA is not stable in solution, which precludes HRMS and determination of N_0, the effective number of valence electrons in this cluster. Work on HRMS for Ag$_{16}$-DNA is ongoing in our group. Future HRMS studies of Ag$_N$-DNA and their comparisons to crystallographically resolved sizes may also discern the role(s) of accessory Ag$^+$ on Ag$_N$-DNA properties. The crystal structures of the Ag$_8$-DNA and the Ag$_{16}$-DNAs contain additional Ag$^+$ that do not interact with the nanocluster core but are involved in non-WC metal-mediated base pairings and crystal packing. Gambucci et al. suggested the existence of such Ag$^+$–DNA interactions in solution-phase Ag$_N$-DNAs [87]. Provided that these "accessory" Ag$^+$ ions are tightly bound to the Ag$_N$-DNA, they can also be counted by HRMS. Currently, it remains unknown whether these accessory Ag$^+$ ions are counted by HRMS.

The puckering conformation of the sugar moiety alters the relative orientation of the phosphate backbone and nucleoside [88, 89]. This leads to variations in the overall structure, flexibility, and functions of a nucleic acid. The DNA backbone is flexible enough to accommodate both C2′-endo and C3′-endo, whereas RNA can only adopt C3′-endo conformation. Recent crystal structure of Ag_{16}-DNA reported by Cerretani et al. found that the sugar moieties in the template DNA strand can adopt both C2′-endo and C3′-endo sugar puckering, suggesting that Ag_{16} nanocluster cannot be stabilized by the corresponding RNA sequence [42]. Thus, modulating the ribofuranose ring to manipulate the overall structure and folding of a nucleic acid strand will allow to explore new exciting and novel nucleic acids-stabilized silver nanoclusters with new functionalities.

Ag_N-DNA crystal structures have dramatically advanced the current understanding on the structural features of Ag_N-DNA and key interactions involved in stabilizing the Ag_N-DNA. (1) These structures confirm that Ag_N-DNA adopts anisotropic rod-like shapes as first proposed by Schultz et al. [22], rather than the globular shapes that are common for monolayer-protected metal nanoclusters. These findings point to the unique properties of DNA as a multidentate ligand for nanocluster stabilization. (2) The abundance of G–Ag^+–G, C–Ag^+–C, and A–Ag^+–A metal-mediated base pairs in reported crystal structures reveals that the interactions of Ag^+ with different nucleobases play a key role in stabilizing Ag_N-DNAs. None of the crystal structures showed the presence of Ag^+-mediated thymine base pairs, although thymines were found to offer flexibility required for specific folding of DNA structures. This points to the roles of differential affinity of nucleobases for Ag^+ ions and arrangement of adjacent nucleobases into multi-base motifs, i.e., sequential placement of nucleobases, in governing the folding of DNA strands around the Ag_N-DNA. (3) The presence of novel non-WC-type H-bonding interactions contributes to the stability of these Ag_N-DNAs. (4) The antiparallel strand orientation of canonical WC-type B-form duplexes is interrupted due to interactions with Ag^+ ions, and noncanonical strand orientations feature prominently in Ag_N-DNAs. (6) Not all nucleotides interact with the nanocluster core, and mutations at these positions can leave the structure and properties of the Ag_N-DNA unchanged. As new Ag_N-DNA crystal structures continue to emerge, our understanding of Ag_N-DNA structure-property relations will be revolutionized, with exciting potential for development of applications of these nanoclusters.

3.2 Ag^+-DNA Interaction – A Prerequisite for Ag_N-DNA Formation

Interactions between Ag^+ and nucleobases are critical for understanding Ag_N-DNA formation and structure, and it is useful to consider what is known about DNA–Ag^+ complexes in light of the recently emerging Ag_N-DNA crystal structures. Nucleobase-specific interactions of DNA with Ag^+ are well documented [90]. Ag^+ can even unravel the highly stable G-quadruplex [47] and i-motif structures to form Ag^+-mediated dsDNA. Ag_N-DNA synthesis begins with incubation of DNA strands in the presence of silver cations prior to chemical reduction, and CD spectra of Ag$_N$-DNA bear similarity with their corresponding Ag$^+$–DNA precursors. HRMS spectra of HPLC-purified Ag$_N$-DNA show that the cluster core contains both silver cations and neutral silver atoms, and recent crystal structures show significant interactions between nucleobases and Ag$^+$ ions. Hence, we discuss how understanding the interaction of Ag$^+$ with the oligonucleotide helps to elucidate the structure-property relations of Ag$_N$-DNA.

At neutral pH, Ag$^+$ interacts preferentially with N's on the nucleobases instead of the O-rich, negatively charged phosphate backbone [91]. Ag$^+$ is known to strongly interact with cytosine (C) to form C–Ag$^+$–C base pairs, and this has been harnessed to form Ag$^+$-mediated dsDNA duplexes containing C-C mismatches [92], Ag$^+$-mediated i-motif formation [93], Ag$^+$-crosslinked DNA hydrogels [94], and other DNA-based sensors [95]. The different affinities of A, C, G, and T for Ag$^+$ are established [46] and silver can "flip" strand alignment in duplexes of C–Ag$^+$–C and G–Ag$^+$–G [47]. For a complex mixed-base sequence, Ag$^+$ can form uninterrupted metallo-DNA nanowires containing only silver-mediated base pairs [96]. This silver-mediated base pairing has potential to expand the utilization of DNA as building blocks for DNA nanotechnology.

While C is well-known for its interaction with Ag$^+$, G is found to exhibit highest affinity toward Ag$^+$, with the order of affinity G > C > A > T. Ag$^+$–mediates the formation of highly stable homoduplexes of C and G over the WC-paired C–G DNA duplexes. On the other hand, the interaction of Ag$^+$-facilitates the formation of A–Ag$^+$–T heteroduplex while replacing the WC A–T base pairs [46]. Quantum chemical calculations further support the higher stability of Ag$^+$-mediated C and G homoduplexes compared to A and T. The calculation showed that nearly planar arrangement of C–Ag$^+$–C and G–Ag$^+$–G contributes to the higher stability relative to A–Ag$^+$–A and T–Ag$^+$–T. Although the A–Ag$^+$–T pair is non-planar, the size difference between A and T and the ability of A to engage in stacking interactions promote stability. The recently solved crystal structures by Cerretani et al. [40–42], showed that thymines are not interacting with the nanocluster core and thus support the lowest affinity of T toward Ag$^+$.

DFT and QM/MM calculations of a Ag$^+$-mediated 5'-d(CC)-3' tetramer, the shortest possible Ag$^+$-mediated DNA duplex of C-homobase strands, predicted that this homoduplex adopts parallel strand orientation, which is further stabilized by novel interplanar H-bonds between cytosines of neighboring C–Ag$^+$–C pairs and π-stacking interactions [97]. Analogous results were obtained for Ag$^+$-mediated guanine homoduplexes [98]. Calculations of longer C-based homoduplexes up to 20 bases long predicted higher stabilities for parallel strand orientation and found that the antiparallel duplex is highly untwisted. The Ag$^+$–C interaction, formation of planar and novel interplanar H-bonds, and base-stacking interactions play key roles in dictating the overall strand orientation [99]. These computational findings were validated by experiments utilized Förster resonance energy transfer (FRET) experiments to elucidate strand orientation, finding parallel duplex structure for (C–Ag$^+$–C)$_{20}$ and (G–Ag$^+$–G)$_{15}$ (Figure 7a and b) [47]. Ion mobility spectrometry (IMS) coupled with DFT calculations of collisional cross

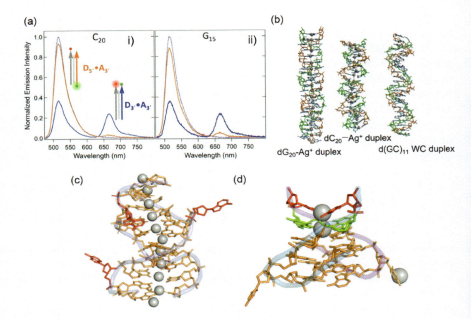

FIGURE 7 (a) Förster resonance energy transfer (FRET) clearly demonstrates that Ag$^+$-mediated pairing of homoduplexes of dC$_{20}$ (A$_{3'}$: 5′-d(T$_5$C$_{20}$T$_5$)-[Alexa 647]-3′, D$_{3'}$: 5′-d(T$_2$C$_{20}$T$_2$)-[Alexa 488]-3′, and D$_{5'}$: 5′-[Alexa 488]-d(T$_2$C$_{20}$T$_2$)-3′) and dG$_{15}$ (A$_{3'}$: 5′-d(T$_4$G$_{15}$T$_4$)-[Alexa 647]-3′, D$_{3'}$: 5′-d(T$_2$G$_{15}$T$_2$)-[Alexa 488]-3′, and D$_{5'}$: 5′-[Alexa 488] d(T$_2$G$_{15}$T$_2$)-3′) arranges strands in a parallel orientation. The dotted blue curve is D$_{3'}$ without Ag$^+$. The solid blue curve is the purified Ag$^+$-paired D$_{3'}$·A$_{3'}$. The solid orange curve is the purified Ag$^+$-paired D$_{5'}$·A$_{3'}$. (b) Structures, optimized by density functional theory (DFT), of Ag$^+$–DNA duplexes of dG$_{20}$ and dC$_{20}$ compared to WC duplexes of a mixed-base dG$_{11}$·dC$_{11}$ [47]. (Adapted from Swasey et al. [47], with permission from the American Chemical Society. Copyright 2018.) (c) Crystal structure of an Ag$^+$-paired DNA duplex with antiparallel orientation. End-to-end assembly of these duplexes forms uninterrupted nanowires [96]. Silver atoms and protruding adenines are shown in gray and red, respectively. Image created from PDB ID 5IX7 with PyMOL. (d) Structure of a dimer of 5′-d(GCACGCGC)-3′ (blue and purple backbone) paired by two Ag$^+$ (gray). The cytosines and guanines involved in metallo-base pair formation are shown in red and green, respectively. The third Ag$^+$ (bottom right of structure) supports supramolecular assembly of the structure during crystallization [100]. Image created from PDB ID 5XJZ with PyMOL.

section (CCS) was used to confirm that Ag$^+$-mediated C or G homoduplexes have higher aspect ratios than antiparallel WC-paired duplexes, bimolecular i-motifs, and bimolecular G-quadruplex structures. The presence of additional H-bonding interactions between nucleobases and the phosphate backbone in the G–Ag$^+$–G duplex leads to higher rigidity as compared to the C–Ag$^+$–C duplex.

The vast majority of Ag$_N$-DNAs are stabilized by mixed-base DNA strands, motivating the need to understand Ag$^+$–DNA interactions for heterobase DNA strand(s). Swasey et al. characterized silver-DNA interactions for ten noncomplementary 11-base DNA strands with sequences formed by single-base mutations of dC_{11} and dG_{11} homobase strands [45], complexes were formed by thermal annealing in the presence of Ag^+ ions and characterized by CD and HRMS. Introduction of single-base mutations in dC_{11} increases the distribution of attached Ag^+ ions, whereas mutations in dG_{11} increase the average number of Ag^+ by up to eight Ag^+ per homoduplex. These differences in Ag^+ recruitment by DNA strands may partly explain how the emission properties of Ag_N-DNA depend on DNA sequence (Section 4).

While $G-Ag^+-G$ and $C-Ag^+-C$ duplexes adopt parallel strand orientations, the manner in which mixed-base strands form complexes with Ag^+ appears more complex. Kondo et al. reported a crystal structure showing that a 12-base DNA strand of all four natural nucleobases forms Ag^+-mediated base pairs to assemble into remarkable uninterrupted Ag^+-DNA nanowires up to 0.1 mm long (Figure 7c). These continuous "wires" form because paired DNA strands have a one-base shift in alignment, allowing higher-order assembly of duplexes in long continuous "nanowires" within the crystal. The structure contains $C-Ag^+-C$, $G-Ag^+-G$, $C-Ag^+-G$, and even $T-Ag^+-T$ base pairings. Interestingly, adenines protrude outwards and contribute to crystal packing through formation of $AT-Ag^+-T$ triples and stacking interactions. Although the strand orientation is antiparallel, the system does not obey WC pairing, since G is bonded through N1 position (Hoogsteen pairing) in the $C-Ag^+-G$ and twist angles are larger than for WC pairing [96].

Mixed-base sequences can also lead to parallel strand alignment. X-ray crystallography showed that the oligomer 5'-d(GCACGCGC)-3' forms silver-mediated complexes that are attached by $G-Ag^+-G$ and $C-Ag^+-C$ bonds with parallel strand orientation (Figure 7d) [100]. The homobase pairs in this complex are less planar than predicted by DFT calculations [46]. Surprisingly, this 8-base sequence was later predicted using ML methods to design templates for hosting fluorescent Ag_N-DNAs [101].

Silvers can interact with multiple sites on DNA. Generally, Ag^+ ions interact with N3 of pyrimidines and N7 of the purine nucleobases [90]. However, crystal structures of Ag_{16}-DNAs also showed additional interaction sites: N1 of A and N1 and O6 of G interact with Ag^+ [40–42]. Ag^+-DNA complexes, as precursors for chemical reduction of fluorescent Ag_N-DNAs, are expected to play a key role in stabilizing the Ag_N-DNA and to drive the sequence-dependent structure/properties. Interactions between Ag^+ and DNA nucleobases can drive reorganization of secondary and tertiary structures of WC-type dsDNA under appropriate conditions and upon reduction can evolve into fluorescent cluster core [48]. As knowledge of metal-nucleic acid complexes increases, these precursors could open up exciting new ways to control the formation of nucleic acid-templated nanoclusters.

4 PHOTOPHYSICAL PROPERTIES

Well before the unique nature of Ag_N-DNA structure was understood, the bright, sequence-tuned luminescence of Ag_N-DNAs attracted intense attention from researchers. Section 3.1 demonstrated how DNA serves as a versatile multidentate ligand for silver nanoclusters with a diversity of different sizes and unique rod-shaped cluster cores. Here, we discuss how these DNA-imbued structural properties are intimately connected to the photophysical properties of Ag_N-DNAs. We mainly constrain this discussion to photophysical properties that can be understood based on currently understood DNA-silver interactions and Ag_N-DNA structure. Other photophysical properties of interest are briefly noted for the reader and described elsewhere in a detailed review [17].

4.1 ANATOMY OF THE Ag_N-DNA FLUORESCENCE SPECTRUM

A compositionally pure Ag_N-DNA solution typically possesses a fluorescence excitation spectrum with two dominant peaks and an emission spectrum with one single peak (Figure 8a). The ultraviolet (UV) excitation peak at ~260 nm corresponds to excitation of the nucleobases. An additional visible to NIR excitation peak is tuned by the cluster core's composition and structure. This size, shape, and charge-dependent excitation peak was the first piece of evidence for rod-like Ag_N-DNA structure [22], agreeing with calculations of silver nanorod clusters that show similar transitions due to longitudinal oscillations of effective valence electrons along the length of the neutral silver core [74]. For purified Ag_N-DNAs, the visible to NIR excitation peak and absorbance peak are coincident. The UV excitation band is "universal" to all fluorescent Ag_N-DNAs, and compositionally pure solutions of Ag_N-DNAs exhibit the same fluorescence emission spectrum when excited indirectly through the nucleobases or directly at the cluster's

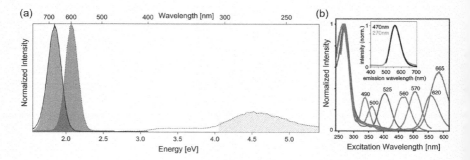

FIGURE 8 (a) Prototypical excitation (dashed black line) and emission (solid black line) spectra for an Ag_N-DNA with single excitation and emission peaks. The emission spectrum is generally fitted by a single Gaussian (shaded). The excitation spectrum is generally composed of two major peaks, one in the visible-NIR region (Gaussian fit shaded), and one in the UV [77]. (b) Ag_N-DNA excitation spectra exhibit a dominant peak in the visible to NIR spectral range and a UV excitation band corresponding to the DNA template strand. Fluorescence spectra of Ag_N-DNA excited via the DNA bases at ~260 nm (inset, gray) have the same shapes as spectra excited at the cluster's unique visible to NIR transition (inset, black) [102]. (Adapted with permission from O'Neill et al. [102], the American Chemical Society. Copyright 2011.)

compositionally dependent excitation peak (Figure 8b) [102]. For this reason, universal UV excitation allows high-throughput analysis of Ag_N-DNA fluorescence emission with a single excitation wavelength (Section 4). While most Ag_N-DNA excitation spectra are dominated by only two transitions, smaller transitions at energies between the nucleobase excitation and the lowest energy transition can vary in strength depending on the Ag_N-DNA. These transitions are, in some cases, significant, which may indicate cluster cores that deviate from linear rod shapes [77].

4.2 Time-Resolved Studies of Ag_N-DNA Excited State Dynamics

The vast majority of Ag_N-DNAs luminesce by fluorescence-like radiative decay, as supported by 1–4 ns fluorescence decay times and high quantum yields (~5%–93%) [20, 22, 23, 43, 103]. This contrasts with the longer decay times and larger Stokes shifts that are characteristic of phosphorescence (less allowed/forbidden luminescent decay), which is more commonly reported for ligand-protected metal nanoclusters [3, 50, 104]. While Ag_N-DNAs can possess quantum yields that are competitive with common organic fluorophores, Ag_N-DNA Stokes shifts are typically several times larger than their molecular counterparts [77], suggesting fundamental differences in the excited state dynamics of these two types of fluorophores. Single-molecule characterization of Ag_N-DNAs shows that these nanoclusters behave as single emitters [7, 105]. Notably, Ag_N-DNAs with longer-lived, μs-scale luminescence have recently been reported, pointing to the potential diversity of photophysical properties of these nanoclusters [106–108].

The fluorescence process of Ag_N-DNAs is not fully described by the simple Jablonski diagram of common organic fluorophores. Femtosecond spectroscopy showed that one Ag_{20}-DNA undergoes rapid 100 fs-scale relaxation from the initial Franck-Condon excited state to a lower-energy emissive state [109], in qualitative agreement with earlier work [110]. This Ag_{20}DNA also exhibits quantum beating of frequency similar to Ag–Ag bond vibration [109]. Ag_N-DNA absorption/excitation and emission spectra lack the vibronic shoulders that are characteristic of organic fluorophores (Figure 8a and b). For a chromophore center that consists of only Ag–Ag and Ag–ligand bonds, this vibronic shoulder is not expected due to the lower vibrational energies of bonds that incorporate high-Z elements as compared to only lighter elements. Ag_N-DNAs also exhibit intriguing dark-state properties, as discussed below, and do not obey the Lippert–Mataga model for solvatochromism of fluorophores, pointing to the complex DNA ligand environment of the fluorescent silver cluster core [111].

Ultrafast studies of several Ag_N-DNAs probed by nanosecond and femtosecond transient absorption measurements, single-molecule blinking experiments, and time-resolved single-photon counting (TRSPC) have aided to establish a phenomenological model for Ag_N-DNA excited state photophysics (Figure 9a) [7, 103, 108, 110, 112]. Femtosecond absorption measurements show that upon photoexcitation of Ag_N-DNA to the initial excited state (Franck-Condon state), a

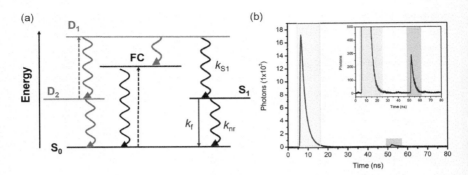

FIGURE 9 (a) General phenomenological model for Ag$_N$-DNAs. S$_0$ and S$_1$ represent ground and emissive state respectively. D$_1$ and D$_2$ are dark states. FC represents the initially excited Franck-Condon (FC) state. Wavy arrows indicate non-radiative decay. Bold, straight line indicates radiative (fluorescence) decay. Dashed lines indicate excitation. (b) Fluorescence signal as a function of time due to primary pulsed excitation at 560 nm (light gray-shaded region) and due to secondary pulsed excitation at 803 nm (gray-shaded region). Inset: Magnification of the 630 nm fluorescence resulting from the 803 nm pulsed secondary excitation after dark-state preparation by pulsed primary excitation at 560 nm. Both primary- and secondary-excited fluorescence exhibit 2.2 ns fluorescence lifetimes [116]. (Reproduced from Fleischer et al. [116], the American Chemical Society, Copyright 2017.)

fraction of the population returns to the ground state within hundreds of fs. On a similar timescale, an additional fraction decays to form a longer-lived emissive state that then fluoresces back to the ground state on a few nanosecond timescale [110]. Nanosecond-microsecond transient absorption spectroscopy [110] and single-molecule blinking experiments [7] also show the presence of a dark state with a μs decay time. No emission from this state has been observed, suggesting that this state decays nonradiatively. The dark states are believed to form from the initial Franck-Condon state [113].

The bulky DNA oligomer template may also affect excited state dynamics. Several HPLC-purified Ag$_N$-DNAs display multiexponential fluorescence decay, despite their compositional purity [19, 20, 103]. This multiexponential decay has been attributed to "slow" relaxation on the time scale of fluorescence decay [103]. Normalized time-resolved emission spectra (TRES) of Ag$_N$-DNAs show a continuous red-shift of emission spectrum on a nanosecond time scale, supporting this slow spectral relaxation process. Due to this slow spectral relaxation, the average decay time increases as emission wavelength increases. Temperature and viscosity of the medium can influence this slow spectral relaxation [23, 103]. The length of the DNA template may play a role in the timescale of spectral relaxation, as this process is typically not observed for Ag$_N$-DNAs stabilized by shorter DNA strands (9–10 bases long), which may undergo relaxation faster than the instrument response function associated with most fluorescence lifetime measurements.

4.3 Dark Excited State Behavior

Vosch et al. first reported μs-lived dark states in Ag$_N$-DNAs [7]. The dark-state quantum yield formation is estimated at a few percent to 25% and shortens with increased excitation intensity. The dark state has been assigned as a triplet state because eliminating molecular oxygen from the environment prolongs its decay time. Its origin is proposed to be due to charge transfer to the DNA template upon photoexcitation [110]. Formation of μs-lived dark states leads to the blinking of Ag$_N$-DNAs [7].

While fluorophore blinking is often a limitation for fluorescence imaging, this behavior can be advantageous when the long-lived dark state can be modulated to "call back" fluorescence at a later time. This has been shown to be possible with Ag$_N$-DNAs. Co-illumination with an intensity-modulated low energy secondary excitation depopulates the primarily excited dark state, returning the Ag$_N$-DNAs to the emissive state and thereby producing fluorescence (Figure 9) [29, 114–116]. The ability to "call back" Ag$_N$-DNA fluorescence from the dark state has been used to achieve optically activated delayed fluorescence (OADF), whereby a longer-wavelength secondary laser repumps the emissive state population from the long-lived dark states back into the initial excited state, generating delayed ns-lived fluorescence (Figure 9b). Because this delayed fluorescence is gated by secondary NIR excitation of the μs-lived dark state, Ag$_N$-DNA fluorescence can be "called back" many microseconds after the fluorescence due to primary excitation [116]. Autofluorescence of biological compounds in tissues often hinders high contrast bioimaging, and OADF is a promising approach to suppress autofluorescence and provide a background-free signal [28, 112, 113].

4.4 Evidence for Initial Collective Electronic Excitation

Because metal nanoclusters represent an intermediate class of materials between traditionally understood molecules and bulk metals, it is not surprising that certain electronic properties of nanoclusters are neither strictly molecule-like nor precisely bulk-like. One major question in metal nanocluster science is the transition from single electron, exciton-like excited state behavior to collective, plasmon-like excited state behavior [117–119]. Computational studies find that elongated or rod-like nanoclusters are ideal systems to study plasmon emergence at the nanocluster scale [119], making Ag$_N$-DNAs important experimentally realizable model systems to investigate this fundamental question.

The dependence of Ag$_N$-DNA peak absorbance wavelength on cluster size can be described by Mie-Gans theory, a simple model describing how plasmonic excitations in metal nanoparticles depend on particle aspect ratio and other factors [120, 121]. While a simple classical theory, Mie-Gans theory captures the peak excitation wavelengths computed by time-dependent density functional theory (TDDFT) for linear chains of $N_0 = 2$–20 neutral silver atoms, where the cluster aspect ratio is a function of N_0. The excitation spectra of these computationally modeled "nanowires" feature a main longitudinal oscillation peak corresponding to the HOMO-LUMO transition along the nanocluster chain, a transverse oscillation peak, and low amplitude d bands. The longitudinal peak red-shifts as aspect ratio increases. Although the transverse peak's energy remains constant, the contribution from the d band scales with higher aspect ratio, i.e., larger N_0 [74]. Purified Ag$_N$-DNAs display similar trends but for rods whose aspect ratios are smaller than linear atomic chains of equal N_0 [30]. Extinction coefficients of Ag$_N$-DNAs also scale linearly with N_0, as expected for plasmon-like excitations in nanoclusters [74, 122, 123]. Together with low-temperature spectroscopy of Ag$_N$-DNAs, which found unusually broad spectral linewidths preserved at 2 K [124], these findings support the notion that Ag$_N$-DNA fluorescence begins with a collective excitation of the effective valence electrons in the cluster core. This initial excited state would then be expected to rapidly relax, perhaps into the luminescent state that displays nanosecond-lived fluorescence. Rapid initial relaxation is supported by ultrafast spectroscopy [109], and this notion could be tested further by determination of N_0 for Ag$_N$-DNAs with reported crystal structures, which would allow full calculations of their excited state properties [119].

4.5 Alignment of Excitation and Emission Transition Dipole Moments

Ag$_N$-DNAs are also notable for their aligned excitation and emission transition dipole moments. Polarization-resolved excitation and emission measurements of single Ag$_N$-DNA emitters linearly polarized emission, which is consistent an emitter with a well-defined emission transition dipole moment [125]. Later, Hooley et al. used defocused polarized wide-field microscopy to simultaneously investigate excitation and emission polarization characteristics of dC$_{24}$-templated Ag$_N$-DNAs immobilized in polyvinyl alcohol (PVA) film, finding that excitation and emission transition dipole moments were co-aligned [126]. Time-resolved anisotropy measurements, which also probe alignment of excitation and emission transition dipoles, support similar alignment in purified solutions of three different Ag$_N$-DNAs [19, 23, 127].

4.6 Large-Scale Studies of Ag$_N$-DNA Stokes Shift

While it is ideal to study the photophysical properties of compositionally pure Ag$_N$-DNA solutions, these studies are limited to one or several Ag$_N$-DNAs due to the practical challenges of purification. Furthermore, many Ag$_N$-DNAs do not survive HPLC. High-throughput fluorimetry of 10^3 Ag$_N$-DNAs can provide complementary information about the scope of possible spectral properties of these nanoclusters without requiring harsh purification. We collected the UV-excited fluorescence emission spectra of 1,880 Ag$_N$-DNAs synthesized by robotic liquid handling (Figure 10) [77]. For those whose emission spectra were characteristic of a single emissive Ag$_N$-DNA, i.e., fitted to a single Gaussian as a function of energy, excitation spectra were then collected. We identified 305

Nucleic Acid-Templated Metal Nanoclusters

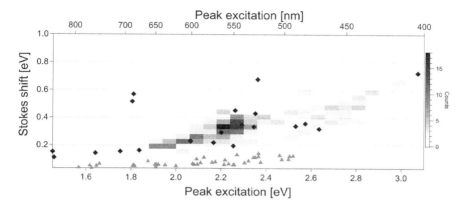

FIGURE 10 Stokes shift versus peak excitation energy for spectrally pure solutions of Ag$_N$-DNAs (gray heatmap shows the abundance of Stokes shift and peak excitation energy values), previously characterized HPLC-purified Ag$_N$-DNAs black diamonds), and commonly used organic fluorophores to label oligonucleotides (gray triangles) [77].

Ag$_N$-DNAs with both singly-peaked visible-to-NIR excitation and emission spectra, whose spectral purity is consistent with a single fluorescent species in solution. These studies showed that the distributions of both peak excitation and emission energies are multimodal, consistent with known magic numbers of Ag$_N$-DNAs. Moreover, Ag$_N$-DNA Stokes shift generally increases as excitation energy increases, but Stokes shifts for a given excitation energy vary widely. Due to the correlation of excitation energy with Stokes shift, it is challenging to separate the roles of nucleobase sequence in selecting these two parameters. Prominent nucleobase sequence features are correlated with excitation energy, and subtler sequence features appear to cause variations in Stokes shift for a given excitation energy [77].

These studies also provide insights into the structures of Ag$_N$-DNAs. First, the distribution of excitation energies and Stokes shift energies of the 305 spectrally pure Ag$_N$-DNAs shows two distinct classes of emitters, corresponding roughly to values of known $N_0=4$ and $N_0=6$ Ag$_N$-DNAs. We hypothesized that these distinct classes represent a transition from planar Ag$_N$ geometry for green-emissive $N_0=4$ nanoclusters to cylindrical Ag$_N$ geometry for red- and NIR-emissive $N_0=6$ nanoclusters. Second, we observed 88 Ag$_N$-DNAs with singly-peaked emission spectra yet multiple excitation peaks >370 nm. Due to the prevalence of these multi-peaked excitation spectra, we hypothesized that these represent Ag$_N$-DNAs possessing curvatures or other deformations from rod-like cluster core structures [77]. Computational studies of electronic excitations in silver atomic chains show that as curvature increases, the longitudinal electronic excitation diminishes in strength while the lower-wavelength transverse excitation grows in strength [82], supporting this claim. Further crystallographic studies will be needed to test these hypotheses.

4.7 Two-Photon Excitation

Dickson and coworkers first reported two-photon induced fluorescence for three unpurified Ag_N-DNAs, emitting at 660, 680, and 710 nm [128]. The emission intensity of these samples depended quadratically on excitation intensity, indicating two-photon excitation (TPE). One-photon excitation (OPE) and TPE had indistinguishable emission energies and fluorescence lifetimes, indicating that emission occurred from the same emissive state for both excitation routes. The reported two-photon cross sections ranged from 35,000 to 60,000 GM, comparable to quantum dots (60,000 GM) and surpassing values for typical organic dyes. The excitation maxima for TPE was blue shifted with respect to OPE maxima, suggesting that TPE can access higher excited states. Yau et al. also detected TPE for an "NCB" Ag_N-DNA templated by ssDNA that becomes highly fluorescent in proximity to a guanine-rich DNA enhancer sequence. This Ag_N-DNA exhibited two-photon fluorescence emission at 630 nm when excited at 800 nm, with a two-photon cross section of 3,000 GM [129].

TPE cross section is a function of the number of participating electrons, the energy of OPE and TPE transitions, and the refractive index of the medium [130]. Highly polarized free movement of electrons within a non-spherical Ag_N-DNA may account for higher two-photon absorption of these nanoclusters, with exciting potential applications. Future investigations on purified Ag_N-DNAs are required to understand the origin of high two-photon cross sections.

4.8 Environmental and Stimulus Effects on Emission Properties

The photophysical properties of certain Ag_N-DNAs are sensitive to changes in their solvent environment or other solutes. These effects have been exploited for biosensing applications that rely on changes in emission intensity or color to signal interaction with the analyte [9, 25, 26]. Currently, the underlying fundamental mechanisms of these changes remain poorly understood. Here, we review some fundamental studies that may shed light on these effects.

Swasey et al. reported that a purified Ag_{10}-DNA stabilized by a 19-base oligomer exhibits a solvent-driven equilibrium between a dark and fluorescent form upon titration with methanol or sucrose [82]. The fluorescent form has 490 nm peak absorbance and 560 nm peak emission, and the dark form has 400 nm peak absorbance. A well-defined isodichroic point at 390 nm in both CD and absorbance spectra supports that dark and fluorescent forms are distinct clusters with the same overall silver content. Similar transformations in Ag_N-DNA structure may be at play in some light-up Ag_N-DNA sensing schemes.

Ag_N-DNAs show a complex range of spectral sensitivities to solvent environment. Studies of four purified Ag_N-DNAs showed diverse changes in Stokes shift behavior as a function of changing ethanol and methanol concentration, with most behavior inconsistent with a simple Onsager-based model where the fluorophore interacts with the solvent exclusively through dipolar interactions with solvent molecules that can freely reorient. Instead, changes in DNA conformation or solvent dielectric in the local vicinity of the Ag_N may play a larger role in governing the excited state properties of Ag_N-DNAs [111]. Studies of purified Ag_N-DNAs in aqueous solvents of various refractive indices as tuned by glycerol, which changes refractive index without perturbing DNA structure, also show a range of sensitivities depending on the specific Ag_N-DNA species [30]. These studies point to the complexity and diversity of possible fluorophore behaviors based on the local nucleic acid environment.

A recent study of a red-emissive Ag_N-DNA provides insights into the sensitivity of Ag_N-DNA optical properties to various biomolecules. At neutral pH, this Ag_N-DNA demonstrated diminished, blue-shifted fluorescence and absorbance intensity for negatively charged biomolecules (ssDNA and bovine serum albumin (BSA)), and fluorescence decay time and rotational correlation coefficient were unaffected [131]. In the presence of positively charged lysine, by contrast, Ag_N-DNA absorption and emission intensity remained unchanged while rotational correlation coefficients increased, implying electrostatic interactions between the positively charged lysine and negatively charged Ag_N-DNA. BSA and ssDNA are known to interact with silver cations and may extract silver ions from the Ag_N-DNA [46, 132]. This observation further supports the importance of purification before Ag_N-DNA photophysical characterization to rule out effects from other unintended or uncontrolled solutes.

Exchanging D_2O with H_2O generally increases luminescence quantum yield and excited state decay time for known ns-lived fluorophores [133] and μs–ms lived lanthanoides [134]. However, trends in changes in photophysical properties vary for different Ag_N-DNAs. Vosch and coworkers studied the effects on the photophysical properties of two Ag_N-DNAs, the Ag_{16}-DNA whose crystal structure has been reported [42] and an Ag_N-DNA with 721 nm peak emission [135]. While the latter displayed the usual trend of increased fluorescence quantum yield and excited state decay times upon D_2O exchange, Ag_{16}-DNA showed a shortened ns-decay time and lowered fluorescence quantum yield. For Ag_{16}-DNA, D_2O exchange enhanced the formation of a red-shifted μs-lived state with increased quantum yield and decay time. These differences may again point to the variation in possible responsive behaviors of Ag_N-DNAs due to subtle differences in their local ligand environments.

4.9 DNA Ligand Effects on Emission Properties

A single-base mutation can be sufficient to tune the photophysical properties of Ag_N-DNAs. 18-base 5′-d(CCCCACCCCTCCCXTTTT)-3′ with X=guanosine and inosine (an analog of guanosine lacking C2-NH_2) form an identical green-emitting Ag_{10}^{6+} nanocluster. However, the guanosine-containing Ag_N-DNA is dimmer, and exhibits diminished fluorescence quantum yield and shorter fluorescence lifetime compared to inosine [136]. Guanosine is correlated with a seven-fold higher non-radiative lifetime yet a similar radiative lifetime than inosine. The higher non-radiative lifetime for guanosine is possibly due to stronger coordination of guanine with the Ag_N, causing tighter orbital overlap and boosting charge transfer and non-radiative relaxation. The absence of C2-NH$_2$ in inosine may imply weaker interaction with the cluster core.

Certain Ag$_N$-DNAs can also exhibit light-up behavior when brought into proximity with guanine-rich DNA oligomers by base pairing [13]. This phenomenon forms the basis of NCB sensors for detection of single polymorphisms in DNA oligomers and nucleobase methylation [64, 137–139]. It is important to note that these light-up effects may be caused by transformations of the nanocluster structure itself and cannot simply be assigned as an electronic-only interaction between an unchanged Ag$_N$ structure and proximal guanines. The affinity of guanines for silver supports that structural changes may occur upon binding of a guanine-rich DNA strand to an Ag$_N$-DNA [46].

5 MACHINE LEARNING-GUIDED STUDIES OF Ag$_N$-DNAs

DNA ligands imbue Ag$_N$-DNAs with sequence-dependent photophysical properties that originate from the nucleobase-specific interactions of DNA with Ag⁺. This programmability is unique among metal nanoclusters and reflects the advantages of employing DNA as multidentate ligands for nanocluster stabilization. One can imagine that by decoding how nucleobase sequence tunes Ag$_N$-DNA structure and properties, it will become possible to achieve designer nanoclusters whose structure-property relations are dictated to atomic precision by their nucleic acid ligands. To harness Ag$_N$-DNAs as programmable functional nanomaterials, we must determine how the immense DNA oligomer sequence space encodes Ag$_N$-DNA properties. Computational models for Ag$_N$-DNAs are still in development [83] and cannot yet simulate Ag$_N$-DNA structures for arbitrary DNA ligands. Due to the combinatorial nature of DNA sequence, ML provides a promising alternative to learn how DNA ligand sequence controls Ag$_N$-DNA properties by experimentally observing many instances of Ag$_N$-DNA ligand sequences in well-controlled experiments and training ML algorithms to extract sequence-to-color trends (Figure 11a). Certain ML models can also be interpreted using feature selection [140], an approach that has provided new chemical insights into how DNA sequence selects Ag$_N$-DNA properties [60]. Here, we present the supervised ML approaches we have pioneered to learn "sequence-structure-property relations" of Ag$_N$-DNAs and guide their discovery.

We first briefly introduce the concept of supervised ML in the specific context of modeling the DNA sequence-to-Ag$_N$-DNA color connection. (Others have written excellent broader reviews on ML for chemical sciences [141, 142], to which the reader is directed for further information.) Supervised ML concerns the problem of learning to map input data onto associated output data by learning from a set of labeled training data, i.e., a set of inputs that are correlated to known outputs. For Ag$_N$-DNAs, we seek to map DNA ligand sequences onto Ag$_N$-DNA properties using known DNA sequences and their associated Ag$_N$-DNAs (Figure 11a). In addition to labeled training data, one must also choose how to represent input data to the ML algorithm. These representations are n-dimensional feature vectors, and the choice of features is referred to as feature engineering, featurization,

Nucleic Acid-Templated Metal Nanoclusters 323

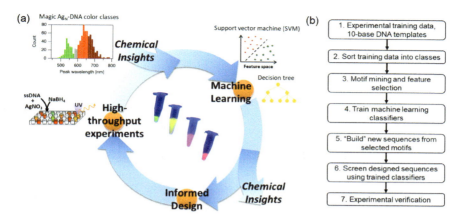

FIGURE 11 Schematic of ML-enabled approach to understand Ag_N-DNA sequence-to-color relations and design DNA ligand sequences for Ag_N-DNAs with targeted properties. High-throughput experiments link 10^3 DNA oligomer sequences to the fluorescence emission spectra of Ag_N-DNAs they stabilize. Then, the ML problem is defined in a chemically motivated manner, by grouping Ag_N-DNAs with similar magic numbers into color classes to ensure that ML classifiers learn to distinguish DNA sequences that select for the same structural class of Ag_N-DNAs. The use of simple ML models also allows feature analysis to shed light on the sequence motifs that select for Ag_N-DNA color. ML models also guide design of new DNA ligand sequences for Ag_N-DNA with targeted fluorescence properties. (b) Workflow for ML-guided design of Ag_N-DNAs. (Adapted from Copp et al. [61].)

or descriptor engineering. ML works best when features are correlated with the trend one seeks to learn. For Ag_N-DNAs, ML will be most accurate if we represent DNA sequence in a manner that allows the ML algorithm to distinguish Ag_N-DNA optical properties. Because these correlations are often unknown for chemical systems, feature selection is a challenging yet critical step in successful ML for chemical sciences.

To understand the "sequence-structure-property relations" of Ag_N-DNAs, it is necessary to obtain high-quality experimental training data that connects Ag_N-DNA ligand sequence to fluorescence properties for a large number of DNA sequences. While the literature harbors a plethora of DNA template sequences that select Ag_N-DNAs with various emission colors, fluorescence quantum yields, and photo- and chemical stabilities, experimental conditions vary across studies, making it challenging to isolate the role of DNA sequence from other factors. Also, most studies only report successful Ag_N-DNA design and omit DNA sequences that are not correlated to brightly fluorescent Ag_N-DNAs. These "dark" DNA sequences make up about 75% of 10-base DNA oligomers [59] and must be included in training data to discriminate for brightly fluorescent Ag_N-DNAs. Data libraries for ML can be obtained by high-throughput experiments discussed in Section 2.1. We have used this approach to correlate ~3,000 DNA template sequences to the fluorescence brightness and emission colors of the Ag_N-DNAs they stabilize. We focused ML studies specifically on training data acquired 1 week after Ag$_N$-DNA synthesis, to capture only time-stable products. We also primarily investigated 10-base DNA oligomers because a reasonable fraction of these (~0.1%) can be synthesized by robotic liquid handling.

The first ML models for Ag$_N$-DNA ligand design were trained to assign fluorescence intensity (output) from input DNA sequence [62]. The general workflow for all Ag$_N$-DNA models is shown in Figure 11b. A training data set of 684 random 10-base DNA sequences and the integrated fluorescence intensities ("brightnesses") of their associated Ag$_N$-DNAs was separated into two classes: "Bright" sequences that stabilized Ag$_N$-DNAs with the top 30% of integrated intensities and "Dark" sequences associated with the bottom 30% of integrated intensities (i.e., no detectable fluorescence); the middle 40% was omitted from training data to avoid choosing a single arbitrary threshold for bright. Bright-associated sequences were rich in C and G, while Dark-associated sequences were rich in T (Figure 12c). A simple ML classifier, the support vector machine (SVM), was trained to sort sequences into Bright and Dark classes. We found that proper feature engineering was critical to the accuracy of this classifier. Feature vectors that directly encode DNA sequence in simple numerical form resulted in

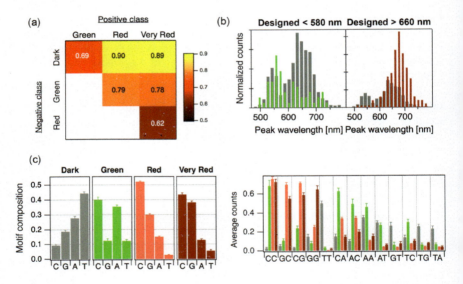

FIGURE 12 (a) Accuracy heat map, representing the ten-fold cross-validation scores of all one-versus-one SVM classifiers for pairs of color classes. (b) Normalized histograms of Ag$_N$-DNA peak emission wavelength of training data (gray) as compared to ML-guided designs for Green Ag$_N$-DNAs (green) and Very Red Ag$_N$-DNAs (dark red). (c) Average composition of motifs identified by feature selection to be correlated to select color classes: dark or nonfluorescent (gray), Green < 580 nm (green), 600 nm < Red < 660 nm (red), and Very Red > 660 nm (dark red). Average number of neighboring pairs of nucleobases per motif is sorted left-to-right by color selectivity, i.e., standard deviation of the four bars per nucleobase pair. (Adapted with permission from Copp et al. [60].)

poor classification accuracy (a measure of the fraction of DNA sequences that a ML classifier properly sorts into classes). Classification accuracy significantly improved for feature vectors representing the presence or absence of select DNA subsequences, or "motifs", identified by motif mining [143] to occur more frequently in one class than the other. These motifs were 3–5 nucleobases in length, with all four canonical nucleobases represented. The trained model, together with identified motifs, were used to design new DNA templates for brightly fluorescent Ag_N-DNAs with 78% success, a three-fold increase over random selection. However, this model had no predictivity for Ag_N-DNA color and selected red-fluorescent Ag_N-DNAs with greater prevalence than green-fluorescent Ag_N-DNAs (Figure 12c).

To learn the sequence-color correlation of Ag_N-DNAs, we defined a multi-class ML problem motivated by the known magic numbers of Ag_N-DNA [60]. Ag_N-DNAs with $N_0=4$ neutral silver atoms have green fluorescence, and Ag_N-DNAs with $N_0=6$ neutral silver atoms have red fluorescence [59]. A ML classifier that learns to distinguish green- and red-emissive Ag_N-DNAs is therefore learning to distinguish DNA sequences that sculpt fundamentally different Ag_N-DNAs. Sequences from an expanded training data set of 10^3 DNA sequences were sorted into color classes defined by peak fluorescence wavelength: Green<580nm, 600nm<Red<660nm, and Very Red>660nm. Dark Sequences were preserved as a fourth class. DNA sequences were represented to the classifier as sets of color-correlated motifs that were identified by motif mining followed by feature selection. (This step is critical for achieving predictive ML classification – without feature selection, ML models can suffer from problematic overfitting.) Then, an ensemble of six one-*versus*-one SVMs was trained to discriminate each pair of the four color classes (Figure 12a). This ML model increased experimental selection of Ag_N-DNA color by up to 330%, a substantial advance over simple combinatorial screening (Figure 12b) [60]. Importantly, these ML models also retain predictivity for DNA template sequences up to 16 bases in length, pointing to a degree of universality in nucleobase patterns that select for Ag_N-DNAs of specific sizes [61].

Our ML model for Ag_N-DNA color prediction also provided new insights into how nucleobase sequence selects Ag_N-DNA size and color. Because feature selection identifies the nucleobase motifs that contribute most to discrimination of Ag_N-DNA color classes, these motifs can be analyzed to gain chemical insights. Figure 12c shows the prevalence of each nucleobase and pairs of neighboring nucleobases in feature-selected motifs. While the full role of DNA sequence for Ag_N-DNA color selection is complex (motivating the use of ML models rather than a simple set of rules for DNA ligand design), several trends become clear. Cytosines and CC are correlated with bright fluorescence in general, while the presence of adenines and guanines appears to discriminate between Green, Red, and Very Red Ag_N-DNAs. Adenines appear to select more for smaller, greener Ag_N-DNAs while GG selects strongly for Very Red; this is in agreement with studies by Swasey and Gwinn on the recruitment of Ag^+ to DNA duplexes as a function of nucleobase sequence [45]. Additionally, thymines are strongly correlated with Dark DNA sequences that do not stabilize fluorescent Ag_N-DNAs, in agreement with the known lack of Ag^+–thymine interaction at neutral pH [46]. Current efforts are ongoing to advance these ML models using emerging information about Ag_N-DNA structure and to expand the color window of ML prediction to encompass newly discovered NIR-emissive Ag_N-DNAs [18].

6 APPLICATIONS AND FUTURE OPPORTUNITIES

The unique properties of Ag_N-DNAs, as imbued by their nucleic acid ligands, have enabled researchers to develop a number of applications reviewed in detail by others [14, 15, 144–148]. Because these applications (Figure 13) have been developed in parallel with the growing fundamental understanding of Ag_N-DNAs, the underlying mechanisms of many remain to be well-understood. Here, we briefly describe promising Ag_N-DNA applications as well as outstanding fundamental

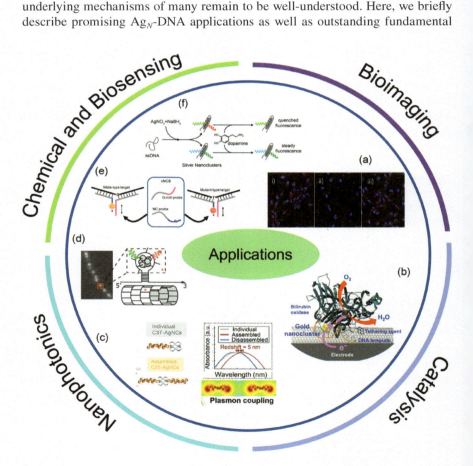

FIGURE 13 Summary of various applications of DNA-stabilized metal nanoclusters in bioimaging (a) [201], catalysis (b) [50] nanophotonics (c, d) [180, 202], and chemical and biomolecular sensing (e, f) [64, 168]. (Figures are reproduced with permission from the American Chemical Society.)

challenges and future opportunities for nucleic acid-templated nanoclusters. This discussion is not meant to be comprehensive but rather to inspire researchers in the field of nucleic acid-metal interactions, whose expertise may contribute to advancing the development of functional applications of DNA-stabilized metal nanoclusters.

6.1 Sensing

The most prevalent application of Ag_N-DNAs is in the area of biomolecular and chemical sensing. As chromophores that are directly scaffolded by nucleic acids, Ag_N-DNAs can respond sensitively to perturbation of the DNA template. This property, discussed in the fundamental context in Section 4, was recognized very early on and exploited for a number of uses.

Ag_N-DNAs can act as both the recognition and the signal output unit, with interactions between analyte and Ag_N-DNA leading to enhanced or restored fluorescence emission or quenching. Petty and coauthors have studied the sensitivity of various Ag_N-DNAs to target DNA strands in detail, finding a variety of optical changes depending on the specific emitter and DNA architecture [21, 149]. In particular, they have shown that nonfluorescent Ag_N-DNAs with violet 400 nm absorption can transform into NIR-emissive or green-emissive Ag_N-DNAs, with NIR products expected to contain twice the number of silver atoms as the violet product [21, 70, 150] and green products expected to contain the same number of silver atoms as the violet product [79, 151, 152]. HRMS shows that these violet and nonfluorescent Ag_N-DNAs are Ag_{10}^{6+} with compact structures [78, 153]. The emissive green Ag_N-DNA is also a Ag_{10}^{6+} but with more extended cluster structure [154]. Swasey et al. also showed a transformation between a green-emissive and a non-emissive Ag_N-DNA tuned by solvent composition, suggesting the prevalence of this phenomenon [82]. These findings present the exciting possibility of using predictable structural transformations of Ag_N-DNAs to sense local changes in DNA conformation.

A well-studied Ag_N-DNA sensing system is the NCB, which employs a "dark", i.e., very weakly green-fluorescent, Ag_N-DNA that "lights up" upon binding to a second DNA strand [13]. The dark Ag_N-DNA, formed by typical chemical reduction, is presumed to be confined to a cytosine-rich region of a long DNA strand, whose longer half is a "tail" of A's and T's. The activator strand also has two regions: an A-T region complementary to the dark Ag_N-DNA's tail and a second "light-up" region that is typically rich in guanines. Because the light-up sequence affects the intensity and color of resulting Ag_N-DNA fluorescence, NCBs can provide a colorimetric readout of the activator strand. By incorporating the NCB into a three-way junction scheme [155], Yeh et al. demonstrated detection of single nucleotide polymorphisms (SNPs) due to colorimetric changes in NCB spectra based on a specific alignment of the dark and light-up components [64]. This method has also been used to detect methylation state of adenine [156], enhance Rolling Circle Enhanced Enzyme Activity Detection (REEAD) [157], and detect telomerase activity [158]. The design of NCBs is challenging due to the large DNA sequence space and lack of target specificity. Strand displacement schemes [159] and high-throughput screening methods [160] may improve the performance of these sensors.

Ag_N-DNAs have also been used by others for SNP detection [161] and other DNA sensing schemes [162–165], as well as to detect miRNAs [9, 25, 166], metal ions including Hg^{2+}, Cu^{2+}, and Pb^{2+}, and small molecules [145, 167, 168]. Additionally, some Ag_N-DNAs display sensitivity to solution refractive index [30], which may have utility for near-field sensing of biomolecular environments with high spatial precision. While the vast majority of the mechanisms that enable these sensing schemes are not understood, the established correlation between Ag_N-DNA structure and optical properties (Section 3) supports that optically signaled analyte detection likely results from local perturbations to DNA structure that produce geometric changes and/or size changes in the Ag_N-DNA. As fundamental understanding of Ag_N-DNAs continues to grow, it may become possible to engineer highly precise Ag_N-DNA sensors that are customized to a specific analyte.

6.2 Bioimaging

Ag_N-DNAs are tunable fluorophores that can possess high quantum yields, high extinction coefficients, innate compatibility with DNA, and (in some cases) high photostabilities and/or low toxicities as compared to conventional fluorophores. These traits are desirable for biolabels for fluorescence microscopy. Early work by the Dickson group pioneered these applications [148]. Shortly after the initial report of Ag_N-DNA synthesis [6], avidin-dC_{24} conjugates were used to template Ag_N-DNA synthesis, followed by cell surface labeling through biotin-avidin binding [169]. They later demonstrated transfection of HeLa cells by Ag_N-DNAs, reporting low toxicity of the nanoclusters [170], and demonstrated cell staining for two cell types, with both live and fixed cells, and intracellular staining was accomplished by conjugation to a cell-penetrating peptide [171]. Others have labeled prions with Ag_N-DNAs, for intracellular labeling. Transfer of low emissive poly(acrylic acid)-templated silver nanoclusters to anti-actin antibody-conjugated dC_{12} resulted in ten-fold brighter cellular imaging compared to the organic dye, Cy3 [172]. The localization of dark Ag_N-DNA in the cell nucleus led to the *in situ* activation of luminescence [173]. This site-specific enhancement in luminescence in nuclei may be due to the presence of G-rich telomeres.

It is notable that the properties of certain Ag_N-DNAs that make them suitable sensors are often undesirable features for fluorescence microscopy. Cellular environments are highly complex and likely to expose Ag_N-DNAs to a huge range of biomolecules, small molecules, and varying ionic strength conditions. Uncontrolled transformation of Ag_N-DNAs under these conditions could preclude identification and/or tracking during fluorescence microscopy. Significant work is needed to develop Ag_N-DNAs or their conjugates that are either ultrastable or have highly controlled and predictable transformations for bioimaging applications.

Despite the challenges of engineering bright and stable Ag_N-DNAs, the unique photophysics of Ag_N-DNAs are highly promising for novel imaging modalities.

In particular, the dark-state properties of certain Ag_N-DNAs enable OADF [29, 108, 116] (Section 4), a promising phenomenon for low-background fluorescence imaging. In combination with emerging NIR-emissive Ag_N-DNAs, these advances may enable new imaging technologies that are of critical importance for biological sciences.

6.3 New NIR-Emitting Ag_N-DNAs

Ag_N-DNAs with NIR luminescence are highly promising for imaging in the so-called NIR tissue transparency windows (750–1,700 nm), where relatively few bright fluorophores exist [36]. Biological tissues are much more transparent at these wavelengths, but conventional NIR organic fluorophores suffer from low probe intensity, poor photostability, and oxygen sensitivity. Quantum dots resolve many of these challenges but are often toxic, larger in size, and suffer from power-law blinking, hindering their application in *in-vivo* and *in-vitro* imaging dynamic studies [34, 35]. Ag_N-DNAs have potential to overcome many of these challenges.

NIR Ag_N-DNAs have been reported since Vosch et al. [7], in 2007, but reports of NIR-emissive Ag_N-DNAs have remained rarer than their visibly fluorescent counterparts [10, 115, 150]. Recently, Swasey et al. developed a custom NIR well plate reader equipped with an InGaAs detector [174] for high-throughput searches for NIR Ag_N-DNA emission. This method uncovered hundreds of previously unidentified NIR-emitting Ag_N-DNAs [18]. Two of these newly discovered Ag_N-DNAs included one with the longest emission wavelength reported to date, 999 nm, and the largest Ag_N-DNA to date, containing 30 Ag atoms (with 12 Ag^0 and 18 Ag^+), which is bright enough to be detected at the single-molecule level [175]. Vosch and coworkers have also reported several NIR-emissive Ag_N-DNAs with highly favorable quantum yields [22, 23]. As more NIR-emissive Ag_N-DNAs are uncovered, their suitability as fluorophores in the NIR tissue transparency windows can be further explored. Furthermore, coupling high-throughput NIR screening with the ML approaches that we have developed (Section 5) can expedite NIR Ag_N-DNA discovery.

6.4 DNA-Directed Nanocluster Architectures

The exquisite programmability of DNA has been used to self-assemble a wide variety of nanostructures, forming the basis of structural DNA nanotechnology [176–178]. Merging this field with DNA-based metal nanoclusters is promising for realizing unprecedented spatial and orientational arrangement of nanocluster arrays. Metal nanocluster assembly, a major goal in the field of atomically precise materials, is of fundamental interest for studying the properties of nanocluster arrays and for realizing ultraprecise control over their emergent properties. At present, these studies are largely confined to computational methods [147, 179]. Such arrays also have exciting potential for applications such as photonics, sensing, and catalysis.

Ag$_N$-DNAs have been synthesized directly onto DNA nanostructures. O'Neill et al. first reported synthesis of fluorescent Ag$_N$-DNAs on a DNA nanostructure [180]. These fluorescent Ag$_N$-DNAs were formed on ssDNA hairpin loops protruding from the nanotube. DNA nanotubes without hairpin loops were unable to host fluorescent nanoclusters, consistent with earlier reports that ssDNA (without WC-type H-bonding) is a more suitable Ag$_N$-DNA template [8]. The authors noted an important issue that must be addressed to merge structural DNA nanotechnology and Ag$_N$-DNAs: DNA nanostructure folding often requires buffers such as Tris or phosphate-buffered saline (PBS) to stabilize the WC duplex, and these buffers can be incompatible with high chemical yield of Ag$_N$-DNAs. For this reason, the DNA nanotubes were folded in a solution of ammonium acetate and magnesium acetate. The resulting labeling efficiency was estimated to be 45%, an extremely high chemical yield for an Ag$_N$-DNA, although it should be noted that a second green-emissive Ag$_N$-DNA developed on the nanotubes over days to weeks [180]. Orbach et al. also demonstrated synthesis of Ag$_N$-DNAs on self-assembled micrometer long DNA nanowires whose formation was triggered by hybridization chain reaction [181]. Ag$_N$-DNAs have also been incorporated into DNA hydrogels [182]. Interestingly, the color of the Ag$_N$-DNA in the hydrogel varied with salt concentration, again pointing to the importance of considering ionic conditions when synthesizing Ag$_N$-DNAs.

Ag$_N$-DNA synthesis generally suffers from low chemical yield and often produces a heterogeneous mixture of products. This inhibits high labeling efficiency by direct synthesis of Ag$_N$-DNAs. Purification of Ag$_N$-DNAs prior to labeling of DNA nanostructures can partly overcome this challenge. Schultz et al. used this approach to form dual-cluster pairs of red and green Ag$_N$-DNAs joined by a WC duplex DNA clamp (Figure 14a) [183]. These Ag$_N$-DNAs were suitable donor and acceptor Förster resonance energy transfer (FRET) pairs, and binding of donor and acceptor produced characteristic FRET behavior [183]. Zhao et al. later developed an approach to measure the diameter of an inverse micelle "nanocage" using *in situ* synthesis of Ag$_N$-DNA FRET pairs from a single-emitting species [184].

It is nontrivial to design bifunctional DNA strands that stabilize the Ag$_N$-DNA in one region and leave a second "tail" free for WC pairing. We presented a strategy to design such modular DNA templates, forming atomically precise arrays of Ag$_N$-DNAs on DNA nanotubes (Figure 14b) [31]. These DNA templates are designed by choosing (1) a DNA sequence known to host a fluorescent HPLC-purifiable Ag$_N$-DNA of known atomic size and (2) a "dark" DNA sequence that does not stabilize any silver nanocluster and can therefore serve as an appended linker sequence to tether the Ag$_N$-DNA to the DNA nanotube *via* WC-type base pairing. We chose dark candidate linkers from our large experimental data libraries. Modular templates are experimentally screened to ensure that Ag$_N$-DNA structural and photophysical characteristics were unaltered. Because the structure and emission wavelengths of Ag$_N$-DNA are highly correlated [59], unaltered spectral characteristics strongly support that the HPLC-purified Ag$_N$-DNAs remain unchanged with the linker attached, as well as unaffected upon binding to programmed sites on DNA nanotubes [31]. Further studies are needed to

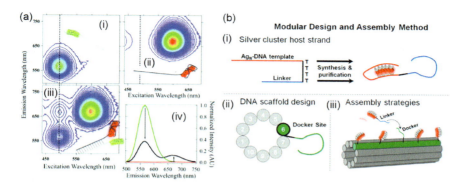

FIGURE 14 (a) Development of dual-cluster pair containing Ag$_{10}$ and Ag$_{15}$ nanoclusters: Contour map of emission intensity from the purified solution of paired clusters shows the expected peaks for direct excitation of Ag$_{10}$ (i) and Ag$_{15}$ (ii), and FRET: emission from Ag$_{15}$ due to excitation of Ag$_{10}$ (iii, iv), via radiationless energy transfer [183]. (b) Schemes to design atomically precise array of Ag$_N$-DNAs on DNA nanorods: (i) The silver cluster host strand contains DNA template that hosts silver nanocluster (red) and is appended to a non-interacting linker sequence (blue), (ii) The docker (green), complementary to the linker (blue), is appended to one of the strands that form the DNA nanotube (gray) and extrudes from the DNA nanotube (end-view schematic), (iii) DNA nanotube decoration is mediated by Watson-Crick base pairing between linkers (blue) and extruding dockers (green) [31]. (Figures reproduced with permission from the American Chemical Society.)

quantitatively assess labeling efficiency of these and other methods for decoration of DNA nanostructures by Ag$_N$-DNAs.

6.5 Catalysis

Metal nanoclusters offer unique advantages as catalysts due to their high surface-to-volume ratios, unsaturated active sites, unique electronic structures, and distinctive structure-induced functionalities [185]. Nanoclusters are also model systems to study the correlation between catalytic efficiency and structure at the atomic level [186]. Zhou et al. synthesized DNA-templated bimetallic nanoclusters to enhance the catalytic activity of Ag$_N$-DNAs toward 4-nitrophenol reduction. The catalytic activity of Ag$_N$-DNAs encapsulated by different template DNA strands was found to be comparable [187].

Guo et al. studied the catalytic activity of Ag$_N$-DNAs templated by C-rich DNA strands of different lengths for reduction of 4-nitrophenol. Adsorption of DNA oligomers onto Ag$_N$-DNAs was found to inhibit their catalytic efficiency, with the extent of inhibition depending on the type of nucleobases, length, and overall conformation of the adsorbed DNA oligomer. Different inhibition effects suggested differential adsorption affinity of homopolymers toward Ag$_N$-DNAs as follows: poly-dA > poly-dG > poly-dC > poly-dT. The catalytic activity of Ag$_N$-DNAs recovered in the presence of triplex dT$_{30}$·dA$_{30}$·dT$_{30}$, whereas single-stranded dA$_{30}$ and ds dA$_{30}$·dT$_{30}$ inhibited catalytic activity. This recovery in catalytic activity in the presence of triplex dT$_{30}$·dA$_{30}$·dT$_{30}$ suggests that N7 of adenines interact with the active site of the Ag$_N$-DNA. Formation of triplex dT$_{30}$·dA$_{30}$·dT$_{30}$ involves hydrogen bonding between N7 of adenine and N3 of thymine and thus masks the N7 site of adenine from interacting with the active site of the catalyst. This study showed that the catalytic activity of Ag$_N$-DNAs can be tuned based on the coordination interactions between Ag$_N$-DNAs and DNA strands and the stimuli-responsive transition between different conformations of DNA [188].

Chakraborty et al. showed that a particular DNA-stabilized gold nanocluster (Au$_N$-DNA) was electrochemically active and enhanced the enzymatic activity of bilirubin oxidase (BOD)-catalyzed oxygen reduction reaction (ORR) through lowering the overpotential and improving the electron transfer between the electrode and active site of the enzyme [50]. Following this, they presented the synthesis of a gold nanocluster stabilized by the DNA analog, phosphorodiamidate morpholino oligomer (PMO) [189]. Unlike the Au$_N$-DNA, this PMO-stabilized nanocluster is not an efficient enzymatic reaction enhancer. Further studies of Au$_N$-DNAs and Ag$_N$-DNAs are needed to understand their structure-property relations and their potential applications for electron transfer.

6.6 Future Opportunities and Outlook

Significant advancements in experimental and computational methods have been made in recent years to understand the sequence-structure-property relations of Ag$_N$-DNAs. Here, we discuss future opportunities and challenges in the field of DNA-stabilized metal nanoclusters.

6.7 Structural Details

Undeniably, recent X-ray crystallography breakthroughs have provided critical new details on the geometry of Ag$_N$-DNAs and key interactions that drive their formation and stabilization. However, because few crystal structures have been reported, it is unknown how representative these structures are of Ag$_N$-DNAs in general. To continue to advance understanding of Ag$_N$-DNA solution-phase structure, it will be critical to grow high-quality crystals that preserve the spectral line shapes of HPLC-purified Ag$_N$-DNAs, as was done in the case of Ag$_{16}$DNAs [40–42]. This approach helps to ensure that the crystallized structure preserves the key features of the atomically precise Ag$_N$-DNA in the solution phase. Understanding the solution-phase structures is key to developing these novel nanomaterials. Additionally, it is important to determine the solution-phase roles played by additional silver ions that only participate in crystal packing and are not involved in the nanocluster core. The relevance of these "accessory silvers" in solution remains unknown.

6.8 Ag$_N$-DNA Photophysics

Combined experimental and computational studies are essential for detailed understanding of the photophysical processes that occur in these nanoclusters.

For example, major questions remain about the nature of the fluorescence excited state(s), the relaxation processes resulting in diverse Stokes shift behavior, the existence of dark-state behavior and microsecond-lived luminescence, and the role of nanocluster core and DNA nucleobases in modulating the excited state properties. One major unanswered question is the nature of the universal UV excitation process, which remains poorly understood, and the related interactions between nucleobase and nanocluster. Recent TRIR spectroscopy studies show that vibrational modes of the nucleobases, which are typically excited in the UV, can be excited by visible excitation of the nanocluster and decay on the same timescale as the visible luminescence [81]. Additionally, the potential of Ag_N-DNAs as experimental manifestations of rod-like nanoclusters for understanding collective electronic excitations is highly promising. Furthermore, changes in optical properties in the presence of biomolecules and analytes are essential to customizing DNA sequences to host novel Ag_N-DNAs for biosensing and bioimaging applications. Vosch et al. have recently studied the influence of differently charged biomolecules such as protein and nucleic acids on the photophysical properties of Ag_N-DNA as mentioned in Section 3.1 [131].

6.9 Improved Chemical and Photostability

Many Ag_N-DNAs undergo degradation in biologically relevant buffers. For example, the presence of ions such as chloride in PBS can quench emission intensity. This lack of stability limits the application of Ag_N-DNAs for bioimaging and biosensing. Additionally, integration of Ag_N-DNAs into DNA architectures such as DNA origami [190] can require high ionic strengths that hamper the stability of Ag_N-DNAs [191]. For real-world biological studies, these limitations must be overcome. One strategy that has recently been pursued is silica encapsulation, which stabilizes Ag_N-DNAs in PBS [192]. This and similar encapsulation strategies may allow researchers to retain the special properties of Ag_N-DNAs but with higher chemical stabilities.

6.10 Purity

The separation of compositionally pure Ag_N-DNAs prior to characterization has been essential to progress in understanding structure-property relations. Future studies should not overlook the importance of purification to avoid polydispersity or interactions with other DNA strands that may affect Ag_N-DNA properties. A single template DNA may host multiple fluorescent nanoclusters, and even chromatographic separation may fail to isolate single compositionally pure Ag_N-DNA species from the mixture containing Ag_N-DNAs with comparable compositions and/or conformations. For example, Schultz et al. found that despite HPLC isolation, a well-studied emissive Ag_N-DNA was a mixture of Ag_{15} and Ag_{16} products [193], pointing to the importance and challenge of precisely characterizing solutions by HRMS and other methods.

6.11 Artificial Nucleic Acids

The conformation of the DNA molecule around the Ag_N-DNA plays a critical role in sculpting the nanocluster. Chemically modified nucleic acids may expand the space of possible DNA-stabilized metal nanoclusters. A plethora of chemically modified nucleic acids known as Xeno nucleic acids (XNAs) have been developed to improve stability against nuclease degradation, bioavailability, cellular uptake, and pharmacokinetics and to reduce immunogenicity and toxicity [194]. These modifications include changes to the phosphate backbone, sugar, and/or nucleobases to introduce desirable functionalities. Feng et al. incorporated aptamers sequence linked to a L-DNA that templates silver nanoclusters, promoting specific target recognition and cell imaging [195].

Artificial nucleobases are known to facilitate formation of site-specific silver-mediated base pairs [196, 197]. Léon et al. reported the synthesis of fluorescent Ag_N-DNAs from DNA templates containing artificial nucleobases [48]. Introduction of fluorescent nucleobases may shift the UV excitation to the blue region of visible spectrum, modulating the emission attributes of Ag_N-DNAs. Further studies are required to understand how XNAs can expand the sequence-dependent optical properties of silver nanoclusters beyond natural DNA/RNA.

6.12 Beyond Silver

Compared to other nucleic acid-stabilized nanoclusters, Ag_N-DNAs have received special attention due to their unique sequence-encoded photophysical properties. However, nucleobases possess a strong affinity toward multiple transition metal ions beyond silver, such as gold, copper, mercury, and platinum [90, 91, 198, 199]. Synthesis of DNA-templated metal nanoclusters containing these metal ions may dramatically expand the properties of nanoclusters.

6.13 Cellular Uptake and Cytotoxicity

Ag_N-DNAs appear to be biocompatible alternatives to commonly used organic dyes and quantum dots. Ag^+ is much less toxic than heavy metal colloidal quantum dots, and some studies suggest that certain Ag_N-DNAs lack cytotoxicity [200]. However, to date, no detailed toxicological studies of Ag_N-DNAs have been performed. These studies are urgently needed to address the cellular uptake, modes of clearance, and toxicity for advancement in biomedical applications.

7 CONCLUDING REMARKS

Nucleic acids are remarkably versatile molecular scaffolds for stabilizing metal nanoclusters, allowing the formation of a rich space of nanoclusters with sequence-encoded structure-property relationships. This chapter has presented a review of what is known about the compositions, structures, and properties of these nanoclusters, with a focus on the well-studied DNA-stabilized silver nanocluster (Ag_N-DNA). DNA imbues silver nanoclusters with unique rod-like structures and complex photophysical properties that arise from the intimate connection between nucleobase and nanocluster. Because of the importance of metal ion-nucleic acid interactions for stabilizing silver nanoclusters, we have placed these nanoclusters in the context of relevant silver ion-nucleic acid interactions, which are key to the structure-property relations of Ag_N-DNAs. Finally, we have highlighted key promising potential applications of Ag_N-DNAs and other nucleic acid-templated nanoclusters.

Much of the work on nucleic acid-templated metal nanoclusters has been empirically driven. However, the enormous sequence space of nucleic acids and the complexity of metal-nucleic acid interactions clearly demonstrate the limitations of such an approach. We hope that this chapter inspires researchers in the field of nucleic acid chemistry to develop new atomically precise nucleic acid-templated nanoclusters by rational design of their polydentate nucleic acid ligands. Together with this fundamental understanding of metal-ligand interactions, emerging high-throughput experimental studies together with data-driven ML models may expedite the discovery of these sequence-encoded nanoclusters, with significant potential to contribute to new innovations in sensing and diagnostics, bioimaging, photonics, and catalysis.

ACKNOWLEDGMENTS

The authors acknowledge support from the National Science Foundation NSF-CBET-2025790 and Air Force Office of Scientific Research FA9550-21-1–0163.

ABBREVIATIONS AND DEFINITIONS

Ag_N-DNA	DNA-stabilized silver nanocluster
Au_N-DNA	DNA-stabilized gold nanocluster
BOD	bilirubin oxidase
BSA	bovine serum albumin
CD	circular dichroism
DFT	density functional theory
ds	double-stranded
ESI	electrospray ionization
EXAFS	extended X-ray absorption fine structure
FRET	Förster resonance energy transfer
GM	Goeppert-Mayer units (1 GM = 10^{-50} cm^4 s molecules^{-1} photons^{-1})
HPLC	high-performance liquid chromatography
HRMS	high-resolution mass spectrometry
ICP-AES	inductively coupled plasma-atomic emission spectroscopy
MD	molecular dynamics
ML	machine learning
NC	nanoclusters
NCB	nanocluster beacon
NGS	next-generation sequencing
NIR	near-infrared

OADF	optically activated delayed fluorescence
OPE	one photon excitation
ORR	oxygen reduction reaction
PBS	phosphate-buffered saline
PMO	phosphorodiamidate morpholino oligomer
PVA	poly(vinyl alcohol)
QM/MM	quantum mechanics/molecular mechanics
ss	single-stranded
SVM	support vector machine
TCSPC	time-correlated single photon counting
TDDFT	time-dependent density functional theory
TEM	transmission electron microscopy
TPE	two-photon excitation
TRES	time-resolved emission spectrum
TRIR	time-resolved infrared
WC	Watson-Crick
XANES	X-ray absorption near edge structure
XNA	xeno nucleic acids
XPS	X-ray photoelectron spectroscopy

REFERENCES

1. W. A. de Heer, *Rev. Mod. Phys.* **1993**, *65*, 611–676.
2. H. Häkkinen, *Chem. Soc. Rev.* **2008**, *37*, 1847–1859.
3. R. Jin, C. Zeng, M. Zhou, Y. Chen, *Chem. Rev.* **2016**, *116*, 10346–10413.
4. I. Díez, R. H. A. Ras, in *Advanced Fluorescence Reporters in Chemistry and Biology II: Molecular Constructions, Polymers and Nanoparticles*, Ed A. P. Demchenko, Springer, Berlin Heidelberg, **2010**, pp. 307–332.
5. I. Díez, R. H. A. Ras, *Nanoscale* **2011**, *3*, 1963–1970.
6. J. T. Petty, J. Zheng, N. V. Hud, R. M. Dickson, *J. Am. Chem. Soc.* **2004**, *126*, 5207–5212.
7. T. Vosch, Y. Antoku, J.-C. Hsiang, C. I. Richards, J. I. Gonzalez, R. M. Dickson, *Proc. Natl. Acad. Sci. U.S.A.* **2007**, *104*, 12616–12621.
8. E. G. Gwinn, P. O'Neill, A. J. Guerrero, D. Bouwmeester, D. K. Fygenson, *Adv. Mater.* **2008**, *20*, 279–283.
9. S. W. Yang, T. Vosch, *Anal. Chem.* **2011**, *83*, 6935–6939.
10. J. T. Petty, B. Sengupta, S. P. Story, N. N. Degtyareva, *Anal. Chem.* **2011**, *83*, 5957–5964.
11. W. Guo, J. Yuan, E. Wang, *Chem. Commun.* **2011**, *47*, 10930–10932.
12. M. Yang, X. Chen, Y. Su, H. Liu, H. Zhang, X. Li, W. Xu, *Front. Chem.* **2020**, *8*, 1–8.
13. H.-C. Yeh, J. Sharma, J. J. Han, J. S. Martinez, J. H. Werner, *Nano Lett.* **2010**, *10*, 3106–3110.
14. J. M. Obliosca, C. Liu, R. A. Batson, M. C. Babin, J. H. Werner, H.-C. Yeh, *Biosensors* **2013**, *3*, 185–200.
15. J. M. Obliosca, C. Liu, H.-C. Yeh, *Nanoscale* **2013**, *5*, 8443–8461.
16. J. Liu, *Trends Analyt. Chem.* **2014**, *58*, 99–111.
17. A. Gonzàlez-Rosell, C. Cerretani, P. Mastracco, T. Vosch, S. M. Copp, *Nanoscale Adv.* **2021**, *3*, 1230–1260.

18. S. M. Swasey, S. M. Copp, H. C. Nicholson, A. Gorovits, P. Bogdanov, E. G. Gwinn, *Nanoscale* **2018**, *10*, 19701–19705.
19. S. A. Bogh, M. R. Carro-Temboury, C. Cerretani, S. M. Swasey, S. M. Copp, E. G. Gwinn, T. Vosch, *Methods Appl. Fluoresc.* **2018**, *6*, 024004.
20. C. Cerretani, T. Vosch, *ACS Omega* **2019**, *4*, 7895–7902.
21. J. T. Petty, B. Giri, I. C. Miller, D. A. Nicholson, O. O. Sergev, T. M. Banks, S. P. Story, *Anal. Chem.* **2013**, *85*, 2183–2190.
22. D. Schultz, K. Gardner, S. S. R. Oemrawsingh, N. Markešević, K. Olsson, M. Debord, D. Bouwmeester, E. Gwinn, *Adv. Mater.* **2013**, *25*, 2797–2803.
23. V. A. Neacşu, C. Cerretani, M. B. Liisberg, S. M. Swasey, E. G. Gwinn, S. M. Copp, T. Vosch, *Chem. Commun.* **2020**, *56*, 6384–6387.
24. T. Li, L. Zhang, J. Ai, S. Dong, E. Wang, *ACS Nano* **2011**, *5*, 6334–6338.
25. P. Shah, A. Rørvig-Lund, S. B. Chaabane, P. W. Thulstrup, H. G. Kjaergaard, E. Fron, J. Hofkens, S. W. Yang, T. Vosch, *ACS Nano* **2012**, *6*, 8803–8814.
26. P. Shah, S. W. Choi, H.-j. Kim, S. K. Cho, Y.-J. Bhang, M. Y. Ryu, P. W. Thulstrup, M. J. Bjerrum, S. W. Yang, *Nucleic Acids Res.* **2015**, *44*, e57–e57.
27. J. Wang, C. Du, P. Yu, Q. Zhang, H. Li, C. Sun, *Biosens. Bioelectron.* **2021**, *348*, 130707.
28. S. Krause, M. R. Carro-Temboury, C. Cerretani, T. Vosch, *Chem. Commun.* **2018**, *54*, 4569–4572.
29. C. I. Richards, J.-C. Hsiang, D. Senapati, S. Patel, J. Yu, T. Vosch, R. M. Dickson, *J. Am. Chem. Soc.* **2009**, *131*, 4619–4621.
30. S. M. Copp, D. Schultz, S. M. Swasey, A. Faris, E. G. Gwinn, *Nano Lett.* **2016**, *16*, 3594–3599.
31. S. M. Copp, D. E. Schultz, S. Swasey, E. G. Gwinn, *ACS Nano* **2015**, *9*, 2303–2310.
32. N. de Souza, *Nat. Methods* **2007**, *4*, 540–540.
33. C. Eggeling, J. Widengren, R. Rigler, C. A. M. Seidel, *Anal. Chem.* **1998**, *70*, 2651–2659.
34. M. Nirmal, B. O. Dabbousi, M. G. Bawendi, J. J. Macklin, J. K. Trautman, T. D. Harris, L. E. Brus, *Nature* **1996**, *383*, 802–804.
35. B. A. Kairdolf, A. M. Smith, T. H. Stokes, M. D. Wang, A. N. Young, S. Nie, *Annu. Rev. Anal. Chem.* **2013**, *6*, 143–162.
36. G. Hong, A. L. Antaris, H. Dai, *Nat. Biomed. Eng.* **2017**, *1*, 0010.
37. C. Zhu, Z. Chen, S. Gao, B. L. Goh, I. B. Samsudin, K. W. Lwe, Y. Wu, C. Wu, X. Su, *Prog. Nat. Sci.: Mater. Int.* **2019**, *29*, 628–640.
38. E. Oh, R. Liu, A. Nel, K. B. Gemill, M. Bilal, Y. Cohen, I. L. Medintz, *Nat. Nanotechnol.* **2016**, *11*, 479–486.
39. D. J. E. Huard, A. Demissie, D. Kim, D. Lewis, R. M. Dickson, J. T. Petty, R. L. Lieberman, *J. Am. Chem. Soc.* **2019**, *141*, 11465–11470.
40. C. Cerretani, J. Kondo, T. Vosch, *RSC Adv.* **2020**, *10*, 23854–23860.
41. C. Cerretani, J. Kondo, T. Vosch, *CrystEngComm* **2020**, *22*, 8136–8141.
42. C. Cerretani, H. Kanazawa, T. Vosch, J. Kondo, *Angew. Chem. Int. Ed.* **2019**, *58*, 17153–17157.
43. C. I. Richards, S. Choi, J.-C. Hsiang, Y. Antoku, T. Vosch, A. Bongiorno, Y.-L. Tzeng, R. M. Dickson, *J. Am. Chem. Soc.* **2008**, *130*, 5038–5039.
44. B. Sengupta, C. M. Ritchie, J. G. Buckman, K. R. Johnsen, P. M. Goodwin, J. T. Petty, *J. Phys. Chem. C* **2008**, *112*, 18776–18782.
45. S. M. Swasey, E. G. Gwinn, *New J. Phys.* **2016**, *18*, 045008.
46. S. M. Swasey, L. E. Leal, O. Lopez-Acevedo, J. Pavlovich, E. G. Gwinn, *Sci. Rep.* **2015**, *5*, 10163.
47. S. M. Swasey, F. Rosu, S. M. Copp, V. Gabelica, E. G. Gwinn, *J. Phys. Chem. Lett.* **2018**, *9*, 6605–6610.

48. J. C. Léon, D. González-Abradelo, C. A. Strassert, J. Müller, *Chem. Eur. J.* **2018**, *24*, 8320–8324.
49. D. Schultz, E. Gwinn, *Chem. Commun.* **2011**, *47*, 4715–4717.
50. S. Chakraborty, S. Babanova, R. C. Rocha, A. Desireddy, K. Artyushkova, A. E. Boncella, P. Atanassov, J. S. Martinez, *J. Am. Chem. Soc.* **2015**, *137*, 11678–11687.
51. Z. Luo, X. Yuan, Y. Yu, Q. Zhang, D. T. Leong, J. Y. Lee, J. Xie, *J. Am. Chem. Soc.* **2012**, *134*, 16662–16670.
52. V. W.-W. Yam, E. C.-C. Cheng, Z.-Y. Zhou, *Angew. Chem. Int. Ed.* **2000**, *39*, 1683–1685.
53. N. Tiwari, R. K. Mishra, S. Gupta, R. Srivastava, S. Aggarwal, P. Bandyopadhyay, M. Munde, *Langmuir* **2021**, *37*, 9385–9395.
54. A. Rotaru, S. Dutta, E. Jentzsch, K. Gothelf, A. Mokhir, *Angew. Chem. Int. Ed.* **2010**, *49*, 5665–5667.
55. Y. Lai, X. Teng, Y. Zhang, H. Wang, P. Pang, C. Yang, C. J. Barrow, W. Yang, *Anal. Methods* **2019**, *11*, 3584–3589.
56. X. Shao, L. Zhu, Y. Zhang, Z. Du, C. Sun, W. Xu, *Sens. Actuators B Chem.* **2020**, *325*, 128769.
57. T. Ye, Y. Peng, M. Yuan, H. Cao, J. Yu, Y. Li, F. Xu, *Microchim. Acta* **2019**, *186*, 760.
58. J. Pang, Y. Lu, X. Gao, L. He, J. Sun, F. Yang, Z. Hao, Y. Liu, *Microchim. Acta* **2019**, *186*, 364.
59. S. M. Copp, D. Schultz, S. Swasey, J. Pavlovich, M. Debord, A. Chiu, K. Olsson, E. Gwinn, *J. Phys. Chem. Lett.* **2014**, *5*, 959–963.
60. S. M. Copp, A. Gorovits, S. M. Swasey, S. Gudibandi, P. Bogdanov, E. G. Gwinn, *ACS Nano* **2018**, *12*, 8240–8247.
61. S. M. Copp, S. M. Swasey, A. Gorovits, P. Bogdanov, E. G. Gwinn, *Chem. Mater.* **2020**, *32*, 430–437.
62. S. M. Copp, P. Bogdanov, M. Debord, A. Singh, E. Gwinn, *Adv. Mater.* **2016**, *28*, 3043.
63. Y.-A. Kuo, O. S. Zhao, S. Hong, T. D. Nguyen, Y.-I. Chen, H.-C. Li, T. Yeh, *Biophys. J.* **2021**, *120*, 272a.
64. H.-C. Yeh, J. Sharma, I.-M. Shih, D. M. Vu, J. S. Martinez, J. H. Werner, *J. Am. Chem. Soc.* **2012**, *134*, 11550–11558.
65. D. Schultz, E. G. Gwinn, *Chem. Commun.* **2012**, *48*, 5748–5750.
66. E. Largy, A. König, A. Ghosh, D. Ghosh, S. Benabou, F. Rosu, V. Gabelica, *Chem. Rev.* **2021**, *122*, 7720–7839.
67. K. Koszinowski, K. Ballweg, *Chem. Eur. J.* **2010**, *16*, 3285–3290.
68. E. Gwinn, D. Schultz, S. M. Copp, S. Swasey, *Nanomaterials* **2015**, *5*, 180–207.
69. V. Gabelica, *Acc. Chem. Res.* **2021**, *54*, 3691–3699.
70. J. T. Petty, S. P. Story, S. Juarez, S. S. Votto, A. G. Herbst, N. N. Degtyareva, B. Sengupta, *Anal. Chem.* **2012**, *84*, 356–364.
71. H. Hirai, S. Ito, S. Takano, K. Koyasu, T. Tsukuda, *Chem. Sci.* **2020**, *11*, 12233–12248.
72. M. Walter, J. Akola, O. Lopez-Acevedo, P. D. Jadzinsky, G. Calero, C. J. Ackerson, R. L. Whetten, H. Grönbeck, H. Häkkinen, *Proc. Natl. Acad. Sci. U.S.A.* **2008**, *105*, 9157–9162.
73. M. Harb, F. Rabilloud, D. Simon, A. Rydlo, S. Lecoultre, F. Conus, V. Rodrigues, C. Félix, *J. Chem. Phys.* **2008**, *129*, 194108.
74. E. B. Guidez, C. M. Aikens, *Nanoscale* **2012**, *4*, 4190–4198.
75. J. Duan, K. Park, R. I. MacCuspie, R. A. Vaia, R. Pachter, *J. Phys. Chem. C* **2009**, *113*, 15524–15532.
76. R. R. Ramazanov, A. I. Kononov, *J. Phys. Chem. C* **2013**, *117*, 18681–18687.

77. S. M. Copp, A. Gonzàlez-Rosell, *Nanoscale* **2021**, *13*, 4602–4613.
78. J. T. Petty, O. O. Sergev, M. Ganguly, I. J. Rankine, D. M. Chevrier, P. Zhang, *J. Am. Chem. Soc.* **2016**, *138*, 3469–3477.
79. J. T. Petty, O. O. Sergev, A. G. Kantor, I. J. Rankine, M. Ganguly, F. D. David, S. K. Wheeler, J. F. Wheeler, *Anal. Chem.* **2015**, *87*, 5302–5309.
80. I. L. Volkov, A. Smirnova, A. A. Makarova, Z. V. Reveguk, R. R. Ramazanov, D. Y. Usachov, V. K. Adamchuk, A. I. Kononov, *J. Phys. Chem. B* **2017**, *121*, 2400–2406.
81. Y. Zhang, C. He, J. T. Petty, B. Kohler, *J. Phys. Chem. Lett.* **2020**, *11*, 8958–8963.
82. S. M. Swasey, N. Karimova, C. M. Aikens, D. E. Schultz, A. J. Simon, E. G. Gwinn, *ACS Nano* **2014**, *8*, 6883–6892.
83. X. Chen, M. Boero, O. Lopez-Acevedo, *Phys. Rev. Mater.* **2020**, *4*, 065601.
84. H. Schmidbaur, A. Schier, *Angew. Chem. Int. Ed.* **2015**, *54*, 746–784.
85. A. Bondi, *J. Phys. Chem. B* **1964**, *68*, 441–451.
86. C. Eaborn, Vol. 282 of *Structural Inorganic Chemistry*, Ed A. F. Wells, 5th ed., Oxford University Press, Oxford, **1985**.
87. M. Gambucci, C. Cerretani, L. Latterini, T. Vosch, *Methods Appl. Fluoresc.* **2019**, *8*, 014005.
88. S. Neidle, M. Sanderson, *Principles of Nucleic Acid Structure*, Elsevier Science & Technology, San Diego, **2021**.
89. W. Saenger, in *Principles of Nucleic Acid Structure* Ed W. Saenger, Springer, New York, **1984**, pp. 51–104.
90. J. Müller, *Coord. Chem. Rev.* **2019**, *393*, 37–47.
91. R. M. Izatt, J. J. Christensen, J. H. Rytting, *Chem. Rev.* **1971**, *71*, 439–481.
92. P. Scharf, J. Müller, *ChemPlusChem* **2013**, *78*, 20–34.
93. H. A. Day, C. Huguin, Z. A. E. Waller, *Chem. Commun.* **2013**, *49*, 7696–7698.
94. W. Guo, X.-J. Qi, R. Orbach, C.-H. Lu, L. Freage, I. Mironi-Harpaz, D. Seliktar, H.-H. Yang, I. Willner, *Chem. Commun.* **2014**, *50*, 4065–4068.
95. H. Torigoe, A. Ono, T. Kozasa, *Nucleosides, Nucleotides & Nucleic Acids* **2007**, *26*, 1635–1639.
96. J. Kondo, Y. Tada, T. Dairaku, Y. Hattori, H. Saneyoshi, A. Ono, Y. Tanaka, *Nat. Chem.* **2017**, *9*, 956–960.
97. L. A. Espinosa Leal, A. Karpenko, S. Swasey, E. G. Gwinn, V. Rojas-Cervellera, C. Rovira, O. Lopez-Acevedo, *J. Phys. Chem. Lett.* **2015**, *6*, 4061–4066.
98. X. Chen, E. Makkonen, D. Golze, O. Lopez-Acevedo, *J. Phys. Chem. Lett.* **2018**, *9*, 4789–4794.
99. X. Chen, A. Karpenko, O. Lopez-Acevedo, *ACS Omega* **2017**, *2*, 7343–7348.
100. H. Liu, F. Shen, P. Haruehanroengra, Q. Yao, Y. Cheng, Y. Chen, C. Yang, J. Zhang, B. Wu, Q. Luo, R. Cui, J. Li, J. Ma, J. Sheng, J. Gan, *Angew. Chem. Int. Ed.* **2017**, *56*, 9430–9434.
101. J. Zheng, P. R. Nicovich, R. M. Dickson, *Annu. Rev. Phys. Chem.* **2007**, *58*, 409–431.
102. P. R. O'Neill, E. G. Gwinn, D. K. Fygenson, *J. Phys. Chem. C* **2011**, *115*, 24061–24066.
103. C. Cerretani, M. R. Carro-Temboury, S. Krause, S. A. Bogh, T. Vosch, *Chem. Commun.* **2017**, *53*, 12556–12559.
104. J. Zheng, J.-N. Wang, T. Wang, K. Wu, R.-J. Wei, W. Lu, D. Li, *J. Phys. Chem. C* **2021**, *125*, 9400–9410.
105. E. N. Hooley, V. Paolucci, Z. Liao, M. R. Carro Temboury, T. Vosch, *Adv. Opt. Mater.* **2015**, *3*, 1109–1115.
106. J. T. Petty, S. Carnahan, D. Kim, D. Lewis, *J. Chem. Phys.* **2021**, *154*, 244302.
107. V. Rück, C. Cerretani, V. A. Neacşu, M. B. Liisberg, T. Vosch, *Phys. Chem. Chem. Phys.* **2021**, *23*, 13483–13489.
108. M. B. Liisberg, S. Krause, C. Cerretani, T. Vosch, *Chem. Sci.* **2022**, *13*, 5582–5587.

109. E. Thyrhaug, S. A. Bogh, M. R. Carro-Temboury, C. S. Madsen, T. Vosch, D. Zigmantas, *Nat. Commun.* **2017**, *8*, 15577.
110. S. A. Patel, M. Cozzuol, J. M. Hales, C. I. Richards, M. Sartin, J.-C. Hsiang, T. Vosch, J. W. Perry, R. M. Dickson, *J. Phys. Chem. C* **2009**, *113*, 20264–20270.
111. S. M. Copp, A. Faris, S. M. Swasey, E. G. Gwinn, *J. Phys. Chem. Lett.* **2016**, *7*, 698–703.
112. S. Krause, C. Cerretani, T. Vosch, *Chem. Sci.* **2019**, *10*, 5326–5331.
113. S. Krause, M. R. Carro-Temboury, C. Cerretani, T. Vosch, *Phys. Chem. Chem. Phys.* **2018**, *20*, 16316–16319.
114. J. T. Petty, C. Fan, S. P. Story, B. Sengupta, A. S. Iyer, Z. Prudowsky, R. M. Dickson, *J. Phys. Chem. Lett.* **2010**, *1*, 2524–2529.
115. J. T. Petty, C. Fan, S. P. Story, B. Sengupta, M. Sartin, J. C. Hsiang, J. W. Perry, R. M. Dickson, *J. Phys. Chem. B* **2011**, *115*, 7996–8003.
116. B. C. Fleischer, J. T. Petty, J. C. Hsiang, R. M. Dickson, *J. Phys. Chem. Lett.* **2017**, *8*, 3536–3543.
117. S. Malola, L. Lehtovaara, J. Enkovaara, H. Häkkinen, *ACS Nano* **2013**, *7*, 10263–10270.
118. A. D. Dillon, R. L. M. Gieseking, *J. Chem. Phys.* **2022**, *156*, 074301.
119. E. B. Guidez, C. M. Aikens, *Nanoscale* **2014**, *6*, 11512–11527.
120. G. Mie, *Ann. Phys.* **1908**, *330*, 377–445.
121. R. Gans, *Ann. Phys.* **1912**, *342*, 881–900.
122. F. Ding, E. B. Guidez, C. M. Aikens, X. Li, *J. Chem. Phys.* **2014**, *140*, 244705.
123. J. Yan, S. Gao, *Phys. Rev. B* **2008**, *78*, 235413.
124. S. S. R. Oemrawsingh, N. Markešević, E. G. Gwinn, E. R. Eliel, D. Bouwmeester, *J. Phys. Chem. C* **2012**, *116*, 25568–25575.
125. N. Markešević, S. S. R. Oemrawsingh, D. Schultz, E. G. Gwinn, D. Bouwmeester, *Adv. Opt. Mater.* **2014**, *2*, 765–770.
126. E. N. Hooley, M. R. Carro-Temboury, T. Vosch, *J. Phys. Chem. A* **2017**, *121*, 963–968.
127. M. Gambucci, C. Cerretani, L. Latterini, T. Vosch, *Methods Appl. Fluoresc.* **2019**, *8*, 014005.
128. S. A. Patel, C. I. Richards, J.-C. Hsiang, R. M. Dickson, *J. Am. Chem. Soc.* **2008**, *130*, 11602–11603.
129. S. H. Yau, N. Abeyasinghe, M. Orr, L. Upton, O. Varnavski, J. H. Werner, H.-C. Yeh, J. Sharma, A. P. Shreve, J. S. Martinez, T. Goodson III, *Nanoscale* **2012**, *4*, 4247–4254.
130. M. G. Kuzyk, *J. Chem. Phys.* **2003**, *119*, 8327–8334.
131. M. Gambucci, G. Zampini, G. Quaglia, T. Vosch, L. Latterini, *ChemPhotoChem* **2021**, *5*, 369–375.
132. A. S. Patel, T. Mohanty, *J. Mater. Sci.* **2014**, *49*, 2136–2143.
133. L. Stryer, *J. Am. Chem. Soc.* **1966**, *88*, 5708–5712.
134. J. L. Kropp, M. W. Windsor, *J. Chem. Phys.* **1963**, *39*, 2769–2770.
135. C. Cerretani, G. Palm-Henriksen, M. B. Liisberg, T. Vosch, *Chem. Sci.* **2021**, *12*, 16100–16105.
136. Y. Zhang, C. He, K. de La Harpe, P. M. Goodwin, J. T. Petty, B. Kohler, *J. Chem. Phys.* **2021**, *155*, 094305.
137. J. M. Obliosca, M. C. Babin, C. Liu, Y. L. Liu, Y. A. Chen, R. A. Batson, M. Ganguly, J. T. Petty, H. C. Yeh, *ACS Nano* **2014**, *8*, 10150–10160.
138. Y.-A. Chen, J. M. Obliosca, Y.-L. Liu, C. Liu, M. L. Gwozdz, H.-C. Yeh, *J. Am. Chem. Soc.* **2015**, *137*, 10476–10479.
139. X. Yan, J. Sun, X. E. Zhao, R. Wang, X. Wang, Y. N. Zuo, W. Liu, R. Kong, S. Zhu, *Microchim. Acta* **2018**, *185*, 403.

140. A. Costine, P. Delsa, T. Li, P. Reinke, P. V. Balachandran, *Int. J. Appl. Phys.* **2020**, *128*, 235303.
141. K. T. Butler, D. W. Davies, H. Cartwright, O. Isayev, A. Walsh, *Nature* **2018**, *559*, 547–555.
142. A. L. Ferguson, *J. Phys. Condens. Matter* **2017**, *30*, 043002.
143. C. Vens, M.-N. Rosso, E. G. J. Danchin, *Bioinformatics* **2011**, *27*, 1231–1238.
144. S. Zhan, J. Jiang, Z. Zeng, Y. Wang, H. Cui, *Coord. Chem. Rev.* **2022**, *455*, 214381.
145. C. Song, J. Xu, Y. Chen, L. Zhang, Y. Lu, Z. Qing, *Molecules* **2019**, *24*, 4189.
146. Y. Chen, M. L. Phipps, J. H. Werner, S. Chakraborty, J. S. Martinez, *Acc. Chem. Res.* **2018**, *51*, 2756–2763.
147. F. Alkan, C. M. Aikens, *Phys. Chem. Chem. Phys.* **2019**, *21*, 23065–23075.
148. S. Choi, R. M. Dickson, J. Yu, *Chem. Soc. Rev.* **2012**, *41*, 1867–1891.
149. J. T. Petty, B. Sengupta, S. P. Story, N. N. Degtyareva, *Anal. Chem.* **2011**, *83*, 5957–5964.
150. J. T. Petty, D. A. Nicholson, O. O. Sergev, S. K. Graham, *Anal. Chem.* **2014**, *86*, 9220–9228.
151. M. Ganguly, C. Bradsher, P. Goodwin, J. T. Petty, *J. Phys. Chem. C* **2015**, *119*, 27829–27837.
152. J. T. Petty, O. O. Sergev, D. A. Nicholson, P. M. Goodwin, B. Giri, D. R. McMullan, *Anal. Chem.* **2013**, *85*, 9868–9876.
153. J. T. Petty, M. Ganguly, I. J. Rankine, E. J. Baucum, M. J. Gillan, L. E. Eddy, J. C. Léon, J. Müller, *J. Phys. Chem. C* **2018**, *122*, 4670–4680.
154. J. T. Petty, M. Ganguly, I. J. Rankine, D. M. Chevrier, P. Zhang, *J. Phys. Chem. C* **2017**, *121*, 14936–14945.
155. H.-C. Yeh, C. M. Puleo, Y.-P. Ho, V. J. Bailey, T. C. Lim, K. Liu, T.-H. Wang, *Biophys. J.* **2008**, *95*, 729–737.
156. E. M. Harcourt, T. Ehrenschwender, P. J. Batista, H. Y. Chang, E. T. Kool, *J. Am. Chem. Soc.* **2013**, *135*, 19079–19082.
157. S. Juul, J. M. Obliosca, C. Liu, Y.-L. Liu, Y.-A. Chen, D. M. Imphean, B. R. Knudsen, Y.-P. Ho, K. W. Leong, H.-C. Yeh, *Nanoscale* **2015**, *7*, 8332–8337.
158. M. Peng, N. Na, J. Ouyang, *Chem. Eur. J.* **2019**, *25*, 3598–3605.
159. Y.-A. Chen, H. T. Vu, Y.-L. Liu, Y.-I. Chen, T. D. Nguyen, Y.-A. Kuo, S. Hong, Y.-A. Chen, S. Carnahan, J. T. Petty, H.-C. Yeh, *Chem. Commun.* **2019**, *55*, 462–465.
160. Y.-A. Kuo, C. Jung, Y.-A. Chen, J. R. Rybarski, T. D. Nguyen, Y.-A. Chen, H.-C. Kuo, O. S. Zhao, V. A. Madrid, Y.-I. Chen, Vol. 10893 of *Reporters, Markers, Dyes, Nanoparticles, and Molecular Probes for Biomedical Applications XI*, SPIE, **2019**, pp. 31–42.
161. W. Guo, J. Yuan, Q. Dong, E. Wang, *J. Am. Chem. Soc.* **2010**, *132*, 932–934.
162. J. T. Del Bonis-O'Donnell, D. Vong, S. Pennathur, D. K. Fygenson, *Nanoscale* **2016**, *8*, 14489–14496.
163. J. T. Del Bonis-O'Donnell, D. K. Fygenson, S. Pennathur, *Analyst* **2015**, *140*, 1609–1615.
164. Y. Zhang, C. Zhu, L. Zhang, C. Tan, J. Yang, B. Chen, L. Wang, H. Zhang, *Small* **2015**, *11*, 1385–1389.
165. K. Zhang, K. Wang, X. Zhu, M. Xie, F. Xu, *RSC Adv.* **2016**, *6*, 99269–99273.
166. Y.-Q. Liu, M. Zhang, B.-C. Yin, B.-C. Ye, *Anal. Chem.* **2012**, *84*, 5165–5169.
167. R. Wang, X. Yan, J. Sun, X. Wang, X.-E. Zhao, W. Liu, S. Zhu, *Anal. Methods* **2018**, *10*, 4183–4188.
168. J. T. Del Bonis-O'Donnell, A. Thakrar, J. W. Hirschberg, D. Vong, B. N. Queenan, D. K. Fygenson, S. Pennathur, *ACS Chem. Neurosci.* **2018**, *9*, 849–857.
169. J. Yu, S. Choi, C. I. Richards, Y. Antoku, R. M. Dickson, *Photochem. Photobiol.* **2008**, *84*, 1435–1439.

170. Y. Antoku, J.-i. Hotta, H. Mizuno, R. M. Dickson, J. Hofkens, T. Vosch, *Photochem. Photobiol. Sci.* **2010**, *9*, 716–721.
171. S. Choi, J. Yu, S. A. Patel, Y.-L. Tzeng, R. M. Dickson, *Photochem. Photobiol. Sci.* **2011**, *10*, 109–115.
172. J. Yu, S. Choi, R. M. Dickson, *Angew. Chem. Int. Ed.* **2009**, *48*, 318–320.
173. D. Li, Z. Qiao, Y. Yu, J. Tang, X. He, H. Shi, X. Ye, Y. Lei, K. Wang, *Chem. Commun.* **2018**, *54*, 1089–1092.
174. S. M. Swasey, H. C. Nicholson, S. M. Copp, P. Bogdanov, A. Gorovits, E. G. Gwinn, *Rev. Sci. Instrum.* **2018**, *89*, 095111.
175. M. B. Liisberg, Z. Shakeri Kardar, S. M. Copp, C. Cerretani, T. Vosch, *J. Phys. Chem. Lett.* **2021**, *12*, 1150–1154.
176. N. C. Seeman, H. F. Sleiman, *Nat. Rev. Mater.* **2017**, *3*, 17068.
177. M. Madsen, K. V. Gothelf, *Chem. Rev.* **2019**, *119*, 6384–6458.
178. Y. Ke, C. Castro, J. H. Choi, *Annu. Rev. Biomed. Eng.* **2018**, *20*, 375–401.
179. F. Alkan, C. M. Aikens, *J. Phys. Chem. C* **2021**, *125*, 12198–12206.
180. P. R. O'Neill, K. Young, D. Schiffels, D. K. Fygenson, *Nano Lett.* **2012**, *12*, 5464–5469.
181. R. Orbach, W. Guo, F. Wang, O. Lioubashevski, I. Willner, *Langmuir* **2013**, *29*, 13066–13071.
182. W. Guo, R. Orbach, I. Mironi-Harpaz, D. Seliktar, I. Willner, *Small* **2013**, *9*, 3748–3752.
183. D. Schultz, S. M. Copp, N. Markešević, K. Gardner, S. S. R. Oemrawsingh, D. Bouwmeester, E. Gwinn, *ACS Nano* **2013**, *7*, 9798–9807.
184. Y. Zhao, S. Choi, J. Yu, *J. Phys. Chem. Lett.* **2020**, *11*, 6867–6872.
185. J. D. Aiken, R. G. Finke, *J. Mol. Catal. A Chem.* **1999**, *145*, 1–44.
186. Y. Du, H. Sheng, D. Astruc, M. Zhu, *Chem. Rev.* **2020**, *120*, 526–622.
187. W. Zhou, Y. Fang, J. Ren, S. Dong, *Chem. Commun.* **2019**, *55*, 373–376.
188. Y. Guo, M. Lv, J. Ren, E. Wang, *Small* **2021**, *17*, 2006553.
189. S. Chakraborty, R. C. Rocha, A. Desireddy, K. Artyushkova, T. C. Sanchez, A. T. Perry, P. Atanassov, J. S. Martinez, *RSC Adv.* **2016**, *6*, 90624–90630.
190. F. Hong, F. Zhang, Y. Liu, H. Yan, *Chem. Rev.* **2017**, *117*, 12584–12640.
191. P. O'Neill, P. W. K. Rothemund, A. Kumar, D. K. Fygenson, *Nano Lett.* **2006**, *6*, 1379–1383.
192. S. M. Jeon, S. Choi, K. Lee, H.-S. Jung, J. Yu, *J. Photochem. Photobiol. A: Chem.* **2018**, *355*, 479–486.
193. D. Schultz, R. G. Brinson, N. Sari, J. A. Fagan, C. Bergonzo, N. J. Lin, J. P. Dunkers, *Soft Matter* **2019**, *15*, 4284–4293.
194. C. Chen, Z. Yang, X. Tang, *Med. Res. Rev.* **2018**, *38*, 829–869.
195. G.-M. Han, Z.-Z. Jia, Y.-J. Zhu, J.-J. Jiao, D.-M. Kong, X.-Z. Feng, *Anal. Chem.* **2016**, *88*, 10800–10804.
196. S. Naskar, R. Guha, J. Müller, *Angew. Chem. Int. Ed.* **2020**, *59*, 1397–1406.
197. B. Jash, J. Müller, *Chem. Eur. J.* **2017**, *23*, 17166–17178.
198. L. A. Espinosa Leal, O. Lopez-Acevedo, *Nanotechnol. Rev.* **2015**, *4*, 173–191.
199. J. V. Burda, J. Šponer, J. Leszczynski, *Handbook of Computational Chemistry* Ed J. Leszczynski, Springer, Dordrecht, Netherlands, **2012**, pp. 1277–1308.
200. N. Bossert, D. de Bruin, M. Götz, D. Bouwmeester, D. Heinrich, *Sci. Rep.* **2016**, *6*, 37897.
201. D. Lyu, J. Li, X. Wang, W. Guo, E. Wang, *Anal. Chem.* **2019**, *91*, 2050–2057.
202. Q. Wu, C. Liu, C. Cui, L. Li, L. Yang, Y. Liu, H. Safari Yazd, S. Xu, X. Li, Z. Chen, W. Tan, *J. Am. Chem. Soc.* **2021**, *143*, 14573–14580.

13 G-Quadruplex Nucleic Acids and the Role of Metal Ions
Insights from Quantum Chemical Bonding Analyses

*Celine Nieuwland and Célia Fonseca Guerra**
Department of Theoretical Chemistry, Amsterdam
Institute of Molecular and Life Sciences (AIMMS),
Amsterdam Center of Multiscale Modeling (ACMM),
Vrije Universiteit Amsterdam, De Boelelaan
1083, 1081 HV Amsterdam, The Netherlands
c.nieuwland@vu.nl, c.fonsecaguerra@vu.nl

CONTENTS

1   Introduction 344
   1.1   G-Quadruplexes: Their Regulatory Roles in Biology and
       Applications 344
   1.2   Understanding G-Quadruplexes Using Computations 345
   1.3   Computational Tools 346
       1.3.1   Level of Theory 346
       1.3.2   Activation Strain Model 347
       1.3.3   Energy Decomposition Analysis 347
       1.3.4   Voronoi Deformation Density Analysis 348
2   Structure and Stability of G-Quadruplex Nucleic Acids 349
   2.1   The G-Quadruplex Building Block: The G-Quartet 349
   2.2   G-Quadruplex Formation 353
   2.3   G-Quadruplex RNA vs. DNA 355
3   The Role of Alkali Metal Cations in G-Quadruplexes 357
   3.1   Origin of Cation Coordination 357
   3.2   Alkali Metal Cation Affinities 358
   3.3   Cation Affinities in Multi-layer G-Quadruplexes 361

---

* Corresponding author

DOI 10.1201/9781003270201-13

4	G-Quadruplexes and Pollution Metals	363
5	General Conclusions	366
Acknowledgments		367
Abbreviations and Definitions		367
References		368

ABSTRACT

G-quadruplexes are biologically occurring non-canonical nucleic acid structures that self-assemble by forming stacks of successive quartets of guanine bases (the G-quartet), stabilized by hydrogen bonds, base stacking, and metal cation coordination. G-quadruplexes are detectable in human cells and are involved in several vital cellular processes at the DNA and RNA levels, such as in telomere homeostasis and gene expression. This chapter outlines some of the available state-of-the-art theories and computational methods that enable the understanding of the physical principles that dictate the structure and stability of G-quadruplexes and other classes of nucleic acids. Furthermore, it demonstrates how experimental questions and phenomena regarding the structure and stability of G-quadruplexes and their interaction with metal ions can nowadays be understood from accurate quantum chemical computations.

KEYWORDS

DNA; Density Functional Computations; G-Quadruplexes; Metal Ions; Nucleic Acids; Pollution Metals; RNA; Quantum (Bio)chemistry

1 INTRODUCTION

1.1 G-QUADRUPLEXES: THEIR REGULATORY ROLES IN BIOLOGY AND APPLICATIONS

Guanine quadruplexes (G-quadruplexes or GQs) are non-canonical nucleic acid structures that are located in regions of the genome that have high concentrations of guanine residues, such as telomeres and promoter regions [1] (see Figure 1). G-quadruplexes are encountered for deoxyribonucleic acid (DNA) and ribonucleic acid (RNA) sequences and are not only formed *intramolecularly* from a guanine-rich nucleic acid single strand but can also form *intermolecular* adducts from two or more individual guanine-rich strands. Depending on the relative orientation of the four-pillared helices and how the G-quartets are connected by the exterior loops, a wide range of topologies is observed for G-quadruplexes (e.g., parallel, anti-parallel, and hybrid topologies) [1].

G-quadruplexes play an essential role in all kinds of regulatory processes involving DNA and RNA inside and outside the cell nucleus, such as DNA transcription, DNA replication, telomere homeostasis, and RNA translation [2]. As such, GQs have a high potential for therapeutic applications [3–6] and the understanding of the structure and stability of G-quadruplexes represents a thriving field in biological and medicinal chemistry. For example, the prominent role of GQs in DNA and RNA processes has led to a field devoted to the rational design

G-Quadruplex Nucleic Acids and the Role of Metal Ions

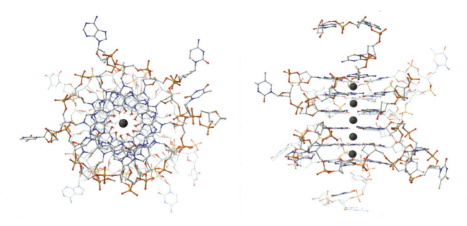

FIGURE 1 Top (left) and side (right) views of a crystal structure of a DNA G-quadruplex hosting K[+] ions in the central cavity (PDBID: 5UA3; [132]).

of so-called *GQ ligands* as a strategy for the development of selective anticancer drugs and treatments [7–18]. These GQ ligands, which can be small organic molecules but also transition metal complexes, have the potential to selectively interact with and stabilize GQs with selective toxicity toward oncogenes. Besides therapeutic purposes, GQs have found many other applications, for instance, as ion conductors [19, 20] and (ion) biosensors [21–25].

1.2 Understanding G-Quadruplexes Using Computations

As highlighted in the previous section, G-quadruplexes have raised considerable attention in the field of bio- and medicinal chemistry and also serve applications in many other fields. Nevertheless, the mechanisms leading to the assembly and stabilization of these non-canonical nucleic acid structures are still under debate, and the understanding of this represents an active field in chemistry. Besides the stabilizing (non-)covalent interactions between the guanine bases, metal cations are found to stabilize GQs upon coordination with the central cavity but also small organic molecules and transition metal complexes can interact and subsequently stabilize quadruplexes. As such, qualification and understanding of these intermolecular interactions represent a relevant topic for medical applications [3–5]. To get an understanding of all kinds of issues related to the formation and function of GQs and their interaction with small molecules and metal ions, a synergy between experimental and theoretical studies is essential [26].

As G-quadruplexes are biomolecules of significant size, classical computational methods based on force fields, such as molecular dynamics (MD), that allow for long-timescale simulations are quite popular in modeling the dynamic motions of nucleic acids [27, 28]. However, such classical methods have shown to be unable to qualify and quantify the phenomena taking place on the electronic level which are essential to understand and correctly predict the structure and stability of G-quadruplexes and their interactions with molecules and metal ions [29–32]. Therefore, one needs to assess quantum chemical methods that take into account the electronic structure of the molecular system (e.g., semi-empirical, quantum mechanics/molecular mechanics (QM/MM), and density functional theory (DFT) methods). Although quantum chemical computations also have limitations, mainly the inability for long-timescale conformational sampling and the approximate description of solvation, they can substantially improve the quality of classical computational methods relying solely on force fields. In particular, dispersion-corrected DFT (DFT-D) computations of G-quadruplexes immersed in a continuum aqueous solution have been shown to correctly reproduce trends and structures in line with experiment [29, 31–35]. In this chapter, we outline some of the available state-of-the-art quantum chemical theories and computational methods, mainly based on DFT-D computations that enable the understanding of experimental questions and phenomena regarding the structure and stability of G-quadruplexes. This chapter is not intended to give a complete overview of all available quantum chemical methods and theories for the analysis of G-quadruplex structures. Instead, we hope to provide a balanced set of examples of how quantum chemical analyses can be employed to answer biochemical questions and thereby stimulate the application of quantum chemical computations in the field of pharmaceutical and medicinal chemistry.

1.3 Computational Tools

1.3.1 Level of Theory

Quantum chemical methods, such as DFT computations, are essential to accurately model G-quadruplexes. In this subsection, we highlight some state-of-the-art computational tools for studying the chemistry of G-quadruplexes based on relativistic DFT-D computations. For the sake of brevity, not all computational setting details are mentioned explicitly in this chapter but can be found in the given references. Nevertheless, most of the computations outlined in this chapter are performed with the Amsterdam Density Functional (ADF) software package [36–38] at the zeroth-order regular approximation (ZORA) [39]-BLYP-D3(BJ) [40–44]/TZ2P [45] level of theory using the conductor-like screening model (COSMO) [46–48] to simulate solvation in water. The BLYP-D3(BJ) functional is our recommendation for DFT modeling of G-quadruplexes, as it has been demonstrated to yield reliable geometries and bond energy trends in line with experimental data [24, 33–35, 49, 50]. Furthermore, this functional outperforms more recently developed meta-hybrid functionals, such as M06-2X, in terms of the accuracy/cost ratio [51, 52] which is preferred for the description of these nucleic acid structures of significant size. The TZ2P basis set is of triple-ζ quality for all atoms and has been augmented with two sets of polarization functions [45]. However, a recent benchmark study has shown that for the description of GQs, a TZP basis set for the guanine bases and metal ions in combination with the smaller DZ basis set for the sugar-phosphate backbone provides accurate geometries and energies but reduces the computation time significantly (by almost three times compared to the TZ2P basis set) which is desired for these large systems [33].

1.3.2 Activation Strain Model

The first computational method that we want to highlight is the activation strain model (ASM) [53, 54] of chemical reactivity and bonding which is a powerful method for analyzing and understanding the stability and reactivity of molecular complexes. Using a fragment-based approach, the ASM relates the bond energy of a molecular complex to two distinct factors, namely, (1) the strain energy (ΔE_{strain}) needed to deform the molecular fragments from their optimum geometry to the geometry they adopt in the interacting complex and (2) the interaction energy (ΔE_{int}) between these deformed fragments, as formulated in Equation 1.

$$\Delta E_{bond} = \Delta E_{strain} + \Delta E_{int} \quad (1)$$

Although the activation strain analysis (ASA) can be used in combination with many quantum chemical software packages, we advise using the ADF software package for this purpose [36–38]. The main advantage of using the ADF program is that the ASA can be extended with (1) a compatible energy decomposition analysis (EDA, *vide infra*), which decomposes the interaction energy (obtained by the ASA) into a number of physically intuitive and meaningful terms, and (2) a coherent Kohn–Sham molecular orbital (MO) analysis, in which the EDA terms can be directly correlated to the MOs of the interacting molecular fragments.

1.3.3 Energy Decomposition Analysis

To get more insight into the trends of interaction energies between molecular fragments, one can perform as an extension to the ASA, an energy decomposition analysis (EDA) [55, 56]. The canonical EDA scheme decomposes the total interaction energy ΔE_{int} based on Kohn–Sham MO theory into four energy terms: the Pauli repulsion, electrostatic interaction, orbital interaction, and dispersion (Equation 2).

$$\Delta E_{int} = \Delta E_{Pauli} + \Delta V_{elstat} + \Delta E_{oi} + \Delta E_{disp} \quad (2)$$

The Pauli repulsion, ΔE_{Pauli}, constitutes the destabilizing interaction between overlapping occupied orbitals and is responsible for any steric repulsion. The electrostatic interaction energy, ΔV_{elstat}, is the classic Coulomb interaction between the unperturbed charge distributions of the deformed fragments and is usually attractive. The orbital interaction energy, ΔE_{oi}, comprises polarization (empty–occupied orbital mixing on one fragment because of the presence of another fragment) and charge transfer (donor–acceptor interactions between occupied orbitals on one fragment and unoccupied orbitals on the other, including highest occupied molecular orbital (HOMO)–lowest unoccupied molecular orbital (LUMO) interactions). The ΔE_{oi} term can be further decomposed into the contributions from each irreducible representation (irrep) of the symmetry point group of the regarded system. For example, the analysis of planar molecular structures (e.g., C_s symmetric), allows for the decomposition of ΔE_{oi} into contributions originating from the σ and π molecular orbitals (Equation 3).

$$\Delta E_{oi} = \Delta E_{oi}^{\sigma} + \Delta E_{oi}^{\pi} \quad (3)$$

Finally, the dispersion energy, ΔE_{disp}, accounts for the long-range dispersion interactions when an explicit dispersion correction is included which is the case for the BLYP-D3(BJ) functional.

Although there are more available EDA schemes (e.g., DFT-SAPT [57]), it has been recently shown that different EDA schemes provide very similar results concerning non-covalent interactions, including hydrogen bonds, and insights into the interaction energy components [58, 59]. The main advantage of the canonical EDA scheme is that the energy components directly correlate to the Kohn–Sham MOs of the molecular species studied.

1.3.4 Voronoi Deformation Density Analysis

Finally, useful information can be obtained from atomic charge analyses. The Voronoi deformation density (VDD) method allows for the chemically intuitive and meaningful analysis of the electronic redistributions within atomic or molecular fragments when a chemical interaction is present between these fragments, for example, to study the interaction between G-quadruplexes and metal ions [60, 61].

The VDD atomic charge Q_A of atom A is given by Equation 4. Equation 4 uses numerical integration over the deformation density $[\rho(\mathbf{r}) - \Sigma_B \rho_B(\mathbf{r})]$ which is the density change going from a superposition of atomic densities, that is a fictitious promolecule, to the density in the final molecular system. This promolecule density is defined as the sum over the (spherically averaged) ground-state atomic densities $\Sigma_B \rho_B(\mathbf{r})$. The Voronoi cell of an atom is the space defined by the bond midplanes on and perpendicular to all bond axes between the nucleus and its neighboring nuclei.

$$Q_A = -\int_{\text{Voronoi cell of A}} [\rho(\mathbf{r}) - \Sigma_B \rho_B(\mathbf{r})] d\mathbf{r} \quad (4)$$

The VDD analysis can also be used for studying the bonding between molecular fragments. Here the charge rearrangement (ΔQ_A) compared to the initial density of the polyatomic fragments is measured and gives insight into the change in electronic density as a consequence of the chemical interaction (see Equation 5). ΔQ_A is an indication of the number of electrons that flows into ($\Delta Q_A < 0$) or out of ($\Delta Q_A > 0$) the Voronoi cell of a nucleus A as the result of the interaction between the two fragments.

$$\Delta Q_A = -\int_{\text{Voronoi cell of A in molecule}} [\rho_{\text{molecule}}(\mathbf{r}) - \Sigma_{\text{subsystems},i}\rho_i(\mathbf{r})]d\mathbf{r} \quad (5)$$

To analyze the charge rearrangements caused by charge transfer within orbitals belonging to different irreps, ΔQ_A, can be further decomposed into the contributions of each irrep (Equation 6).

$$\Delta Q_A^\Gamma = -\int_{\text{Voronoi cell of A in molecule}} [\rho_{\text{molecule}}^\Gamma(\mathbf{r}) - \rho_{\text{Fragment1}}^\Gamma(\mathbf{r}) - \rho_{\text{Fragment2}}^\Gamma(\mathbf{r})]d\mathbf{r} \quad (6)$$

The density ρ^Γ is the sum of the occupied MO densities within a particular irrep Γ. For example, in the case of planar systems, one could decompose the total change in atomic charge ΔQ, into the contributions from charge shifts within the σ (ΔQ^σ) and π (ΔQ^π) electronic system.

2 STRUCTURE AND STABILITY OF G-QUADRUPLEX NUCLEIC ACIDS

2.1 THE G-QUADRUPLEX BUILDING BLOCK: THE G-QUARTET

The quantum chemical exploration of G-quadruplexes naturally begins with the analysis of the basic building block of a G-quadruplex: the G-quartet (G_4), which consists of four guanine bases interconnected by Hoogsteen-type hydrogen bonding (see Figure 2a). The natural guanine nucleobases are superior in forming quartet structures and form more stable quartets than substituted analogs or other nucleobases [62, 63]. There are, however, several examples that demonstrate that the guanines in G_4 can be substituted by other nucleobases or molecules and can be tolerated if stabilized by additional G-quartets [64–67].

The hydrogen bonding between the guanine residues in G_4 is, next to metal cation binding (*vide infra*), one of the main driving forces for G-quadruplex formation [1]. The nature of the hydrogen bonds between DNA bases has been under debate for quite some time [68–71]. Hydrogen bonds were long believed to be purely non-covalent electrostatic interactions, where a δ^- hydrogen-bond *acceptor* (e.g., O or N) interacts with a δ^+ hydrogen-bond *donor* (e.g., (N)H) [72]. However, it has been demonstrated that in hydrogen-bond interactions, thus also between DNA bases, the covalent character is of equal importance [73, 74].

In G-quartets electronic density is donated from the lone-pair σ_{LP} orbital of the O6 or N7 hydrogen-bond acceptor to the σ^*_{NH} orbital of the interacting NH hydrogen-bond donors through donor–acceptor interactions, or so-called charge-transfer interactions (see Figure 2b) [75]. Furthermore, temporary dipoles give rise to attractive dispersion interactions in the G-quartet, but also repulsive interactions are present that arise from overlapping filled orbitals of the hydrogen-bond donor and acceptor (i.e., steric Pauli repulsion).

Gilli et al. [70, 71] proposed that hydrogen bonds between unsaturated molecules, such as the guanine residues in G_4, are reinforced by π-assistance

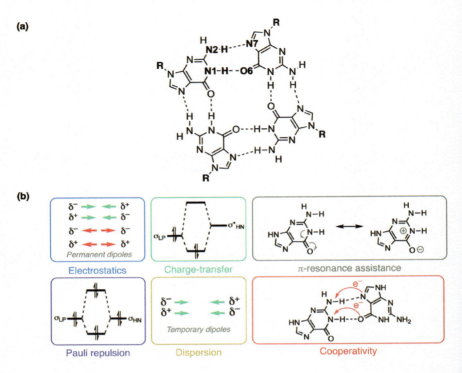

FIGURE 2 (a) Structure of the guanine quartet (G_4) and (b) relevant interactions present in G_4.

(Figure 2b), a phenomenon called π-resonance-assisted hydrogen bonding (RAHB). It was confirmed in previous computational work that the π electrons provide a small additional stabilizing component to hydrogen bonds but not as important as the covalent component in the hydrogen bonds [76].

It was also established that the hydrogen bonds in the G-quartet encounter *cooperativity* (Figure 2b) [77–80]. As such, the computed hydrogen-bond energy, that is the strength, of G_4 was found to be substantially more stabilizing than four times the hydrogen-bond energy of one guanine dimer (G_2) although G_4 has four times the number of hydrogen bonds as G_2 [75]. This phenomenon was originally ascribed to the resonance assistance of the hydrogen bonds by the π-electrons in the G-quartet [77]. However, computational analyses revealed that the cooperativity in G-quartets originates from the σ-electrons, and not from the π-electronic system [63, 75]. The conclusions were derived from the analysis of the stepwise assembling of a G-quartet (Figure 3a) in which G_4 is constructed by adding guanine residues (in the geometry of G_4) and decomposition of the subsequent interaction energies. This stepwise approach enables the identification of why and at which point the cooperativity starts. In this analysis, a planar quartet geometry (C_{4h} symmetric) was considered which allows for the

G-Quadruplex Nucleic Acids and the Role of Metal Ions

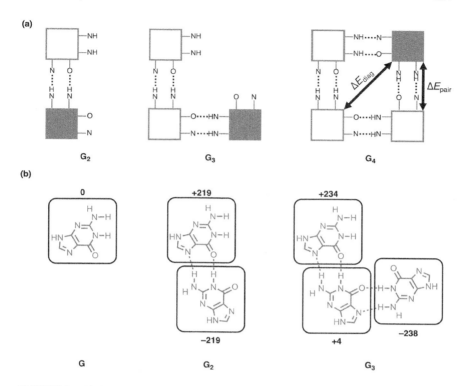

FIGURE 3 (a) Analysis of a planar G-quartet (G₄) in a stepwise manner. (b) Assembling of G₄ induces charge separation in the σ-electronic system. VDD σ-electron charges $Q^σ$ (in milli-electrons) of guanine bases in G, G₂, and G₃ fragments in the geometry of the C_{4h} symmetric G-quartet, computed at ZORA-BLYP-D3(BJ)/TZ2P. (Data taken from Ref. [63].)

discrimination between the σ and π electronic systems (see Sections 1.3.3 and 1.3.4). This approach is justified as the planar quartet furnishes bond energies and hydrogen-bond distances in very good agreement with the S_4 symmetric global minimum geometry.

The cooperativity of the hydrogen bonds in G₄ was computed by comparing the interaction energy (ΔE_{int}) of the stepwise formation of the quartet from four guanine bases (in the geometry of G₄) with the sum of the individual pairwise interactions (ΔE_{sum}) for all possible pairs of bases in the G-quartet (see Equation 7).

$$\Delta E_{sum} = 4 \cdot \Delta E_{pair} + 2 \cdot \Delta E_{diag} \qquad (7)$$

Within ΔE_{sum} the distinction is made between interaction energies between neighboring hydrogen-bonded base pairs (ΔE_{pair}) and between diagonally oriented non-hydrogen-bonded guanine bases (ΔE_{diag}) (see Figure 3a). The cooperativity or *synergy* (ΔE_{syn}) occurring in the quartet is then defined as the difference between the total interaction energy and this summation (Equation 8).

$$\Delta E_{syn} = \Delta E_{int} - \Delta E_{sum} \qquad (8)$$

Here, $\Delta E_{syn} < 0$ indicates a stabilizing cooperative effect so that the stability of the G-quartet is reinforced due to the occurrence of all hydrogen bonds simultaneously.

The results of the energy decomposition analysis (EDA) of the stepwise assembling of G_4 are reported in Table 1. The interaction energy $\Delta E_{int}(G_n)$ becomes more stabilizing when the fragment size increases (from -16.5 to -23.0, to -51.1 kcal mol^{-1}, for $n=2, 3$, and 4, respectively). Important to note is that from the decomposition of ΔE_{int} follows that the hydrogen bonds in G_4 indeed contain a large orbital interaction component as ΔE_{oi} is of the same order of magnitude as the electrostatic interaction term ΔV_{elstat}. Furthermore, the stabilizing ΔE_{oi} is crucial to overcome the significant destabilizing steric Pauli repulsion (ΔE_{Pauli}). In line with previous work into the nature of hydrogen bonds [73], ΔE_{oi} stems mainly from charge transfer within the σ electronic system (ΔE_{oi}^σ), and the remaining follows from charge rearrangements (i.e., polarization) of the π electrons (ΔE_{oi}^π) [63, 75]. This polarization of the π system is the so-called resonance-assistance stabilization of the hydrogen bonds in G_4. However, the π electrons contribute with a small synergy of -3.1 kcal mol^{-1} for ΔE_{oi}^π not significantly to the total synergy of -20.9 kcal mol^{-1} encountered in G_4. ΔE_{syn} follows primarily from the synergy in the electrostatic interactions ΔV_{elstat} (-9.4 kcal mol^{-1}) and σ-electron charge transfer ΔE_{oi}^σ (-8.2 kcal mol^{-1}). It was computationally established that

TABLE 1
Energy Decomposition (in kcal mol^{-1}) of the Cooperative Stepwise Assembling of the G-Quartet (G_4)[a, b]

	G_2	G_3	G_4	G_2^{diag}	ΔE_{sum}	ΔE_{syn}[c]
ΔE_{oi}^σ	-14.7	-16.4	-36.1	-0.1	-59.1	-8.2
ΔE_{oi}^π	-1.8	-2.4	-6.2	-0.1	-7.3	-3.1
ΔE_{oi}	-16.5	-18.8	-42.3	-0.2	-66.4	-11.3
ΔE_{Pauli}	30.9	31.4	61.3	0.1	123.8	-0.2
ΔV_{elstat}	-26.4	-30.9	-60.9	-1.6	-108.8	-9.4
ΔE_{disp}	-4.5	-4.7	-9.1	-0.2	-18.3	0.0
$\Delta E_{int}(G_n)$	-16.5	-23.0	-51.1	-1.9	-69.7	-20.9

[a] Computed at ZORA-BLYP-D3(BJ)/TZ2P for frozen (fragments of) C_{4h}-symmetric G_4.
[b] Data taken from Ref. [63].
[c] Overall synergy in each energy term is defined as: $\Delta E(G_2) + \Delta E(G_3) + \Delta E(G_4) - 4\,\Delta E(G_2) - 2\,\Delta E(G_2^{diag})$.

the origin of the synergy in the G_4 hydrogen bonds (i.e., ΔE_{syn}) lies in the charge separation that occurs through the donor–acceptor interactions in the σ-electronic system (Figure 3b) [75]. This charge separation induces cooperative effects by (1) enhancing the σ orbital interactions ($\Delta E_{oi}{}^\sigma$), by raising the energy of the O6 and N7 lone-pair like σ_{HOMOs} and lowering the energy of the σ^*_{NH} LUMOs of the NH hydrogen-bond donors thereby reducing the HOMO–LUMO gap, and (2) by increasing the electrostatic attraction with an incoming guanine base (ΔV_{elstat}). Moreover, it was demonstrated that the cooperativity of the G-quartet persists in biologically relevant structures such as telomeres, that is, in a stack of G-quartets with Na^+ or K^+ ions coordinated in between the layers [63, 75]. Inspired by the cooperativity of the hydrogen bonds in biological systems like G-quadruplexes, cooperative hydrogen bonding has found its application nowadays in the field of supramolecular chemistry and material sciences where cooperativity can be used to tune the geometrical or thermodynamic properties of hydrogen-bonded supramolecular assemblies [81–84].

2.2 G-Quadruplex Formation

Although the detailed analysis of the G_4 building block is the first step in understanding G-quadruplex chemistry, the direct connection to biochemical and pharmaceutical applications requires the consideration of these structures as how they occur in cells. Under physiological conditions, G-quartets can assemble into larger G-quadruplex structures by the lateral stacking of two or more G_4 layers (see Figure 1) driven by stabilizing electrostatic and dispersion interactions [1, 63, 75, 85]. The sugar-phosphate groups of the guanosine monomers define the outer backbone of GQs and enhance their stability. A central channel defined by the carbonyl O6 atoms of the guanine bases surpasses the whole length of the G-quadruplex and hosts under biological conditions monovalent alkali metal cations such as K^+ and Na^+.

GQ structures have a very rich topological diversity as loops of various lengths and sequences connect the pillars of the G-quadruplex [86, 87]. The polymorphism follows from the different strand stoichiometries (1–4 nucleic acid strands), but also from the relative orientation of the strands constituting the quadruplex pillars that can run in the same direction (parallel) or in opposite directions (antiparallel), and also hybrid topologies are reported. While GQ-DNA occurs in various topologies [87], RNA G-quadruplexes almost exclusively appear as parallel-stranded due to the strong preference for the anti-conformation of glycosidic bonds in ribonucleosides [88, 89]. Following the topology of the sugar-phosphate backbone also the relative orientation of the stacked G-quartets can vary [87, 90]. The hydrogen bonds of the stacked G_4 layers can either point all in the same direction (in the parallel topology) or in opposite directions (in the hybrid/antiparallel topology). The parallel orientation is under physiological conditions the prevalent arrangement for DNA G-quadruplexes [91, 92], while GQ-RNA folds exclusively into the parallel geometry [88, 89].

The formation of G-quadruplexes occurs when guanine-rich DNA or RNA single strands self-assemble in the presence of alkali metal cations. In the simplest example, one can form a double-layered GQ from four guanosine dimers (GG) and a metal cation M^+ (Figure 4). In quantum chemical analyses, the energy of formation (ΔE_{form}) associated with the formation of this double-layered G-quadruplex would be defined by Equation 9.

$$\Delta E_{form} = E(GQ-M^+)_{aq} - 4 \cdot E(GG)_{aq} - E(M^+) = \Delta E_{assemble} + \Delta E_{bond} \qquad (9)$$

Here $E(GQ-M^+)_{aq}$ and $E(GG)_{aq}$ denote the energies of the G-quadruplex ($GQ-M^+$) and the guanosine dimer (GG) in their optimum solvated geometry. $E(M^+)_{aq}$ is the energy of the metal cation (M^+) in aqueous solution (denoted by the subscript 'aq'). DFT analyses established that G-quadruplexes with the sugar-phosphate backbone neutralized by H^+ are computationally more robust than quadruplexes with Na^+ counterions (i.e., backbone neutralization *in vivo*) while displaying identical trends in stability and geometry [49, 93].

To gain more insight into the process of G-quadruplex formation, ΔE_{form} can be regarded as the sum of the energies of two coordination steps (Figure 4 and Equation 9). In this model, the guanosine dimers first assemble into an empty G-quadruplex scaffold (GQ–[ ]) by forming the cooperative Hoogsteen-hydrogen bonds with a stabilizing energy denoted by $\Delta E_{assemble}$. In the second step, the metal cation M^+ binds to the empty GQ cavity, associated with a stabilizing bond energy ΔE_{bond} that depends on the type of cation.

The two-step model of G-quadruplex formation presented in Figure 4 is particularly useful to delineate the role of hydrogen bonding, G_4 stacking, and metal

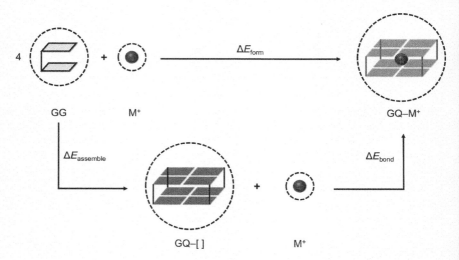

FIGURE 4 Partitioning of the energy of formation ΔE_{form} of a double-layer G-quadruplex. The dashed circles surrounding the structures indicate that the calculation is performed with COSMO to simulate solvation in water.

cation coordination in the formation and overall stability of the G-quadruplex but does not reveal the exact mechanism of formation. *In situ* spectroscopic analyses of GQ formation in organic solvents by González-Rodríguez et al. support a reaction pathway in which the alkali cation shifts the equilibrium toward a G-quartet–M$^+$ transient intermediate, which then can act as a template for G-quadruplex formation [79]. Quantum chemical analyses could help elucidate and confirm their proposed mechanism.

2.3 G-Quadruplex RNA vs. DNA

G-quadruplexes play an essential role in many regulatory processes at the DNA as well as the RNA level [2]. While G-quadruplex RNA shares the main structural characteristics with G-quadruplex DNA (*vide supra*), it has been experimentally observed that GQ-RNA has a higher thermal stability than the DNA analogs [88, 94]. This phenomenon was hypothesized to be the result of the better stacking of the piled G-quartets in GQ-RNA [95] and the presence of additional intermolecular hydrogen-bond networks between the extra 2′-hydroxyl (OH) groups on the RNA ribose rings and the phosphate oxygen atoms of the sugar-phosphate backbone [96].

DFT computations on double-layered G-quadruplexes were performed to test these hypotheses and uncover the origin of the higher thermal stability of GQ-RNA compared to GQ-DNA [93]. In line with experiment, the energy of formation ΔE_{form} was found to be substantially more stabilizing for GQ-RNA complexes compared to the DNA analogs (see Table 2).

TABLE 2
Energy of Formation ΔE_{form} (in kcal mol^{-1}) of Double-Layer RNA and DNA G-Quadruplexes with and without Alkali Metal Cations (M$^+$)[a, b]

M$^+$	$_{RNA}$GQ–M$^+$ ΔE_{form}	$_{DNA}$GQ–M$^+$ ΔE_{form}
No metal	−69.1[c]	−62.2[c]
Li$^+$	−106.2	−100.2
Na$^+$	−120.4	−114.5
K$^+$	−120.8	−115.4
Rb$^+$	−115.4	−111.1
Cs$^+$	−107.7	−103.1

[a] Computed at ZORA-BLYP-D3(BJ)/TZ2P.
[b] Data taken from Ref. [93].
[c] The energy of formation of the empty G-quadruplex (GQ–[ ]) corresponds to $\Delta E_{assemble}$.

By partitioning of ΔE_{form} of the RNA and DNA GQ–M$^+$ complexes (as presented in Figure 4) into contributions of the formation of the empty GQ scaffold ($\Delta E_{assemble}$) and the coordination of the alkali metal cation (ΔE_{bond}) it was established that the enhanced stability of RNA G-quadruplexes results from (1) their higher conformational stability, but also from (2) enhanced electrostatic interactions present between the individual RNA strands [93]. The binding of the alkali metal cations and their order of affinity (K$^+$>Na$^+$>Rb$^+$>Cs+$^+$>Li$^+$, *vide infra*) were found to not discriminate the formation of RNA and DNA quadruplexes.

First of all, the higher conformational stability of GQ-RNA results from the presence of an additional OH group on the 2′ position of the ribose ring (Figure 5a). These 2′-OH groups enable, as predicted by Fraternali and coworkers [96], the formation of intramolecular hydrogen bonds (Figure 5b). These intrastrand hydrogen bonds induce a geometry within the isolated RNA strands that are already closer to the geometry that is required within the G-quadruplex structure than in the case of the DNA single strands that lack the ability to form these intrastrand hydrogen bonds [93]. This preorganization of the RNA strands reduces the energetic cost of deformation upon G-quadruplex formation, leading to a less destabilizing strain (ΔE_{strain}), in the case of GQ-RNA compared to GQ-DNA, and contributes to the higher thermal stability (i.e., more stabilizing ΔE_{form}) of RNA G-quadruplexes.

Besides the better fit of the RNA strands for GQ assembling, the higher stability of GQ-RNA also follows from more stabilizing interstrand interactions. This effect was again attributed to the extra 2′-OH groups. These additional functional groups induce a stronger electrostatic attraction between the four individual nucleic acid strands, associated with a more stabilizing $\Delta E_{assemble}$ for the formation of the empty RNA scaffold GQ–[ ], compared to the DNA analogs that lack the ribosidic 2′-OH functionality.

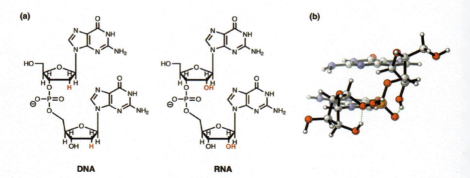

FIGURE 5 (a) Structure of the guanosine-phosphate backbone in DNA and RNA G-quadruplexes (structural differences indicated in red). (b) Ball-and-stick structure of a guanosine-phosphate RNA dimer (neutralized with H$^+$) with the intramolecular hydrogen bonds highlighted by green dotted lines.

3 THE ROLE OF ALKALI METAL CATIONS IN G-QUADRUPLEXES

3.1 Origin of Cation Coordination

The presence of alkali metal cations is requisite for the self-assembly of G-quadruplexes [97, 98] and for maintaining GQ stability even in the presence of damaged nucleobases [99, 100]. Moreover, it was for a long time believed that cation coordination to the central cavity is required for screening of the repulsion between the guanine O6 lone pairs inside the GQ cavity, thereby providing additional stabilization [86, 101]. However, DFT computations at the ZORA-BLYP-D3(BJ)/TZ2P level revealed that the cation in the central cavity is not required to compensate for electrostatic repulsion, as the O6 oxygen atoms do not repel each other [49, 93]. These conclusions were derived from the computation of the total interaction between eight formaldehyde molecules (Figure 6). In this simplified model system, the guanine residues of the GQ scaffold are displaced by formaldehyde residues where the C=O groups are fixed in the position they adopt within the quadruplex. The total interaction energy between the eight formaldehyde molecules was calculated to be only 0–0.6 kcal mol^{-1}, which means that the

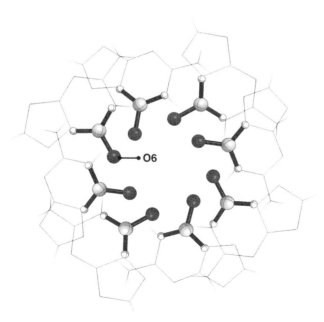

FIGURE 6 Representation of the formaldehyde model system for studying the interaction between the guanine-O6 atoms in the central cavity of a double-layer G-quadruplex.

net repulsion between the central carbonyl oxygen atoms is neglectable and the cation coordination is not required to compensate for any electrostatic repulsion. It is, however, experimentally observed that G-quadruplexes do not self-assemble in the absence of metal cations [97, 98] and quantum chemical analyses could provide clarity on this matter.

It was computationally found that cation coordination in G-quadruplexes is essential to overcome the entropic penalty of self-assembly [93], as the cation provides additional stabilization through electrostatic and donor–acceptor orbital interactions (*vide infra*). Computation of the Gibbs free energy of formation (ΔG_{form}) of double-layer G-quadruplexes in water at the ZORA-BLYP-D3(BJ)/DZP level indicated a positive ΔG_{form} in the absence of cations but a strongly negative ΔG_{form} in the presence of K^+ ions ($\Delta G_{form} = +7.6$ and -45.3 kcal mol^{-1} for $_{RNA}$GQ–[ ] and $_{RNA}$GQ–K^+, respectively). Therefore, only in the presence of metal cations, the interactions within the G-quadruplex structure are stabilizing enough to overcome the entropic cost of self-assembly. These findings support the experimental observations by González-Rodríguez et al. that suggest a cation-templated mechanism for the formation of G-quadruplexes [79].

3.2 Alkali Metal Cation Affinities

Under physiological conditions, G-quadruplexes host monovalent alkali metal cations inside the central channel defined by the guanine O6 atoms [1]. The experimentally observed cation affinity sequence of G-quadruplexes toward alkali metal cations in water is $K^+ > Na^+$, $Rb^+ >> Li^+$ [102–105] and many studies have tried to shed light on the origin of this cation affinity trend. Early experimental work in 1989 by Williamson et al. [106] suggested that the observed alkali metal cation affinity order and the ability to promote G-quadruplex formation follow directly from the size of the cavity relative to the cationic radii and the relatively snug fit of some cations. Others [107, 108] later proposed that the affinity order could be explained by the relative Gibbs free energy of solvation (ΔG_{solv}) of the various cations (as the cations need to be desolvated completely upon entering the central cavity). For a long time, there was no consensus on the origin of the observed cation affinity trend, but in 2016, it was computationally established that both factors (i.e., cation radius and ΔG_{solv}) are of almost equal importance for determining the cation affinity order in G-quadruplexes [33, 49]. This followed from DFT analyses (at the ZORA-BLYP-D3(BJ)/TZ2P level) of double-layer G-quadruplexes interacting with the monovalent alkali metal cations ($M^+ = Li^+$, Na^+, K^+, and Rb^+) in aqueous solution. For these analyses the bond energy ΔE_{bond} (i.e., cation affinity) was defined as the energy change related to the binding of an alkali metal cation M^+ to the central cavity of the empty quadruplex scaffold (GQ–[ ]) thereby forming a double-layer G-quadruplex (GQ–M^+), all occurring in water solution (denoted by 'aq') (see Equation 10 and Figure 7).

$$\Delta E_{bond} = E(GQ-M^+)_{aq} - E(GQ-[\ ])_{aq} - E(M^+)_{aq} \quad (10)$$

G-Quadruplex Nucleic Acids and the Role of Metal Ions

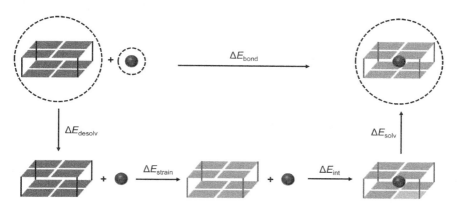

FIGURE 7 Partitioning of ΔE_{bond} of a metal cation (black sphere) binding to the central cavity of a double-layer G-quadruplex. The dashed circles surrounding the structures indicate that the calculation is performed with COSMO to simulate solvation in water.

These quantum chemical computations reproduced the experimental order of affinity with ΔE_{bond} becoming more stabilizing in the order $Li^+ < Rb^+ < Na^+ < K^+$ and obtained accurate G-quadruplex geometries in line with experimental geometrical parameters (e.g., hydrogen-bond and O6–M^+ distances). To understand the different components that determine the trend in the cation affinity, the bond energy was further decomposed into various energy terms as formulated by Equation 11 (see Figure 7 for a graphical representation of the energy terms).

$$\Delta E_{bond} = \Delta E_{desolv} + \Delta E_{strain} + \Delta E_{int} + \Delta E_{solv} \quad (11)$$

In this decomposition, solvation effects that may contribute to the observed affinity trend can be studied computationally by the sum of the desolvation energy (ΔE_{desolv}) of the separated M^+ and GQ–[ ] fragments and the solvation energy (ΔE_{solv}) of the final GQ–M^+ complex. The role of the effective size of the alkali metal cations can herein be evaluated by the strain energy (ΔE_{strain}) and the interaction energy (ΔE_{int}) term. ΔE_{strain} is a measure for the required deformation of the GQ cavity to host a specific metal cation M^+. Finally, the strength of the stabilizing interactions present between M^+ and the deformed empty scaffold GQ–[ ] are covered in the interaction energy term (ΔE_{int}).

The partitioning of the ΔE_{bond}, as presented in Figure 8a, revealed that the overall desolvation ($\Delta E_{desolv} + \Delta E_{solv}$) and the effective size ($\Delta E_{int} + \Delta E_{strain}$) of the cation are of equal importance in determining the cation affinity order. Descending Group 1 of the Periodic Table from Li^+ to Rb^+, the overall desolvation energy of the cation (represented by $\Delta E_{desolv} + \Delta E_{solv}$) gradually becomes less destabilizing but at the same time, the stabilizing interactions (ΔE_{int}) between the cation and the G-quadruplex cavity also diminish. The deformation ΔE_{strain} of the G-quadruplexes is small but decreases with increasing radius of M^+, that is,

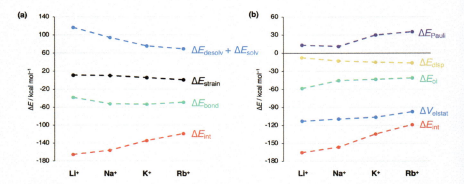

FIGURE 8 Partitioning of the (a) bond energy ΔE_{bond} and (b) interaction energy ΔE_{int} (in kcal mol^{-1}) for the binding of different alkali metal cations to the central cavity of a double-layer G-quadruplex. (Data taken from Ref. [49].)

from Li$^+$ to Rb$^+$, because the size of the larger alkali cations matches better with the size of the vacant cavity in GQ–[ ] which in turn needs to deform less to host the cation. The counteracting energy terms translate into a shallow minimum of ΔE_{bond} and thus the highest cation affinity for K$^+$, followed closely by Na$^+$ (+1 kcal mol^{-1}).

A subsequent energy decomposition analysis (EDA) of the total interaction energy ΔE_{int} between M$^+$ and GQ–[ ], shown in Figure 8b, revealed that the stabilizing interaction between the alkali cations and the quadruplex follows primarily from attractive electrostatic interactions (ΔV_{elstat}), but also the orbital interaction (ΔE_{oi}) is a large contributor to the GQ–M$^+$ stability. The latter involves charge-transfer interactions between mainly the σ lone-pair type orbitals of the O6 atoms and the lowest unoccupied orbitals (LUMOs) of M$^+$ (see Section 4 for more details).

Although K$^+$ has among the alkali cations the highest binding affinity toward G-quadruplexes, its interaction energy ΔE_{int} is surprisingly much less stabilizing than for the smaller ions Na$^+$ and Li$^+$ (Figure 8). The most important reason for the significantly weaker interaction for GQ–K$^+$ compared to GQ–Na$^+$ is the Pauli repulsion (ΔE_{Pauli}), which is more destabilizing for the larger and more diffuse potassium ion (Figure 8b). This higher steric repulsion for larger cations is in line with computational investigations by, among others, Villani [109, 110] and Van Mourik [111] that identified that the larger cation K$^+$ prefers a more central position in between two G-quartets while the smaller ions Na$^+$ and Li$^+$ can move more freely through the central channel because they encounter various minima positions connected by low-energy barriers. The smallest alkali cation, Li$^+$, even prefers coordination in the middle of one of the quartet layers. Note that because the small Li cation resides within one of the quartet layers, ΔE_{Pauli} for Li$^+$ is slightly more destabilizing than for Na$^+$ which prefers (like the larger alkali cations) a central position in between the two G-quartets (Figure 8b).

While the bond energy analysis presented in Figure 8 concerns parallel-stranded double-layer G-quadruplexes with a sugar-phosphate backbone neutralized by H[+], DFT computations showed that G-quadruplexes with parallel and the anti-parallel stacking topologies, as well as DNA and RNA based G-quadruplexes, and G-quadruplexes with Na[+] counterions, furnish identical cation binding mechanisms and affinity trends [49, 93]. Moreover, it was found that GQ model systems *without* the sugar-phosphate backbone give rise to the same alkali metal cation binding affinity sequence as the counterparts with backbone and are therefore considered excellent G-quadruplex model systems for studying cation affinities [33, 49]. The significant reduction in system size upon removal of the backbone enables the analysis of multi-layer G-quadruplex structures, which will be addressed in the next section.

3.3 Cation Affinities in Multi-layer G-Quadruplexes

The previous section demonstrated that the origin of the experimental GQ alkali metal cation affinity order could be traced by quantum chemical investigations of double-layer G-quadruplexes interacting with the various alkali metal cations. However, naturally occurring GQs are often encountered as larger structures containing multiple stacked G-quartets, so one could wonder how well these results extend to G-quadruplexes with more than two layers that include the repulsive interaction between metal cations in adjacent cavities. Computational investigations of the alkali metal cation affinities in multi-layer GQs, using the same bond energy decomposition scheme as presented in Figure 7, showed that the order of affinity (K[+] < Na[+] < Rb[+] < Li[+]) is preserved in triple-layer G-quadruplexes (GQ–K[+]–M[+], with M[+] = Li[+], Na[+], K[+], Rb[+]) and that again the desolvation energy and the effective size of the alkali cations are equally responsible for the binding affinity order [33]. So, the conclusions of the double-layered systems do turn over to multiple-layer quadruplexes in which M[+]···M[+] interactions are regarded.

The presence of such inter-cation repulsion could lower the propensity for binding of two cations in adjacent GQ-cavities, possibly resulting in an alternating pattern of vacant and occupied centers. Nevertheless, quantum chemical investigations, at the ZORA-BLYP-D3(BJ)/TZP level, using COSMO to simulate solvation in water, revealed that the binding strength of alkali cations in successive layers in multi-layer G-quadruplexes is roughly constant [33]. The magnitude of the bond energy ΔE_{bond} for an incoming cation, for instance K[+], is ca. constant for the first, second, and third binding event in double-, triple-, and quadruple-layered G-quadruplexes, respectively (Figure 9a). This was found to be the consequence of two counteracting forces: (1) for the incoming metal cation M[+] the interaction energy (ΔE_{int}) with the quadruplex is becoming *less stabilizing* but at the same time (2) the overall desolvation effect ($\Delta E_{desolv} + \Delta E_{solv}$) becomes *less destabilizing* compared to the proceeding binding event, overall leading to a constant ΔE_{bond} for successive cation binding events.

First of all, the interaction energy ΔE_{int} between the incoming cation and the rest of the quadruplex becomes less stabilizing for successive binding events of

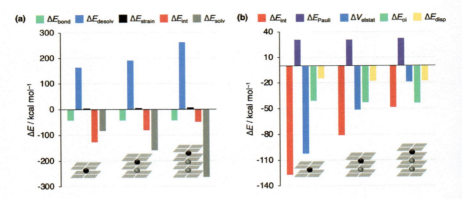

FIGURE 9 Partitioning of the (a) bond energy ΔE_{bond} and (b) interaction energy ΔE_{int} (in kcal mol^{-1}) for successive binding events of incoming K$^+$ cations (black spheres) in multi-layer G-quadruplexes. Gray spheres depict precoordinated K$^+$ cations. (Data taken from Ref. [33].)

K$^+$ in double-, triple-, and quadruple-layered GQs, respectively (Figure 9). The decomposition of the interaction energy (ΔE_{int}) in Figure 9b shows that it is the decrease in electrostatic attraction (ΔV_{elstat}) that is responsible for the observed decrease in ΔE_{int}, as the energy terms ΔE_{Pauli}, ΔE_{oi}, and ΔE_{disp} remain constant. The diminishing electrostatic attraction of the K$^+$ cations toward the GQ cavity is the result of the Coulombic repulsion between the incoming cation and the precoordinated cation(s) in the G-quadruplex. That the decrease in ΔV_{elstat} scales with the number of precoordinated cations implies that the electrostatic repulsion operates not only locally, that is, between directly neighboring cations, but also over longer distances, that is, for non-neighboring cations.

The analysis in Figure 9a demonstrates that at the same time the overall desolvation effect ($\Delta E_{desolv} + \Delta E_{solv}$) becomes less destabilizing for successive K$^+$ binding events. This is a consequence of the stabilizing solvation energy ΔE_{solv} of the GQ–M$^+$ complex that increases faster than the destabilizing desolvation energy ΔE_{desolv} of the separate cation M$^+$ and the GQ scaffold comprising the vacant site. For example, the gain in solvation energy for going from a double-layer GQ–K$^+$ complex (total charge of +1) to a triple-layer GQ–K$^+$–K$^+$ complex (total charge of +2) is larger than the increase in solvation energy for going from GQ–[ ] (neutral) and K$^+$ (charge of +1) to GQ–K$^+$–[ ] (total charge of +1) and K$^+$ (charge of +1). In other words, the solvation energy of molecular species scales non-linearly with the charge of the individual species. In practice, this means that solvation effects become increasingly important in highly charged systems, which has implications for the stability of biomolecular structures, as demonstrated here, but also for synthetic supramolecular assemblies.

The computational results shown above demonstrate that the binding of multiple alkali metal cations to a G-quadruplex does not alter the affinity order nor the absolute binding strength. However, the mutual cation repulsion can influence their precise location within the GQ cavity [86], in particular for the smaller cations (e.g., Li⁺ and Na⁺) that can move more easily within the central channel [109–112].

4 G-QUADRUPLEXES AND POLLUTION METALS

Although the alkali metal cations Na⁺ and K⁺ bind to G-quadruplexes under physiological conditions, chronic or acute exposure to pollution metals is a threat to human health as the cations of these elements can bind strongly to G-quadruplex structures [113–115] thereby causing genomic instability [116–118]. Examples of such pollution metal cations are the divalent cations of cadmium (Cd²⁺), mercury (Hg²⁺), and lead (Pb²⁺) which represent some of the most widespread heavy metal pollutants [116]. Although it is well established that divalent metal cations (i.e., ionic charge of +2) generally bind G-quadruplexes more strongly than monovalent cations (i.e., ionic charge of +1) [1, 119, 120], their relative binding strength had for a long time no experimental consensus nor a fully understood theoretical explanation [121–127].

In a recent computational study [34], the affinity of G-quadruplex DNA toward divalent cations was examined using DFT-D computations at the ZORA-BLYP-D3(BJ)/TZ2P level with COSMO to simulate aqueous solvation. They analyzed the interaction of G-quadruplexes with divalent cations of alkaline earth metals (Group 2: Mg²⁺, Ca²⁺, Sr²⁺, and Ba²⁺), Group 12 metals (Zn²⁺, Cd²⁺, and Hg²⁺), and a post-transition metal (Group 14: Pb²⁺) relative to the monovalent alkali metal cations (Group 1: Li⁺, Na⁺, K⁺, and Rb⁺). By computing the bond energies ΔE_{bond} (recall Figure 7) of the various metal cations binding to the internal channel site of double-layered G-quadruplexes it was observed that divalent cations generally bind to the GQ cavity more strongly than monovalent alkali metal cations of Group 1 (Table 3). This demonstrates that most of the divalent (pollution) metal cations can potentially displace K⁺ and Na⁺ *in vivo* and can induce genotoxic effects by perturbation of telomeric and promoter regions of the genome.

To pinpoint what factors contribute to the higher affinity of G-quadruplex DNA toward divalent cations, ΔE_{bond} was partitioned within the framework of the ASM of reactivity and bonding (see Figure 7 for the partition scheme and Table 3 for the results).

The bond energy ΔE_{bond}, that is the cation affinity, results from the balance between a large stabilizing interaction energy (ΔE_{int}) and a large destabilizing overall desolvation ($\Delta E_{desolv} + \Delta E_{solv}$). Although the strain energy (ΔE_{strain}) varies relatively minorly for the various cations, smaller ions induce a more shrinkage of the cavity upon coordination thereby demanding a higher deformation strain. Furthermore, smaller cations face a more destabilizing desolvation energy, but can simultaneously induce more favorable interactions with the GQ interior. Overall, this leads among the studied metal cations to an optimum and thus the highest affinity for K⁺ (Group 1), Sr²⁺ (Group 2), Hg²⁺ (Group 12), and Pb²⁺ (Group 14), with ΔE_{bond} values of −53.2, −69.3, −71.1, and −74.2 kcal mol⁻¹, respectively. Compared to the monovalent alkali cations, the divalent cations bind more

TABLE 3
Partitioning of the Bond Energy ΔE_{bond} (in kcal mol⁻¹) of Metal Cation M^{n+} Coordination to the Internal Channel Site of a Double-Layered G-Quadruplex[a, b]

Group	M^{n+}	ΔE_{bond}	ΔE_{desolv}	ΔE_{strain}	ΔE_{int}	ΔE_{solv}	$\Delta E_{desolv}+\Delta E_{solv}$
1	Li⁺	−37.9	251.8	11.3	−165.7	−135.2	116.5
1	Na⁺	−52.2	225.8	10.4	−156.6	−131.8	94.0
1	K⁺	−53.2	208.1	5.7	−134.7	−132.2	75.9
1	Rb⁺	−48.8	204.0	0.9	−119.1	−134.6	69.4
2	Mg²⁺	−44.4	575.3	22.0	−441.4	−200.4	375.0
2	Ca²⁺	−69.1	497.8	28.7	−421.4	−174.2	323.7
2	Sr²⁺	−69.3	467.8	17.3	−377.5	−177.0	290.9
2	Ba²⁺	−68.2	436.8	14.4	−345.7	−173.7	263.1
12	Zn²⁺	−59.0	605.0	22.0	−491.4	−194.6	410.4
12	Cd²⁺	−56.7	557.0	22.3	−461.4	−174.6	382.4
12	Hg²⁺	−71.1	557.4	17.8	−471.4	−174.9	382.5
14	Pb²⁺	−74.2	478.0	13.5	−388.7	−177.0	301.0

[a] Computed at COSMO(H₂O)-ZORA-BLYP-D3(BJ)/TZ2P.
[b] Data taken from Refs. [34, 49].

strongly (i.e., more stabilizing ΔE_{bond}) to the central G-quadruplex channel. With ΔE_{strain} and $\Delta E_{desolv}+\Delta E_{solv}$ becoming more destabilizing for the divalent cations, this enhanced affinity originates entirely from the more stabilizing interactions (ΔE_{int}) they induce.

The interaction of G-quadruplex DNA with divalent cations is more stabilizing compared to monovalent cations as the former can participate in more stabilizing electrostatic (ΔV_{elstat}) and orbital interactions (ΔE_{oi}), as follows from the results of the energy decomposition analysis (EDA) in Table 4. The Pauli repulsion (ΔE_{Pauli}) and dispersion energy (ΔE_{disp}) do not contribute to the more stabilizing interaction of the GQ cavity with the divalent ions, as ΔE_{Pauli} becomes more *destabilizing* and ΔE_{disp} changes barely when switching from M^+ to M^{2+}. The enhanced ΔV_{elstat} can be rationalized by the increased ionic charge from +1 to +2, where the double positively charged metal nuclei will interact more strongly with the partially negatively charged carbonyl oxygen atoms in the G-quadruplex cavity. The source of the more stabilizing ΔE_{oi} was traced through a Kohn–Sham MO analysis of a representative model system that was generated by replacing the guanine residues in the GQ–M^{n+} complex with formaldehyde molecules in which the C=O coordinates are fixed in the geometry of the original GQ–M^{n+} complex (see Figure 10a for a representative example).

By computation of the metal cation virtual atomic orbital (that is, LUMO) energies and the corresponding gross Mulliken populations (i.e., a measure for the number of electrons donated to a specific orbital), it was found that the *s*, *p*, and *d* LUMOs of the metal cations are all involved in donor–acceptor interactions

TABLE 4
Energy Decomposition Analysis of the Interaction Energy ΔE_{int} (in kcal mol^{-1}) between Metal Cations M^{n+} and the Internal Channel Site of a Double-Layered G-Quadruplex[a,b]

Group	M^{n+}	ΔE_{int}	ΔE_{Pauli}	ΔV_{elstat}	ΔE_{oi}	ΔE_{disp}
1	Li$^+$	−165.7	13.2	−112.8	−58.3	−7.7
1	Na$^+$	−156.6	11.1	−109.3	−45.2	−13.2
1	K$^+$	−134.7	29.9	−106.2	−43.2	−15.2
1	Rb$^+$	−119.1	35.2	−97.1	−40.9	−16.5
2	Mg^{2+}	−442.2	46.9	−246.9	−230.0	−12.2
2	Ca^{2+}	−421.4	57.2	−250.9	−209.1	−18.7
2	Sr^{2+}	−377.6	75.5	−240.3	−192.1	−20.6
2	Ba^{2+}	−345.8	98.3	−240.0	−181.0	−23.6
12	Zn^{2+}	−491.5	80.0	−282.8	−276.1	−12.7
12	Cd^{2+}	−461.5	50.6	−256.3	−233.8	−22.0
12	Hg^{2+}	−468.8	56.7	−251.9	−251.0	−22.5
14	Pb^{2+}	−388.7	97.3	−245.8	−211.4	−28.8

[a] Computed at ZORA-BLYP-D3(BJ)/TZ2P.
[b] Data taken from Refs. [34, 49].

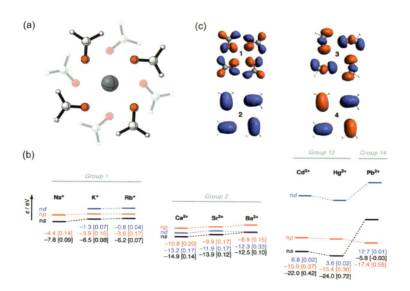

FIGURE 10 (a) Carbonyl oxygen atoms of the formaldehyde model system interacting with Pb^{2+}. (b) Metal cation M^{n+} s, p, and d LUMO energy levels (in eV), and gross Mulliken populations (in electrons between brackets) resulting from the interaction with the formaldehyde cavity, computed at ZORA-BLYP-D3(BJ)/DZ. (c) Examples of HOMOs (isosurfaces at 0.03 a.u.) of one layer of the formaldehyde model system that are involved in the interaction with the metal s, p, and d LUMOs. (Data taken from Ref. [34].)

upon coordination to the G-quadruplex internal channel site (Figure 10b). From this analysis, it became evident that compared to the monovalent cations of Group 1, the metal cation LUMOs are lowered in energy for the divalent alkaline earth metal cations (Group 2) and even further for the (post-)transition metal cations (Group 12 and 14). This orbital energy lowering is coherent with the higher ionic charge and the increasing electronegativity along this trend in the Periodic Table. The low-energy LUMOs of Group 2, 12, and 14 can accept more readily electronic density from the G-quadruplex, reflected by their higher gross Mulliken populations, thereby leading to more stabilizing orbital interactions compared to the Group 1 alkali metal cations.

Figure 10b also shows that the s, p, and d unoccupied orbitals of Group 1 and 2 metal cations are all involved in donor–acceptor interactions with the occupied orbitals of the carbonyl cavity (see the gross populations), but only the s and p LUMOs of Cd^{2+} and Hg^{2+} of Group 12 are populated, as the unoccupied d orbitals are too high in energy to accept a significant number of electrons. For Group 14 Pb^{2+}, only the p level is populated, with the highly destabilized s and d levels playing no significant role in the cation coordination to the GQ cavity.

The reason why the s, p, and d unoccupied atomic orbitals can all engage in donor–acceptor interactions is that the HOMOs of the formaldehyde monomers form different in-phase and out-of-phase combinations (see Figure 10c for examples), which allows the formation of both σ and π-type bonds between the cavity and the cation. These lone-pair-like HOMOs with a large coefficient on the carbonylic oxygen atoms make up the key electron-donating orbitals to interact with the metal cations since they have sufficient overlap with the M^{n+} LUMOs. For example, HOMO number 1 in Figure 10c has all the filled formaldehyde orbitals in phase in the central cavity, which makes it a suitable partner for overlapping with the spherical s orbitals of a metal cation. This concept can be extended to stacks of quartets where the carbonyl-localized HOMOs of the guanine residues make bonding and antibonding combinations that are either suitable for orbital interactions with s, p, or d metal LUMOs.

These computational results reveal the bonding mechanisms of metal cations to G-quadruplexes and explain the experimental observation that divalent cations, especially Hg^{2+} and Pb^{2+}, induce the formation of G-quadruplexes and coordinate with high affinities to the central cavity, possibly leading to the irreversible displacement of K^+ and Na^+ *in vivo* and thus to genotoxic effects.

5 GENERAL CONCLUSIONS

G-quadruplexes are non-canonical nucleic acid structures that form in guanine-rich regions of the genome and are involved in several vital cellular processes at the DNA and RNA levels. The understanding of the mechanisms leading to the self-assembly of G-quadruplexes and their stabilization by metal ions represents an active field in chemistry. Over the years, it has become evident that this field requires synergy between experimental and theoretical studies and that quantum chemical methods are essential in the accurate description of the interactions within G-quadruplexes and their interactions with metal ions and molecules.

This chapter outlines some of the available state-of-the-art quantum chemical theories and computational methods based on DFT computations and provides a balanced set of examples of how these methods can be used to tackle experimental questions and phenomena regarding the structure and stability of G-quadruplexes and their interactions with metal ions.

We want to emphasize that the exploration of these quantum chemical computational methods is not limited to studying G-quadruplexes and the interaction with metal ions but has also shown to be a helpful tool in the analysis of other classes of nucleic acid structures, such as B-DNA [128–131]. As such, quantum chemical analyses can be employed to answer a wide scope of biochemical questions related to the structure and function of biomolecules, which highlights the growing importance of the application of quantum chemical computations in the field of pharmaceutical and medicinal chemistry.

ACKNOWLEDGMENTS

The authors acknowledge the financial support of the Netherlands Organization for Scientific Research (NWO). Molecular structures in this chapter are visualized using ChemDraw21.0.0 (schematic structures) and CYLview20 (ball-and-stick structures).

ABBREVIATIONS AND DEFINITIONS

$\Delta E_{assemble}$	energy of assembly of the empty G-quadruplex scaffold
ΔE_{bond}	cation bond energy
ΔE_{disp}	dispersion energy
ΔE_{form}	energy of formation
ΔE_{int}	interaction energy
ΔE_{oi}	orbital interaction energy
ΔE_{Pauli}	Pauli repulsion energy
ΔE_{strain}	strain energy
ΔG_{form}	Gibbs free energy of formation
ΔQ	change in VDD atomic charge
ΔV_{elstat}	electrostatic interaction
ADF	Amsterdam Density Functional (program)
aq	aqueous solution
ASA	activation strain analysis
ASM	activation strain model
BJ	Becke–Johnson damping
BLYP	Becke exchange/Lee-Yang-Parr correlation functional
COSMO	conductor-like screening model
D3	Grimme's D3 dispersion correction
DFT	density functional theory

DFT-D	dispersion-corrected density functional theory
DNA	deoxyribonucleic acid
DZ	double-ζ (basis set)
DZP	double-ζ + one polarization function (basis set)
EDA	energy decomposition analysis
G	guanine
G$_2$	guanine dimer
G$_3$	guanine trimer
G$_4$	guanine quartet
gas	gas phase
GG	guanosine dimer
GQ–[ ]	empty G-quadruplexes scaffold
GQ–M^{n+}	G-quadruplex hosting a metal cation M^{n+} with charge $n+$
GQ(s)	guanine quadruplex(es)
HOMO	highest occupied molecular orbital
Irrep	irreducible representation
LUMO	lowest unoccupied molecular orbital
M$^+$	monovalent (alkali) metal cation
M^{2+}	divalent metal cation
MD	molecular dynamics
MM	molecular mechanics
MO	molecular orbital
Q	VDD atomic charge
QM	quantum mechanics
RAHB	resonance-assisted hydrogen bonding
RNA	ribonucleic acid
TZ2P	triple-ζ+two polarization functions (basis set)
TZP	triple-ζ+one polarization function (basis set)
VDD	Voronoi deformation density
ZORA	zeroth-order regular approximation

REFERENCES

1. S. Neidle, S. Balasubramanian, in *Quadruplex Nucleic Acids*, Royal Society of Chemistry, Cambridge, **2006**.
2. D. Rhodes, H. J. Lipps, *Nucleic Acids Res.* **2015**, *43*, 8627–8637.
3. J. Xu, H. Huang, X. Zhou, *JACS Au* **2021**, *1*, 2146–2161.
4. S. Balasubramanian, S. Neidle, *Curr. Opin. Chem. Biol.* **2009**, *13*, 345–353.
5. S. Neidle, in *Therapeutic Applications of Quadruplex Nucleic Acids*, Elsevier Academic Press, **2011**.
6. T. Hagen, A. Laski, A. Brü, A. Pruš, V. Schlösser, A. Cléry, F. H.-T. Allain, R. Zenobi, S. Bergmann, J. Hall, *J. Am. Chem. Soc.* **2021**, *143*, 15120–15130.
7. R. Guha, D. Defayay, A. Hepp, J. Müller, *ChemPlusChem* **2021**, *86*, 662–673.
8. A. Schmidt, R. Guha, A. Hepp, J. Müller, *J. Inorg. Biochem.* **2017**, *175*, 58–66.
9. I. Pont, Á. Martínez-Camarena, C. Galiana-Roselló, R. Tejero, M. T. Albelda, J. González-García, R. Vilar, E. García-España, *ChemBioChem* **2020**, *21*, 1167–1177.

10. C. L. Ruehl, A. H. M. Lim, T. Kench, D. J. Mann, R. Vilar, *Chem. Eur. J.* **2019**, *25*, 9691–9700.
11. Á. Sánchez-González, N. A. G. Bandeira, I. O. de Luzuriaga, F. F. Martins, S. Elleuchi, K. Jarraya, J. Lanuza, X. Lopez, M. J. Calhorda, A. Gil, *Molecules* **2021**, *26*, 4737.
12. S. Neidle, *Pharmaceuticals* **2021**, *15*, 7.
13. R. Bonsignore, A. Terenzi, A. Spinello, A. Martorana, A. Lauria, A. M. Almerico, B. K. Keppler, G. Barone, *J. Inorg. Biochem.* **2016**, *161*, 115–121.
14. R. Bonsignore, F. Russo, A. Terenzi, A. Spinello, A. Lauria, G. Gennaro, A. M. Almerico, B. K. Keppler, G. Barone, *J. Inorg. Biochem.* **2018**, *178*, 106–114.
15. G. Farine, C. Migliore, A. Terenzi, F. Lo Celso, A. Santoro, G. Bruno, R. Bonsignore, G. Barone, *Eur. J. Inorg. Chem.* **2021**, *2021*, 1332–1336.
16. A. Terenzi, H. Gattuso, A. Spinello, B. K. Keppler, C. Chipot, F. Dehez, G. Barone, A. Monari, *Antioxidants* **2019**, *8*, 472.
17. S. Naskar, R. Guha, J. Müller, *Angew. Chem. Int. Ed.* **2020**, *59*, 1397–1406.
18. K. T. McQuaid, S. Takahashi, L. Baumgaertner, D. J. Cardin, N. G. Paterson, J. P. Hall, N. Sugimoto, C. J. Cardin, *J. Am. Chem. Soc.* **2022**, *144*, 5956–5964.
19. S.-H. Kang, K. M. Lee, S.-K. Cho, J. E. Lee, D. Won, S.-Y. Lee, S. K. Kwak, C. Yang, *ChemSusChem* **2022**, *15*, e202102201.
20. G. I. Livshits, A. Stern, D. Rotem, N. Borovok, G. Eidelshtein, A. Migliore, E. Penzo, S. J. Wind, R. Di Felice, S. S. Skourtis, J. Carlos Cuevas, L. Gurevich, A. B. Kotlyar, D. Porath, *Nat. Nanotechnol.* **2014**, *9*, 1040–1046.
21. S. Xu, X. Chen, G. Peng, L. Jiang, H. Huang, *Anal. Bioanal. Chem.* **2018**, *410*, 5879–5887.
22. H. Yang, Y. Zhou, J. Liu, *Trends Anal. Chem.* **2020**, *132*, 116060.
23. M. Nishio, K. Tsukakoshi, K. Ikebukuro, *Biosens. Bioelectron.* **2021**, *178*, 113030.
24. T. van der Wijst, C. Fonseca Guerra, M. Swart, F. M. Bickelhaupt, B. Lippert, *Angew. Chem. Int. Ed.* **2009**, *48*, 3285–3287.
25. N. Busto, P. Calvo, J. Santolaya, J. M. Leal, A. Guédin, G. Barone, T. Torroba, J. L. Mergny, B. García, *Chem. Eur. J.* **2018**, *24*, 11292–11296.
26. I. Ortiz De Luzuriaga, X. Lopez, A. Gil, *Annu. Rev. Biophys.* **2021**, *50*, 209–243.
27. S. Roy, A. Ali, S. Bhattacharya, *J. Phys. Chem. B* **2021**, *125*, 5489–5501.
28. S. Pal, S. Paul, *J. Phys. Chem. B* **2020**, *124*, 3123–3136.
29. J. Šponer, A. Mládek, N. Špačková, X. Cang, T. E. Cheatham, III, S. Grimme, *J. Am. Chem. Soc.* **2013**, *135*, 9785–9796.
30. M. Krepl, M. Zgarbová, P. Stadlbauer, M. Otyepka, P. Banáš, J. Koča, T. E. Cheatham, III, P. Jurečka, J. Šponer, *J. Chem. Theory Comput.* **2012**, *8*, 2506–2520.
31. K. Gkionis, H. Kruse, J. Šponer, *J. Chem. Theory Comput.* **2016**, *12*, 2000–2016.
32. K. Gkionis, H. Kruse, J. A. Platts, A. Mládek, J. Koča, J. Šponer, *J. Chem. Theory Comput.* **2014**, *10*, 1326–1340.
33. C. Nieuwland, F. Zaccaria, C. Fonseca Guerra, *Phys. Chem. Chem. Phys.* **2020**, *22*, 21108–21118.
34. F. Zaccaria, S. C. C. van der Lubbe, C. Nieuwland, T. A. Hamlin, C. Fonseca Guerra, *ChemPhysChem* **2021**, *22*, 2286–2296.
35. I. Ortiz de Luzuriaga, S. Elleuchi, K. Jarraya, E. Artacho, X. Lopez, A. Gil, *Phys. Chem. Chem. Phys.* **2022**, *24*, 11510–11519.
36. G. te Velde, F. M. Bickelhaupt, E. J. Baerends, C. Fonseca Guerra, S. J. A. van Gisbergen, J. G. Snijders, T. Ziegler, *J. Comput. Chem.* **2001**, *22*, 931–967.
37. C. Fonseca Guerra, J. G. Snijders, G. te Velde, E. J. Baerends, *Theor. Chem. Acc.* **1998**, *99*, 391–403.

38. *ADF*, SCM, Theoretical Chemistry, Vrije Universiteit, Amsterdam, The Netherlands, www.scm.com.
39. E. van Lenthe, A. Ehlers, E.-J. Baerends, *J. Chem. Phys.* **1999**, *110*, 8943–8953.
40. A. D. Becke, *Phys. Rev. A* **1988**, *38*, 3100.
41. C. Lee, W. Yang, R. G. Parr, *Phys. Rev. B* **1988**, *37*, 789.
42. S. Grimme, *J. Comput. Chem.* **2004**, *25*, 1463–1473.
43. S. Grimme, *J. Comput. Chem.* **2006**, *27*, 1787–1799.
44. S. Grimme, S. Ehrlich, L. Goerigk, *J. Comput. Chem.* **2011**, *32*, 1456–1465.
45. E. van Lenthe, E. J. Baerends, *J. Comput. Chem.* **2003**, *24*, 1142–1156.
46. A. Klamt, G. Schüürmann, *J. Chem. Soc., Perkin Trans. 2* **1993**, 799–805.
47. A. Klamt, *J. Phys. Chem.* **1995**, *99*, 2224–2235.
48. C. C. Pye, T. Ziegler, *Theor. Chem. Acc.* **1999**, *101*, 396–408.
49. F. Zaccaria, G. Paragi, C. Fonseca Guerra, *Phys. Chem. Chem. Phys.* **2016**, *18*, 20895–20904.
50. C. Fonseca Guerra, T. van der Wijst, J. Poater, M. Swart, F. M. Bickelhaupt, *Theor. Chem. Acc.* **2010**, *125*, 245–252.
51. N. Mardirossian, M. Head-Gordon, *Mol. Phys.* **2017**, *115*, 2315–2372.
52. R. Sedlak, T. Janowski, M. Pitoňák, J. Řezáč, P. Pulay, P. Hobza, *J. Chem. Theory Comput.* **2013**, *9*, 3364–3374.
53. P. Vermeeren, S. C. C. van der Lubbe, C. Fonseca Guerra, F. M. Bickelhaupt, T. A. Hamlin, *Nat. Protoc.* **2020**, *15*, 649–667.
54. F. M. Bickelhaupt, K. N. Houk, *Angew. Chem. Int. Ed.* **2017**, *56*, 10070–10086.
55. F. M. Bickelhaupt, E. J. Baerends, *Rev. Comput. Chem.* **2000**, *15*, 1–86.
56. T. A. Hamlin, P. Vermeeren, C. Fonseca Guerra, F. M. Bickelhaupt, in *Complementary Bonding Analyses*, Ed S. Grabowsky, De Gruyter, Berlin, **2021**, pp. 199–212.
57. A. Heßelmann, G. Jansen, M. Schütz, *J. Chem. Phys.* **2004**, *122*, 014103.
58. M. Ernst, G. Gryn'ova, *ChemPhysChem* **2022**, *23*, e202200098.
59. O. A. Stasyuk, R. Sedlak, C. Fonseca Guerra, P. Hobza, *J. Chem. Theory Comput.* **2018**, *14*, 3440–3450.
60. C. Fonseca Guerra, J.-W. Handgraaf, E. J. Baerends, F. M. Bickelhaupt, *J. Comput. Chem.* **2004**, *25*, 189–210.
61. O. A. Stasyuk, H. Szatylowicz, T. M. Krygowski, C. Fonseca Guerra, *Phys. Chem. Chem. Phys.* **2016**, *18*, 11624–11633.
62. D. A. Megger, P. M. Lax, J. Paauwe, C. Fonseca Guerra, B. Lippert, *J. Biol. Inorg. Chem.* **2018**, *23*, 41–49.
63. L. P. Wolters, N. W. G. Smits, C. Fonseca Guerra, *Phys. Chem. Chem. Phys.* **2015**, *17*, 1585–1592.
64. V. V. Cheong, C. J. Lech, B. Heddi, A. T. Phan, *Angew. Chem. Int. Ed.* **2016**, *55*, 160–163.
65. V. V. Cheong, B. Heddi, C. J. Lech, A. T. Phan, *Nucleic Acids Res.* **2015**, *43*, 10506–10514.
66. R. V. Brown, T. Wang, V. R. Chappeta, G. Wu, B. Onel, R. Chawla, H. Quijada, S. M. Camp, E. T. Chiang, Q. R. Lassiter, C. Lee, S. Phanse, M. A. Turnidge, P. Zhao, J. G. N. Garcia, V. Gokhale, D. Yang, L. H. Hurley, *J. Am. Chem. Soc.* **2017**, *139*, 7456–7475.
67. B. Heddi, N. Martín-Pintado, Z. Serimbetov, T. M. A. Kari, A. T. Phan, *Nucleic Acids Res.* **2016**, *44*, 910–916.
68. C. Fonseca Guerra, F. M. Bickelhaupt, J. G. Snijders, E. J. Baerends, *Chem. Eur. J.* **1999**, *5*, 3581–3594.

69. C. Fonseca Guerra, F. M. Bickelhaupt, J. G. Snijders, E. J. Baerends, *J. Am. Chem. Soc.* **2000**, *122*, 4117–4128.
70. P. Gilli, V. Bertolasi, V. Ferretti, G. Gilli, *J. Am. Chem. Soc.* **2000**, *122*, 10405–10417.
71. G. Gilli, F. Bellucci, V. Ferretti, V. Bertolasi, *J. Am. Chem. Soc.* **1989**, *111*, 1023–1028.
72. Eds A. D. McNaught, A. Wilkinson, *IUPAC. Compendium of Chemical Terminology (the "GoldBook")*, Blackwell Scientific Publications, Oxford, **1997**.
73. S. C. C. van der Lubbe, C. Fonseca Guerra, *Chem. Asian J.* **2019**, *14*, 2760–2769.
74. C. Nieuwland, C. Fonseca Guerra, *Chem. Eur. J.* **2022**, e202200755.
75. C. Fonseca Guerra, H. Zijlstra, G. Paragi, F. M. Bickelhaupt, *Chem. Eur. J.* **2011**, *17*, 12612–12622.
76. R. Kurczab, M. P. Mitoraj, A. Michalak, T. Ziegler, *J. Phys. Chem. A* **2010**, *114*, 8581–8590.
77. R. Otero, M. Schöck, L. M. Molina, E. Lægsgaard, I. Stensgaard, B. Hammer, F. Besenbacher, *Angew. Chem. Int. Ed.* **2005**, *44*, 2270–2275.
78. A. Taylor, J. Taylor, G. W. Watson, R. J. Boyd, *J. Phys. Chem. B* **2010**, *114*, 9833–9839.
79. M. Martín-Arroyo, A. del Prado, R. Chamorro, N. Bilbao, D. González-Rodríguez, *Angew. Chem. Int. Ed.* **2020**, *59*, 9041–9046.
80. T. van Mourik, A. J. Dingley, *J. Phys. Chem. A* **2007**, *111*, 11350–11358.
81. G. Vantomme, G. M. Ter Huurne, C. Kulkarni, H. M. M. Ten Eikelder, A. J. Markvoort, A. R. A. Palmans, E. W. Meijer, *J. Am. Chem. Soc.* **2019**, *141*, 18278–18285.
82. L. de Azevedo Santos, D. Cesario, P. Vermeeren, S. C. C. van der Lubbe, F. Nunzi, C. Fonseca Guerra, *ChemPlusChem* **2022**, *87*, e202100436.
83. C. Kulkarni, E. W. Meijer, A. R. A. Palmans, *Acc. Chem. Res.* **2017**, *50*, 1928–1936.
84. D. Serrano-Molina, C. Montoro-García, M. J. Mayoral, A. de Juan, D. González-Rodríguez, *J. Am. Chem. Soc.* **2022**, *144*, 5450–5460.
85. Y. P. Yurenko, J. Novotný, R. Marek, *Chem. Eur. J.* **2017**, *23*, 5573–5584.
86. E. Largy, J.-L. Mergny, V. Gabelica, Vol. 16 of *The Alkali Metal Ions: Their Role for Life. Metal Ions in Life Sciences*, Eds A. Sigel, H. Sigel, R. K. O. Sigel, Springer, Cham, **2016**, pp. 203–258.
87. H. L. Lightfoot, T. Hagen, N. J. Tatum, J. Hall, *FEBS Lett.* **2019**, *593*, 2083–2102.
88. A. Joachimi, A. Benz, J. S. Hartig, *Bioorg. Med. Chem.* **2009**, *17*, 6811–6815.
89. K. Halder, J. S. Hartig, Vol. 9 of *Structural and Catalytic Roles of Metal Ions in RNA. Metal Ions in Life Sciences*, Eds A. Sigel, H. Sigel, R. K. O. Sigel, **2011**, pp. 125–139.
90. C. J. Lech, B. Heddi, A. T. Phan, *Nucleic Acids Res.* **2013**, *41*, 2034–2046.
91. E. Largy, A. Marchand, S. Amrane, V. V. Gabelica, J.-L. Mergny, *J. Am. Chem. Soc.* **2016**, *138*, 2780–2792.
92. J. Chen, M. Cheng, G. F. Salgado, P. Stadlbauer, X. Zhang, S. Amrane, A. Guédin, F. He, J. Šponer, H. Ju, J. L. Mergny, J. Zhou, *Nucleic Acids Res.* **2021**, *49*, 9548–9559.
93. F. Zaccaria, C. Fonseca Guerra, *Chem. Eur. J.* **2018**, *24*, 16315–16322.
94. A. Arora, S. Maiti, *J. Phys. Chem. B* **2009**, *113*, 10515–10520.
95. C. M. Olsen, L. A. Marky, *J. Phys. Chem. B* **2009**, *113*, 9–11.
96. B. Pagano, C. A. Mattia, L. Cavallo, S. Uesugi, C. Giancola, F. Fraternali, *J. Phys. Chem. B* **2008**, *112*, 12115–12123.
97. J. T. Davis, *Angew. Chem. Int. Ed.* **2004**, *43*, 668–698.
98. G. Gottarelli, S. Masiero, E. Mezzina, G. P. Spada, P. Mariani, M. Recanatini, *Helv. Chim. Acta* **1998**, *81*, 2078–2092.

99. T. Miclot, C. Corbier, A. Terenzi, C. Hognon, S. Grandemange, G. Barone, A. Monari, *Chem. Eur. J.* **2021**, *27*, 8865–8874.
100. C. Hognon, A. Gebus, G. Barone, A. Monari, *Antioxidants* **2019**, *8*, 337.
101. W. Xu, Q. Tan, M. Yu, Q. Sun, H. Kong, E. Lægsgaard, I. Stensgaard, J. Kjems, J. G. Wang, C. Wang, F. Besenbacher, *Chem. Commun.* **2013**, *49*, 7210–7212.
102. A. Wong, G. Wu, *J. Am. Chem. Soc.* **2003**, *125*, 13895–13905.
103. C. Detellier, P. Laszlo, *J. Am. Chem. Soc.* **1980**, *102*, 1135–1141.
104. T. J. Pinnavaia, C. L. Marshall, C. M. Mettler, C. L. Fisk, H. T. Miles, E. D. Becker, *J. Am. Chem. Soc.* **1978**, *100*, 3625–3627.
105. R. Ida, G. Wu, *J. Am. Chem. Soc.* **2008**, *130*, 3590–3602.
106. J. R. Williamson, M. K. Raghuraman, T. R. Cech, *Cell* **1989**, *59*, 871–880.
107. N. V. Hud, F. W. Smith, F. A. L. Anet, J. Feigon, *Biochemistry* **1996**, *35*, 15383–15390.
108. J. Gu, J. Leszczynski, *J. Phys. Chem. A.* **2002**, *106*, 529–532.
109. G. Villani, *ACS Omega* **2018**, *3*, 9934–9944.
110. G. Villani, *New J. Chem.* **2017**, *41*, 2574–2585.
111. T. van Mourik, A. J. Dingley, *Chem. Eur. J.* **2005**, *11*, 6064–6079.
112. S. Balasubramanian, S. Senapati, *J. Phys. Chem. B* **2020**, *124*, 11055–11066.
113. I. V Smirnov, F. W. Kotch, I. J. Pickering, J. T. Davis, R. H. Shafer, *Biochemistry* **2002**, *41*, 12133–12139.
114. Y. Wu, Y. Shi, S. Deng, C. Wu, R. Deng, G. He, M. Zhou, K. Zhong, H. Gao, *Food Chem.* **2021**, *343*, 128425.
115. V. G. Kanellis, C. G. dos Remedios, *Biophys. Rev.* **2018**, *10*, 1414.
116. T. C. Hutchinson, K. M. Meema, *Lead, Mercury, Cadmium, and Arsenic in the Environment*, John Wiley and Sons, Chichester, **1987**.
117. N. Coen, C. Mothersill, M. Kadhim, E. G. Wright, *J. Pathol.* **2001**, *195*, 293–299.
118. V. I. Mitkovska, H. A. Dimitrov, T. G. Chassovnikarova, *Ecotoxicol. Environ. Saf.* **2020**, *194*, 110413.
119. A. Włodarczyk, P. Grzybowski, A. Patkowski, A. Dobek, *J. Phys. Chem. B* **2005**, *109*, 3594–3605.
120. J. S. Lee, *Nucleic Acids Res.* **1990**, *18*, 6060.
121. C. C. Hardin, T. Watson, M. Corregan, C. Bailey, *Biochemistry* **1992**, *31*, 833–841.
122. E. A. Venczel, D. Sen, *Biochemistry* **1993**, *32*, 6220–6228.
123. J. A. Mondragón-Sánchez, J. Liquier, R. H. Shafer, E. Taillandier, *J. Biomol. Struct. Dyn.* **2004**, *22*, 365–373.
124. H. Guiset Miserachs, D. Donghi, R. Börner, S. Johannsen, R. K. O. Sigel, *J. Biol. Inorg. Chem.* **2016**, *21*, 975–986.
125. B. I. Kankia, L. A. Marky, *J. Am. Chem. Soc.* **2001**, *123*, 10799–10804.
126. S. Pal, S. Paul, *Int. J. Biol. Macromol.* **2019**, *121*, 350–363.
127. X. Li, A. Sánchez-Ferrer, M. Bagnani, J. Adamcik, P. Azzari, J. Hao, A. Song, H. Liu, R. Mezzenga, *Proc. Natl. Acad. Sci. U. S. A.* **2020**, *117*, 9832–9839.
128. G. Barone, C. Fonseca Guerra, F. M. Bickelhaupt, *ChemistryOpen* **2013**, *2*, 186–193.
129. C. Nieuwland, T. A. Hamlin, C. Fonseca Guerra, G. Barone, F. M. Bickelhaupt, *ChemistryOpen* **2022**, *11*, e202100231.
130. T. A. Hamlin, J. Poater, C. Fonseca Guerra, F. M. Bickelhaupt, *Phys. Chem. Chem. Phys.* **2017**, *19*, 16969–16978.
131. M. A. Van Bochove, G. Roos, C. Fonseca Guerra, T. A. Hamlin, F. M. Bickelhaupt, *Chem. Commun.* **2018**, *54*, 3448–3451.
132. M. Meier, A. Moya-Torres, N. J. Krahn, M. D. McDougall, G. L. Orriss, E. K. S. McRae, E. P. Booy, K. McEleney, T. R. Patel, S. A. McKenna, J. Stetefeld, *Nucleic Acids Res.* **2018**, *46*, 5319–5331.

14 Transition Metal-Binding G-Quadruplex DNA

*Lukas M. Stratmann and Guido H. Clever**
Department of Chemistry and Chemical Biology, TU Dortmund University, Otto-Hahn Str. 6, D-44227 Dortmund, Germany
lukas.stratmann@tu-dortmund.de,
guido.clever@tu-dortmund.de

CONTENTS

1	Introduction	374
	1.1 DNA G-Quadruplex Structures and Their Topological Diversity	374
	1.2 Biological Relevance of G-Quadruplexes	376
	1.3 G-Quadruplex Structural Motifs in DNA Nanotechnology	376
	1.4 Metal-Mediated Base Pairing in DNA	377
2	Transition Metal-Binding in Loop Regions of G-Quadruplexes	378
3	The Metal-Mediated Base Tetrad	380
	3.1 Metal-Mediated Base Tetrads in Tetramolecular G-Quadruplexes	380
	3.2 Metal-Mediated Base Tetrads in Unimolecular G-Quadruplexes	384
4	Fine-Tuned Coordination Environments in G-Quadruplexes	386
5	Transition Metal-Binding G-Quadruplexes in Catalysis	388
6	Cu(Pyridine)$_4$ Tetrads as Paramagnetic EPR Spin Labels	390
7	Conclusion and Future Prospects	393
Acknowledgment		394
Abbreviations		394
References		395

ABSTRACT

G-quadruplexes represent an important class of nucleic acid secondary structures. They are formed by guanine-rich sequences and are composed of π-stacked tetrads of circularly hydrogen-bonded guanines. Since the recent discoveries proving their formation *in vivo*, G-quadruplexes are evidenced to have high biological relevance, for example in the regulation of key biological processes such as replication and transcription. Hence, G-quadruplexes have been identified as promising drug targets, especially in anticancer research.

---

* Corresponding author

DOI 10.1201/9781003270201-14

In addition, the G-quadruplex structural motif has frequently been exploited in the field of DNA nanotechnology as a useful complement to duplex DNA. A powerful strategy to incorporate new functionality into DNA assemblies for nanotechnological applications is the covalent implementation of transition metal complexes, acting as Lewis acids, redox-active centers, or stabilizing structural nodes. In this respect, much effort has been put into the development of metal-mediated base pairs, where suitable transition metal complexes substitute canonical Watson-Crick base pairs in duplex DNA.

In recent years, following a similar approach, G-quadruplexes have been decorated with covalently bound metal complexes. Typically, artificial ligand-carrying nucleobase surrogates, named 'ligandosides', are installed in DNA sequences via solid-phase oligonucleotide synthesis. Addition of metal ions results in metal complex formation which can be exploited to stabilize a particular secondary structure. In this way, stimuli-responsive control can be gained over G-quadruplex folding and unfolding, or over their adopted topology. Transition metal complexes attached to G-quadruplexes have additionally been used as catalytic centers in asymmetric catalysis or as a rigid paramagnetic spin labels for precise distance measurements in higher-order DNA structures such as non-covalent dimers and sandwiches. This chapter illustrates the approach of covalently incorporating transition metal complexes inside G-quadruplex motifs and gives an overview over recent developments in this field.

KEYWORDS

DNA; G-Quadruplex; Transition Metal; Stimuli-Responsive; DNAzyme; Spin Label; DNA Nanotechnology

1 INTRODUCTION

1.1 DNA G-Quadruplex Structures and Their Topological Diversity

The key function of DNA is the storage of genetic information in all living organisms, bearing the blueprints for protein biosynthesis. DNA itself is kept in the nucleus and mostly adopts the well-known double-helical structure, where two complementary oligonucleotides are connected *via* specific Watson-Crick base pairs. In the last decades, however, several additional secondary DNA structure types were discovered, such as hairpin and cruciform folds, three-way and four-way junctions, triple helices, i-motifs, and G-quadruplexes (G4s) [1]. The latter are four-stranded and formed from guanine-rich sequences. In each repetitive unit of this structural motif, four circularly arranged guanine residues interact with each other *via* Hoogsteen hydrogen bonding forming a planar G-tetrad (also named G-quartet). Several G-tetrads π-stack on top of each other, building a helical structure called G-quadruplex (Figure 1). Metal ions such as K^+ or Na^+ typically reside in a central channel between the stacked G-quartets to compensate the negative partial charges resulting from the inward-pointing carbonyl oxygen atoms [2].

G4s show a high structural diversity concerning G-tetrad count, type of stabilizing alkali metal ion, and number of involved DNA strands (i.e., uni-, bi-, tetramolecular structures). Furthermore, the folding of bi- and unimolecular

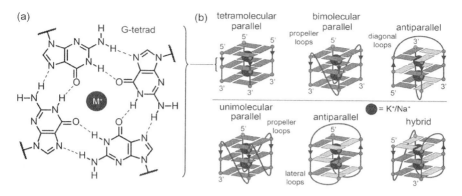

FIGURE 1 (a) Structure of a planar G-tetrad with Hoogsteen hydrogen bonding. (b) Examples of different G-quadruplex structures, including tetra-, bi-, and unimolecular constructs with parallel, antiparallel or hybrid topologies. Different loop motifs are indicated. The N-glycosidic bond conformations in the guanosine residues are denoted with dark gray (*anti*) or light gray (*syn*) tiles. These schematic illustrations allow a clear demonstration of different folding topologies. However, it should be kept in mind, that the structure's distinct (usually right-handed) helicity is omitted for clarity.

G4s results in loop regions which can differ in length, nucleobase composition, and connectivity (diagonal, lateral, and propeller shape, Figure 1b). Different loop arrangements lead to distinct directionalities of the four G-tracts in the G4 stem which can be parallel or antiparallel with respect to each other. As a direct consequence, the N-glycosidic bonds in the guanosine residues must adopt either *syn* or *anti* conformations dictated by the overall structural topology [3].

Often, a single oligonucleotide can adopt several G4 topologies of similar energy which coexist next to each other. Factors like nature and concentration of electrolyte, pH, DNA concentration and molecular crowding, cosolvents, or the presence of G4-binding small molecules or proteins can shift the equilibrium toward one topology or the other. For example, the extensively investigated htel sequence found in the human telomeres can adopt a parallel topology in the solid state [4] and several topologies in solution [5–7]. In addition, G4s tend to form higher-order structures like long G-wires [8] or simple dimers [9] interacting with each other via π-stacking of terminal G-tetrads.

To understand the biological relevance of G4 species, G4 structure elucidation is of high importance. This is a challenging task, though, due to the aforementioned structural diversity, tendency to form higher-order aggregates, and variety of interactions with G4 binders. Structural information with atomic resolution can be provided by X-ray diffraction (XRD) (in the solid state), NMR spectroscopy, and cryo-electron microscopy (cryo-EM) (in liquid or frozen solution, respectively). However, these methods are relatively time-consuming and have individual drawbacks. Complementary methods that give less direct atom-by-atom structural insight but still deliver precious information about properties such as thermal stability toward unfolding, number and type of bound metal cations, and to some extent the folding topology and glycosidic bond orientations include temperature-dependent UV-vis and circular dichroism (CD) spectroscopy, (ion mobility) mass spectrometry and gel electrophoresis.

1.2 Biological Relevance of G-Quadruplexes

In terms of biological relevance, recent studies showed that potential G4-forming sequences are positioned non-randomly in different genomes [10, 11]. Evidence for the G4 formation *in vivo* was obtained through specific antibody staining techniques [12]. For example, a large number of directly neighboring G4s is found in telomeric single-stranded overhangs at the end of chromosomes. They are involved both in the protection of the chromosomes from DNA-damage-response pathways and in the regulation of the telomere maintenance by the enzyme telomerase. Moreover, a significant number of usually isolated G4s is found in promoter regions of several onco- and tumor suppressor genes where they are thought to influence gene expression, e.g., by engaging in specific interactions with DNA-binding proteins, a field of study that is currently rapidly expanding [13].

Due to their regulatory roles in several biological processes, G4s have been identified as promising drug targets [14]. The stabilization of G4 structures leads for example to the inhibition of telomerase which is upregulated in most human cancers. Many small molecules [15] and transition metal complexes [16] have been found in recent years to bind and stabilize G4s, thereby acting as potential anticancer drugs. They are often positively charged and possess large π-surfaces suitable for π-stacking interactions with terminal G-tetrads. Important challenges are the selective binding of G4s with respect to other DNA structures as well as achieving selectivity for a specific G4 topology. Recently, also targeting strategies have been suggested that aim at specific destabilization of certain G4s in noncoding regulatory regions with respective downstream effects that are hoped to avoid problems concerning genome instability that can arise from the G4 stabilization approach [17, 18].

1.3 G-Quadruplex Structural Motifs in DNA Nanotechnology

Beyond their biological function, nucleic acids have been extensively used in the field of nanotechnology for the self-assembly of complex 2D and 3D architectures. Pioneered by Seeman [19–22] in the 1980s and significantly influenced by Rothemund in 2006 with the development of DNA origami [23], DNA nanotechnology has evolved into an influential branch of research. The unique molecular properties of DNA such as its highly predictable and programmable association and its remarkable binding specificity have been exploited for the design of nanodevices used for the transport of cargo, in molecular switches, machines, and more [24–27].

While most work in this area is based on the typical duplex DNA structure with canonical Watson-Crick base pairing, also other secondary structure types have been applied which often show lower susceptibility to enzymatic degradation, are less flexible or show a higher sensitivity to external chemical stimuli. Examples for the latter are the strong pH sensitivity of i-motifs and the alkali metal cation sensitivity of G-quadruplexes [28]. Hence, the G-quadruplex structural motif is frequently used in nanodevices such as switches [29–31], logic gates [32], and motors [33] as well as in materials such as supramolecular hydrogels [34–36] or catalytic DNA species (DNAzymes) [37–40]. Several sensors have been designed based on this secondary structure, which often benefit from well-established detection strategies revealing G-quadruplex formation [41–43]. One strategy applies G-quadruplex binders as fluorescent light-up probes upon binding to a terminal G-quartet [44–46]. A second strategy exploits the specific DNAzyme activity of a non-covalent hemin-G-quadruplex complex. Here, the π-stacking of hemin (an iron-porphyrin complex) onto an accessible G-tetrad results in a catalytic system that promotes peroxidase-like oxidation of different substrates in the presence of hydrogen peroxide [47–51]. The catalytic activity is exploited to generate a chromophore, thus giving an easily detectable readout indicating G-quadruplex formation.

1.4 METAL-MEDIATED BASE PAIRING IN DNA

Base pairing in natural DNA is conveyed by the specific hydrogen bonding patterns formed between the complementary nucleobases (A with T and G with C). The substitution of protons in hydrogen bonds between oligonucleotides by metal ions of suitable (linear) coordination geometry leading to an ordered duplex structure was demonstrated (at least) as early as 1980 by Eichhorn and coworkers, applying X-ray fiber diffraction methods, among others [52]. The authors also revealed the generation of a tetrastranded assembly of poly(I) in the presence of Ag^+ ions. In the early 2000s, the question arose whether hydrogen bonding is required at all within the π-stacked double-stranded assembly (leading to the field of hydrophobic base pairs [53, 54]) or whether it could be replaced by other dynamic interactions such as coordinate bonds to selected transition metals. This idea, shaped and extended by Tanaka, Shionoya, Schultz, Romesberg, Meggers, Ono, Carell, Müller, and others led to vibrant activity toward the development of nucleobase surrogates that pair via metal coordination within the stack of double-stranded DNA equipped with these base modifications by means of automated DNA solid phase synthesis. This research founded the field of DNA metal-mediated base pairing based on artificial ligands [55–59] (see also Chapter 11 in this book). Motivation for replacing hydrogen-bonded Watson–Crick base pairs came from several directions, including the quest for an expanded or alternative genetic alphabet [53], the desire to make base pairing stimuli-responsive [60], and the idea to use metal-containing DNA as an electron or hole conductor in DNA-based nanoelectronic devices [61].

Besides a wide variety of artificial base modifications developed to form metal-mediated base pairs in duplex DNA, also some natural nucleobases were found to be stabilized by specific coordinative interactions. Most prominently, the T–Hg–T base pair has been extensively investigated as a highly versatile motif containing solely canonical nucleobases as ligand functionalities. It was shown that duplexes bearing **TT** mismatches are highly stabilized upon the addition of Hg^{2+} ions due to the formation of **T–Hg–T** complexes inside the base pair stack of double-stranded DNA [62–65].

G-quadruplex DNA was not considered in terms of transition metal-base pairing in the above sketched early developments in this field. Only later, first attempts aimed at specifically incorporating transition metal cations within G4 constructs were reported. All examples discussed below, however, differ from most of the above-mentioned DNA double strands containing metal-base pairs in the fact that metal-base pairs in duplex DNA can often be designed to be flat and thus perfectly incorporate into the base stack of largely undisturbed B-type helical DNA. The design of a flat metal complex coordinated by four nucleobase surrogates that mimics a G-tetrad and tightly integrates into the base stack of a G-quadruplex, however, is not so straightforward as many ligands known to form square-planar complexes, i.e., ones based on N-heterocycles such as pyridines, have sizes that do not allow a flat arrangement around the central metal ion, but rather lead to a propeller-shaped arrangement that cannot fit snugly into a dense π-stacked quadruplex stem. On the other hand, it was realized that metal binding to the less constraint ends of tetramolecular G4s as well as the less densely packed loop regions of folded G4s also leads to highly interesting new assemblies with a variety of applications as detailed below.

2 TRANSITION METAL-BINDING IN LOOP REGIONS OF G-QUADRUPLEXES

Unimolecular chair-type G4 structures possess two neighboring lateral loops with opposite directionality (Figure 2a). To some extent, this loop region therefore resembles a duplex DNA motif with two neighboring antiparallel DNA strands. Inspired by the metal-mediated T–Hg–T base pair previously observed in duplex DNA structures, Mergny et al. designed G4 species containing a single thymidine residue each in both neighboring lateral loops (5′-d(G$_3$**AA**TG$_3$CAG$_3$**AA**TG$_3$)) [66]. In the absence of Hg^{2+} ions, two distinct structural conformations were adopted, as evidenced by two sets of ^{1}H NMR signals corresponding to the imino protons of the guanosine residues involved in G-tetrad formation. In the presence of Hg^{2+} ions, however, only one distinct set of signals was observed. In addition, UV-based melting experiments (detection at 295 nm) revealed a higher melting temperature of the overall secondary structure in the presence of Hg^{2+} ions ($\Delta T_m = 2.4°C$). In analogy to previous results in duplex DNA, the increased thermal stability can be explained by the formation of a **T–Hg–T** complex cross-linking the two lateral loops in the G4 structure (Figure 2a). Mass spectrometry was performed to confirm the stoichiometric binding of one Hg^{2+} ion per G-quadruplex. Apparently, the stabilizing metal-mediated base pair can only form in one distinct G4 conformation and hence reduces the structural polymorphism found for this G4-forming sequence.

In a different study, Sugimoto et al. modified the loop regions of a G-quadruplex by incorporating 2,2′-bipyridine (bipy) ligand functionalities for transition metal

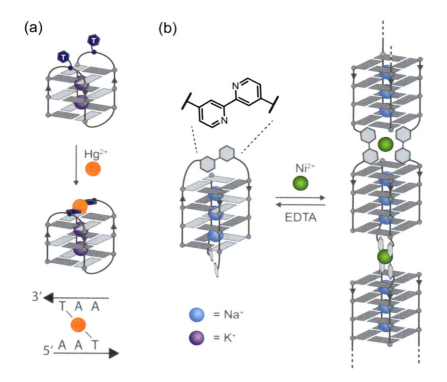

FIGURE 2 (a) The presence of one thymidine each in two neighboring lateral loops of a unimolecular antiparallel G-quadruplex allows the formation of a **T–Hg–T** metal-mediated base pair, cross-linking the loops thereby stabilizing the overall secondary structure [66]. (b) Incorporation of bipy ligands in the loop regions of a bimolecular G-quadruplex allows for a reversible transition metal-dependent switch to a higher-order G-wire structure [67]. CD-spectroscopic evidence points to a switch from an antiparallel to a parallel strand re-configuration upon metal-triggered formation of the 1D wire assembly.

binding [67]. They synthesized the respective modified oligonucleotide by solid-phase DNA synthesis using a bipy-based phosphoramidite. Inspired by the G4-forming sequence 5'-d(G$_4$T$_4$G$_4$), all four thymidine residues were substituted by a single bipy unit (5'-d(G$_4$-bipy-G$_4$)).

In the presence of Na$^+$ ions, the canonical sequence folds into a bimolecular antiparallel G4 topology and also the ligand-modified oligonucleotide forms the respective structural motif, confirmed by CD spectroscopy suggesting that both bipy units reside in the loop regions at opposite sides of the G4 structure (Figure 2b). Interestingly, in the presence of transition metal ions such as Zn^{2+}, Co^{2+}, or Ni^{2+}, CD spectra of the bipy-containing species showed patterns indicating parallel-oriented G4 topologies. This effect is not observed for the unmodified species. The CD data demonstrate a transition metal-induced structural transition from an antiparallel to a parallel G4 topology and an interaction between the metal ions and the bipy units.

The Ni^{2+}-DNA adduct was subsequently investigated in more detail. Formation of a Ni^{2+}-bipy complex was confirmed by absorption spectroscopy, and slower migrating, smearing bands in polyacrylamide gel electrophoresis (PAGE) experiments revealed the transition metal-G4 species to be a heterogenous mixture of a series of higher-order structures. Finally, long linear polymeric structures with an average length of 73 nm were visualized by atomic force microscopy (AFM). The experimental data support the transition metal-induced formation of a so-called G-wire, an interlocked nanowire with stacked parallel G4 units [8, 68]. A reasonable structural model suggests Ni^{2+}-bipy complexes residing between the single G4 units within the G-wire (Figure 2b).

A key finding of this study was the reversibility of the transition metal-induced switching from a distinct antiparallel bimolecular G-quadruplex to a polymeric parallel G-wire structure. The addition of ethylenediaminetetraacetic acid (EDTA) as a strong chelating agent to the Ni^{2+}-containing G-wire resulted in a transition back to the distinct bimolecular structure, again confirmed by CD spectroscopy, PAGE, and AFM. Hence the bipy-modified G-quadruplex functions as a structural switch interchanging between a distinct G4 and higher-order G-wires, controlled by Ni^{2+} ions and EDTA as chemical stimuli. The reversible switching was demonstrated over multiple cycles with a high cycling efficiency.

Both examples described in this section deal with ligand functionalities in loop regions of G-quadruplexes used for transition metal binding. The metal binding was either exploited for thermal stabilization and reduction of polymorphism of the secondary structures or as a chemical stimulus for a structural switch to a higher-order G-wire structure.

3 THE METAL-MEDIATED BASE TETRAD

The four-stranded nature of G4 structures suggests the incorporation of square-planar transition metal complexes carrying four monodentate ligands (ligandosides) into the G-rich secondary architectures. Formally substituting a full G-tetrad, the resulting "metal-mediated base tetrad" (termed in analogy to metal-mediated base pairs in duplex DNA) connects all four DNA strands. As mentioned above, however, the non-planar character of so far realized examples of this structural motif (even if the metal coordination environment is square-planar, the ligand structures usually extend above and below the plane), only allows incorporation at the 3′- or 5′-ends of the G-stack.

3.1 Metal-Mediated Base Tetrads in Tetramolecular G-Quadruplexes

In a first approach to form a metal-base tetrad, Clever et al. covalently attached pyridine donors (L^C) at the 5′-end of short G-rich oligonucleotides (d($L^C G_n$), $n=3-5$) using a pyridine-based phosphoramidite for standard solid-phase DNA synthesis (Figure 3a) [69].

Transition Metal-Binding G-Quadruplex DNA

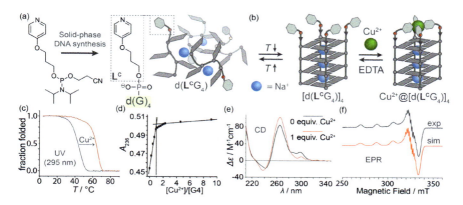

FIGURE 3 (a) Ligandoside-modified G-rich oligonucleotides are synthesized by standard solid-phase DNA synthesis using a pyridine-based phosphoramidite. (b) In the presence of Na+ ions, tetramolecular G-quadruplexes form resulting in a preorganized ligand environment suitable for complexation of transition metal ions such as Ni^{2+} or Cu^{2+}. The formation of a Cu(pyridine)$_4$ tetrad (evidenced by UV titration and EPR spectroscopy, (d) and (f)) increases the thermal stability of the overall structure (c) without changing the overall topology of the G-quadruplex core (e). (Reproduced with permission from Ref. [69]. © 2013 Wiley-VCH Verlag GmbH & Co. KGaA, Weinheim.)

At a high concentration of Na+ ions, formation of tetramolecular G4s ([d(**L**^{C}**G**$_n$)]$_4$, n=4–5) was observed, evidenced by UV-based melting analysis monitored at 295 nm (Figure 3c) and thermal difference spectra. As usual for tetramolecular species, a characteristic pattern in the CD spectrum showing a positive Cotton effect with a maximum at around 260 nm and a minimum around 240 nm revealed a parallel G4 topology (Figure 3e). This distinct folding arrangement of the pyridine-modified DNA strands resulted in a prearranged chelating ligand environment at the 5′-face suitable for binding of transition metal cations. Addition of 1 equiv. of Ni^{2+} ions caused a strong thermal stabilization of the secondary structure with an increased denaturation temperature ($\Delta T_{1/2}$=15 °C for Ni^{2+}@[d(**L**^{C}**G**$_4$)]$_4$). An even larger stabilization was observed upon addition of 1 equiv. of Cu^{2+} ions ($\Delta T_{1/2}$=20 °C for Cu^{2+}@[d(**L**^{C}**G**$_4$)]$_4$, Figure 3b and c). Importantly, the overall G4 structure remained intact, evidenced by only minor changes in the CD spectrum upon Ni^{2+} or Cu^{2+} addition (Figure 3e). The specific interaction of the metal ions with the pyridine ligandosides residing at the 5′-face was confirmed by analysis of a control G4 species that carried phenyl groups instead of pyridine rings, hence, lacking the N-donor functionality. No increased stability was observed upon transition metal addition for this species.

The Cu^{2+} binding mode to the pyridine-modified G4s was further investigated by UV-based titration proving a 1:1 stoichiometry (Figure 3d), and by EPR spectroscopy suggesting Cu^{2+} coordination by four pyridine donors in a square-planar geometry, resulting in a Cu(pyridine)$_4$ tetrad (probably with loosely bound axial

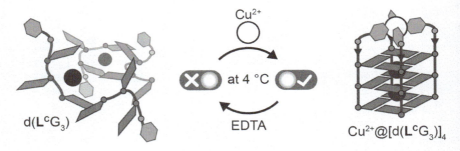

FIGURE 4 Cu^{2+}-dependent switching between hybridization and denaturation of ligand-modified tetramolecular G-quadruplexes [69].

water ligands in a Jahn–Teller distorted octahedral or square-pyramidal environment, Figure 3f).

EDTA was used as a strong chelating agent to seize the transition metal ion from the G4 adduct, regenerating the transition metal-free G4 species with its initial stability. Several cycles of alternating stabilization (Cu^{2+} addition) and destabilization (EDTA addition) showcased the reversibility of the transition metal-induced thermal G4 stabilization. This metal-dependent switch was exploited to gain control over G4 de- and renaturation with a short G4 species (Figure 4) that was unstable at 4°C in the transition metal-free state ($T_{1/2}$ <4 °C for [d(L^{C}G$_3$)]$_4$), but stable in the metal-bound state ($T_{1/2}$ = 17°C for Cu^{2+}@[d(L^{C}G$_3$)]$_4$) at a given electrolyte concentration.

In a subsequent systematic study, both the stability of transition metal-free G4s and the degree of Cu^{2+}-induced G4 stabilization could be adjusted by the length of the linkers connecting the pyridine ligandosides to the oligonucleotide backbones at the 5′-end (L^{A-D}, Figure 5a) [70]. Melting temperatures in

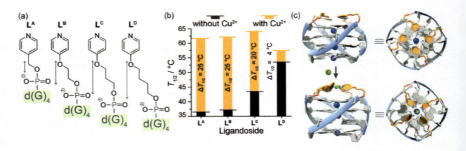

FIGURE 5 (a) Linker lengths of pyridine ligandosides L^A–L^D. (b) Melting temperatures of G-quadruplexes in absence and presence of Cu^{2+} ions depending on the linker length. (c) Structural models of ligand-modified tetramolecular G-quadruplexes containing L^C (highlighted in orange) derived from MD simulations. In the Cu^{2+}-free state, pyridines π-stack to the top G-tetrad, which is abolished upon Cu^{2+}-binding. (Adapted with permission from Ref. [70]. © 2018 Wiley-VCH Verlag GmbH & Co. KGaA, Weinheim.)

the Cu^{2+}-free state strongly increase with longer linkers ($T_{1/2}$=36.5°C for [d(L^{A}G$_4$)]$_4$, $T_{1/2}$=37.0°C for [d(L^{B}G$_4$)]$_4$, $T_{1/2}$=43.5°C for [d(L^{C}G$_4$)]$_4$, and $T_{1/2}$=53.5 °C for [d(L^{D}G$_4$)]$_4$). On the other hand, stabilities of the Cu^{2+}-bound species with various linker lengths are quite similar ($T_{1/2}$=57°C–64°C for Cu^{2+}@[d(L^{A-D}G$_4$)]$_4$, Figure 5b). As a direct consequence, the Cu^{2+}-induced stabilization strongly depends on the linker length. To explain these findings, Cu^{2+}-free and Cu^{2+}-bound G4 species have been modeled with the help of molecular dynamics (MD) simulations (Figure 5c). Longer linkers allow attractive π-stacking interactions between the aromatic pyridine residues and the top 5'-G-tetrad and, hence, stabilize the Cu^{2+}-free G4 structure. π-stacking is prevented upon Cu^{2+} coordination because the pyridine donors have to adopt a propeller-like arrangement around the metal center due to steric hindrance. This effect explains the lower Cu^{2+}-induced stabilization for species with longer linkers, since attractive π-stacking is exchanged for metal coordination in these cases whereas constructs with shorter linkers do not give up any stabilization upon metal addition.

In the following step, the donor functionalities attached to the 5'-face of tetramolecular G4s were changed to imidazole groups, which again allowed to complex Cu^{2+} and Ni^{2+} ions, but also Co^{2+} and Zn^{2+} ions [71]. Unprecedentedly strong transition metal-induced thermal stabilization of up to $\Delta T_{1/2}$=51°C (for Cu^{2+}) was observed. Electrospray ionization (ESI) mass spectrometry was applied to study the folded metal-G4 species in the gas phase and confirmed the 1:1 stoichiometry of transition metal complexation.

Furthermore, the effect of transition metal ion addition on the folding kinetics of imidazole-modified G4s was examined. Cu^{2+} ions likely serve as a template by preorganizing the four oligonucleotides due to ligandoside coordination and allow rapid G-tetrad formation. This phenomenon results in about 100 times higher association rates of G4 formation compared to hybridization in the absence of Cu^{2+} ions. In contrast to G4s carrying the Cu(pyridine)$_4$ tetrad, transition metal-G4 adducts bearing imidazole ligandosides are preserved in the presence of EDTA, highlighting the remarkable kinetic stability of the Cu(imidazole)$_4$ complex within the G4 environment [71].

The described investigations introduced a robust and synthetically feasible approach to covalently incorporate transition metal complexes into tetramolecular G-quadruplexes that stabilize the overall secondary DNA structure. As demonstrated, variation of the donor groups, metal ions, and linker lengths allows fine-tuning of the G4's overall stability, the degree of transition metal-induced stabilization, and reversibility of metal binding.

In a recent similar approach, histidine ligands (L^{His}) were covalently incorporated into G-rich sequences (d(G$_2$L^{His}$_2$G$_2$)) by Sugiyama et al. via solid-phase DNA synthesis [72]. CD spectra confirmed the formation of a parallel G4 topology ([d(G$_2$L^{His}$_2$G$_2$)]$_4$) in the presence of K$^+$ ions. The most reasonable structure is an arrangement with two G-quartets each at the 5'-end and the 3'-end of a tetramolecular species creating a preorganized ligand environment containing eight histidine groups in its center. Interestingly, the addition of one equivalent of various transition metal ions resulted in different topology changes due to metal complexation. While the parallel topology is maintained upon Cu^{2+} addition, Co^{2+} and Ni^{2+} ions induced a rearrangement to an antiparallel structure, and the addition of Zn^{2+} ions resulted in either a hybrid topology or a mixture of different conformations.

3.2 Metal-Mediated Base Tetrads in Unimolecular G-Quadruplexes

The second generation of ligandosides designed by Clever et al. was based on a glycol backbone in analogy to glycol nucleic acids (GNA) introduced by Meggers et al. [73]. These new building blocks allow internal ligandoside installation into oligonucleotide sequences by solid-phase DNA synthesis. Hence, this design enables the covalent incorporation of transition metal complexes into unimolecular G4s, folded from a single G-rich strand, by formally replacing one G-quartet with a metal-mediated quartet (e.g., a Cu(pyridine)₄ tetrad). Importantly, the ligandosides contain a chiral carbon atom and can be installed either in the (R) or (S) configuration, giving rise to diastereomeric DNA constructs (Figure 6a).

At first, a unimolecular G4-forming sequence found in htel22 was modified [74]. Four pyridine-based ligandosides were covalently installed (htel22-L_4), substituting four guanosines which in the wild-type G4 are involved in G-tetrad formation. In the presence of K^+ ions, the CD spectrum revealed a typical pattern for an antiparallel G4 arrangement with chair-type topology, which was supported by MD simulation results. Interestingly, the configuration of the incorporated ligandosides (either $4 \times S$ or $4 \times R$) substantially impacts the thermal stability of the resulting G-quadruplexes (Figure 6c). The two respective diastereomeric G4s show melting temperatures of $T_m = 18$ °C (for htel22-(R)-L_4) and $T_m = 13$ °C (for htel22-(S)-L_4). As already discussed for tetramolecular species, the stability difference might be explained with attractive π-stacking interactions between the pyridine groups and the top G-tetrad, somehow facilitated by the (R)-configured ligandosides.

In accordance with previously studied ligandoside-modified tetramolecular G4s [69, 71], the addition of 1 equiv. of Cu^{2+} ions per unimolecular G-quadruplex results in a strong thermal stabilization of the secondary structure without changing the overall topology due to Cu(pyridine)₄ tetrad formation ($\Delta T_m = 15$ °C for Cu^{2+}@htel22-(R)-L_4, $\Delta T_m = 23$ °C for Cu^{2+}@htel22-(S)-L_4). Metal binding was observed to be very fast, and equilibrium is already reached within 1 min at 25 °C (or within 5 min at 4°C). Subsequently, Cu^{2+} ions were used as a trigger to initiate rapid unimolecular G4 formation from the unfolded oligonucleotide at 25 °C as monitored by CD spectroscopy. Addition of EDTA induces fast denaturation due to removal of the stabilizing Cu^{2+} ion from the G4 structure (Figure 6b, d, and e). This experiment showcases the transition metal-induced switching between folded and unfolded unimolecular G4 structures.

A second G4 system was designed based on a sequence found in *Tetrahymena* telomeric DNA (ttel24) [74]. Four pyridine-based ligandosides were incorporated into an oligonucleotide forming a mixture of hybrid-type G4 topologies. The positions of the pyridine residues were assumed not to be all on the same face of the

Transition Metal-Binding G-Quadruplex DNA

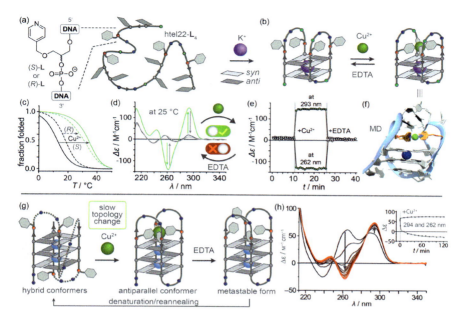

FIGURE 6 (a) Long oligonucleotide htel22-L_4 containing four glycol-based pyridine ligandosides either all in (R) or all in (S) configuration. (b) In presence of K$^+$ ions, a unimolecular G-quadruplex is formed adopting an antiparallel topology. The four ligandosides form a binding site for Cu^{2+} complexation. (c) The Cu^{2+}-induced thermal stabilization (monitored at 295 nm) is dependent on the ligandosides' configuration (solid: (S) configuration, dashed: (R) configuration, black: without Cu^{2+}, green: with Cu^{2+}). (d, e) Cu^{2+}-dependent switching between hybridization and denaturation of ligand-modified unimolecular G-quadruplexes at 25 °C monitored by CD spectroscopy. (e) MD-derived structural model of Cu^{2+}@hte122-(S)-L_4. (g) Oligonucleotide ttel24-(S)-L_4 forms a mixture of hybrid-type topologies, which rule out the formation of a Cu(pyridine)$_4$ quartet due to the distribution of the pyridine ligands over both G4 faces. Upon addition of Cu^{2+} ions, a slow topology change toward an antiparallel conformation can be observed by CD spectroscopy (h). Removal of the Cu^{2+} ion from the Cu(pyridine)$_4$ complex results in a metastable antiparallel topology which can be transferred back into the initial state by thermal denaturation and reannealing. (Reproduced with permission from Ref. [74]. © 2017 Wiley-VCH Verlag GmbH & Co. KGaA, Weinheim.)

metal-free quadruplex, so that most probably two ligandosides reside on one side of the G-tetrad core while the other two ligands are positioned at the opposite end (ttel24-(S)-L_4; note that the exact folding topology could not be unambiguously determined, as expressed by the gray dashed backbone lines in the structural suggestion depicted in Figure 6g). This arrangement does not allow Cu(pyridine)$_4$ tetrad formation. Interestingly, upon Cu^{2+} addition, a slow change in topology to an antiparallel structure was monitored by CD spectroscopy (Figure 6h), and equilibrium was reached after 2 h at 25 °C (or after 7 h at 4°C). In the antiparallel topology, all four pyridine ligandosides reside on the same side of the G-tetrad core and, hence, Cu(pyridine)$_4$ quartet formation is possible. If the Cu^{2+} ion is removed by the addition of EDTA, the antiparallel G4 arrangement is preserved as a metastable species which can be transformed back into the original hybrid-type topology by thermal de- and renaturation.

In both discussed G4 systems, Cu^{2+} ions are exploited as a trigger for Cu^{2+}-induced topology switching. They can either be used to quickly switch between the unfolded oligonucleotide and folded G4 species (htel22-**L**$_4$) or to induce a slow topology change from a mixture of hybrid conformers to a single antiparallel G4 structure (ttel24-**L**$_4$).

4 FINE-TUNED COORDINATION ENVIRONMENTS IN G-QUADRUPLEXES

A detailed look into metalloproteins discloses a wide variety of metal complex environments in terms of ligand count, position, and types, usually of heteroleptic nature. The metal ions are typically involved in fixing the desired protein structure or serve as catalytic centers or redox cofactors. For example, about 50% of all enzymes contain metal cofactors and several metals are therefore essential elements for living organisms [75]. Interestingly, only around a dozen different metal ions can be frequently found in proteins, but they are part of numerous differing metal complexes comprising a wide range of functions with fine-tuned properties. It becomes directly clear that not only the nature of the metal ion itself but also its coordination environment determines those complex properties. There are several organic (and inorganic) cofactors that function as ligands (e.g., tetrapyrroles). More often, however, ligand functionalities are provided by amino acid side chains of the surrounding protein. In proteinogenic amino acids, several different donor groups can be found, ranging from hard Lewis bases such as carboxylates (glutamate and aspartate) and phenol (tyrosine), borderline Lewis donors like imidazole (histidine) to soft Lewis bases like sulfur-containing ligands (methionine and cysteine). Metal complexes in metalloproteins are usually heteroleptic. The choice and number of distinct ligands in combination with the coordination geometry determined by the peptide framework mainly define the complex properties [75].

One goal of bioinorganic chemists is to investigate and understand the role of metal ions in metalloproteins and to mimic their structure and function in model complexes [76, 77]. In the field of protein engineering, scientists try to improve reaction rates of natural enzymes or even design artificial enzymes for xenobiotic reactions [78–80]. In addition to approaches such as directed evolution and *de novo* protein design, another strategy exploits DNA instead of peptides as scaffold to bring together ligand functionalities that form active metal complexes. Nucleic acid secondary structures are better predictable and programmable compared to peptides and proteins, which might allow easier structural design. Furthermore, they can be embedded into larger devices utilizing advances in DNA nanotechnology [81, 82]. In this context, the approach of covalently installing transition metal complexes into G-quadruplexes by incorporation of ligandosides into G4-forming sequences, described in the previous section, might pave the way to mimic functional metal complexes, found in metalloproteins, inside a DNA environment.

The number and position of ligandosides within the loop regions of unimolecular G4s can be easily varied due to the ease of sequence modification in solid-phase DNA synthesis. This modular approach allows for the controlled design of distinct coordination environments with fine-tuned transition metal affinities. In the first attempt, the number of imidazole-based ligandosides was varied within an antiparallel G-quadruplex. Three to seven ligandosides were incorporated into the loops of a G4-forming oligonucleotide and G4 formation resulted in a preorganized ligand arrangement [83]. The number of offered ligands resulted in varying transition metal affinity. For example, Cu^{2+} ions which are usually coordinated in a square-planar fashion show a higher affinity to G-quadruplexes containing four imidazole ligandosides. On the other hand, Ni^{2+} ions prefer binding to G4 structures offering six ligands, as judged by their stabilizing effect on the overall secondary structure (Figure 7a).

A second adjustable parameter is the position of the ligands within the G-quadruplex loops, which is easily programmable by varying the G-quadruplex-forming DNA sequence. Two G4s with an arrangement of four imidazole ligandosides either in a square-planar or in a tetrahedral fashion were designed (Figure 7b). As expected, Cu^{2+} ions favor coordination to a square-planar oriented ligand environment ($\Delta T_m = 23°C$) over the tetrahedral geometry ($\Delta T_m = 21°C$).

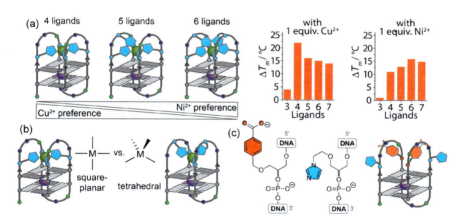

FIGURE 7 (a) The number of imidazole-based ligandosides in G4s fine-tunes metal binding affinity. While Cu^{2+} ions prefer a coordination environment containing four imidazole residues, as judged by their stabilizing effect on the G4 structure, Ni^{2+} ions show a higher affinity to G4s offering six ligands. (b) Variation of the ligandosides' positions within the G4-forming DNA sequence allows adjustment of the offered coordination geometry. While Cu^{2+} ions prefer a square-planar ligand arrangement, Zn^{2+} ions show a much higher affinity to G4s offering a tetrahedral coordination geometry [83]. (c) Combination of different ligandosides within the G4-forming sequence results in heteroleptic coordination environments and allows further control over metal affinity [84].

In contrast, Zn^{2+} ions strongly prefer coordination to a tetrahedral ligand environment (ΔT_m = 21°C) over the square-planar geometry (ΔT_m = 3°C) [83].

Further fine-tuning of coordination environments could be achieved by combining different ligand functionalities leading to heteroleptic coordination environments preorganized within the G4 structure. To test this idea, and with the ligand diversity found in metalloproteins in mind, a novel benzoate-based ligandoside was designed [84]. In contrast to the previously utilized pyridine and imidazole residues, the new ligand represents a hard donor according to the HSAB (hard and soft acids and bases) concept and brings an additional negative charge at physiological pH. Various G4-forming oligonucleotides containing different ratios of benzoate- and imidazole-based ligands were synthesized (Figure 7c). Complexation of transition metal ions such as Cu^{2+}, Ni^{2+}, or Zn^{2+} within the G4s was confirmed by CD and UV spectroscopy and native ESI mass spectrometry. An effect on transition metal affinity due to different ligand compositions was found, although the direct involvement of the benzoates in the metal coordination remained unclear.

The described examples showcase the possibility of fine-tuning ligand environments by varying both number and position of the ligandosides and by combining different donor groups within a modified, G4-forming oligonucleotide sequence. This modular approach of incorporating ligandosides into unimolecular G-quadruplexes is suitable to easily build tailored ligand environments resulting in transition metal complexes with tunable properties. It will pave the way for the custom-made design of heteroleptic metal complexes with various properties and opens possibilities for mimicking active metal complexes found in metalloproteins in a DNA-based environment.

5 TRANSITION METAL-BINDING G-QUADRUPLEXES IN CATALYSIS

Similar to nature's strategy of incorporating metal cofactors with distinct coordination environments into metalloproteins, the idea to install metal complexes into DNA nanostructures aims at introducing additional functionality to the otherwise passive assemblies. The approach merges the high programmability of DNA structures on the nanoscale with specific metal complex properties, which are promising prerequisites for catalysis [85]. The concept of using transition metal-containing DNA architectures for asymmetric catalysis was pioneered by Roelfes and Feringa who exploited Cu^{2+} complexes that non-covalently bind to duplex DNA. In this way, the chirality of DNA was transferred directly to organic bond-forming transformations such as Diels-Alder reactions, Michael additions, or Friedel–Crafts reactions, and high enantiomeric excesses were obtained [86–89].

In addition to duplex DNA or hairpin loops, also G4 motifs have been utilized to design metal-containing DNA architectures for enantioselective catalysis. First, very similar approaches exploited either planar transition metal complexes non-covalently π-stacked to G-tetrads or directly coordinated transition metal ions as catalytic centers, and various reaction types could be catalyzed in this way

[90–92]. Interestingly, although using the same oligonucleotide, the enantioselectivity could be reversed from one preferred enantiomer to the other by changing the G4 topology e.g., by varying the electrolyte composition [31, 93].

The first attempt to covalently attach transition metal complexes as catalytic centers to G4 structures for asymmetric catalysis was reported by Jäschke et al. [94–96]. In contrast to previous non-covalent adducts of catalytic metal complexes and chiral DNA, which were usually poorly structurally characterized, the covalent approach aims to understand and gain control over the structural basis of the asymmetric catalytic activity. A bipyridine ligand for Cu^{2+} complexation was covalently and site-selectively attached into a loop position of a unimolecular G-quadruplex via synthetic nucleobase modification. Corresponding Cu^{2+}-G4 complexes were applied in asymmetric Michael reactions and variation of parameters such as the nature of the ligand or the length of the linker connecting the G4 and the Cu^{2+} complex allowed to control both the rate acceleration and the enantioselectivity. Remarkably, moving the position of the nucleobase modification carrying the Cu^{2+} complex by only two positions in the G4-forming sequence resulted in an inversion of the stereoselectivity.

Even more control over the exact localization and orientation of the catalytic center in transition metal-containing DNA architectures was provided by the incorporation of monodentate ligands as described above for creating a metal-mediated base tetrad. The carefully designed incorporation of several ligands within the G4-forming oligonucleotide sequence with predictable folding topology was shown to allow for a rational development of hybrid catalysts. This modular approach was pursued by Clever et al. and a Michael addition was catalyzed as a model reaction [97]. Therefore, two or three imidazole-based ligandosides were incorporated into the G4 structures and addition of Cu^{2+} ions led to Lewis-acidic, coordinatively unsaturated Cu^{2+} complexes with catalytic activity within the chiral DNA environment (Figure 8; note that G4s chelating the Cu^{2+} ions by four ligandosides did not show any significant catalytic activity). Iterative rounds of rational sequence design resulted in tailored metallo-DNAzymes generating

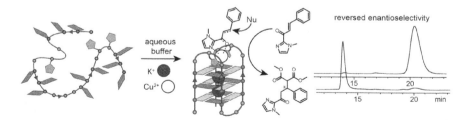

FIGURE 8 Rational positioning of two or three imidazole-based ligandosides in the loops of G4-forming DNA sequences allows for controlling the orientation and activity of the catalytic Cu^{2+} complex in a G4-based metallo-DNAzyme. Michael additions can be catalyzed with excellent enantioselectivities, which can be inverted by changing the number and position of the ligandosides within the oligonucleotide sequence. (Adapted with permission from Ref. [97]. © 2021 American Chemical Society.)

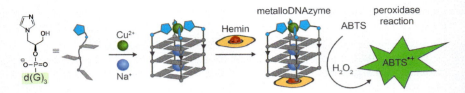

FIGURE 9 The Cu^{2+}-induced G4 hybridization of an imidazole-modified tetramolecular G-quadruplex was exploited to design a Cu^{2+}-activated DNAzyme based on the well-known hemin-G4 adduct with peroxidase activity. As readout for catalytic activity, the oxidation of ABTS (2,2′-azino-bis(3-ethylbenzothiazoline-6-sulfonic acid) with H_2O_2 to its strongly green colored radical was monitored spectroscopically [71].

both high conversions and stereoselectivities. Interestingly, varying the number and position of the imidazole ligandosides in the G4-forming oligonucleotide sequence provided control over the observed enantioselectivity.

In addition to directly serving as catalytically active centers, transition metals have also been used as a trigger to gain control over other catalytically active species. The hemin-G4 adduct is a well-known metallo-DNAzyme with peroxidase activity [37, 49]. The iron cation in the hemin cofactor serves as a catalytic center and only shows activity when π-stacked onto a terminal G-quartet of a G4 structure. Clever et al. exploited the previously described Cu^{2+}-dependent control over hybridization and denaturation of ligand-modified tetramolecular G-quadruplexes and designed a Cu^{2+}-dependent hemin-G4 DNAzyme (Figure 9) [71].

Also, the thrombin-binding DNA aptamer (tba) that adopts a G4 structure was modified by incorporation of pyridine ligandosides to enable Cu^{2+}-dependent switching between hybridization and denaturation. Noteworthy, tba only binds to the target enzyme thrombin in its folded state and thereby inhibits the hydrolysis of fibrinogen to fibrin. The ligand-modified tba species was then shown to control thrombin binding using Cu^{2+} ions as a stimulus. In this way the enzymatic activity was put under the control of the transition metal [74].

6 Cu(PYRIDINE)$_4$ TETRADS AS PARAMAGNETIC EPR SPIN LABELS

An important principle in biology states that structure determines function, known as structure-function relationship. Consequently, structure elucidation of biomolecules such as nucleic acids or proteins is crucial for the understanding of their biological function. Particular interest lies also in understanding the dynamics of biomolecules and in the question, how structural changes affect their function. Several different techniques are available for the structure elucidation of biomolecules, each with advantages and disadvantages. It is important to choose the right method for investigating a certain species in a specific environment (in particular *in vivo* studies are challenging) and the more orthogonal techniques support a structural result, the more reliable it is.

In addition to single-crystal XRD [98], nuclear magnetic resonance (NMR) spectroscopy [99], and cryo-EM [100] that can all provide atomic resolution structural data for biomolecules, pulsed dipolar electron paramagnetic resonance (PDEPR) spectroscopy can be used as an orthogonal method for relatively noise-free intra- and intermolecular distance measurements. It closes gaps where other techniques are not applicable to gain structural information. It is frequently used to support the elucidation of structure and dynamics of biomolecules, especially proteins [101–104]. The technique requires two or more paramagnetic spin labels attached to the structure of interest and distances between them in a range of about 1.5–10 nm can be detected. If no paramagnetic groups are present in the analyte, they can be installed at suitable positions by site-directed spin labeling (SDSL) [105]. Paramagnetic metal complexes or organic radicals (usually nitroxides) are frequently used for this purpose.

PDEPR has also been used to study nucleic acid structures [106–109]. A variety of spin labels has been developed mostly based on nucleobase or backbone modifications [107, 109–111]. While mostly organic radicals like nitroxide spin labels have been used, there are also examples for Cu^{2+}-based alternatives [109, 112, 113]. While most studies so far aimed at investigating the conformational flexibility of duplex structures, few reports describe PDEPR-based examinations on other secondary nucleic acid structures. Among these, G-quadruplex topologies of human telomeric sequences were probed [114–116], including an in-cell investigation scheme [117, 118]. Other studies explored the formation of G-quadruplex-metal complex adducts [119, 120]. However, these G-quadruplex investigations resulted in very broad distance distributions which were caused either by flexible spin labels (often attached via floppy chains) or by their installation in very flexible structural regions such as loop regions in unimolecular G-quadruplexes.

Recently, the intrinsic paramagnetic property of d^9-configured Cu^{2+}(pyridine)$_4$ complexes introduced into tetramolecular G4s was exploited as EPR-active spin labels. In a first attempt, one transition metal complex each was attached at both the 5'- and the 3'-ends of tetramolecular G4s with varying G-tetrad counts in-between the metal complexes (2Cu^{2+}@[d(LG$_n$LT)]$_4$, n=3–5). This arrangement allowed the determination of intramolecular $Cu^{2+}\cdots Cu^{2+}$ distances within the secondary DNA structures with unprecedented accuracy by PDEPR techniques such as DEER (double electron-electron resonance) and RIDME (relaxation-induced dipolar modulation enhancement). The planar four-point attachment of the square-planar Cu(pyridine)$_4$ complexes results in a rigid and coplanar orientation of the two magnetic $d_{x^2-y^2}$ orbitals separated by the stacked G-quartets (Figure 10a–c). This arrangement reduces the conformational flexibility of the spin labels, which enables taking orientation selectivity into account and thus provides additional information on geometrical parameters [121].

In the next step, the new spin label was exploited to investigate G4 dimers, a simple representative for higher-order G4 structures, with PDEPR. Tetramolecular G4s containing a terminal G-tetrad at either the 5'- or the 3'-end was labeled with a single Cu(pyridine)$_4$ complex at the opposite side. The formation of

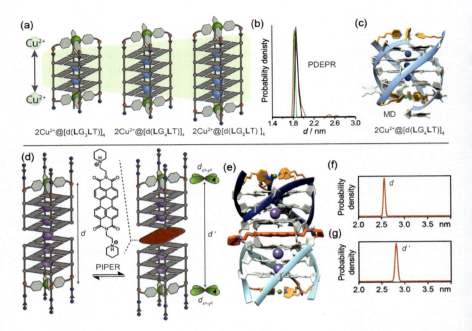

FIGURE 10 (a) Tetramolecular G4s containing Cu(pyridine)$_4$ spin labels both at the 5'- and 3'-ends (2Cu^{2+}@[d(LG$_n$LT)]$_4$, $n=3$–5). b) Extremely narrow Cu^{2+}⋯Cu^{2+} distance distributions obtained for 2Cu^{2+}@[d(LG$_4$LT)]$_4$ by different PDEPR spectroscopy methods. (c) Experimentally obtained Cu^{2+}⋯Cu^{2+} distances were in good agreement with MD simulation results. (Reproduced from Ref. [121] with permission from the Royal Society of Chemistry.) (d) Spin-labeled G4 monomers in π-stacked G4 dimers allow intermolecular Cu^{2+}⋯Cu^{2+} distance measurements by PDEPR methods. PIPER intercalates in between the two monomers of a dimer, resulting in a so-called sandwich complex confirmed by an increased Cu^{2+}⋯Cu^{2+} distance. (e) MD-derived molecular model of sandwich complex PIPER@(Cu^{2+}@[d(T$_2$LG$_3$)]$_4$)$_2$. (f)-(g) PDEPR-derived Cu^{2+}⋯Cu^{2+} distance distributions obtained for the G4 dimer and its sandwich complex [122].

head-to-head and tail-to-tail oriented G4 dimers of different spatial dimensions by π-stacking of the terminal G-quartets was confirmed with DEER-based intermolecular Cu^{2+}⋯Cu^{2+} distance measurements (e.g., (Cu^{2+}@[d(T$_2$LG$_3$)]$_4$)$_2$ and (Cu^{2+}@[d(G$_3$LT$_2$)]$_4$)$_2$, Figures 10d–g). Unprecedentedly narrow distance distributions were again attributed to the high rigidity of both the G4 structure and the Cu^{2+}-based spin labels fixated by four pyridine ligandosides. Obtained geometry parameters, e.g., the rigid and colinear alignment of the z-axes of the two Cu^{2+} complexes, support a tight π-stacking interface between the terminal G-quartets of the two G4 monomers [122].

The approach of spin-labeling both monomers in G4 dimers with Cu(pyridine)$_4$ tetrads was applied to investigate the interaction of different G4 binders (often referred to as G4-binding ligands) such as drug-like PIPER (*N,N'*-bis[2-(1-piperidino)ethyl]-3,4,9,10-perylenetetracarboxylic diimide) or natural product telomestatin with the G4 dimers. Both small molecules were shown to intercalate in-between the two monomers of a tail-to-tail stacked dimer, proven by an increase in the observed $Cu^{2+}\cdots Cu^{2+}$ separation by one π-stacking distance (e.g., PIPER@$(Cu^{2+}@[d(T_2LG_3)]_4)_2$, Figure 10d–g). Previously unknown binding motifs, i.e., for telomestatin, could thus be revealed. In addition, untethered G-quartets composed of four free guanine or guanosine residues added to the samples were shown to intercalate into G4 dimers (e.g., guanine$_4$@$(Cu^{2+}@[d(T_2LG_3)]_4)_2$). All experimentally obtained distance data were in excellent agreement with structural models derived from MD simulations [122].

In comparison to other published approaches of incorporating spin labels into G4 structures, the high rigidity of the Cu(pyridine)$_4$ tetrad is an unprecedented advancement. Common organic spin labels often suffer from flexible linkers or are incorporated into flexible G4 loop regions, hence permitting many different conformations and resulting in broad distance distributions obtained with PDEPR-based measurements [114–116]. This is also true for non-covalently attached spin labels [120]. The extremely narrow distance distributions obtained with the rigid Cu^{2+}-based label (Figure 10f and g) allow for resolving very small length differences and are therefore well suited to detect small structural changes. Furthermore, the Cu^{2+} ion is spatially fixed so that EPR orientation selectivity can be considered, providing an additional set of valuable geometric parameters. These advantages of PDEPR open new possibilities in the precise elucidation of structure and dynamics of higher-order DNA architectures ranging from biologically relevant telomeric folds over G4-drug adducts and DNA-protein complexes to bio-hybrid DNA nanodevices and dynamic DNA origami systems.

7 CONCLUSION AND FUTURE PROSPECTS

The concept of covalently incorporating transition metal complexes into DNA G-quadruplex structures aims at introducing additional functionality to the nucleic acid architectures. Usually, artificial ligand residues are incorporated via phosphoramidite-based DNA synthesis. Coordinating donor groups can be attached in the flexible loop regions of a G4 structure, or four ligandosides replace four guanosine residues substituting a full G-tetrad at the 3′- or 5′-end of the quadruplex stack. Subsequently, transition metal salts are added to the ligand-modified G4s to form the desired metal complexes.

As demonstrated for several examples, transition metal-binding results in a thermal stabilization of the overall secondary structure, as the formed metal complex cross-links different parts of the G4 fold. Often, but not always, the transition metal ion can be removed again using strong chelating agents such as EDTA. Variation of the donor groups, metal ions, and linker lengths allows fine-tuning of the G4's overall stability, the degree of transition metal-induced stabilization (up to $\Delta T_{1/2}=51°C$), and reversibility of metal binding. The metal-induced stabilizing effect can be exploited for the design of transition metal-triggered G4 switches. Different studies demonstrated transition metal-dependent switching between unfolded oligonucleotide and folded G4, between different topologies of discrete G4 folds (e.g. from hybrid-type to antiparallel structure), and between discrete G4 structures and polymeric G-wires. Such transition metal-dependent G4 constructs have the potential to greatly extend the toolbox of DNA nanotechnology to design stimuli-responsive materials and devices.

Due to the straightforward incorporation of ligandosides into oligonucleotides, the approach was extended to develop fine-tuned ligand environments within the G-quadruplex environment. The variation of type, number, and positioning of the ligandosides within a sequence forming unimolecular G-quadruplexes results in distinct heteroleptic coordination environments. The modular approach allows the design of tailored coordination spheres for transition metal complexes with distinct properties and might allow transferring a plethora of metal complexes with various functions from metalloproteins to nucleic acid environments.

The first step in this direction was made by exploiting the Lewis acidity of transition metal complexes incorporated into chiral G-quadruplex structures for enantioselective catalysis. In this way, Michael additions in aqueous medium with high conversions and excellent enantioselectivities (≥99%) were achieved. Notably, the variation of the number and positions of the ligandosides in the DNA sequence allowed to control the enantioselectivity resulting in one or the other enantiomeric reaction product to be formed. The concept will be expanded to other types of reactions catalyzed by G4-based metallo-DNAzymes.

Copper complexes covalently incorporated into G-quadruplexes were additionally applied as paramagnetic spin labels for EPR-based distance measurements. The extraordinary rigidity of the Cu(pyridine)$_4$ quartets residing in the G4 structures enabled unprecedentedly precise Cu-Cu distance measurements within G4 structures and higher-order G4 architectures such as dimers as well as sandwich-like G4-small molecule adducts. The Cu-binding G4 constructs bear the potential as universal spin labels of high rigidity, applicable also for the structural investigation of larger nucleic acid architectures.

ACKNOWLEDGMENT

We thank the Deutsche Forschungsgemeinschaft (DFG, project CL489/4-1) for support.

ABBREVIATIONS

ABTS	2,2′-azino-bis(3-ethylbenzothiazoline-6-sulfonic acid
AFM	atomic force microscopy
bipy	2,2′-bipyridine
CD	circular dichroism
cryo-EM	cryo-electron microscopy
DEER	double electron-electron resonance
DNAzyme	catalytic DNA
EDTA	ethylenediaminetetraacetic acid

EPR	electron paramagnetic resonance
ESI	electrospray ionization
G4	guanine quadruplex
GNA	glycol nucleic acid
HSAB	hard and soft acids and bases
htel22	human telomeric DNA sequence
I	inosine
L[A-C]	ligands with covalently attached pyridine donors
MD	molecular dynamics
PAGE	polyacrylamide gel electrophoresis
PDEPR	pulsed dipolar electron paramagnetic resonance
RIDME	relaxation-induced dipolar modulation enhancement
SDSL	site-directed spin labeling
XRD	X-ray diffraction

REFERENCES

1. J. Choi, T. Majima, *Chem. Soc. Rev.* **2011**, *40*, 5893–5909.
2. M. L. Bochman, K. Paeschke, V. A. Zakian, *Nat. Rev. Genet.* **2012**, *13*, 770–780.
3. H. L. Lightfoot, T. Hagen, N. J. Tatum, J. Hall, *FEBS Lett.* **2019**, *593*, 2083–2102.
4. G. N. Parkinson, M. P. H. Lee, S. Neidle, *Nature* **2002**, *417*, 876–880.
5. K. N. Luu, A. T. Phan, V. Kuryavyi, L. Lacroix, D. J. Patel, *J. Am. Chem. Soc.* **2006**, *128*, 9963–9970.
6. K. W. Lim, S. Amrane, S. Bouaziz, W. Xu, Y. Mu, D. J. Patel, K. N. Luu, A. T. Phan, *J. Am. Chem. Soc.* **2009**, *131*, 4301–4309.
7. B. Heddi, A. T. Phan, *J. Am. Chem. Soc.* **2011**, *133*, 9824–9833.
8. K. Bose, C. J. Lech, B. Heddi, A. T. Phan, *Nat. Commun.* **2018**, *9*, 1959.
9. Y. Kato, T. Ohyama, H. Mita, Y. Yamamoto, *J. Am. Chem. Soc.* **2005**, *127*, 9980–9981.
10. A. K. Todd, M. Johnston, S. Neidle, *Nucleic Acids Res.* **2005**, *33*, 2901–2907.
11. J. L. Huppert, S. Balasubramanian, *Nucleic Acids Res.* **2005**, *33*, 2908–2916.
12. G. Biffi, D. Tannahill, J. McCafferty, S. Balasubramanian, *Nat. Chem.* **2013**, *5*, 182–186.
13. D. Rhodes, H. J. Lipps, *Nucleic Acids Res.* **2015**, *43*, 8627–8637.
14. H. Han, L. H. Hurley, *Trends Pharmacol. Sci.* **2000**, *21*, 136–142.
15. T. V. T. Le, S. Han, J. Chae, H.-J. Park, *Curr. Pharm. Des.* **2012**, *18*, 1948–1972.
16. S. N. Georgiades, N. H. Abd Karim, K. Suntharalingam, R. Vilar, *Angew. Chem. Int. Ed.* **2010**, *49*, 4020–4034.
17. J. Mitteaux, P. Lejault, F. Wojciechowski, A. Joubert, J. Boudon, N. Desbois, C. P. Gros, R. H. E. Hudson, J.-B. Boulé, A. Granzhan, D. Monchaud, *J. Am. Chem. Soc.* **2021**, *143*, 12567–12577.
18. P. Lejault, J. Mitteaux, F. R. Sperti, D. Monchaud, *Cell Chem. Biol.* **2021**, *28*, 436–455.
19. N. R. Kallenbach, R.-I. Ma, N. C. Seeman, *Nature* **1983**, *305*, 829–831.
20. J. E. Mueller, S. M. Du, N. C. Seeman, *J. Am. Chem. Soc.* **1991**, *113*, 6306–6308.
21. J. Chen, N. C. Seeman, *Nature* **1991**, *350*, 631–633.
22. E. Winfree, F. Liu, L. A. Wenzler, N. C. Seeman, *Nature* **1998**, *394*, 539–544.
23. P. W. K. Rothemund, *Nature* **2006**, *440*, 297–302.
24. C. Mao, W. Sun, Z. Shen, N. C. Seeman, *Nature* **1999**, *397*, 144–146.

25. E. S. Andersen, M. Dong, M. M. Nielsen, K. Jahn, R. Subramani, W. Mamdouh, M. M. Golas, B. Sander, H. Stark, C. L. P. Oliveira, J. S. Pedersen, V. Birkedal, F. Besenbacher, K. V. Gothelf, J. Kjems, *Nature* **2009**, *459*, 73–76.
26. C. K. McLaughlin, G. D. Hamblin, H. F. Sleiman, *Chem. Soc. Rev.* **2011**, *40*, 5647–5656.
27. N. C. Seeman, H. F. Sleiman, *Nat. Rev. Mater.* **2017**, *3*, 17068.
28. J.-L. Mergny, D. Sen, *Chem. Rev.* **2019**, *119*, 6290–6325.
29. X. Wang, J. Huang, Y. Zhou, S. Yan, X. Weng, X. Wu, M. Deng, X. Zhou, *Angew. Chem. Int. Ed.* **2010**, *49*, 5305–5309.
30. F. Wang, X. Liu, I. Willner, *Angew. Chem. Int. Ed.* **2015**, *54*, 1098–1129.
31. C. Wang, G. Jia, Y. Li, S. Zhang, C. Li, *Chem. Commun.* **2013**, *49*, 11161–11163.
32. T. Li, E. Wang, S. Dong, *J. Am. Chem. Soc.* **2009**, *131*, 15082–15083.
33. Q. Y. Yeo, I. Y. Loh, S. R. Tee, Y. H. Chiang, J. Cheng, M. H. Liu, Z. S. Wang, *Nanoscale* **2017**, *9*, 12142–12149.
34. X. Liu, J. Zhang, M. Fadeev, Z. Li, V. Wulf, H. Tian, I. Willner, *Chem. Sci.* **2018**, *10*, 1008–1016.
35. J. S. Kahn, Y. Hu, I. Willner, *Acc. Chem. Res.* **2017**, *50*, 680–690.
36. C.-H. Lu, X.-J. Qi, R. Orbach, H.-H. Yang, I. Mironi-Harpaz, D. Seliktar, I. Willner, *Nano Lett.* **2013**, *13*, 1298–1302.
37. P. Travascio, Y. Li, D. Sen, *Chem. Biol.* **1998**, *5*, 505–517.
38. I. Willner, B. Shlyahovsky, M. Zayats, B. Willner, *Chem. Soc. Rev.* **2008**, *37*, 1153–1165.
39. T. D. Canale, D. Sen, *Biochim. Biophys. Acta Gen. Subj.* **2017**, *1861*, 1455–1462.
40. J. H. Yum, S. Park, H. Sugiyama, *Org. Biomol. Chem.* **2019**, *17*, 5947–5961.
41. B. Ruttkay-Nedecky, J. Kudr, L. Nejdl, D. Maskova, R. Kizek, V. Adam, *Molecules* **2013**, *18*, 14760–14779.
42. H. Li, J. Liu, Y. Fang, Y. Qin, S. Xu, Y. Liu, E. Wang, *Biosens. Bioelectron.* **2013**, *41*, 563–568.
43. W. Zhou, R. Saran, J. Liu, *Chem. Rev.* **2017**, *117*, 8272–8325.
44. B. R. Vummidi, J. Alzeer, N. W. Luedtke, *ChemBioChem* **2013**, *14*, 540–558.
45. S.-B. Chen, W.-B. Wu, M.-H. Hu, T.-M. Ou, L.-Q. Gu, J.-H. Tan, Z.-S. Huang, *Chem. Commun.* **2014**, *50*, 12173–12176.
46. A. Laguerre, L. Stefan, M. Larrouy, D. Genest, J. Novotna, M. Pirrotta, D. Monchaud, *J. Am. Chem. Soc.* **2014**, *136*, 12406–12414.
47. Y. Cheng, M. Cheng, J. Hao, G. Jia, D. Monchaud, C. Li, *Chem. Sci.* **2020**, *11*, 8846–8853.
48. Y. Guo, J. Chen, M. Cheng, D. Monchaud, J. Zhou, H. Ju, *Angew. Chem. Int. Ed.* **2017**, *129*, 16863–16867.
49. J. Kosman, B. Juskowiak, *Anal. Chim. Acta* **2011**, *707*, 7–17.
50. D. Sen, L. C. H. Poon, *Crit. Rev. Biochem. Mol. Biol.* **2011**, *46*, 478–492.
51. D.-M. Kong, N. Wang, X.-X. Guo, H.-X. Shen, *Analyst* **2010**, *135*, 545–549.
52. Y. A. Shin, G. L. Eichhorn, *Biopolymers* **1980**, *19*, 539–556.
53. D. A. Malyshev, F. E. Romesberg, *Angew. Chem. Int. Ed.* **2015**, *54*, 11930–44.
54. M. Kimoto, I. Hirao, *Chem. Soc. Rev.* **2020**, *49*, 7602–7626.
55. G. H. Clever, C. Kaul, T. Carell, *Angew. Chem. Int. Ed.* **2007**, *46*, 6226–6236.
56. G. H. Clever, M. Shionoya, *Coord. Chem. Rev.* **2010**, *254*, 2391–2402.
57. S. Naskar, R. Guha, J. Müller, *Angew. Chem. Int. Ed.* **2020**, *59*, 1397–1406.
58. J. Müller, *Coord. Chem. Rev.* **2019**, *393*, 37–47.
59. I. Sinha, J. Müller, in DNA in Supramolecular Chemistry and Nanotechnology, Eds E. Stulz, G. H. Clever, John Wiley & Sons, Chichester, UK, **2017**, pp. 52–64.

60. S. Johannsen, N. Megger, D. Böhme, R. K. O. Sigel, J. Müller, *Nat. Chem.* **2010**, *2*, 229.
61. S. Liu, G. H. Clever, Y. Takezawa, M. Kaneko, K. Tanaka, X. Guo, M. Shionoya, *Angew. Chem. Int. Ed.* **2011**, *50*, 8886–8890.
62. S. Katz, *Biochim. Biophys. Acta* **1963**, *68*, 240–253.
63. E. Buncel, C. Boone, H. Joly, R. Kumar, A. R. Norris, *J. Inorg. Biochem.* **1985**, *25*, 61–73.
64. Z. Kuklenyik, L. G. Marzilli, *Inorg. Chem.* **1996**, *35*, 5654–5662.
65. A. Ono, H. Togashi, *Angew. Chem. Int. Ed.* **2004**, *43*, 4300–4302.
66. N. M. Smith, S. Amrane, F. Rosu, V. Gabelica, J.-L. Mergny, *Chem. Commun.* **2012**, *48*, 11464–11466.
67. D. Miyoshi, H. Karimata, Z.-M. Wang, K. Koumoto, N. Sugimoto, *J. Am. Chem. Soc.* **2007**, *129*, 5919–5925.
68. T. C. Marsh, J. Vesenka, E. Henderson, *Nucleic Acids Res.* **1995**, *23*, 696–700.
69. D. M. Engelhard, R. Pievo, G. H. Clever, *Angew. Chem. Int. Ed.* **2013**, *52*, 12843–12847.
70. D. M. Engelhard, L. M. Stratmann, G. H. Clever, *Chem. Eur. J.* **2018**, *24*, 2117–2125.
71. P. M. Punt, G. H. Clever, *Chem. Sci.* **2019**, *10*, 2513–2518.
72. S. Park, H. Matsui, K. Fukumoto, J. H. Yum, H. Sugiyama, *RSC Adv.* **2020**, *10*, 9717–9722.
73. L. Zhang, A. Peritz, E. Meggers, *J. Am. Chem. Soc.* **2005**, *127*, 4174–4175.
74. D. M. Engelhard, J. Nowack, G. H. Clever, *Angew. Chem. Int. Ed.* **2017**, *56*, 11640–11644.
75. W. Kaim, B. Schwederski, A. Klein, *Bioinorganic Chemistry: Inorganic Elements in the Chemistry of Life*, 2nd edn., John Wiley & Sons, Chichester, UK, **2013**.
76. A. P. S. Samuel, D. T. Co, C. L. Stern, M. R. Wasielewski, *J. Am. Chem. Soc.* **2010**, *132*, 8813–8815.
77. B. Dicke, A. Hoffmann, J. Stanek, M. S. Rampp, B. Grimm-Lebsanft, F. Biebl, D. Rukser, B. Maerz, D. Göries, M. Naumova, M. Biednov, G. Neuber, A. Wetzel, S. M. Hofmann, P. Roedig, A. Meents, J. Bielecki, J. Andreasson, K. R. Beyerlein, H. N. Chapman, C. Bressler, W. Zinth, M. Rübhausen, S. Herres-Pawlis, *Nat. Chem.* **2018**, *10*, 355–362.
78. P. Srivastava, H. Yang, K. Ellis-Guardiola, J. C. Lewis, *Nat. Commun.* **2015**, *6*, 7789.
79. L. A. Churchfield, F. A. Tezcan, *Acc. Chem. Res.* **2019**, *52*, 345–355.
80. H. M. Key, P. Dydio, D. S. Clark, J. F. Hartwig, *Nature* **2016**, *534*, 534.
81. K. Schlosser, Y. Li, *Chem. Biol.* **2009**, *16*, 311–322.
82. C. E. McGhee, R. J. Lake, Y. Lu, in *Artificial Metalloenzymes and MetalloDNAzymes in Catalysis: From Design to Applications*, Eds. D. Montserrat, J.-E. Bäckvall, P. Oscar, Wiley-VCH, Weinheim, Germany, **2018**, pp. 41–68.
83. P. M. Punt, G. H. Clever, *Chem. Eur. J.* **2019**, *25*, 13987–13993.
84. P. M. Punt, L. M. Stratmann, S. Sevim, L. Knauer, C. Strohmann, G. H. Clever, *Front. Chem.* **2020**, *8*, 26.
85. H. Yang, K. L. Metera, H. F. Sleiman, *Coord. Chem. Rev.* **2010**, *254*, 2403–2415.
86. G. Roelfes, B. L. Feringa, *Angew. Chem. Int. Ed.* **2005**, *44*, 3230–3232.
87. A. J. Boersma, B. L. Feringa, G. Roelfes, *Angew. Chem. Int. Ed.* **2009**, *48*, 3346–3348.
88. J. J. Marek, R. P. Singh, A. Heuer, U. Hennecke, *Chem. Eur. J.* **2017**, *23*, 6004–6008.
89. J. Mansot, J. Lauberteaux, A. Lebrun, M. Mauduit, J. Vasseur, R. M. de Figueiredo, S. Arseniyadis, J. Campagne, M. Smietana, *Chem. Eur. J.* **2020**, *26*, 3519–3523.

90. S. Roe, D. J. Ritson, T. Garner, M. Searle, J. E. Moses, *Chem. Commun.* **2010**, *46*, 4309–4311.
91. J. Hao, W. Miao, Y. Cheng, S. Lu, G. Jia, C. Li, *ACS Catal.* **2020**, *10*, 6561–6567.
92. C. Wang, Y. Li, G. Jia, Y. Liu, S. Lu, C. Li, *Chem. Commun.* **2012**, *48*, 6232–6234.
93. C. Wang, G. Jia, J. Zhou, Y. Li, Y. Liu, S. Lu, C. Li, *Angew. Chem. Int. Ed.* **2012**, *51*, 9352–9355.
94. S. Dey, A. Jäschke, *Angew. Chem. Int. Ed.* **2015**, *54*, 11279–11282.
95. S. Dey, C. L. Rühl, A. Jäschke, *Chem. Eur. J.* **2017**, *23*, 12162–12170.
96. S. Dey, A. Jäschke, *Molecules* **2020**, *25*, 3121.
97. P. M. Punt, M. D. Langenberg, O. Altan, G. H. Clever, *J. Am. Chem. Soc.* **2021**, *143*, 3555–3561.
98. M. Egli, P. S. Pallan, *Annu. Rev. Bioph. Biom.* **2007**, *36*, 281–305.
99. M. Adrian, B. Heddi, A. T. Phan, *Methods* **2012**, *57*, 11–24.
100. S. Raunser, *Angew. Chem. Int. Ed.* **2017**, *56*, 16450–16452.
101. G. Jeschke, *Annu. Rev. Phys. Chem.* **2012**, *63*, 419–446.
102. H. Sameach, S. Ruthstein, *Isr. J. Chem.* **2019**, *59*, 980–989.
103. M. Ji, S. Ruthstein, S. Saxena, *Acc. Chem. Res.* **2013**, *47*, 688–695.
104. Q. Miao, C. Nitsche, H. Orton, M. Overhand, G. Otting, M. Ubbink, *Chem. Rev.* **2022**, *122*, 9571–9642.
105. P. Roser, M. J. Schmidt, M. Drescher, D. Summerer, *Org. Biomol. Chem.* **2016**, *14*, 5468–5476.
106. O. Schiemann, N. Piton, J. Plackmeyer, B. E. Bode, T. F. Prisner, J. W. Engels, *Nat. Protoc.* **2007**, *2*, 904–923.
107. K. Halbmair, J. Seikowski, I. Tkach, C. Höbartner, D. Sezer, M. Bennati, *Chem. Sci.* **2016**, *7*, 3172–3180.
108. M. Heinz, N. Erlenbach, L. S. Stelzl, G. Thierolf, N. R. Kamble, S. T. Sigurdsson, T. F. Prisner, G. Hummer, *Nucleic Acids Res.* **2020**, *48*, 924–933.
109. S. Ghosh, M. J. Lawless, H. J. Brubaker, K. Singewald, M. R. Kurpiewski, L. Jen-Jacobson, S. Saxena, *Nucleic Acids Res.* **2020**, *48*, e49.
110. G. Sicoli, F. Wachowius, M. Bennati, C. Höbartner, *Angew. Chem. Int. Ed.* **2010**, *49*, 6443–6447.
111. A. M. Popova, T. Kálai, K. Hideg, P. Z. Qin, *Biochemistry* **2009**, *48*, 8540–8550.
112. D. Abdullin, N. Florin, G. Hagelueken, O. Schiemann, *Angew. Chem. Int. Ed.* **2014**, *54*, 1827–1831.
113. B. E. Bode, J. Plackmeyer, T. F. Prisner, O. Schiemann, *J. Phys. Chem.* **2008**, *112*, 5064–5073.
114. V. Singh, M. Azarkh, T. E. Exner, J. S. Hartig, M. Drescher, *Angew. Chem. Int. Ed.* **2009**, *48*, 9728–9730.
115. V. Singh, M. Azarkh, M. Drescher, J. S. Hartig, *Chem. Commun.* **2012**, *48*, 8258–8260.
116. X. Zhang, C.-X. Xu, R. D. Felice, J. Sponer, B. Islam, P. Stadlbauer, Y. Ding, L. Mao, Z.-W. Mao, P. Z. Qin, *Biochemistry* **2016**, *55*, 360–372.
117. I. T. Holder, M. Drescher, J. S. Hartig, *Bioorg. Med. Chem.* **2013**, *21*, 6156–6161.
118. M. Azarkh, V. Singh, O. Okle, D. R. Dietrich, J. S. Hartig, M. Drescher, *ChemPhysChem* **2012**, *13*, 1444–1447.
119. V. M. Marathias, K. Y. Wang, S. Kumar, T. Q. Pham, S. Swaminathan, P. H. Bolton, *J. Mol. Biol.* **1996**, *260*, 378–394.
120. M. P. Donohue, V. A. Szalai, *Phys. Chem. Chem. Phys.* **2016**, *18*, 15447–15455.
121. D. M. Engelhard, A. Meyer, A. Berndhäuser, O. Schiemann, G. H. Clever, *Chem. Commun.* **2018**, *54*, 7455–7458.
122. L. M. Stratmann, Y. Kutin, M. Kasanmascheff, G. H. Clever, *Angew. Chem. Int. Ed.* **2021**, *60*, 4939–4947.

15 Metabolite Regulation by Riboswitches
The Role of Metal Ions in Folding, Ligand Binding and Functionality

Maria Reichenbach, Sofia Gallo, and Roland K.O. Sigel
Department of Chemistry, University of Zurich, Winterthurerstrasse 190, CH-8057 Zurich, Switzerland
maria.reichenbach@chem.uzh.ch,
sofia.gallo@chem.uzh.ch, roland.sigel@chem.uzh.ch

CONTENTS

1. Introduction 400
2. Metal Ion-Assisted Folding of Riboswitches 402
3. Metal Ion-Assisted Binding Motifs Found across Riboswitch Classes 409
   3.1 Phosphate Recognition by Riboswitches 409
   3.2 Carboxylate Recognition by Riboswitches 412
   3.3 Fluoride Sensing by Riboswitches 414
   3.4 Purine-Recognizing Riboswitches 415
4. Metallo Cofactor and Metal Ion-Responsive Riboswitches 417
   4.1 Metallo Cofactor-Binding Riboswitch Classes 417
      4.1.1 Cobalamin-Responsive Riboswitches 417
      4.1.2 Moco- and Wco-Responsive Riboswitches 420
   4.2 Riboswitches Responsive to Metal Ions 422
      4.2.1 Na$^+$ 422
      4.2.2 Li$^+$ 422
      4.2.3 Mg^{2+} 422
      4.2.4 Mn^{2+} 424
      4.2.5 Transition Metals Ni^{2+}, Co^{2+} and Fe^{2+} 426
5. General Conclusions 427

Acknowledgments 428
Abbreviations 428
References 429

DOI: 10.1201/9781003270201-15

ABSTRACT

Metal ions in association with RNA fulfill numerous functions and are vital for structure formation and functionality. K^+ and Mg^{2+} are the most crucial, being the most abundant freely available metal ions in the cell. These ions not only shield the negative charges derived from the phosphate sugar backbone, but also allow the formation of highly complex, functional structures by mediating specific tertiary interactions. In ribozymes, specifically bound Mg^{2+} additionally promotes catalytic activity by metal ion-assisted RNA self-cleavage. In the context of riboswitches, metal ions take up further roles. Riboswitches are natural RNA aptamers involved in gene regulation by directly binding cellular metabolites or ions. In addition to their role in RNA folding, metal ions are often the key element for ligand binding allowing negatively charged moieties like phosphates, carboxylates, or even the single atomic fluoride to be recognized and bound by the RNA. Additionally, some riboswitch classes respond to metal ion-containing cofactors like molybdenum cofactor or cobalamins, while others are sensitive to single metal ions. For the latter, the RNA needs to discriminate between the correct metal ion and other, more abundant metal ions, a very difficult task to achieve in a cellular environment. For all these purposes riboswitches evolved elaborate binding pockets exploiting the different properties and binding strategies metal ions (and their ligands) can offer: size, softness/hardness, inner- and outer-sphere binding through an intricate H-bond pattern of coordinated water molecules as well as the inclusion of all functional moieties of the binding ligand. In this chapter, we discuss the different roles executed by metal ions for the proper functioning of riboswitches. Besides the general role during structure formation, we present different metal ion-dependent recognition modes, as well as metallo cofactor- and metal ion-binding riboswitches in more detail.

KEYWORDS

Riboswitches; Metal Ions; Aptamers; RNA; Gene Regulation

1 INTRODUCTION

The contribution to gene regulation by small non-coding RNAs has gathered interest for many years [1–3]. About two decades ago it was found that gene regulation can take place without the involvement of additional protein or oligonucleotide cofactors [4–6]. These findings sparked the idea that mRNA could act as a direct sensor for small molecules to regulate their cellular concentration. For a better understanding of gene regulation solely by RNA particular focus was laid on RNAs known to bind specific molecules with high specificity and affinity, i.e., aptamers. A strategic search of the genome yielded numerous conserved RNA sequences that bind specific metabolites, leading to the identification of natural aptamers [7, 8]. In 2002, such aptamers were shown to be involved directly in gene regulation and hence the term "riboswitch" was coined [9–11]. Riboswitches are regulatory mRNA elements located in the 5′-UTR of mRNA and have since been identified in all three domains of life, although predominantly in bacteria.

Metabolite Regulation by Riboswitches: The Role of Metal Ions

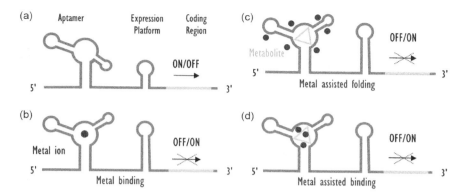

FIGURE 1 Schematic representation of the functioning of riboswitches and the respective role of metal ions. (a) Riboswitch composed of an aptamer and an expression platform. The arrow represents the translation of the coding region. In general, in the absence of a specific metabolite the gene expression downstream of the riboswitch is turned on. (b) A switched structure upon specific metal ion (sphere) coordination recognized by the riboswitch. (c) A switched structure where metal ions (spheres) are necessary for the specific metabolite ∇ recognition through preformation of the binding site. The number of metal ions does not represent a relative concentration but is only for visualization. (d) A switched riboswitch where metal ions are necessary for site-specific coordination of the metabolite for specific recognition and binding.

The general riboswitch architecture consists of two parts, the aptamer and the expression platform, which are interlinked with each other.

The aptamer region binds a specific metabolite and is highly conserved across different organisms. Riboswitches that bind the same metabolite are categorized as one family, however, they do not need to employ the same coordination strategy. Riboswitches binding a metabolite with the same core structure are categorized as a class. The binding of a specific metabolite by the aptamer induces a structural change of the expression platform. The expression platform is less conserved and can differ in sequence, structure, and even regulation mechanism within the same class (Figure 1a) [12, 13]. The expression platform interacts or even contains those RNA elements that are involved in gene expression, like the Shine–Dalgarno sequence or a terminator stem. A change in structure of the expression platform leads to modulation of gene expression downstream of the 5′-UTR [14]. Riboswitches regulate gene expression of proteins that manage the cellular concentration and homeostasis of the respective binding metabolite itself, i.e., proteins involved in either transport or biosynthesis [9]. Gene regulation through riboswitches occurs at several levels with transcriptional and translational regulation being the most frequent. An exception is the glmS riboswitch that is regulated *via* self-cleavage. In most cases, ligand binding to the riboswitch inhibits gene expression, but in the case of the guanidine, ppGpp, PRPP, and Mn^{2+} riboswitches ligand binding enhances gene expression [15, 16]. A discussion of the individual riboswitch regulation mechanisms exceeds the scope of this review and will therefore not be discussed. In any case, independent of the employed mechanism, the correct folding of the two mutually exclusive on and off conformations of the riboswitch is crucial and always dependent on metal ions [17].

In order to fulfill their task, riboswitches need to be highly selective within a specific affinity range, to keep the metabolite concentration within the livable boundaries. Many riboswitches sense ligands that are building blocks or derivatives of RNA nucleotides or their precursors [18]. Remarkably, about half of the common cofactors and nucleotide-based signaling molecules have at least one corresponding riboswitch class. The high similarity between these emphasizes the necessity of a specific recognition. The exceptional selectivity for their target metabolite by riboswitches is achieved by the riboswitch domains exploiting many different structural features thereby creating specific binding pockets. In this context, it is interesting to note that organisms evolved different recognition mechanisms for the same metabolite [19]. While most riboswitches guarantee selectivity through tight binding pockets, the glutamine and the THF riboswitch have open binding pockets and guarantee binding specificity by involving every heteroatom of the metabolite [20, 21]. Riboswitches illustrate a remarkably high specificity through the recognition of functional groups of the metabolite [11, 22, 23], atomic charge [24], and stereochemistry [10, 25]. Metal ions are thereby often crucial for the formation of specific binding pockets (Figure 1c). In addition, metal ions can directly bind negatively charged functional groups of the metabolite, as e.g., in the case of the lysine and flavin mononucleotide (FMN) riboswitches, thereby contributing directly to recognition and binding (Figure 1d) [26, 27]. In some cases, specific recognition is only possible through direct metal ion coordination. For example, the lysine riboswitch recognizes its cognate ligand as a K^+ ion chelate with the carboxylate, thus rendering the cation contribution vital [27]. In the second case of metal ion-mediated ligand recognition, the fluoride-dependent riboswitch, F^- is recognized through coordination to Mg^{2+} ions [28].

Below, we discuss the various roles of metal ions in the functionality of riboswitches. Besides their contribution to folding to achieve a metabolite-binding competent form and their assistance in specifically binding the metabolite, we will especially focus on riboswitches that bind metal cofactors and metal ions themselves (Figure 1b).

2 METAL ION-ASSISTED FOLDING OF RIBOSWITCHES

Metal ions are the most important and abundant RNA cofactors and are crucial to obtain a highly complex, spatially tight, and functional three-dimensional structure [29–31]. General charge compensation of the polyanionic backbone is mostly accomplished by loosely bound monovalent metal ions. Pockets within the three-dimensional fold accumulate a highly negative potential, serve as specific M^{n+} binding sites, and are involved in the formation of key structural elements and/or tertiary interactions. These specific binding sites offer intrinsic networks of direct inner-sphere and water-mediated outer-sphere contacts and are mainly occupied by divalent metal ions. Due to their abundance and availability in the cell K^+ and Mg^{2+} are usually associated with RNA, but also other metal ions can coordinate to RNA. Details on this topic are beyond the scope of this chapter and we, therefore, refer to the respective literature [32, 33]. For riboswitches, metal ions play various roles in (1) prefolding the aptamer to adopt a binding-competent fold, (2) metal-assisted ligand binding, and (3) refolding the RNA key elements to transduct ligand binding into regulatory function (Table 1).

The extent of pre-organization of the aptamer and the binding pocket itself can vary between riboswitch classes as does the structural impact of the binding event. Riboswitches are thus classified into two categories, type I and II, depending on the degree of their structural rearrangement upon ligand binding [34]. Type I riboswitches have a single, localized binding pocket supported by a largely pre-established global fold. In this case, ligand binding induces rather small local structural changes [35–41]. Type II riboswitches on the other hand are characterized by local as well as a global restructuration of the aptamer, needed to complete the binding site [39, 42]. Examples of this distinction are the purine and the thiamine pyrophosphate (TPP) riboswitches, which are both organized in a three-way junction and thus have a similar general fold [42, 43]. For the **purine riboswitches,** the junction serves as a binding pocket and no major structural changes occur upon ligand binding, categorizing them as type I. In the case of the **TPP riboswitch**, a type II riboswitch, the loops of the branching helices are part of the binding pocket. A bigger structural rearrangement is therefore observed upon ligand binding. In general, Mg^{2+}-mediated prefolding of the aptamer seems a common requirement for riboswitches independent of the category. In some cases, high salt concentrations can even lead to the formation of a bound-like fold, while ligand binding itself does not require the presence of metal ions. Pre-assembly of the ligand-binding site by Mg^{2+} has thus been observed for several riboswitches, among them the **adenine,** the **glmS,** the **TPP,** and the **glutamine** riboswitch.

The **adenine riboswitch** does not apply M^{n+} to bind its ligand. However, hydrated M^{n+} located within the aptamer help to form a binding-competent structure, capable of accommodating adenine [44, 45]. In contrast, for the **glmS riboswitch**, Mg^{2+} is used in ligand binding [46]. However, also in this case Mg^{2+} has a further role in pre-organization. At high Mg^{2+} concentration, ligand-bound and unbound states are even indistinguishable as observed by hydroxyl radical footprinting and UV crosslinking [47]. Also **TPP riboswitch** prefolding is Mg^{2+} dependent [48], reaching again a bound-like fold solely at high Mg^{2+} concentrations [49] and showing that the role of Mg^{2+} in riboswitch folding is independent of type I or II.

In many cases, metal ion binding goes hand in hand with ligand binding and riboswitch folding. In the case of the **glycine riboswitch**, addition of Mg^{2+} alone yields a significant compaction of the RNA structure, which is then even more compacted in the presence of glycine. In the absence of Mg^{2+} however, glycine cannot trigger a structural change [50]. It was shown that Mg^{2+} facilitates crucial tertiary interactions between aptamer domains necessary for ligand binding [51, 52]. Similarly, solution studies showed that the **cyclic-di-GMP riboswitch** has a strong requirement for Mg^{2+} to adopt the ligand-bound conformation [53]. Mg^{2+} stabilizes an intermediate binding-competent form [54], which then recognizes the

TABLE 1
Overview of the Investigated Influences of Metal Ions on Riboswitches

Category	Metabolite	Riboswitch	Detailed Explanation	No Influence	Required for Binding	Required for Folding	Metal Ions as Trigger
Metallo cofactors	Cobalamins	Cbl-I/II	Mg^{2+} is needed for correct prefolding. Specific Mg^{2+} binding sites facilitate kissing-loop formation.			✓	
	Moco	Moco					
	Wco	Wco					
Other cofactors	FMN		Mg^{2+} directly binds diphosphate moiety of FMN. Prefolding is required for the ligand to bind, induced by divalent metal ions.		✓	✓	
	HMP-PP						
	NAD^+	NAD^+-I	Mg^{2+} directly binds each phosphate group of the ADP moiety of NAD^+. An additional metal ion holds the RNA structure together forming the binding site.		✓	✓	
		NAD^+-II					
	SAH	SAH	In the presence of too high divalent metal ion concentrations the RNA structure collapses.				
	SAM	SAM-I	Divalent metal ions facilitate long-range tertiary interactions and stabilize the hairpin motif.		✓	✓	
		SAM-II	Pre-organization due to Mg^{2+} allows the formation of base triplets needed for the intercalation of SAM.		✓	✓	
		SAM-III/IV/VI					
		SAM-V	Hydrated Mg^{2+} binds carboxyl group site-specifically to the RNA.		✓		
		SAM-SAH					
	THF	THF-I	Long-range tertiary interactions are stabilized by metal ions.				
		THF-II					
	TPP	thi-box	Divalent metal ion assists the pyrophosphate binding. Site-specific Mg^{2+} binding aids the formation of tertiary contacts. High Mg^{2+} concentrations can lead to the formation of the ligand-bound form, without the presence of the ligand.			✓	

Metabolite Regulation by Riboswitches: The Role of Metal Ions

Overview of the Investigated Influences of Metal Ions on Riboswitches

Category		Metabolite	Riboswitch	Influence of Metal Ions — Detailed Explanation	No Influence	Required for Binding	Required for Folding	Metal Ions as Trigger
RNA-related Signaling molecules	Purines	Adenine	Adenine	Mg^{2+} enhances tertiary folding and is necessary.			✓	
		Guanine	Guanine	Mg^{2+} is not necessary for folding or ligand binding.	✓			
		Xanthine	Xanthine	Fold depends on divalent metal ions. Mg^{2+} bridges the ligand oxygen with the phosphate backbone through inner-sphere coordination.		✓		
	Cyclic dinucleotides	Cyclic-di-AMP	c-di-AMP					
		Cyclic-AMP-GMP	c-AMP-GMP					
		Cyclic-di-GMP	c-di-GMP-I	Mg^{2+} required to form a ligand-binding competent form.			✓	
			c-di-GMP-II				✓	
		ppGpp		K^+ associated with pyrophosphate moieties facilitates charge neutralization, but is not necessary for ligand recognition.				
		2′-deoxy-guanosine	dG	Mg^{2+} not necessary, but facilitates prefolding and increases the binding affinity.		✓		
		Guanidine	2′-dG-I/II/III/IV					
	RNA precursors	Prequeuosine-I	PreQ-I	Selectivity is suggested to depend on a tightly bound Ca^{2+}.	✓			
			PreQ-II	Metal ions are needed for tight ligand binding.		✓		
			PreQ-III	Mg^{2+} needed to form a ligand-binding competent form.			✓	
		PRPP		Metal ions bind weakly to the phosphate and more strongly to the pyrophosphate moiety. Third metal ion forms a water-mediated coordination to the 5′-phosphate.		✓		
		ZTP		Mg^{2+} coordinates the carboxyamide oxygen of the Z base and via inner-sphere contact also the backbone phosphates.		✓		

(Continued)

TABLE 1 (Continued)
Overview of the Investigated Influences of Metal Ions on Riboswitches

Category		Metabolite	Riboswitch	Influence of Metal Ions — Detailed Explanation	No Influence	Required for Binding	Required for Folding	Metal Ions as Trigger
Elemental ions	Halogenide	F⁻	F⁻	Three Mg^{2+} ions are essential for F⁻ binding. One K^+ ion assists binding network. Prefolding by Mg^{2+}.		✓	✓	
	Metals	Li⁺	Li⁺-I, Li⁺-II					✓
		Mg^{2+}	Mg^{2+}-I	Mg^{2+} ions stabilize tertiary contacts.				✓
			Mg^{2+}-II					✓
		Mn^{2+}	yybP-ykoY	Moderate stabilization of the Mn^{2+}-free riboswitch by Mg^{2+} binding to the same site.				✓
			mntH					✓
		Na⁺	Na⁺-I, Na⁺-II					✓
		$Ni^{2+}, Co^{2+}, Fe^{2+}$	NiCo					✓
Amino acids		Glutamine	Glutamine-I					
			Glutamine-II	Metal ion is directly coordinated to carboxylate oxygen atom and enforces the ligand selectivity.		✓		
		Glycine	Glycine	Mg^{2+} is needed for glycine to induce structural change and a significant compaction.			✓	
		Lysine	Lysine	K^+ is needed for the recognition of the extended lysine.		✓		
Sugars		GlcN6P	glmS	Fully hydrated Mg^{2+} binds phosphate of GlcN6P to the RNA.		✓		

two purine moieties of cyclic-di-GMP through canonical and non-canonical base pairing and stacking interactions. In response to ligand binding, the riboswitch undergoes a subsequent compaction and large-scale structural rearrangement.

As evident from the above-mentioned examples, some, if not most, riboswitch classes do not follow a linear folding pathway. The typical route needing mono and divalent metal ions to reach the native tertiary structure can aberrate as was observed, e.g., for the M-box riboswitch. Recent experimental developments facilitate the study of dynamic processes as well as of the more flexible, ligand-free aptamers revealing detailed binding mechanisms and softening the strict subdivision into type I and type II [55]. For instance, ligand binding can allow the stabilization of a substructure, which is present already in the free state but in dynamic equilibrium with other substructures. Examples for such a folding pathway are the adenine [45] and the *btuB* adenosylcobalamin (AdoCbl)-specific riboswitches. Today's knowledge of the metal ion-induced folding mechanisms of the M-box riboswitch and the *btuB* riboswitch is discussed in more detail below.

Folding of **Mg^{2+}-sensing M-box riboswitch** is strictly and only dependent on divalent metal ions [56]. Although four K$^+$ ions were found in its crystal structure, the correct Mg^{2+}-bound form could be reached without addition of monovalent ions. In contrast, folding in high K$^+$ concentration but in absence of Mg^{2+} did not result in the correct compact tertiary conformation. Among divalent ions, the M-box riboswitch is relatively unselective since also Mn^{2+}, Ca^{2+}, Sr^{2+}, or Co^{2+} can induce the correct compacted structure [56]. Nevertheless, as an actual metal sensor, *in vivo* the M-box riboswitch can discriminate between the different divalent ions despite its rather low affinity toward Mg^{2+} with an EC$_{50}$ in the range of 0.2–2.7 mM [56]. In the cell, Mg^{2+} is the only divalent metal ion freely accessible in this concentration range making binding to the other mostly protein-bound and/or tightly regulated divalent metal ions insignificant. As is discussed in Section 4.2.3, the M-box riboswitch responds to Mg^{2+} by binding to three distinct cores able to host a total of nine specific Mg^{2+} ions [57]. This multiple and highly cooperative binding mode was proposed to allow a fast genetic response to minor Mg^{2+} fluctuations.

In the case of the AdoCbl-responding *btuB* riboswitch, instead of full restructuration of the aptameric [58] region, ligand binding induces only local changes [58, 59]. The additionally observed global compaction upon ligand binding [59] most probably results from stabilization of key tertiary interactions when AdoCbl is bound, and can be explained by the enclosure of the binding pocket by a peripheral extension (PE1) or a specific kissing loop (KL) (Section 4.1.1) [58, 60]. Mg^{2+} was found crucial for correctly prefolding the aptamer *in vitro*. In-line probing revealed two distinct conformations (Figure 2): The first is formed only in the presence of K$^+$ ions and is retained at low Mg^{2+} concentrations. This fold is unable to bind AdoCbl. At 0.5 mM Mg^{2+}, reorganization into a so-called binding-competent form finally enables the aptamer to bind the ligand [59]. This fold is highly pre-organized and very similar to the final, ligand-bound structure with key tertiary interactions

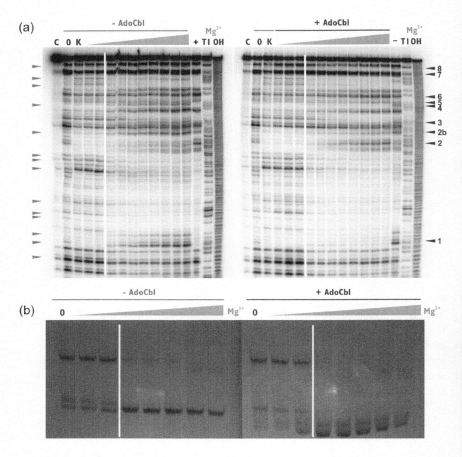

FIGURE 2 Mg^{2+}-dependent folding of the *btuB* riboswitch of *E. coli* in the absence (left) and in the presence (right) of 0.5 mM AdoCbl visualized by either in-line probing using 5′-end labeled RNA (a) or by native PAGE and UV-shadowing (b). The white lines mark the Mg^{2+}-dependent refolding step which takes place in the same concentration range independent of AdoCbl. C: Unreacted RNA, 0: RNA incubated in solely buffer, K: RNA incubated in the presence of 100 mM K^+. Mg^{2+} concentrations were (a): 0.05–20 mM, or (b): 0.1–50 mM. (+): RNA incubated in the presence of 20 mM Mg^{2+} and 0.5 mM AdoCbl, (−): RNA incubated in the presence of 20 mM Mg^{2+} but in the absence of AdoCbl. Gray marks on the left indicate the sites which show the highest Mg^{2+}-dependent intensity changes above 0.1 mM Mg^{2+}. Black marks at the right indicate the nine sites modulated by the addition of AdoCbl. (This figure is taken from Ref. [59] and reproduced with permission (CC-BY-NC).)

including the L4/J6/7 T-loop/T-loop-like interaction and the L5-P13 kissing loop already formed [58, 60–62]. The Mg^{2+}-dependent KL formation is supported by specific Mg^{2+}-binding sites situated in both L5 and L13 [63, 64], a common feature found in KL structures [65, 66]. Specific metal ion sites were determined to correlate with conserved bases [58] and comparison with the crystallized AdoCbl-riboswitches [63, 64] showed a partial match of the metal ion-binding sites found *via* Tb(III) cleavage with the iridium(III) hexaammines in the *Sth* riboswitch crystal structure [64]. Mg^{2+}-binding at these sites therefore very likely facilitates crucial tertiary interactions common to AdoCbl-dependent riboswitches to achieve an active, binding-competent structure. In the absence of ligand, smFRET studies showed the kissing loop in dynamic equilibrium with an "open" form, and only fully stabilized upon ligand binding. In the presence of the cobalamin ligand, the needed Mg^{2+} concentration is thereby lowered from millimolar to a physiological relevant sub-millimolar range. This mechanism of action was observed for several cobalamin riboswitches [61–63] demonstrating that this mode of binding and regulation is most probably typical for the entire family [61].

3 METAL ION-ASSISTED BINDING MOTIFS FOUND ACROSS RIBOSWITCH CLASSES

To date, more than 50 riboswitch classes have been identified and verified [18]. The more seldom a riboswitch motif occurs in nature, the harder it is to identify its binding metabolite because there are fewer sequences that can be compared with respect to the downstream encoded genes. Potential riboswitches with so far unknown metabolites are commonly called orphan-riboswitches. Throughout the so far identified metabolites, several recurring recognition mechanisms have been identified. Frequently metabolites carry an aromatic component and a charged functional group like a phosphate component or another charged functional group on either end. While the aromatic moiety is directly incorporated through intercalation or hydrogen bonding, charged functional groups often require metal ions to facilitate tight and correct binding to the RNA. In general, the knowledge of the influence of metal ions on metabolite recognition by riboswitches is rather scarce, and hence in this review, we summarize the trends and patterns that can be deduced from the existing literature.

3.1 Phosphate Recognition by Riboswitches

Numerous metabolites identified to interact with riboswitches carry a negatively charged phosphate group. Considering the negatively charged backbone of the RNA it is not surprising that metal ions are frequently employed to accommodate

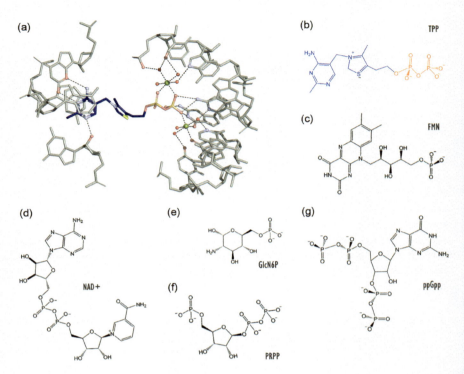

FIGURE 3 Metabolites being recognized by the riboswitch through direct metal ion-mediated coordination. (a) The TPP binding pocket within its riboswitch is shown. The metabolite TPP is shown in blue with the sulfur in yellow and phosphor atoms in orange. Coordinating oxygen and nitrogen atoms are shown as red or blue spheres, respectively. The dark green spheres represent Mg^{2+} involved in the metabolite coordination. Water molecules coordinated to Mg^{2+} are shown in red together with the hydrogen-bonding network indicated by dotted lines. This panel was generated with PyMOL [187] using the PDB ID 2GCI. Further metabolites shown are (b) thiamine pyrophosphate TPP, (c) flavine mononucleotide FMN, (d) nicotinamide adenine dinucleotide NAD^+, (e) glucosamine 6-phosphate GlcN6P, (f) α-5'-phosphoribosyl-1'-pyrophosphate PRPP, and (g) 5'-diphosphate 3'-diphosphate guanosine ppGpp.

these additional phosphate moieties in the binding pockets. In fact, optimal binding to the polyanionic RNA is often achieved by metal ion coordination as observed for the redox cofactors TPP, FMN, and NAD^+, the alarmone ppGpp, the metabolic intermediate PRPP, and the sugar Glc6NP to name just a few (Figure 3). The binding of these phosphate-carrying metabolites to their respective riboswitch is discussed in more detail below.

TPP is bound in an extended conformation, with the pyrimidine moiety embedded within an intercalating pocket formed by a helix, and the pyrophosphate moiety within a separate binding pocket of another helical region. Neither the thiazole ring nor the ethylene bridge is bound allowing for a rather flexible structure even in the bound state [67]. Footprinting experiments revealed that while thiamine monophosphate and thiamin are also recognized by the riboswitch, the binding affinity is 1,000-fold weaker, emphasizing the importance of the pyrophosphate group [67]. TPP is tightly bound to the riboswitch by an intrinsic network of inner- and outer-sphere contacts including two partially hydrated Mg^{2+} ions coordinated to the diphosphate moiety in addition to four direct contacts of non-bridging PP-oxygen atoms to the RNA (Figure 3) [68]. Co-crystallization with various metal ions showed that not only Mg^{2+} can stabilize TPP in the binding pocket, but also Mn^{2+}, Ca^{2+}, and Ba^{2+} [69].

A similar case is observed for the **FMN** riboswitch. The riboswitch consists of a six-stem junction, which adopts a butterfly-like scaffold, stapled together but opposingly directed and nearly identically folded peripheral domains. The cofactor is bound asymmetrically, the isoalloxazine ring system lying outside the central binding pocket and its phosphate group coordinated *via* a Mg^{2+} by inner-sphere interactions with a non-bridging phosphate oxygen and the N7 nitrogen of a guanine base [26, 70]. Binding studies highlight the importance of the phosphate group for coordination: The unphosphorylated form of FMN, riboflavin, binds to the RNA 100 times weaker in the presence of physiological concentrations of monovalent and divalent ions. The additional removal of the ribityl moiety (resulting in lumiflavin) further decreases the binding affinity only by a factor of 2 [26]. As in the case of TPP, this effect is not limited to Mg^{2+} but is also observed in the presence of the divalent ions Ba^{2+}, Ca^{2+}, and Mn^{2+} [26].

NAD⁺ is one of the larger riboswitch-binding metabolites. The aptamer region appears in a tandem conformation and first it was believed that only domain one binds NAD⁺ [71]. A later study demonstrated that also domain two binds NAD⁺ with the same coordination pattern but a much lower binding affinity [72]. Metabolite binding relies entirely on the recognition of the adenosine diphosphate moiety [44]. Co-crystallization showed two Mg^{2+}, one coordinating in an inner-sphere fashion to two non-bridging phosphate oxygen atoms, and the second in an outer-sphere fashion to the pyrophosphates but inner-sphere to the riboswitch. A third Mg^{2+} participates in folding of the binding pocket but is not directly interacting with NAD⁺ [72].

The guanidine riboswitch motif has two subcategories, namely the **PRPP riboswitch** and the **ppGpp** riboswitch that are both heavily reliant on their phosphate moieties for selective coordination. The overall structure of both riboswitches is very similar but the orientation of the corresponding metabolite within the binding pocket is inverted [15, 73]. The **PRPP** aptamer recognizes its ligand through a shifted and extended helical ligand-binding region, allowing the retention of bound metal ions and extensive hydrogen bond donation to phosphate groups. Two crystal structures show a slightly different contribution of M^{2+} coordination. Knappenberg et al. suggest the participation of two Mg^{2+} in direct coordination and one through its hydration shell. The 5′-phosphate binds weakly to one Mg^{2+} whereas the pyrophosphate moiety more strongly coordinates the second. A third Mg^{2+} forms a water-mediated coordination to the 5′-phosphate [15, 74].

Peselis et al. suggest the coordination of three metal ions, two Ba^{2+} (present in the crystallization buffer) and one Mg^{2+} [73]. A single mutation of the PRPP riboswitch aptamer, namely G96A, renders the aptamer capable of recognizing ppGpp selectively and with high affinity [15].

A crystal structure of the **ppGpp** riboswitch suggests that the 5′-pyrophosphate moiety is held in place by numerous hydrogen bonds from amino groups of conserved nucleobases. Several metal ions close by were assigned to be K^+ ions [15]. In a different study, however, direct Mg^{2+} coordination of the riboswitch to the ppGpp was observed [73], probably due to the differing conditions. Given that Mg^{2+} is the major player in phosphate recognition and binding [33], the second coordination pattern seems more plausible. However, it is also well known that charge screening by metal ions from a distance is a crucial effect on both proteins and RNAs [29].

The *glmS* riboswitch recognizes glucosamine-6-phosphate (Glc6NP) and self-cleaves upon binding, making it also a ribozyme [75]. The metabolite binds to a rigid, pre-organized riboswitch structure in an open, solvent-accessible pocket adjacent to the cleavable phosphodiester. The Glc6NP amino group contacts the scissile phosphate, while the Glc6NP phosphate makes hydrogen bonds to G1 of the riboswitch (just 3′ of the cleavage site) and also coordinates two fully hydrated Mg^{2+} linking the metabolite to the riboswitch through an extensive hydrogen-bonding network [76, 77].

3.2 Carboxylate Recognition by Riboswitches

Like phosphate groups, also carboxylate groups carry a negative charge at physiological pH. To date, four different families of riboswitches have been identified where the carboxylate functional group of the metabolite is essential for correct binding and recognition, i.e., via metal ion coordination. The metabolites in question are the three amino acids lysine, glutamine and glycine, as well as the sulfonium-betaine cofactor *S*-adenosyl methionine (SAM).

The **lysine riboswitch** is built up of a three-helix bundle and a two-helix bundle radiating from a five-way junction, whereby the ligand-free and the ligand-bound structures were found to be remarkably similar [78]. The lysine riboswitch adopts essentially indistinguishable three-dimensional structures in the presence or absence of the amino acid and presumably even in the absence of Mg^{2+}. Nevertheless, Mg^{2+} stabilizes tertiary interactions and therefore enhances selectivity and is crucial for metabolite binding [79]. Lysine is bound in an extended conformation with the carboxylate as well as both ammonium moieties involved in efficient binding [80]. In this case, K^+ is not only used for the "usual" charge compensation, but the riboswitch recognizes lysine through an indispensable K^+ ion chelate with the carboxylate (Figure 4a). Removal of the carboxylate group of lysine makes it impossible for the riboswitch to bind [25], and the replacement of K^+ with Na^+ or Mg^{2+} leads to a decrease in affinity by a factor of 50–100, emphasizing the specificity of this coordination motif [27].

Metabolite Regulation by Riboswitches: The Role of Metal Ions 413

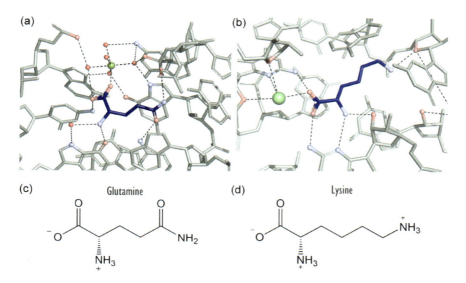

FIGURE 4 Depiction of the carboxylate-metal ion-assisted binding motifs found in riboswitches. The hydrogen-bonding and coordination network is indicated around the metabolite (in blue), with the oxygen atoms shown as red spheres. Metal ions are shown as green spheres. The binding pockets of the glutamine riboswitch (a) and the lysine riboswitch (b) are shown, with the structure of the two amino acids shown underneath. The panels have been prepared with PyMOL [187] using the PDB IDs 5DDP and 3D0U.

The **glutamine** and **glycine** riboswitch both coordinate the carboxylate moiety *via* a specifically bound Mg^{2+} in an otherwise open binding pocket [81]. To prevent loss in binding capacity, an intricate hydrogen-bonding network of direct or water-mediated contacts involves every heteroatom of the metabolite (Figure 4b) leading to very high selectivity. Any modification of the hydrogen-bonding network or the absence of Mg^{2+} results in a loss of selectivity and affinity, as was also shown by HMQC NMR studies [81]. In the presence of Mg^{2+} the apo-riboswitch is in conformational equilibrium between a flexible tuning fork and a minor conformation similar but not identical to the ligand-bound L-shape. Upon addition of glutamine, a larger structural change of the RNA is observed [81].

The **glycine riboswitch** functions similarly to the glutamine riboswitch. A three-helical bundle originating from a three-way junction accommodates the glycine in a bulge-containing binding pocket above the junction. Two Mg^{2+} are employed to recognize the carboxylate moiety. One coordinates directly, the second one stabilizes the correct fold of the binding pocket but does not directly interact with glycine [82]. Like the lysine riboswitch, the ligand-free and the ligand-bound glycine riboswitch structures are remarkably similar [27, 82].

The **SAM riboswitch** family is exemplary for how different RNA motifs can bind the same metabolite and that a specific moiety does not implicate a specific coordination mechanism. Six distinct classes have been identified to target S-adenosyl methionine [83]. In addition, related SAH riboswitches have been identified, binding SAH (S-adenosyl-L-homocysteine) selectively or, as the SAH/SAM riboswitch, not distinguishing between the two molecules. The structures of the six known riboswitch classes recognizing SAM are very different, and still, they exploit similar molecular strategies to recognize individual moieties and functional groups of their common target [83]. The adenine base is involved in base stacking and base-triple interactions in all SAM riboswitches. The positively charged sulfonium moiety is recognized through favorable electrostatic interactions, usually with one or two O4 carbonyl oxygen atoms from surrounding uracil residues. The recognition of the positive charge allows for the distinction between SAM and SAH. The largest difference among SAM riboswitches is to what extent they involve the methionine tail in metabolite recognition. SAM-I and SAM-IV have a very similar coordination motif. They completely engulf SAM in a pocket between two helical stacks. The methyl group itself is not critical in SAM-I [24]. SAM-II riboswitches adopt a classical H-type pseudoknot and enclose SAM inside an RNA triple helix. They appear to directly or indirectly recognize every available functional group [84, 85]. SAM-III intercalates SAM into a tight pocket in a three-way junction and seems not to recognize the methionine tail at all [86].

While Mg^{2+} was shown to enhance the folding of all SAM riboswitch classes [87], only SAM-V was shown to use a metal ion for direct metabolite recognition, most probably Mg^{2+}. The aminoacyl group is hydrogen bonded to an adenine residue and the carboxylate is hydrogen bonded to inner-sphere water molecules of a metal ion that is site specifically bound to the RNA backbone [88].

3.3 Fluoride Sensing by Riboswitches

Aside from metabolites of various sizes and metal ions, which are well known to interact with RNA, also a rather unexpected ligand was discovered about ten years ago, fluoride. The fluoride-binding motif is unique throughout riboswitches, being able to sense a small atomic anion. Fluoride riboswitches upregulate mainly fluoride transporters and ion channels to prevent toxic levels of this anion [89]. F^- is bound with a K_D of ~60 µM, while the riboswitch disregards other halides or small anions/Lewis bases such as hydroxide, carbon monoxide, or nitric oxide. F^- recognition is strongly Mg^{2+}-dependent with similar affinities at 5 or 1 mM Mg^{2+} but no binding in the absence of Mg^{2+}. The Mg^{2+} requirement becomes obvious from the crystal structure revealing a central binding pocket small enough to sense exclusively F^- (Figure 5): Three partially hydrated Mg^{2+} organized in planar position coordinate concomitantly to a central F^-, which protrudes from the plane by around 0.5 Å [28]. Five inwardly pointing backbone phosphates constitute an outer shell of ligands anchoring the binding pocket to the RNA. Three phosphate groups coordinate to Mg^{2+} with bidentate coordination while two phosphates are involved in monodentate coordination donating a total of eight oxygen atom ligands. At the same time, these phosphates together

Metabolite Regulation by Riboswitches: The Role of Metal Ions

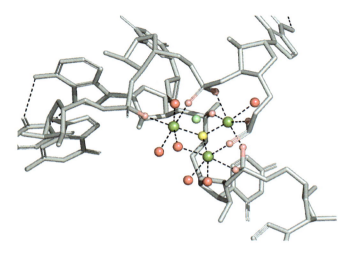

FIGURE 5 The binding pocket of the fluoride riboswitch depicting the two-shelled coordination site of the ligand. Three Mg^{2+} (dark green spheres) coordinate the central F^- (yellow sphere), and a nearby K^+ (light green sphere) helps keeping the phosphate groups in place. Coordinating phosphoryl oxygen atoms from the RNA are marked in red while the larger red spheres represent coordinating water molecules. This panel was generated with PyMOL [187] using the PDB ID 4ENC.

with a nearby K^+ bring two different domains of the RNA close in space, locking the riboswitch tertiary fold upon F^- binding.

The folding pathway was studied in detail by chemical-exchange saturation transfer NMR, co-transcriptional SHAPE, and smFRET [90–96] and was consistently shown to be Mg^{2+}-dependent to form a binding-competent form able to bind F^-. The pseudoknotted apo-structure of the riboswitch is already very similar to the F^--bound fold, but dynamic, populating two distinct states. One of these is a short-lived excited state [94], but both come together to a single stable conformation upon F^--binding by stabilizing a crucial long-range single-base interaction (A40·U48) [95, 96]. The here observed decisive impact of a single long-range interaction stabilized by ligand-binding stands in contrast to other pseudoknotted riboswitches [97] and is so far unique for the F^- riboswitch.

3.4 PURINE-RECOGNIZING RIBOSWITCHES

Most metabolites triggering riboswitches are in some way derived from nucleobases. The purine moieties adenine and guanine are thus not only very frequently part of riboswitch-triggering metabolites but are also crucial for recognition by the riboswitches through a network of hydrogen bonds and π-stacking/intercalation.

Both purine nucleobases adenine and guanine bind to their specific riboswitch, both being rather similar in secondary structure showing a three-way junction.

The two riboswitches differ in three nucleotides situated in the junction region. One specific mutation, namely C74 to a U74, converts the guanine to an adenine riboswitch, each ensuring Watson-Crick base pairing with the respective nucleobase as the decisive factor [41, 98]. The strong specificity relies on an extensive hydrogen-bonding network and shape complementarity (Figure 6). Substantial loss of affinity was associated with alteration of every functional group on the guanine ring, indicating that the guanine is completely encapsulated within the RNA fold [99]. In addition, the kissing-loop interaction between the hairpin loops in the purine riboswitches appears to be critical for both global scaffold formation and binding pocket architecture, and thereby mediates long-range effects on ligand binding and release [35].

Despite their similarity in purine recognition, the two riboswitches differ distinctly in the structure of the ligand-free states and their metal ion-induced folding. In the case of the **adenine riboswitch**, the apo-riboswitch shows conformational heterogeneity, and only upon addition of Mg^{2+} a homogeneously folded RNA along with stabilization of the loop-loop interaction is formed [100]. Further studies report a pre-organization of long-range tertiary interactions upon addition of Mg^{2+} and monovalent ions [45].

The **guanine riboswitch** on the other hand shows pre-organization of long-range interactions independent of the presence of Mg^{2+} [38, 101]. Despite the different prefolding behavior, ligand binding is detected for both purine-sensing riboswitches in the absence of Mg^{2+} even though the tertiary interaction is only partially formed in the adenine-sensing riboswitch.

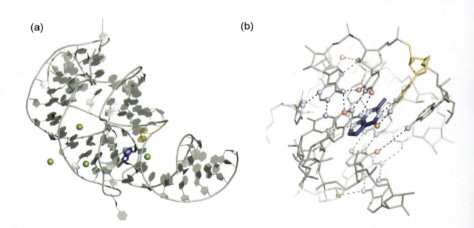

FIGURE 6 (a) Adenine riboswitch with the green spheres representing Mg^{2+} ions, the metabolite adenine in blue within the binding pocket and the nucleotide C74 in yellow. (b) The guanine riboswitch-binding pocket with the same color coding as in (a). The light blue spheres indicate the nitrogen atoms involved in hydrogen bonding and the light red spheres indicate the oxygen atoms involved in hydrogen bonding. This panel was generated with PyMOL [187] using the PDB IDs 1Y26 and 1Y27.

While most purine moieties are exclusively interacting *via* intercalation, in the case of the third respective riboswitch family, **xanthine** is recognized in a rod-like fold within an intriguing binding pocket that is critically dependent on Mg^{2+} bridging xanthine O6 and a backbone phosphate oxygen atom through inner-sphere coordination. The key recognition feature is the insertion of the xanthine pyrimidine moiety between an opened G-U base pair, thus enabling shape complementarity and simultaneous recognition of the C2 urea substructure *via* a maximum of four hydrogen bonds [102].

4 METALLO COFACTOR AND METAL ION-RESPONSIVE RIBOSWITCHES

4.1 Metallo Cofactor-Binding Riboswitch Classes

Numerous enzymatic cofactors are regulated by riboswitches, the most prominent representatives being the TPP, SAM, and cobalamin riboswitches [103]. Enzymatic cofactors are very versatile and such are their respective riboswitches, which vary in size, structure, and binding strategy in order to fit their ligand. Among these riboswitch-binding cofactors, two are metallo cofactors which are each rather described as a molecular family of derivatives. The first is the cobalamin family with cofactor B_{12} and vitamin B_{12} as the most common derivatives, whereas the second family comprises molybdenum cofactor, tungsten cofactor, and potentially also derivatives thereof.

4.1.1 Cobalamin-Responsive Riboswitches

The B_{12} cofactor family comprises some of the largest and most complex of all coenzymes. These cofactors are composed of a corrin ring substituted with seven amide side chains and a central Co^{3+} (Figure 7). Three side chains, the acetamide groups *a*, *c*, and *g* point upwards with respect to the corrin plane (β-side), while the four propionamide sidechains *b*, *d*, *e*, and the linking sidechain *f* are directed downwards (α-side). The coordination sphere of Co^{3+} is completed by an α-ligand which mostly is linked to sidechain *f*, and a versatile β-ligand. B_{12} cofactors are considered to be the evolutionary most ancient protein cofactors [104–106] and possibly originate from the so-called RNA world [107]. Natural B_{12} derivatives comprise around a dozen variants, out of which two, AdoCbl and MeCbl, act as cofactors in enzymatic reactions. Both have in common a unique organometallic and light-sensitive Co^{3+}–C bond to either 5′-deoxyadenosine (AdoCbl) or methyl (MeCbl). Further, naturally occurring analogs possess modifications at either the α- or β-side. Three derivatives often used in studies with cobalamin riboswitches, aquacobalamin (AqCbl), hydroxocobalamin (HyCbl), and cyanocobalamin, better known as vitamin B_{12} (CNCbl), all lack the organometallic bond and have only a small substituent.

Cobalamin riboswitches, also called Cbl or B_{12} riboswitches, are the second most widespread riboswitch class, exceeded only by the TPP riboswitches [108]. The cobalamin riboswitch family was among the first described [109, 110], and in

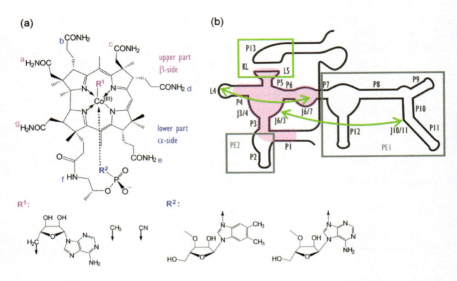

FIGURE 7 (a) Schematic view of the corrin ring system common to cobalamin derivatives. The acetamide sidechains *a*, *c*, and *g* pointing to the β-side as well as the upper variable ligand R^1 are market in magenta. The propionamide sidechains *b*, *d*, *e*, and *f* and the lower ligand R^2 are marked in purple. Some examples of R^1 and R^2 are shown below. (b) Secondary structure of the *btuB* riboswitch of *E. coli* as a representative of a class I Cbl riboswitch. The central binding core for cobalamin is marked in magenta, the variable regions PE1 and PE2 are boxed in gray and the key tertiary interactions are indicated in green (KL=kissing loop).

2021 over 14,600 representatives were known out of which 9,000 are of bacterial origin from over 5,000 species. 36 of these bacterial strands are human pathogens, raising the interest of cobalamin riboswitches as potential new targets for antimicrobial drugs [111–113]. Situated upstream of mostly B$_{12}$ transporters or of proteins involved in B$_{12}$ biosynthesis, the cobalamin riboswitches regulate gene expression at both transcriptional and/or translational levels [110]. While transcription termination is predominant in Gram-positive bacteria, the translation regulation upon ribosome binding site (RBS) sequestration is the mode of choice in Gram-negative bacteria and is generally more common [110, 114]. Some Cbl riboswitches, such as for example the *btuB* riboswitch of *E. coli*, regulate at both levels [4, 115].

Unlike the other riboswitch classes [35, 116], the Cbl riboswitch class is not restricted to a single ligand. It rather shows a broad spectrum of selectivity toward different cobalamins [117–121] which could derive from adaptation to the natural conditions the organisms are facing, e.g., light exposure which degrades the organometallic B$_{12}$ derivatives. Acceptance of different B$_{12}$ derivatives would therefore ensure the correct functionality throughout the daily cycle [63, 118], which is otherwise only achieved by having several copies of Cbl riboswitches within the genome – a condition which is more or less common and/

or pronounced depending on the bacterial strain [110, 122, 123]. Depending on which B_{12} derivative they respond to, cobalamin riboswitches are roughly subdivided into two classes: Cbl-I and Cbl-II. Cbl-I riboswitches show high affinity to the large AdoCbl, and Cbl-II representatives bind more specifically to the smaller derivatives. Due to structural variations and the resulting ligand preferences, class Cbl-II is further subdivided into the subclasses Cbl-IIa, which is strongly linked to the small B_{12} derivatives, and Cbl-IIb, whose members show a fainter selectivity [118].

Like other riboswitches, cobalamin riboswitches are composed of a conserved, ligand-binding aptamer and a regulatory platform which are connected by a variable linker. This linker shows no sequence conservation but contains a stemloop structure (Figure 7b, P13). The aptameric part encompasses around 200 nucleotides and belongs to the largest and most complex aptamers found in riboswitches. Its global fold is composed of two coaxial stacks with P1-P3-P6 and P4-P5-P13 linked together *via* a T-loop/T-loop-like interaction between L4 and J6/7. Stack P4-P5-P13 contains a well-organized kissing-loop (L5-P13) connecting the aptamer to the linker region [63, 64, 120]. This L5-P13 kissing-loop interaction was proposed to be important for high-affinity binding since early on [123] and was later demonstrated to be indeed crucial for regulation, although not for binding *per se* [63, 64, 124].

To date five structures of Cbl riboswitches are available. Two are Cbl-I riboswitches bound to AdoCbl: the *Thermoanaerobacter tengcongensis* (*Tte*) riboswitch which includes also P13 and thus the kissing-loop interaction [63] and the *Symbiobacterium thermophilum* (*Sth*) riboswitch [64]. The second pair of structures derives from the same class II riboswitch from an environmental metagenome (*env8*) [63]. Env8 originates from the ocean surface where cobalamins are predominantly found as hydrolyzed AqCbl. Both structural derivatives of *env8* were crystallized bound to AqCbl, one including the extension containing P13, the other without. The fifth structure is from an atypical cobalamin riboswitch from *Bacillus subtilis* (*Bsu*) [120], which lies in the middle of classes I and II with regard to structure and selectivity. While it possesses a shortened PE1 typical for class II, its PE2 resembles that of class I, and hence this riboswitch interacts equally with either AdoCbl, MeCbl, or HyCbl, but not with CNCbl. Although its uncommon secondary structure was noted already in one of the first studies on B_{12} riboswitches [123], it is only now that its structural variations can be placed in the context of ligand binding and selectivity explaining its promiscuous behavior [120, 125].

Metal ions seem to play a minor role in the recognition of the B_{12} derivative. The B_{12} binding site is composed of joining strands of J3/4 and J6/3 of the highly conserved central core, which is buried within and is flanked by the class-specific peripheral extensions. Van-der-Waals-interactions as well as shape complementarity are the primary binding criteria for the interaction to the respective cobalamin derivative, supplemented by hydrogen bonds. In all five structures, the β-sidechains *a* and *c* are involved in H-bonding. This explains why modification of sidechain *c* was found to have such a severe impact on the *btuB* riboswitch, preventing it from correctly folding [126]. In AdoCbl, the upper adenosyl ligand interacts *via* H-bonding and stacking. In this region of the binding site, a metal ion was found only in the *B. subtilis* riboswitch structure [120]. Here a missing adenosyl nucleotide, otherwise present and H-bonding to the adenosyl ligand of AdoCbl, is replaced by a cobalt hexaammine molecule, most likely substituting for hydrated Mg^{2+}, which in turn binds to the sugar-phosphate backbone of the riboswitch. On the α-side of the cobalamin plane, the picture is different: only sidechain *b* was consistently found to be involved in hydrogen bonds. In none of the crystal structures, sidechain *d* is involved in binding, which does not correlate with earlier results which showed incomplete switching of the *btuB* riboswitch by applying CNCbl derivatives modified at sidechains *b*, *d*, and *e* [126]. This difference could either derive from the experimental method or from the riboswitch itself, as not all Cbl riboswitches are equally sensitive to structural changes of the ligand [121].

The linking sidechain *f* with its bridging sugar-phosphate and benzimidazole ligand is very scarcely involved in RNA interactions. This correlates to earlier findings, where adenosylcobinamide, which lacks the α-ligand, -phosphate, and -sugar, induced a very similar switch as AdoCbl but was found to bind with a more than 1,000-fold decreased affinity [117]. As revealed later by the crystal structures [63], the L5-P13 kissing loop encloses the α-side shaping a binding pocket ideal to host a base-on constitution of the lower ligand and contributing to the stability of the interaction [61, 62, 121, 124, 127]. Although the preference of a base-on constitution seems widespread, differences between individual Cbl-riboswitch representatives are possible as also base-off derivatives were already shown to interact similar to AdoCbl [117]. Coordination of a riboswitch-derived nucleobase to the Co^{3+} center of corrinoids of any constitution similar to the "base-off/His-on"-binding scheme of cobalamin-dependent enzymes [128] was so far not detected and can most probably be excluded as binding strategy of Cbl riboswitches.

No metal ion-binding site was found in the α-side when it was enclosed by a kissing loop [63, 120]. In the absence of the L5-P13 kissing loop, the α-side is completely exposed while the Cbl-derivative interacts only through its β-side [63]. That such a binding scheme is sufficient to provide high affinity was demonstrated by the synthetic CNCbl-aptamer which binds its ligand with a K_D value of 90 nM [129], which is in the range of natural aptamers of riboswitches. For the shortened *Sth* riboswitch a Mg^{2+} ion was found undergoing cation-π-stacking [130] to the α-benzimidazole. The close proximity of this Mg^{2+} to the amides of sidechains *g* and *b* as well as to the 2′-sugar oxygen atoms of sidechain *f* and of G64 within P4 could point to the involvement of this ion in a larger network, which was however not resolved in the crystal structure. This metal ion-binding site could however well be an artifact due to lack of the kissing-loop interaction.

4.1.2 Moco- and Wco-Responsive Riboswitches

The molybdenum cofactor (Moco) riboswitch with 176 representatives known as yet was identified through computational sequence alignment. The high oxygen sensitivity of Moco makes experimental work highly challenging, which is the reason that to date there is still no unambiguous proof if Moco alone, or in combination with protein cofactor(s), is responsible for the functional switch of the RNA [71, 131]. Moco and its tungsten analog (Wco) are crucial cofactors for several enzymes and are involved in key steps of the carbon, nitrogen, and sulfur metabolisms [132, 133]. The Moco (and Wco) scaffold is composed of a tricyclic fused pyran and pterin moiety, and the transition metal ion is bound *via* two sulfide groups (Figure 8). Molybdenum and tungsten adopt oxidation states VI, V, and IV, enabling one-electron and two-electron transfers of the enzymes.

While the biosynthesis of Moco is conserved throughout all Moco-dependent organisms [134], the derivatization of Moco before incorporation into the corresponding enzymes differs. In general, the final metabolic product of a biosynthetic pathway is sensed by the respective riboswitch. Accordingly, either Moco itself or an immediate precursor is considered the most likely ligand for the riboswitch. Because of its high oxygen sensitivity, information on the interaction of Moco/Wco with the riboswitch is very scarce [135, 136]. Comparing the molybdenum cofactor to other metabolites suggests that the organic pterin moiety as well as the phosphate are involved in metabolite recognition. In a recent study, it was however shown that neither isolated pterin nor tetrahydrobiopterin are recognized by the riboswitch, showing that further structural elements are required for recognition, such as the molybdenum complex and/or the phosphate group [137]. Tb^{3+} cleavage assays revealed several potential metal ion-binding pockets within the aptamer that might be crucial for ligand recognition [137].

The secondary structure of the Moco riboswitch consists of a conserved five-way junction [136] which undergoes a general compaction in the presence of Mg^{2+} to the presumable ligand-binding form [137]. This recent study describes a K^+- and Mg^{2+}-dependent folding pathway, whereby a high degree of aptamer organization is achieved already at low ion concentration. The different domains of the aptamer are indicated to be important for different purposes. In the *E. coli moaA* riboswitch, P1 presumably contains the ribosomal binding sites, but in other organisms different types of expression platforms were observed for the Moco riboswitch (Figure 8). P2 contains a crucial tetraloop receptor for a long-range interaction with the tetraloop on P4, and P3 is believed to be crucial for

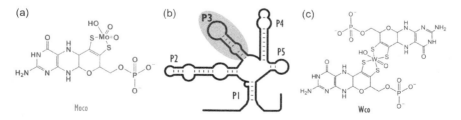

FIGURE 8 The Moco and Wco metabolites together with the schematic riboswitch structure. Moco is found as a monomer or a dimer, while Wco occurs only as dimer in biological systems. The presence of the P3 stem discriminates against Wco and only allows Moco binding.

distinguishing between Moco and Wco [136, 138, 139]. Moco is known to exist as monomer or dimer, while Wco is always found in dimeric form [139]. This makes it unclear whether the selectivity of the riboswitch is based on the nature of the metal ion, or on size and geometry, or both [135, 136]. In this context, it is important to know that in the cell, Moco is always associated with a carrier protein or integrated into an enzyme. This raises the question whether Moco alone or the protein-Moco complex is actually recognized by the riboswitch, or alternatively, a protein-RNA contact is necessary for transfer of the metabolite.

4.2 Riboswitches Responsive to Metal Ions

4.2.1 Na$^+$

Na$^+$-sensing riboswitches were described only very recently and are subdivided into two classes: the Na$^+$-I class with over 300 representatives detected so far and the Na$^+$-II class with only nine known individuals [140]. Na$^+$-I riboswitches seem to be involved in cellular pH-regulation, Na$^+$ detoxification, and cellular energy balance since they were found to be associated to Na$^+$/H$^+$ antiporters and ATPases, respectively. The other representatives are associated with osmotic stress response mechanisms [140].

4.2.2 Li$^+$

Li$^+$ sensing riboswitches have only recently been discovered [18]. These riboswitches are subdivided into two classes and believed to be involved in Li$^+$ homeostasis and detoxification [18].

4.2.3 Mg^{2+}

Mg^{2+} plays an indispensable role in the folding process of RNA in general. In the context of riboswitches, Mg^{2+} in addition enables binding of ligands carrying negatively charged moieties like phosphates or carboxylates (see Section 3), being the intermediary link between ligand and RNA. Given all these important general roles of Mg^{2+} with all RNAs, Mg^{2+}-sensing riboswitches must have evolved unique features to further transduct Mg^{2+}-binding to a regulatory effect.

Mg^{2+}-sensing riboswitches were the first metal ion-responding riboswitches discovered. Two distinct classes are known, which share neither sequence nor structure: the M-box riboswitches mostly found in Gram-positive bacteria and the *mgtA* riboswitch in Gram-negative bacteria. Both classes were discovered and described rather early in riboswitch history [56, 141–143] and both are involved in Mg^{2+} homeostasis and control of intercellular Mg^{2+} concentration by regulating Mg^{2+} efflux proteins, Mg^{2+} importers or P-type ATPases, which couple metal ion transport with ATP hydrolysis. All literature prior to 2011 on Mg^{2+}-responsive riboswitches was discussed previously [144]. At that time, the M-box riboswitch was already well described with a crystal structure at hand [56] but only very little was known regarding the *mgtA* riboswitch. Five years after its first description, neither its Mg^{2+} sensing domain was identified nor its way of action.

Plausible possibilities seemed to be either the Mg^{2+}-mediated transcription termination or the Mg^{2+}-induced targeting for RNase E-dependent mRNA degradation [144–146]. Here, we will therefore summarize the new discoveries from the last decade regarding these two riboswitch classes.

At first, the *mgtA riboswitch* seemed a relatively simple system, switching from stemloop A and terminator stem B at high to stemloops D and C at low Mg^{2+} concentration. However, the length of 264 nt is indicative of a more elaborate mechanism. Early on, it was proposed that apart from Mg^{2+} the *mgtA* leader sequence might be regulated by further, riboswitch-atypical control mechanisms promoting transcription initiation and elongation into the *mgtA* coding region [147]. Several proteins were demonstrated to regulate mgtA transcription and expression, i.e., the transcription regulator Rob [148] as well as inactivation of the RNA chaperone Hfq [149, 150]. Subsequent studies revealed a regulatory role of the 17-residue peptide mgtL on the *mgtA* riboswitch [151, 152], the mgtL peptide being encoded in an open reading frame embedded in the *mgtA* riboswitch loop A. mgtL is therefore only translated at high Mg^{2+} concentrations while a suggested proline dependence remains under dispute. Independently, *in vivo* mgtL translation was shown to be necessary for premature *mgtA* transcription termination, a discovery to add another complex representative to the rising number of riboswitch control mechanisms [153]. Mg^{2+} was later demonstrated to also stimulate Rho-dependent transcription termination *in vivo* and *in vitro*, whereby the single-stranded region between stemloops A and B, formed only at high Mg^{2+} concentration, was proposed to be the most important site for Rho interaction [154]. To our knowledge the *mgtA* riboswitch-based regulatory system is one of the most complex ones known with a multitude of control mechanisms, sometimes influencing each other, and including several protein cofactors, and all of them, as it seems, being Mg^{2+}-dependent.

The so-far-only study on the *mgtA* tertiary structure and its Mg^{2+}-binding properties focused on the antiterminator stemloop C that is formed at low Mg^{2+} concentrations [155]. The solution structure of the simplified construct derived from the *Yersinia enterocolitica mgtA* riboswitch was solved by NMR spectroscopy revealing a high-affinity Mg^{2+} binding site located in a four base-pair long AU stretch within the stem which includes the stop codon of mgtL. At this site the helix bends with a kink widening the major groove and increasing accessibility for Mg^{2+}. The binding mode is most probably fully outer-sphere since line-broadening studies with $MnCl_2$ as mimic for Mg^{2+} inner-sphere binding showed no effect [155].

In 2017 the *mgtA* riboswitch was renamed as class II of the Mg^{2+}-responding riboswitches, with stemloop A as the principal regulatory element [108]. In a new computational search, only 101 representatives were found exclusively distributed in proteobacteria. As it stands, also after more than 15 years after its first description, conclusive information regarding the *mgtA* riboswitch mechanism is still scarce.

The second Mg^{2+}-sensing riboswitch class, the so-called **M-box riboswitch** is structurally much better characterized. Formerly also known as the ykoK motif, this riboswitch is today denominated as a class I Mg^{2+}-responding riboswitch [108]. Its crystal structure shows three closely packed, nearly parallel helices stabilized by six Mg^{2+} within an extensive network of inner- and outer-sphere contacts mediating multiple long-range interactions [56]. Phosphorothioate interference studies demonstrated that all six Mg^{2+} are equally important for structure formation [57]. Four Mg^{2+} reside in an internal core formed by L4, L5, and P2, which is closely packed and inaccessible to solvent. A conserved A-rich internal loop of P4 serves as a second metal binding core for the other two Mg^{2+}. Although positioned in a peripheral location, the latter metal ion-binding site is of equal importance for structure formation. A metal-ion-mediated kink of the helix orients L4 in the right position for long-range interactions participating in central core formation and the sequestration of antiterminator nucleotides [57]. Later results however suggest this site to be a region of structural flexibility due to inconsistent metal ion binding [156].

Further metal ion-binding sites were subsequently identified in the M-box riboswitch. Phosphorothioate studies suggested three Mg^{2+} within a third metal ion core, core 3, near the apex of the fold, most probably facilitating long-range tertiary contacts, but with a generally lower affinity [57]. While in a first crystal structure no Mg^{2+} were identified within core 3, probably due to too low resolution, later co-crystallization of the *B. subtilis mgtE* M-box riboswitch with Mn^{2+} was successful [156]. Mn^{2+} has an intrinsically higher affinity toward phosphate oxygen atoms as well as nitrogen ligands [157, 158] and in this case could be identified within core 3, as well as at six further binding sites. One of these Mn^{2+} binding sites (M10, within core 1) is of special interest because it facilitates interaction of L5 to the P2 helix by coordinating N7 of a L5 guanine as well as the sugar edge of A155 in P2 [156]. Interestingly, M-box riboswitches were also linked to resistance-associated transporters of Mn^{2+} and iron, which makes such a broader selectivity a plausible natural property [108, 159].

A recent comparison of two M-box riboswitches from *B. subtilis* and *M. tuberculosis* [160] revealed differences in ion specificity resulting from small differences in sequence and size of the otherwise well-compatible motifs [161]. Only *M. tuberculosis* M-box recognizes the larger Sr^{2+} instead of Mg^{2+}. While Mg^{2+} has a strictly octahedral geometry, Sr^{2+} also accepts eight ligands and is more flexible to geometrical distortions [162, 163]. While it could just be a chance that Sr^{2+} is recognized, it has also been proposed [161] that, depending on the regulated gene and the organism of origin, some M-box riboswitches could have adapted to sense other divalent metal ions than only Mg^{2+}.

4.2.4 Mn^{2+}

First described in 2004 [159], the Mn^{2+}-responding **yybP–ykoY RNA motif** is one of the most widespread riboswitches sometimes occurring in multiple copies within a genome. It resides upstream of genes encoding cation transport ATPases or membrane proteins. This riboswitch shows an increased response mechanism at basic pH [16] and due to its allegation to ion transporters, the yybP–ykoY motif was initially also hypothesized to act as a pH sensor. Later investigations showed that this riboswitch does neither respond directly to pH [164, 165] nor to any molecules involved in pH homeostasis [166]. Instead, upon binding to Mn^{2+} the yybP–ykoY motif is an up-regulator for gene expression leading to an increased efflux rate of this potentially toxic metal ion [16, 167]. This is in contrast to most riboswitches which primarily down-regulate gene expression.

The yybP–ykoY riboswitch harbors a central four-way helical junction with four helices organized into two coaxially stacked superhelices [168]. The two superhelices create a phosphate-rich and highly conserved tertiary docking site coordinating two metal ions: site M_A accepts both Mg^{2+} or Mn^{2+} whereas site M_B is specific to Mn^{2+} [168]. M_A shows four to five inner-sphere (and two or one outer-sphere) interaction while M_B shows exclusively inner-sphere contacts, five to phosphate oxygen atoms and one to a conserved adenine N7 [168, 169], the latter interaction being crucial for Mn^{2+} selectivity (Figure 9). This rare coordination scheme deprived of intermediary water ligands and the slightly lower energetic penalty for dehydration [163] probably allows the RNA to sense Mn^{2+} over Mg^{2+} and also to discriminate other ions. The coordination of Mn^{2+} to the fully

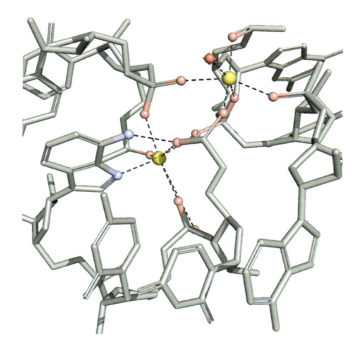

FIGURE 9 The metal ion-binding core of the yybP–ykoY riboswitch. The two ligated metal ions are shown as yellow spheres. The metal on the top right is coordinated to site M_A and can either be Mn^{2+} or Mg^{2+}. The lower left, which includes N7 coordination, is strictly Mn^{2+} bound to site M_B. Coordinating oxygen atoms from the RNA are marked as red spheres while the slightly darker red sphere represents the single coordinating water molecule. Nitrogen atoms of the conserved adenine are marked in blue. This panel was generated with PyMOL [187] using the PDB ID 4Y1I.

dehydrated form was proposed to be a stepwise process, also supported by the crystal structure of a folding intermediate [169]. In the same study, Mg^{2+}-assisted cooperative Mn^{2+} binding was described. In the absence of Mn^{2+}, Mg^{2+} binds to site M_A stabilizing the tertiary fold to a certain extent [168]. Under these conditions, site M_B remains metal free and collapses leading to more flexibility of the riboswitch. The RNA adopts two conformations, the unbound "off-state" and the bound "on-state", which are in dynamic equilibrium and congregate toward the "on-state" at high Mg^{2+}. Only in the presence of 0.1 mM Mn^{2+} (with a background of 1 mM Mg^{2+}) the riboswitch is locked in its "on-state" reflecting Mn^{2+}-binding to site M_B. At high Mn^{2+} concentrations (2.5 mM), both sites, M_B as well as M_A are occupied by Mn^{2+} [169].

Cellular concentration, charge, ligand softness, ionic radius, and coordination scheme provide the necessary selectivity for Mn^{2+} in site M_B. The alkaline earth metal ions Mg^{2+}, Ca^{2+}, or Ba^{2+} do not show a meaningful affinity at physiological conditions [108, 167, 168, 170], having no preference for N7 inner-sphere binding. Selectivity of transition metal ions is vaguer. Besides Mn^{2+}, also Cd^{2+} was found to bind with high affinity [169, 170]. Selectivity toward these two ions was proposed to be facilitated by a so-called pseudo-heptacoordination by including an aqua ligand present in M_B into the coordination sphere of the metal ion [170], leading to a pentagonal bipyramidal geometry, which has been observed previously for Cd^{2+} and Mn^{2+} [171]. Along the same line, it was proposed that some representatives of this riboswitch class have adapted their specificity to other transition metal ions [172].

The *mntH* **riboswitch** is a more recently identified Mn^{2+}-sensing riboswitch [173], regulating the bacterial metal ion import protein MntH [174, 175]. Although in *E. coli* MntH was shown to mediate the import not only of Mn^{2+} but also of Cd^{2+}, Co^{2+}, Fe^{2+}, and Zn^{2+} [174], the *mntH* riboswitch is highly selective for Mn^{2+} over Mg^{2+} or Ca^{2+}.

4.2.5 Transition Metals Ni^{2+}, Co^{2+} and Fe^{2+}

First described to respond to Ni^{2+} and Co^{2+} [176], this so-called **NiCo riboswitch** class is presumably involved in metal homeostasis and detoxification as it is often associated with czcD genes encoding cation diffusion facilitator proteins. Monovalent metal ions alone do not switch the RNA but weak binding to Mn^{2+} was demonstrated early on, pointing to a certain flexibility in divalent metal ion selection [176]. Recently, sensing of cellular Fe^{2+} was demonstrated by this riboswitch class [177, 178]. Depending on the organism and taking into account the labile cellular concentrations of the respective ions, the oxygen-sensitive Fe^{2+} (which oxidizes and precipitates under standard physiological conditions) might even be the primary ligand [177]. In *E. coli*, on the other hand, Fe^{2+} seems not to be detected by this riboswitch class [179].

Coordination of either Fe^{2+}, Ni^{2+}, or Co^{2+} is cooperative with Hill coefficients ranging between 2 and 3, respectively, pointing to multiple metal ion binding [177, 178]. Indeed, the crystal structure of the Co^{2+}-bound aptamer shows four bound Co^{2+}, three of them being tightly bound in the very conserved four-stem junction while the fourth Co^{2+} is possibly an artifact from experimental conditions [176]. The interaction of the three central Co^{2+} ions is characterized by two inner-sphere contacts per Co^{2+} to N7 atoms of five guanines and one adenine. Again, inner-sphere N7 coordination is the most probable key element in metal ion selectivity against Mg^{2+}. This metal ion core links bases from different regions of the RNA, being in good concordance to in-line probing experiments (stabilization of the antiterminator fold) [176] and FRET studies (enhanced rigidity upon Co^{2+} binding) [180]. A second FRET study on NiCo riboswitch folding demonstrated a three-state folding mechanism [181]. Na^+ and Mg^{2+} assist the first folding step toward a long-lived intermediate, which exhibits a pre-organized binding pocket for the transition metal ions. The final folding step is then controlled by Ni^{2+} and Co^{2+}, respectively. This key-lock or "fold-then-bind" mechanism is characterized by a well-structured intermediate, the binding-competent form, able to sense the transition metal ions.

5 GENERAL CONCLUSIONS

In this review, we have summarized the various roles of metal ions in the function of riboswitches. For structure formation, metal ions cover the whole spectrum from "simple" charge compensation during initial folding to the formation of binding-competent intermediates and the stabilization of structural elements as well as tertiary contacts, which can be crucial for either proper structure formation, stabilization of the ligand-binding pocket, transduction of the regulatory information or for a combination thereof. Folding or refolding upon metabolite binding is crucial for the functionality of riboswitches. Besides the correctness of the fold, it is also important that the structure can be adopted in time and with the required thermodynamic stability. It has to be noted that folding and structural studies of riboswitches have almost exclusively been performed under *in vitro* conditions. In the cell however additional factors like crowding [182, 183] influence folding and structure formation of riboswitches. Riboswitch folding occurs also co-transcriptionally and substructures are formed in the order in which they are transcribed and stabilized depending on the presence or absence of the ligand [184]. Transcriptional pausing additionally influences RNA folding and coordinates the structure formation of both the aptamer domain and the expression platform. This might be a general mechanism for coordinated folding and conformational rearrangements in response to environmental cues [185]. The question whether riboswitches are thermodynamically or kinetically controlled has so far only rarely been addressed [186]. In the case of the FMN riboswitch, the mechanism regulating gene expression under high ion concentrations differs from the one at lower concentrations [182]. High ion concentrations thereby might speed up the process, converting a thermodynamically driven system into a kinetically regulated one. An indication for such a mechanism is the adoption of bound-like structures for certain riboswitches at high metal ion concentrations in the absence of the metabolite, as described for the glmS and TPP riboswitches [47, 49].

In the context of metabolite binding, metal ions are not only involved in the formation of the correct binding pocket, but are, depending on the ligand, directly involved in interactions thereof. Metal ions are especially important when it comes to the binding of negatively charged moieties like phosphates or carboxylates – functional moieties which are common in riboswitch-binding ligands, and which are often decisive for specificity.

Some metal ions are the recognized target itself and thus induce the gene-regulatory reorganization of the riboswitch upon binding. Thereby riboswitches take use of diverse strategies to discriminate between very similar ions. To fulfill this task, riboswitches exploit not only the chemical properties of metal ions but also their abundance within the cellular milieu adapting their affinity accordingly. This adaptability of riboswitches might also be exploited by the organism to respond to its specific needs as was observed for cobalamin riboswitches, which accept a broad variety of B_{12} derivatives and the Moco/Wco riboswitch, which adapted according to a molybdenum- or tungsten-based metabolism. The finding that Ni/Co riboswitches in some cases equally, if not exclusively, sense Fe^{2+} is another indication that riboswitches are adaptable. Thus more so far undetected classes might still be discovered.

ACKNOWLEDGMENTS

Financial support from the Swiss National Science Foundation, the European Research Council (ERC Starting Grant MIRNA-259092) as well as within the COST Action CM1105 from the Swiss State Secretariat for Education and Research over the past years is gratefully acknowledged (RKOS). We also acknowledge gratefully the continuous support from the University of Zurich.

ABBREVIATIONS

AdoCbl	5′-desoxyadenosylcobalamin, coenzyme B_{12}
AqCbl	aquacobalamin
CNCbl	cyanocobalamin, vitamin B_{12}
FMN	flavin mononucleotide
Glc6NP	glucosamine-6-phosphate
glms	gene encoding for glutamine-fructose-6-phosphate amidotransferase
HyCbl	hydroxocobalamin
J	linker region (in an RNA)
KL	kissing loop
L	loop region (in an RNA)
MeCbl	methylcobalamin
NAD⁺	nicotinamide adenine dinucleotide (oxidized form)
P	double-stranded stem region (in an RNA)
PE	peripheral extension
ppGpp	5′-diphosphate 3′-diphosphate guanosine

PRPP	α-5′-phosphoribosyl-1′-pyrophosphate
RNA	ribonucleic acid
SAH	S-adenosyl-L-homocysteine
SHAPE	selective 2′-hydroxyl acylation analyzed by primer extension
smFRET	single-molecule fluorescence resonance energy transfer
THF	tetrahydrofolate
TPP	thiamine pyrophosphate
UTR	untranslated region

REFERENCES

1. R. Green, H. F. Noller, *Annu. Rev. Biochem.* **1997**, *66*, 679–716.
2. P. Nissen, J. Hansen, N. Ban, P. B. Moore, T. A. Steitz, *Science* **2000**, *289*, 920–930.
3. K. Kruger, P. J. Grabowski, A. J. Zaug, J. Sands, D. E. Gottschling, T. R. Cech, *Cell* **1982**, *31*, 147–157.
4. X. Nou, R. J. Kadner, *Proc. Natl. Acad. Sci. U.S.A.* **2000**, *97*, 7190–7195.
5. M. Gelfand, A. Mironov, J. Jomantas, Y. I. Kozlov, D. A. Perumov, *Trends Genet.* **1999**, *15*, 439–442.
6. J. Miranda-Rios, M. Navarro, M. Soberon, *Proc. Natl. Acad. Sci. U.S.A.* **2001**, *98*, 9736–9741.
7. J. Cruz-Toledo, M. McKeague, X. Zhang, A. Giamberardino, E. McConnell, T. Francis, M. C. DeRosa, M. Dumontier, *Database* **2012**, *2012*, bas006.
8. A. D. Ellington, J. W. Szostak, *Nature* **1990**, *346*, 818–822.
9. A. S. Mironov, I. Gusarov, R. Rafikov, L. Errais Lopez, K. Shatalin, R. A. Kreneva, D. A. Perumov, E. Nudler, *Cell* **2002**, *111*, 747–756.
10. A. Nahvi, N. Sudarsan, M. S. Ebert, X. Zou, K. L. Brown, R. R. Breaker, *Chem. Biol.* **2002**, *9*, 1043–1049.
11. W. C. Winkler, S. Cohen-Chalamish, R. R. Breaker, *Proc. Natl. Acad. Sci. U.S.A.* **2002**, *99*, 15908–18913.
12. T. Hermann, D. J. Patel, *Science* **2000**, *287*, 820–825.
13. S. D. Gilbert, R. T. Batey, *Cell. Mol. Life Sci.* **2005**, *62*, 2401–2404.
14. W. C. Winkler, R. R. Breaker, *ChemBioChem* **2003**, *4*, 1024–1032.
15. A. J. Knappenberger, C. Wetherington Reiss, S. A. Strobel, *eLife* **2018**, *7*, e36381.
16. M. Dambach, M. Sandoval, T. B. Updegrove, V. Anantharaman, L. Aravind, L. S. Waters, G. Storz, *Mol. Cell* **2015**, *57*, 1099–1109.
17. E. Nudler, A. S. Mironov, *Trends. Biochem. Sci.* **2004**, *29*, 11–17.
18. R. R. Breaker, *Biochemistry* **2022**, *61*, 137–149.
19. E. Poiata, M. M. Meyer, T. D. Ames, R. R. Breaker, *RNA* **2009**, *15*, 2046–2056.
20. J. J. Trausch, P. Ceres, F. E. Reyes, R. T. Batey, *Structure* **2011**, *19*, 1413–1423.
21. L. Huang, J. Wang, A. M. Watkins, R. Das, D. M. J. Lilley, *Nucleic Acids Res.* **2019**, *47*, 7666–7675.
22. W. C. Winkler, A. Nahvi, N. Sudarsan, J. E. Barrick, R. R. Breaker, *Nat. Struct. Biol.* **2003**, *10*, 701–707.
23. S. D. Gilbert, R. K. Montagne, C. D. Stoddard, R. T. Batey, *Cold Spring Harb. Protoc.* **2006**, *71*, 259–268.
24. J. Lim, W. C. Winkler, S. Nakamura, V. Scott, R. R. Breaker, *Angew. Chem. Int. Ed.* **2006**, *45*, 964–968.
25. N. Sudarsan, J. K. Wickiser, S. Nakamura, M. S. Ebert, R. R. Breaker, *Cold Spring Harb. Protoc.* **2003**, *17*, 2688–2697.
26. A. Serganov, L. Huang, D. J. Patel, *Nature* **2009**, *458*, 233–237.

27. A. Serganov, L. Huang, D. J. Patel, *Nature* **2008**, *455*, 1263–1267.
28. A. Ren, K. R. Rajashankar, D. J. Patel, *Nature* **2012**, *486*, 85–89.
29. R. K. O. Sigel, A. M. Pyle, *Chem. Rev.* **2007**, *107*, 97–113.
30. D. E. Draper, *Biophys. J.* **2008**, *95*, 5489–5495.
31. D. E. Draper, D. Grilley, A. M. Soto, *Annu. Rev. Biophys. Biomol. Struct.* **2005**, *34*, 221–243.
32. F. D. Steffen, M. Kier, D. Kowerko, R. A. Cunha, R. Börner, R. K. O. Sigel, *Nat. Commun.* **2020**, *11*, 104.
33. H. Sigel, R. K. O. Sigel, *Comprehensive Inorganic Chemistry*, Eds J. Reedijk, K. R. Poeppelmeier, 3rd ed., Elsevier Ltd., Oxford, UK, pp. 623–660.
34. R. K. Montange, R. T. Batey, *Annu. Rev. Biophys.* **2008**, *37*, 117–133.
35. A. Serganov, Y.-R. Yuan, O. Pikovskaya, A. Polonskaia, L. Malinina, A. T. Phan, C. Höbartner, R. Micura, R. R. Breaker, D. J. Patel, *Chem. Biol.* **2004**, *11*, 1729–1741.
36. S. D. Gilbert, C. D. Stoddard, S. J. Wise, R. T. Batey, *J. Mol. Biol.* **2006**, *359*, 754–768.
37. J.-F. Lemay, J. C. Penedo, R. Tremblay, D. M. J. Lilley, D. A. Lafontaine, *Chem. Biol.* **2006**, *13*, 857–868.
38. J. Noeske, J. Buck, B. Fürtig, H. R. Nasiri, H. Schwalbe, J. Wöhnert, *Nucleic Acids Res.* **2007**, *35*, 572–583.
39. J. Noeske, C. Richter, E. Stirnal, H. Schwalbe, J. Wöhnert, *ChemBioChem* **2006**, *7*, 1451–1456.
40. R. Rieder, K. Lang, D. Graber, R. Micura, *ChemBioChem* **2007**, *8*, 896–902.
41. R. T. Batey, S. D. Gilbert, R. K. Montange, *Nature* **2004**, *432*, 411–415.
42. T. E. Edwards, A. R. Ferré D'Amaré, *Structure* **2006**, *14*, 1459–1468.
43. C. D. Stoddard, S. D. Gilbert, R. T. Batey, *RNA* **2008**, *14*, 675–684.
44. L. Huang, J. Wang, D. M. J. Lilley, *RNA* **2020**, *26*, 878–887.
45. P. St-Pierre, E. Shaw, S. Jacques, P. A. Dalgarno, C. Perez-Gonzalez, F. Picard-Jean, J. C. Penedo, D. A. Lafontaine, *Nucleic Acids Res.* **2021**, *49*, 5891–5904.
46. D. J. Klein, S. R. Wilkinson, M. D. Been, A. R. Ferré D'Amaré, *J. Mol. Biol.* **2007**, *373*, 178–189.
47. K. J. Hampel, M. M. Tinsley, *Biochemistry* **2006**, *45*, 7861–7871.
48. J. Ma, N. Saikia, S. Godar, G. L. Hamilton, F. Ding, J. Alper, H. Sanabria, *RNA* **2021**, *27*, 771–790.
49. S. Kumar, G. Reddy, *J. Phys. Chem. B* **2022**, *126*, 2369–2381.
50. J. Lipfert, R. Das, V. B. Chu, M. Kudaravalli, N. Boyd, D. Herschlag, S. Doniach, *J. Mol. Biol.* **2007**, *365*, 1393–1406.
51. K. M. Ruff, S. A. Strobel, *RNA* **2014**, *20*, 1775–1788.
52. T. V. Erion, S. A. Strobel, *RNA* **2011**, *17*, 74–84.
53. N. Kulshina, N. J. Baird, A. R. Ferré D'Amaré, *Nat. Struct. Mol. Biol.* **2009**, *16*, 1212–1217.
54. S. Wood, A. R. Ferré D'Amaré, D. Rueda, *ACS Chem. Biol.* **2012**, *7*, 920–927.
55. K. C. Suddala, J. Wang, Q. Hou, N. G. Walter, *J. Am. Chem. Soc.* **2015**, *137*, 14075–14083.
56. C. E. Dann, C. A. Wakeman, C. L. Sieling, S. C. Baker, I. Irnov, W. C. Winkler, *Cell* **2007**, *130*, 878–892.
57. C. A. Wakeman, A. Ramesh, W. C. Winkler, *J. Mol. Biol.* **2009**, *392*, 723–735.
58. P. K. Choudhary, S. Gallo, R. K. O. Sigel, *Front. Chem.* **2017**, *5*, 10.
59. P. K. Choudhary, R. K. O. Sigel, *RNA* **2014**, *20*, 36–45.
60. B. Ma, G. Bai, R. Nussinov, J. Ding, Y.-X. Wang, *J. Phys. Chem.* **2021**, *125*, 2589–2596.
61. S. Wang, D. Chen, L. Gao, Y. Liu, *J. Am. Chem. Soc.* **2022**, *144*, 5494–5502.
62. E. D. Holmstrom, J. T. Polaski, R. T. Batey, D. J. Nesbitt, *J. Am. Chem. Soc.* **2014**, *136*, 16832–16843.

63. J. E. Johnson, F. E. Reyes, J. T. Polaski, R. T. Batey, *Nature* **2012**, *492*, 133–137.
64. A. Peselis, A. Serganov, *Nat. Struct. Mol. Biol.* **2012**, *19*, 1182–1184.
65. E. Ennifar, P. Walter, B. Ehresmann, C. Ehresmann, P. Dumas, *Nat. Struct. Biol.* **2001**, *8*, 1064–1068.
66. S. Horiya, X. Li, G. Kawai, R. Saito, A. Katoh, K. Kobayashi, K. Harada, *Chem. Biol.* **2003**, *10*, 645–654.
67. W. Winkler, A. Nahvi, R. R. Breaker, *Nature* **2002**, *419*, 952–956.
68. S. Thore, C. Frick, N. Ban, *J. Am. Chem. Soc.* **2008**, *130*, 8116–8117.
69. A. Serganov, A. Polonskaia, A. T. Phan, R. R. Breaker, D. J. Patel, *Nature* **2006**, *441*, 1167–1171.
70. Q. Vicens, E. Mondragón, F. E. Reyes, P. Coish, P. Aristoff, J. Berman, H. Kaur, K. W. Kells, P. Wickens, J. Wilson, R. C. Gadwood, H. J. Schostarez, R. K. Suto, K. F. Blount, R. T. Batey, *ACS Chem. Biol.* **2018**, *13*, 2908–2919.
71. Z. Weinberg, C. E. Lünse, K. A. Corbino, T. D. Ames, J. W. Nelson, A. Roth, K. R. Perkins, M. E. Sherlock, R. R. Breaker, *Nucleic Acids Res.* **2017**, *45*, 10811–10823.
72. H. Chen, M. Egger, X. Xu, L. Flemmich, O. Krasheninina, A. Sun, R. Micura, A. Ren, *Nucleic Acids Res.* **2020**, *48*, 12394–12406.
73. A. Peselis, A. Serganov, *Nat. Chem. Biol.* **2018**, *14*, 887–894.
74. R. E. Thompson, E. L. Li, H. O. Spivey, J. P. Chandler, A. J. Katz, J. R. Appleman, *Bioinorg. Chem.* **1978**, *9*, 35–45.
75. W. C. Winkler, A. Nahvi, A. Roth, J. A. Collins, R. R. Breaker, *Nature* **2004**, *428*, 281–286.
76. T. J. McCarthy, M. A. Plog, S. A. Floy, J. A. Jansen, J. K. Soukup, G. A. Soukup, *Chem. Biol.* **2005**, *12*, 1221–1226.
77. D. J. Klein, M. D. Been, A. R. Ferré D'Amaré, *J. Am. Chem. Soc.* **2007**, *129*, 14858–14859.
78. A. D. Garst, A. Héroux, R. P. Rambo, R. T. Batey, *J. Biol. Chem.* **2008**, *283*, 22347–22351.
79. A. Serganov, A. Polonskaia, B. Ehresmann, C. Ehresmann, D. J. Patel, *EMBO J.* **2003**, *22*, 1898–1908.
80. K. F. Blount, J. X. Wang, J. Lim, N. Sudarsan, R. R. Breaker, *Nat. Chem. Biol.* **2007**, *3*, 44–49.
81. A. Ren, Y. Xue, A. Peselis, A. Serganov, H. M. Al-Hashimi, D. J. Patel, *Cell Rep.* **2015**, *13*, 1800–1813.
82. L. Huang, A. Serganov, D. J. Patel, *Mol. Cell* **2010**, *40*, 774–786.
83. I. R. Price, J. C. Grigg, A. Ke, *Biochim. Biophys. Acta.* **2014**, *1839*, 931–938.
84. K. A. Corbino, J. E. Barrick, J. Lim, R. Welz, B. J. Tucker, I. Puskarz, M. Mandal, N. D. Rudnick, R. R. Breaker, *Genome. Biol.* **2005**, *6*, R70.
85. S. D. Gilbert, R. P. Rambo, D. van Tyne, R. T. Batey, *Nat. Struct. Mol. Biol.* **2008**, *15*, 177–182.
86. C. Lu, A. M. Smith, R. T. Fuchs, F. Ding, K. Rajashankar, T. M. Henkin, A. Ke, *Nat. Struct. Mol. Biol.* **2008**, *15*, 1076–1083.
87. Z. Weinberg, E. E. Regulski, M. C. Hammond, J. E. Barrick, Z. Yao, W. L. Ruzzo, R. R. Breaker, *RNA* **2008**, *14*, 822–828.
88. L. Huang, D. M. J. Lilley, *Nucleic Acids Res.* **2018**, *46*, 6869–6879.
89. J. L. Baker, N. Sudarsan, Z. Weinberg, A. Roth, R. B. Stockbridge, R. R. Breaker, *Science* **2012**, *335*, 233–235.
90. B. Zhao, A. L. Hansen, Q. Zhang, *J. Am. Chem. Soc.* **2014**, *136*, 20–23.
91. B. Zhao, Q. Zhang, *Curr. Opin. Struct. Biol.* **2015**, *30*, 134–146.
92. B. Zhao, S. L. Guffy, B. Williams, Q. Zhang, *Nat. Chem. Biol.* **2017**, *13*, 968–974.
93. B. Zhao, J. T. Baisden, Q. Zhang, *J. Magn. Reson.* **2020**, *310*, 106642.

94. J. Lee, S.-E. Sung, J. Lee, J. Y. Kang, J.-H. Lee, B.-S. Choi, *Int. J. Mol. Sci.* **2021**, *22*, 3224.
95. K. E. Watters, E. J. Strobel, A. M. Yu, J. T. Lis, J. B. Lucks, *Nat. Struct. Mol. Biol.* **2016**, *23*, 1124–1131.
96. R. Yadav, J. R. Widom, A. Chauvier, N. G. Walter, *Nat. Commun.* **2022**, *13*, 207.
97. C. P. Jones, A. R. Ferré D'Amaré, *Annu. Rev. Biophys.* **2017**, *46*, 455–481.
98. M. Mandal, R. R. Breaker, *Nat. Struct. Mol. Biol.* **2004**, *11*, 29–35.
99. M. Mandal, B. Boese, J. E. Barrick, W. C. Winkler, R. R. Breaker, *Cell* **2003**, *113*, 577–586.
100. J. Noeske, H. Schwalbe, J. Wöhnert, *Nucleic Acids Res.* **2007**, *35*, 5262–5273.
101. M. D. Brenner, M. S. Scanlan, M. K. Nahas, T. Ha, S. K. Silverman, *Biochemistry* **2010**, *49*, 1596–1605.
102. X. Xu, M. Egger, H. Chen, K. Bartosik, R. Micura, A. Ren, *Nucleic Acids Res.* **2021**, *49*, 7139–7153.
103. R. R. Breaker, *CSH Perspect. Biol.* **2012**, *4*, 1–15.
104. N. H. Georgopapadakou, A. I. Scott, *J. Theor. Biol.* **1977**, *69*, 381–384.
105. A. Eschenmoser, *Angew. Chem. Int. Ed. Engl.* **1988**, *27*, 5–39.
106. B. Kräutler, D. Arigoni, B. T. Golding, *Vitamin B12 and B12-Proteins*, Ed G. Radau, Wiley-VCH, Weinheim, Chichester, **1998**.
107. W. Gilbert, *Nature* **1986**, *319*, 618.
108. P. J. McCown, K. A. Corbino, S. Stav, M. E. Sherlock, R. R. Breaker, *RNA* **2017**, *23*, 995–1011.
109. A. Nahvi, N. Sudarsan, M. S. Ebert, X. Zou, K. L. Brown, R. R. Breaker, *Chem. Biol.* **2002**, *9*, 1043–1049.
110. A. G. Vitreschak, D. A. Rodionov, A. A. Mironov, M. S. Gelfand, *RNA* **2003**, *9*, 1084–1097.
111. N. Pavlova, D. Kaloudas, R. Penchovsky, *Gene* **2019**, *708*, 38–48.
112. N. Pavlova, R. Penchovsky, *Expert Opin. Ther. Targets* **2019**, *23*, 631–643.
113. J. Palou-Mir, A. Musiari, R. K. O. Sigel, M. Barceló-Oliver, *J. Inorg. Biochem.* **2016**, *160*, 106–113.
114. J. E. Barrick, R. R. Breaker, *Genome. Biol.* **2007**, *8*, R239.
115. C. V. Franklund, R. J. Kadner, *J. Bacteriol.* **1997**, *179*, 4039–4042.
116. R. K. Montange, E. Mondragón, D. van Tyne, A. D. Garst, P. Ceres, R. T. Batey, *J. Mol. Biol.* **2010**, *396*, 761–772.
117. S. Gallo, M. Oberhuber, R. K. O. Sigel, B. Kräutler, *ChemBioChem* **2008**, *9*, 1408–1414.
118. J. T. Polaski, S. M. Webster, J. E. Johnson, R. T. Batey, *J. Biol. Chem.* **2017**, *292*, 11650–11658.
119. J. Li, Y. Ge, M. Zadeh, R. Curtiss III, M. Mohamadzadeh, *Proc. Natl. Acad. Sci. U.S.A.* **2020**, *117*, 602–609.
120. C. W. Chan, A. Mondragón, *Nucleic Acids Res.* **2020**, *48*, 7569–7583.
121. K. J. Kennedy, F. J. Widner, O. M. Sokolovskaya, V. L. Innocent, R. R. Procknow, K. C. Mok, M. E. Taga, *Microbiologie* **2022**, *13*, e01121-22.
122. P. K. Choudhary, A. Duret, E. Rohrbach-Brandt, C. Holliger, R. K. O. Sigel, J. Maillard, *J. Bacteriol.* **2013**, *195*, 5186–5195.
123. A. Nahvi, J. E. Barrick, R. R. Breaker, *Nucleic Acids Res.* **2004**, *32*, 143–150.
124. A. Lussier, L. Bastet, A. Chauvier, D. A. Lafontaine, *J. Biol. Chem.* **2015**, *290*, 26739–26751.
125. S. R. Lennon, R. T. Batey, *J. Mol. Biol.* **2022**, *434*, 167585.
126. S. Gallo, S. Mundwiler, R. Alberto, R. K. O. Sigel, *Chem. Commun.* **2011**, *47*, 403–405.

127. J. T. Polaski, E. D. Holmstrom, D. J. Nesbitt, R. T. Batey, *Cell Rep.* **2016**, *15*, 1100–1110.
128. K. Gruber, C. Kratky, *Curr. Opin. Chem. Biol.* **2002**, *6*, 598–603.
129. D. Sussman, J. C. Nix, C. Wilson, *Nat. Struct. Biol.* **2000**, *7*, 53–57.
130. J. Schnabl, Studies on the stabilization of RNA structures through metal ions, ion-π interactions and metallo-supramolecular helicates, Zürich.
131. Z. Weinberg, J. E. Barrick, Z. Yao, A. Roth, J. N. Kim, J. Gore, J. X. Wang, E. R. Lee, K. F. Block, N. Sudarsan, S. Neph, M. Tompa, W. L. Ruzzo, R. R. Breaker, *Nucleic Acids Res.* **2007**, *35*, 4809–4819.
132. J. L. Johnson, K. V. Rajagopalan, S. Mukund, M. W. Adams, *J. Biol. Chem.* **1993**, *268*, 4848–4852.
133. R. Hille, *Chem. Rev.* **1996**, *96*, 2757–2816.
134. R. R. Mendel, G. Schwarz, *Crit. Rev. Plant Sci.* **1999**, *18*, 33–69.
135. L. M. Patterson-Fortin, C. A. Vakulskas, H. Yakhnin, P. Babitzke, T. Romeo, *J. Mol. Biol.* **2013**, *425*, 3662–3677.
136. E. E. Regulski, R. H. Moy, Z. Weinberg, J. E. Barrick, Z. Yao, W. L. Ruzzo, R. R. Breaker, *Mol. Microbiol.* **2008**, *68*, 918–932.
137. F. Amadei, M. Reichenbach, S. Gallo, R. K. O. Sigel, *J. Inorg. Biochem.* **2023**, in press (doi: 10.1016/j.jinorgbio.2023.112153).
138. M. K. Chan, S. Mukund, A. Kletzin, M. W. W. Adams, D. C. Rees, *Science* **1995**, *267*, 1463–1469.
139. R. Hille, *Trends. Biochem. Sci.* **2002**, *27*, 360–367.
140. N. White, H. Sadeeshkumar, A. Sun, N. Sudarsan, R. R. Breaker, *Nat Chem Biol* **2022**, *18*, 878–885.
141. M. J. Cromie, Y. Shi, T. Latifi, E. A. Groisman, *Cell* **2006**, *125*, 71–84.
142. E. A. Groisman, M. J. Cromie, Y. Shi, T. Latifi, *CSH Symp. Quant. Biol.* **2006**, *71*, 251–258.
143. S. Brantl, *Trends. Biotechol.* **2006**, *24*, 383–386.
144. A. R. Ferré-D'Amaré, W. C. Winkler, *Met. Ions Life Sci.* **2011**, *9*, 141–173.
145. S. V. Spinelli, L. B. Pontel, E. García Véscovi, F. C. Soncini, *FEMS Microbiol. Lett.* **2008**, *280*, 226–234.
146. A. Ramesh, W. C. Winkler, *RNA Biol.* **2010**, *7*, 77–83.
147. M. J. Cromie, E. A. Groisman, *J. Bacteriol.* **2010**, *192*, 604–607.
148. J. Barchiesi, M. E. Castelli, F. C. Soncini, E. G. Véscovi, *J. Bacteriol.* **2008**, *190*, 4951–4958.
149. N. Figueroa-Bossi, S. Lemire, D. Maloriol, R. Balbontín, J. Casadesús, L. Bossi, *Mol. Microbiol.* **2006**, *62*, 838–852.
150. A. Sittka, S. Lucchini, K. Papenfort, C. M. Sharma, K. Rolle, T. T. Binnewies, J. C. D. Hinton, J. Vogel, *PLoS Genet.* **2008**, *4*, e1000163.
151. G. Zhao, W. Kong, N. Weatherspoon-Griffin, J. Clark-Curtiss, Y. Shi, *EMBO J.* **2011**, *30*, 1485–1496.
152. S.-Y. Park, M. J. Cromie, E.-J. Lee, E. A. Groisman, *Cell* **2010**, *142*, 737–748.
153. L. Bastet, A. Dubé, E. Massé, D. A. Lafontaine, *Mol. Microbiol.* **2011**, *80*, 1148–1154.
154. K. Hollands, S. Proshkin, S. Sklyarova, V. Epshtein, A. Mironov, E. Nudler, E. A. Groisman, *Proc. Natl. Acad. Sci. U.S.A.* **2012**, *109*, 5376–5381.
155. M. M. T. Korth, R. K. O. Sigel, *Chem. Biodivers.* **2012**, *9*, 2035–2049.
156. A. Ramesh, C. A. Wakeman, W. C. Winkler, *J. Mol. Biol.* **2011**, *407*, 556–570.
157. J. Schnabl, R. K. O. Sigel, *Curr. Opin. Chem. Biol.* **2010**, *14*, 269–275.
158. R. K. O. Sigel, H. Sigel, Vol. 3 of *Comprehensive Inorganic Chemistry II*, Eds J. Reedijk, K. R. Poeppelmeier, Elsevier Ltd., Amsterdam, **2013**, 623–659.

159. J. E. Barrick, K. A. Corbino, W. C. Winkler, A. Nahvi, M. Mandal, J. Collins, M. Lee, A. Roth, N. Sudarsan, I. Jona, J. K. Wickiser, R. R. Breaker, *Proc. Natl. Acad. Sci. U.S.A.* **2004**, *101*, 6421–6426.
160. K. Arnvig, D. Young, *RNA Biol.* **2012**, *9*, 427–436.
161. B. Bahoua, S. E. Sevdalis, A. M. Soto, *Biochemistry* **2021**, *60*, 2781–2794.
162. E. Ennifar, P. Walter, P. Dumas, *Nucleic Acids Res.* **2003**, *31*, 2671–2682.
163. M. C. Erat, R. K. O. Sigel, *Met. Ions Life Sci.* **2011**, *9*, 37–100.
164. G. Nechooshtan, M. Elgrably-Weiss, A. Sheaffer, E. Westhof, S. Altuvia, *Genes. Dev.* **2009**, *23*, 2650–2662.
165. G. Nechooshtan, M. Elgrably-Weiss, S. Altuvia, *Nucleic Acids Res.* **2014**, *42*, 622–630.
166. M. M. Meyer, M. C. Hammond, Y. Salinas, A. Roth, N. Sudarsan, R. R. Breaker, *RNA Biol.* **2011**, *8*, 5–10.
167. J. E. Martin, M. T. Le, N. Bhattarai, D. A. Capdevila, J. Shen, M. E. Winkler, D. P. Giedroc, *Nucleic Acids Res.* **2019**, *47*, 6885–6899.
168. I. R. Price, A. Gaballa, F. Ding, J. D. Helmann, A. Ke, *Mol. Cell* **2015**, *57*, 1110–1123.
169. K. C. Suddala, I. R. Price, S. S. Dandpat, M. Janeček, P. Kührová, J. Šponer, P. Banáš, A. Ke, N. G. Walter, *Nat. Commun.* **2019**, *10*, 4304.
170. S. T. Bachas, A. R. Ferré D'Amaré, *Cell Chem. Biol.* **2018**, *25*, 962–973.
171. D. Casanova, P. Alemany, J. M. Bofill, S. Alvarez, *Chem. Eur. J.* **2003**, *9*, 1281–1295.
172. M. E. Sherlock, R. R. Breaker, *RNA* **2020**, *26*, 675–693.
173. Y. Shi, G. Zhao, W. Kong, *J. Biol. Chem.* **2014**, *289*, 11353–11366.
174. H. Makui, E. Roig, S. T. Cole, J. D. Helmann, P. Gros, M. F. Cellier, *Mol. Microbiol.* **2000**, *35*, 1065–1078.
175. T. H. Hohle, M. R. O'Brian, *Mol. Microbiol.* **2009**, *72*, 399–409.
176. K. Furukawa, A. Ramesh, Z. Zhou, Z. Weinberg, T. Vallery, W. C. Winkler, R. R. Breaker, *Mol. Cell* **2015**, *57*, 1088–1098.
177. J. Xu, J. A. Cotruvo, *Biochemistry* **2020**, *59*, 1508–1516.
178. J. Xu, J. A. Cotruvo, *Curr. Opin. Chem. Biol.* **2022**, *68*, 102135.
179. X. Wang, W. Wei, J. Zhao, *Front. Chem.* **2021**, *9*, 631909.
180. S. C. Y. Jeng, R. J. Trachman, F. Weissenboeck, L. Truong, K. A. Link, M. D. E. Jepsen, J. R. Knutson, E. S. Andersen, A. R. Ferré D'Amaré, P. J. Unrau, *RNA* **2021**, *27*, 433–444.
181. H.-L. Sung, D. J. Nesbitt, *J. Phys. Chem.* **2020**, *124*, 7348–7360.
182. A. B. Rode, T. Endoh, N. Sugimoto, *Angew. Chem. Int. Ed.* **2018**, *57*, 6707–6944.
183. W. C. Winkler, R. R. Breaker, *Annu. Rev. Microbiol.* **2005**, *59*, 487–517.
184. B. Lutz, M. Faber, A. Verma, S. Klumpp, A. Schug, *Nucleic Acids Res.* **2014**, *42*, 2687–2696.
185. G. A. Perdrizet, I. Artsimovitch, R. Furman, T. R. Sosnick, T. Pan, *Proc. Natl. Acad. Sci. U.S.A.* **2012**, *109*, 3323–3328.
186. A. Haller, M. F. Soulière, R. Micura, *Acc. Chem. Res.* **2011**, *44*, 1339–1348.
187. The Pymol Molecular Graphics System, Version 2.0 Schrödinger, LLC.

Index

Note: **Bold** page numbers refer to tables; *italic* page numbers refer to figures.

Abasic site, 309
Acetate, 8, 14
Actinoide, 233
Activation strain analysis *see* ASA
Activation strain model *see* ASM
Adenine, *53*, *233*
   acid-base chemistry, 18, 20
   as bridging ligand, *3*, 4, 8–16, 21, 22, 147
   as ligand, *18*, 82, 83, *109*, 126, *135*–137, 139–145, 149, 150, *221*
   rare tautomer, 107, 108
S-Adenosyl-l-homocysteine *see* SAH
S-Adenosyl methionine *see* SAM
ADF-STEM, 220
Adsorption, 8, 9, 13, 14, 22
Aerogel, 54, 71–73
Affibody, *178*, 179
AFM, 66, *67*, *69*, 88, *91*, 92, 95, *96–98*, 197, 380
Alkali metal, 232
Alkaline earth metal, 233
Alpha hemolysin, 222, 223
Alzheimer's disease, 147
2-Aminopurine, 53, 69, 70
Angiogenesis, 161
Anion-π interaction, 106, 107, 123, 124, *125*, **126**, 128
Anisotropy, 318
Annular dark field scanning transmission electron microscopy *see* ADF-STEM
Anthracene, 175
anti conformation, 375
Anticancer drug, 376
Apoptosis, 135, 141
Aptamer, 294, 334, 400, *401*, 403, 407, 411, 412, 419–421, 426, 427; *see also* DNA aptamer
   metal-responsive, 269, 272, 277, 278, 285
   thrombin-binding, 390
Architecture, 46, 71, 73, 380
   2-dimensional, 42, 376
   3-dimensional, 153, 376
   DNA, 80, 231, 327, 333, 388, 389, 393, 394
   functional, 27
   infinite, 53

molecular, 56, 63, 244, 263
nanocluster, 329
riboswitch, 401
secondary, 380
solid-state, 107, 307
supramolecular, *12*, 15–*17*, *19*, 28, *29*, 30, 67, 135
synthetic, 26
Argentophilic interaction, 28, 38, 63, 86, 87, 107, 113, 116, 117, 120, 128
Arginine, 278
Array, 235, 237, 244, 245, 247, 262, 264, 265, 329–331
ASA, 347
ASM, 347, 363
Aspartate, 386
Association constant, 261
Atomic force microscopy *see* AFM
Atomically precise, 301, 329–332, 335
ATP, 277, 278
ATPase, 422, 424
Aurophilic interaction, 107, 116, 120, *121*, 128
Autofluorescence, 317
5-Aza-7-deazapurine, 241
8-Aza-7-deazapurine, 241
Azido ligand, 169, 170
4,4'-Azopyridine, 39, 40, 42

Bacillus subtilis, 419, 420, 424
Band gap, 88, 89, 92
Band structure, 87, 89
Barium, 28, 30, 363–**365**, 411, 412, 426
Beacon, 299
Benzimidazole, 420
Benzoate, 16, *18*, *19*
BET surface area, 4, 6
Bifacial nucleobase, 279–286
Binding pocket, 402, 403, 407, 410, 411, 413–417, 420, 421, 427, 428
Bioavailability, 334
Biofilm, 138
Bioimaging, 107, 294, 317, 326, 328, 329, 333, 335
Biosynthesis, 401, 418, 421
2,2'-Bipyridine, 42–44, 169, 174, *223*, 378–380, 389

435

4,4'-Bipyridine, *39*, 40, 42, 55–58, 64, 65, 68, 69, 71, *72*, 73, *74*
Bottom-up strategy, 231, 244, 245, 247, 249, 250
6-Butyladenine, 6, 7

Cadmium, 9, 33–37, 44, 62, 66, *67*, 70, 126, 363–366, 426
Caffeine, 126, 127, 140–142
Calcium, 28, 30, 106, 110, 123, 363–**365**, **405**, 407, 411, 426
Calf thymus DNA *see* ct-DNA
Calixarene, 38
Cambridge Crystallographic Data Centre *see* CCDC
Cambridge Structural Database *see* CSD
Carbene, 137, 140–142, 146
Carbohydrate, 162
Carbon nanotube, 264, 265
Carboplatin, 150, 161, 164, 168
4-Carboxyimidazole *see* Imidazole-4-carboxylate
Carboxylate, 6, 8, 16, *18*, *53*
  recognition, 412
5-Carboxyuracil, 116, 236, *280*–283, 285, 286
Casp-3, 141
Catalysis, *326*, 329, 335, 388, 389, 394
Cation-π interaction, 106, 107, 121, 123, 126, 128
Cation-π-stacking, 420
Cavity, 8, 11, 30, 31
CCDC, 26, 30, 38, 41
CD, 95, 96, 263–265, 271, 281, 282
  spectroscopy, 173, 174, 180, 241, 246, 248, *306*, 307, 311, 313, 320, 376, 379–385, 388
  spectrum, 192, 195, *196*, 199–*204*, 206, 241–243
Cell lines
  A2780/DDP, 142
  A549, 137, 146
  CH1/DDP, 142
  HeLa, 147, 148, 328
  HOS, 140
  HT-29, 142
  MCF7, 138, 140
  MDA-MB-231, 142
  MS-1, 140
  SKOV3, 150
  T2, 150
Cerium, 70–71
Cesium, 151, 196, **355**–356
Chalcoplatin, 163
Channel, 4, 8, 9, 11, 13, 16, 22, 34, 36–38, 45
Chirality, 26–28, 33, 39, 40, 42–44, 46, 384, 389, 394

Chromatin, 190, 206
Chromium, 18, 169
Chromosome, 376
Circular dichroism *see* CD
Circularly polarized luminescence *see* CPL
Cisplatin, 144, 160, 170, 192, 194, 206
  anticancer drug, 2, 135, 161, 164, 191, 234, 259
  cisplatin prodrug, 163, 167, 168
  cisplatin-sensitive cell lines, 150
  cytotoxicity, 140–142
  DNA interaction, 139, 198, 199
cmc, 201
CMP, 27, 30, 32, *33*, 34, *36*, *37*, 38, *39*–45, 61, 63, *88*, 89, 120
CO, 169
CO_2, 8, 9, 11, 13, 31, 54, 71–73, 145
Cobalamin, 409, 417–420, 428
Cobalt
  Co^{2+}, *8*, 28, *29*, 42, 62, 66, 107, 136, 264, 275, 379, 383–384, **406**–407
  Co^{3+}, 164, 165, 175, 417
  complex, 12–14, 29, 30, 33–34, 39, 40
  hexaammine complex, 123, 198, 206, 420
  M-DNA, 61, 87
  in metal-mediated base pairing, 267
  prodrug, 164, *165*
  riboswitch, 426–428
Cofactor, 386, 388, 390, 400, 402, **404**, 410–412, 417, 420, 421, 423
  B_{12}, 417
Coinage bond *see* Regium bond
Colloids, 67, 68, 75
Complex
  azolato-bridged, 191, 192, 195, 196, 199
  dinuclear, 191, 199, 206
  heteronuclear, 265
Conducting AFM, 88
Conductivity, 54, 59–66, 234, 235, 238
Conductor-like screening model *see* COSMO
Cooperativity, *350*, 351, 353
Coordination environment, 380, 386–388, 304
Coordination polymer, 53–71, 73–75, 82–83, 89, 94–97, 99
Copper
  adenine complex, *8*, *15*, 18
  aerogels, 71
  complexes, *55*, 58, *60*, 63, *64*, 68, *144*, 145, 176, 177, 394, 387–390
  Cu^+, 164–165, 175
  Cu^{2+}, 8, 136, 175, 233
  cytosine complex, 30, 32, *43*, 44, *45*
  dependent DNAzymes, 145, 273–279
  EPR, 391–393

Index

in metal-mediated base pairing, 110, 116,
  145, 236, 238, 259, 260, 263–268,
  273–280, 282, 283, 285–286
MOF, 4, 8, 45, 145
nanocluster, 298, 334
physiological role, 144
prodrugs, 164
in quadruplexes, 381–393
reduction/oxidation of, 165, 285
responsive aptamers, 277, 278
sensor, 328
Corrin, 417, 418
COSMO, 346, 354, 359, 361, 363, **364**
Cotton effect, 195, 196, 202, 381
Coulomb interaction, 347
Coumarin, 170
COX-2, 163, 166
CPL, 94–96, 99
Critical micelle concentration *see* cmc
Cross section, 303, 320
Cryo-electron microscopy, 375, 391
Crystal engineering, 10, 106, 117, 122, 128,
  106, 117, 122, 128
Crystal structure, 261–264, 294–296, 305,
  307–313, 318, 321, 332
CSD, 4, 28
ct-DNA, 169, 177, 195, 196, 199–204
Cubane, 13
Cyclen, 165, 247
Cyclooctadiene, 180, 182
Cyclooxygenase *see* COX-2
Cysteine, 271, 272, 386
Cytidine, 27, 28, 30, *31*, 32, 34, 38, 42, 84, *86*,
  87, *88*, 91, 92, 111, 117, 120
Cytidine monophosphate *see* CMP
Cytochrome *c*, 90
Cytosine, 3, 9, *10*, 27, 28, *29*, 30, 33–37, 41, 42,
  44–46, *53*, 56, 63, 84, *85*, *86*, *135*,
  221, *233*, *240*
Cytotoxicity, 334

DAPI, 177, 179
1-Deazaadenine, 237
7-Deazaadenine, *114*, 138, 139, 149, 232, 238,
  239, *240*, **242**, 245, 250
7-Deazaguanine, 117, 138, 232, 238, 239, *240*,
  241, **242**, 250, 283
DEER, 391, 392
Dehydration, 425
Density functional theory *see* DFT
Density of states *see* DOS
Deoxycytidine, 214, 216
Deoxycytidine monophosphate, 30, 32–40,
  41, 42
Desolvation, 359, 361–363

DFT (calculation of), 73, 95, 110, 111, 123,
  137, 249
band gap, 62, 66
collisional cross section, 311
dispersion-corrected, 346, 363
DOS, 63
electronic structure, 62, 96
magnetic coupling constants, 59
for quadruplex modeling, 346, 354, 355,
  357, 358, 361, 363, 367
structure, 86, 137, 243, 303, 312, 313
TD-DFT, 95
Diastereomer, 384
Dicarboxylate, 8, 9, 16
1,3-Dideazaadenine, *114*, 237
Dielectric, 321
Diels-Alder reaction, 388
Dimethylcarbamate, 11, 12
1,9-Dimethylguanine, 83
1,3-Dimethyluracil, 108, 120
Dipicolinic acid, 71
2,2'-Dipyridylamine, 42, 43
Dispersion, 346–350, 353, 364
DNA, 80–84, 92, *93*, 106, 112, *173*, 175, 176
  A-form, 195, 231
  aptamer, 260, 269, 272, 277, 278, 285
  B-form, 122, 145, 195, 197, 201, 230, 231,
    237, 241, 242, 246, 258, 261, 262,
    281, 282, 310, 367
  C-form, 195, 196, 199, 203, 205
  functional, 260, 265, 268, 269, 273, 275,
    277–279, 282, 285, 286
  human telomeric (htel22), 384–386
  metallization of, 231, 232, *233*, *234*, 235,
    239, 241, 243, 249, 250
  metal-responsive, 260, 263, 265–270,
    272–279, 282–286
  nanotechnology, 231, 249, 260, 263, 278,
    283, 286, 260, 263, 278, 283, 286,
    376, 386, 394
  origami, 231, 232, 333, 376, 393
  replication, 344
  single-stranded, 233, 239, 244–246, 249,
    250, 294, 296, 304, 320, 321, 330
  structures, *81*
  transcription, 344
  Z-form, 124, 195, 231
DNAzyme, 145, 260, 267–279, 285, 377, 389,
  390, 394
  metallo, 389, *390*
  split, 270, 271, 273–276, 285
Dopamine, 151
Doping, 89, 97
DOS, 88, 89
Double electron-electron resonance *see* DEER

Index

Doxorubicin, 178, 180–183
Dynamics, 307, 315, 316

EDA, 347, 348, 352, 360, 364
EDTA, 174, 175, 177, 265, 284, 380, *382*–384, 386, 393
EFM, 66
Electrical conductivity, 59, 61–63, 82, 87, 89, 94, 97, 264–265
Electron microscopy *see* EM
Electrostatic force microscopy *see* EFM
Electrostatic interaction, 347, 349, 352, 356, 360
EM, 219, 220, 222
Emission, 294, 298, 299, 303–305, 313–316, 318–321, 323, 324, 327, 329–331, 333, 334
Enantiomeric excess, 388
Enantioselectivity, 389, 390, 394
Endogenous stimuli, 161
Energy decomposition analysis *see* EDA
Enzyme, 376, 386, 390
EPR spectroscopy, 260, 263, 265, 381
Escherichia coli, 138, 408, 418, 421, 426
ESI mass spectrometry, 245, 246, 248, 300, 301, 383, 388
Ethacraplatin, 162
1,N^6-Ethenoadenine, 138, 146
Ethidium bromide, 177, 179, 246
9-Ethyladenine, 110, 245, 246, *248*, 249
Ethylenediamine, 42, 43
Ethylenediaminetetraacetic acid *see* EDTA
9-Ethylguanine, 193, **194**, 195
Europium, 70, 71, 107
EXAFS, 304, 305
Excitation, 298, 299, 303, 304, 307, 314–320, 331, 333, 334
Expression platform, 401, 421, 427
Extended axial chirality, 40, 42
Extended X-ray absorption fine structure *see* EXAFS

Femtosecond spectroscopy, 315
Fermi
 energy, 63, 88
 wavelength, 92, 293
Ferrocene, 81, 218, 219
Ferromagnetic coupling, 265
Fiber, 91, 92, 95, 96, 98
Fibrin, 390
Fibrinogen, 390
Five-way junction, 412
Fluorescence, 57, 70, 71, 113
 decay, 315, 316, 321
 microscopy (*see* FM)
 spectrum, 294, *314*

Fluoride, 402, 414, 415
Fluorimetry, 298, 318
5-Fluorouracil, 53, 58, 68, 73, *112*, 117, 179
FM, 175, 192, 197, 201, *202*, 205, 294, 299, 328
FMN, 402, **404**, 410, 411, 427
Folding, 190, 197, 201, 205, 206, 402, 403, **405**, 407, 409, 411–413, 415–417, 419, 420, 424, 426, 427
Footprinting, 403, 411
Formaldehyde, 357, 364–366
Förster resonance energy transfer *see* FRET
Four-way junction, 231, 374
Franck-Condon state, 315, 316
FRET, *217*, 311, *312*, 330, 331, 427
Friedel-Crafts reaction, 388
Furan, 220
Fusobacterium nucleatum, 152

Gadolinium, 170, 180, 236, 280–282, 284
Gel electrophoresis, 376, 380
Gelation, 82, 89, 95, 96
Gemcitabine, 179
Gene
 expression, 401, 418, 425, 427
 regulation, 400, 401
Genotyping, 212–214, 219, 224
Glucosamine-6-phosphate, 410, 412
Glutamate, 386
Glycol nucleic acid *see* GNA
GMP, 68, 70, 89, *90*, 92, 193, **194**, 195
GNA, 116, 214, 215, 217, 384
Gold; *see also* Aurophilic interactions
 Au⁺, 121, 126, 142
 Au³⁺, 69, 70
 catalysis, 182
 in metal-mediated base pairing, 82–83, 108–109, 120, 237
 nanocluster, 142, *143*, 298, 332, 334
 nanoparticle, 80, 143–144, 235
 nucleobase complex, 82–84, 97, 99, 120, 121, 127, 128
 in regium bonds, 122, 128
 thiolate complex, 61–63, 96–98
 van der Waals radius, 122
G-quadruplex, 231, 259, 269, 271, 272, 344–346, 348, 349, 353, *354*, **355**, *356*–**364**, **365**, 366, 367, 374, *375*–394
 binding complexes, 128, 163, 164, 171, 177
 dimeric, 122
 metal-ion affinity, 151, 358–366
 RNA, 355
G-quartet, 122, 128, 136, 137, 151, 344, 349, *350*, 351, **352**, 353, 355, 360, 361, 366, 374, 377, 384, 390

Index

Guanine, *3*–4, 9–11, **14**, 22, *53*, 82–83, *135*, 137, 139, 141, 149–151, *233*
  monophosphate (*see* GMP)
  quadruplex (*see* G-quadruplex)
  quartet (*see* G-quartet)
G-wire, 375, 379, 380, 394

Hairpin, 272, 307, 330
Half-life, 194
HDAC, 163, 164
Helix, 87
Hemin, 269, 271, 377, 390
HER2, 179, 180, 182
Heteroleptic, 386–388, 394
1-Hexylcytosine, 28, 86, 87, 117, 118, 121, 122
Higher-order structure, 190–192, 194, 197, 199, 201, 202, 205, 206
High-performance liquid chromatography *see* HPLC
High-throughput, 296, 298, 299, 303, 315, 318, 323, 328, 329, 335
Hill coefficient, 426
Histidine, 174, 175, 383, 386
Histone deacetylase *see* HDAC
Hoechst-33258, 68, 90
HOMO, 318, 347, 353, 365, 366
Homoduplex, 311–313
Hoogsteen
  base pair, 56, 280, 283, 284
  edge, *10*, 11, 15, 22
  face, 243
  hydrogen bond, 349, 354
Horseradish peroxidase, 269–272
HPLC, 71–73, 75, 297, 299, 300, 303, 305–309, 311, 316, 318, 319, 330, 332, 333
HSAB concept, 388
Human epidermal growth factor receptor 2 *see* HER2
Hybrid, 375, 384–386, 389, 393, 394
Hybridization probe, 212, 213, 217–219, 224
Hydration shell, 123, 411
Hydrogel, 89, 90, 92, 94–96, 107, 120, 136, 151, 152, 311, 330, 377
Hydrogen bond, 248, 249, 280, 332, 411, 412, 417, 420
  acceptor, 205, 349
  cooperativity, 351, 353, 354
  distance, 351, 359
  donor, 349, 353, 411
  energy, 348, 350, 353
  in guanine quadruplexes, 353, 349
  in MOFs, 2, 22
  interaction, 2, 10, 11, 13, 15–17, 21, 22, 28, 34, 64, 84, 86, 92, 106, 110, 117, *118*, 150, 206, 230, 244, 419
  intermolecular, 87

interplanar, 311
intramolecular, 11, 13, 22, 85, 109, 110, 177, 246, 356
involving solvent molecules, 13, 150
involving water molecules, 15, 86, 109, 145, 190
network, 116, 355, 410, 413, 415, 416
N–H⋯Cl, 122
N–H⋯N, 111
N–H⋯O, 87, 111
pattern, 377
resonance-assisted stabilization, 350, 352
strength, 350
supported stabilization, 138
Watson-Crick (*see* Watson-Crick hydrogen bond)
Hydrophobic effect, 56
Hydroxido ligand, 13, 18, 19, 21, 22, 44
Hydroxypropylmethacrylamide polymer, 166
3-Hydroxy-4-pyridone *see* Hydroxypyridone
Hydroxypyridone, 238, 259, 263–267, 273–279, 285
5-Hydroxyuracil, 236, 280–285
Hypoxanthine, 124–**126**
Hypoxia, 161, 162, 165, 169

Ibuprofen, 20, *21*
ICS-AES, 301
Imaging
  in vitro, 329
  in vivo, 294, 329
Imidazole, 138, 139, 220, 238, *277*, 387, *389*, *390*
Imidazole-4-carboxylate, 145, 266–268, 273–275, 277, 278, 285
Imidazolocytosine, 218
Imidazophenanthroline, 214, 215, 217, 218
Iminodiacetic acid, 175
i-motif, 41, 110, 231, 310–312, 374, 377
Immune chemotherapy, 163
IMS, 311
in vivo studies, 390
Inductively coupled plasma-atomic emission spectroscopy *see* ICP-AES
Inosine, 305, 306, 321, 322
  monophosphate, 68, 69
Insulator, 63, 65, 66
Interaction energy, 347, 348, 351, 352, 357, 359–363, 365
Intercalation, 175, 180, **404**, 409, 415, 417
Intercalator, 170, 175, 179, 191
Interstrand crosslink, *149*
Intrastrand crosslink, 191, 192, 194
Ion mobility spectrometry *see* IMS
Iridium, 150, *151*, 409

Iron
  coordination polymers, 69
  Fe^{2+}, 62, 66, 275, 426, 428
  Fe^{3+}, 70, 174, 191
  metabolite, **406**
  porphyrin, 377, 390
  prodrug, 164, 165
  sensor, 107
  staircase, 118
  transporter, 424
Irving-Williams series, 267
Isoalloxazine, 411
Isonicotine, 9
Isophthalate, 9
Isothermal titration calorimetry *see* ITC
ITC, 261

Jahn-Teller distortion, 18
Jellium model, 302
Job's plot, 281

Kinetics, 383
Kissing loop, **404**, 416, 419, 420
Kohn-Sham orbital, 306, 347, 348, 364

Langmuir surface area, 9
Lanthanoide, 106, 107, 233, 281, 321
Lead, 328, 363–366
LED, 69, 70
Leucine zipper, 173, 174, 180
Lifetime, 298, 316, 320, 321
Ligandoside, 380–390, 392–394
Light-up behavior, 320, 322, 327
Lippert-Mataga model, 315
Lithium, 123, 151, 195, 196, **355**, 356, 358–361, 363–**365**, **406**, 422
Logic gate, 278, 279, 286, 377
Loop, 375, 378–380, 387–389, 391, 393
Lumiflavin, 411
Luminescence
  of Ag nanoclusters, 294, 307, 313, 315, 328, 329, 333
  of Au^I-thiolate, 98
  circularly polarized (*see* CPL)
  of coordination polymers, 54, 59, 70, 94
  of lanthanoides, 107
  quantum yield, 321
LUMO, 89, 318, 347, 353, 360, 364–366

Machine learning, *295*, 296, 309, 313, 322–326, 329, 335
Magnesium, 259, 269
  acetate, 330
  in cation-π interaction, 121–123
  in C-form DNA, 195
  in coordination polymers, 69
  cytosine-O2 coordination, 28
  dependent folding pathway, 421
  in guanine quadruplexes, 363–365
  Mg^{2+} 106, 404, 137, 190, 206,
  in riboswitches, 402–417, 420–427
  in supramolecular assemblies, 28, *29*
Magnetism, 54, 59, 80
Malonate, 9
Manganese
  in coordination polymers, 69
  cytosine-O2 coordination, 28
  in metal-mediated base pairs, 82, 113, *115*, 236
  in nucleobase complexes, 38–42
  riboswitch, 401, **406**, 407, 424–426
  in riboswitches, 411, 424
  in supramolecular assemblies, 28
Mass spectrometry, 260, 263, 265, 281, 282, *297*, 300, 376, 378, 383, 388; *see also* ESI mass spectrometry
MD, 304, 345, 382–385, 392, 393
M-DNA, *61*, 62, 66
Melting transition, 197
MEP, 124
8-Mercaptoadenine, 144–145
6-Mercaptopurine, *53*, 62, 66, 67
Mercury
  acetate, 220
  in anion-π interactions, 124
  contrast-enhancing agent, 220
  in coordination polymers, 69
  in guanine quadruplexes, 363–366
  in metal-mediated base pairing, 82, 111, 112, 116, 145, 146, 214–216, 219, 233–236, 238, 259–265, 268–273, 275, 283, 285, 377–379
  in nucleobase complexes, 107, 108, 110, 112, 113, 136, 334
  organometallic nucleobase, 215–219
  sensor, 328
Metabolite, 401, 402, **404–406**, 409–414, 416, 421, 422, 427, 428
Metal-assisted ligand binding, 401, 403
Metal-DNA assembly, 249, 250
Metallo-base pair, 231, 232, 234–239, 244, 245, 249, 250
Metallocage, 107
Metallo cofactor, **404**, 417
Metallocycle, 107
Metallogel, 138
Metallophilic interaction, 107; *see also* Argentophilic interaction; Aurophilic interaction
Metalloprotein, 386–388, 394

Index

Metal-mediated base pair (with), 152, 213, 231, 239–244, 250, 259–275, 277–283, 285, 286, 377, 378
    copper, 81, 82, *116*, 145, 236, 238, 259, 263, *264*–268, 274–279
    gadolinium, 236, 280–284
    gold, 82–84
    manganese, 82, 115, 236
    mercury, 81, 82, *116*, 145, *146*, 214–219, 234–236, 259–263, 267, 269, 270
    nickel, 81, 82, 326
    organometallic, 214–218
    palladium, 116, 218, 236, *245*, 246, *247*, 248
    silver, 81–85, 90, 93, 113, 114, *116*–*119*, 138, 139, 217, 237, 238, 240–244, 259–263, 269, 270
    zinc, 236
Metal-mediated base tetrad, 380, 389
Metal-modified base pair, 81, 109, *116*, 119, 128, 213, 231, 237–243, 250, 259
Metal-organic framework *see* MOF
Metal-organic gel, 54, 62, 67–73
Metastasis, 161
Methionine, 386
6-Methoxyadenine, 137
6-Methoxy-9-methylguanine, 83
6-Methyladenine, 139
9-Methyladenine, 56, 83, 107–110, 126, 127
1-Methylcytosine, 28, 29, 83, 87, 88, 109–111, 117
5-Methylcytosine, 149, 150
9-Methylguanine, 56
1-Methylthymine, 110, 111, 113
1-Methyluracil, 83, 110
Micelle, 168, 181
Michael addition, 388, 389, 394
Mie-Gans theory, 317
miRNA, 328
Mitaplatin, 163
Mitochondria, 163, 170
MOF, 2, 4–7, 9, 10, 14, 18, 22, 89, 145, 147
Molecular
    machine, 376
    recognition, 54–56, 58, 63, 66–68, 75
    switch, 376
Molecular beacon, 212, 217, 218
Molecular dynamics *see* MD
Molecular electrostatic potential *see* MEP
Molybdenum, 417, 420, 421, 428
Morphology, 68, 73, 201
Motexafin gadolinium, 170, 180
mRNA, 400, 423
Mulliken population, 364–366
Mycobacterium smegmatis porin A, 222, 223
Mycobacterium tuberculosis, 424

NAD+, **404**, 410, 411
Nanocluster
    gold 142, *143*
    silver, 92, 234, 293–311, 313–315, 317–322, 326–335
Nanodevice, 66, 75, 376, 377, 393
Nanoelectronics, 234, 239, 377
Nanofiber, 67, 68, 72, 73
Nanomachine, 111
Nanomaterials, 136
Nanoparticle, 67–70, 293, 294, 317
    gold, 80, 143
    lanthanoide, 107
    palladium, 180, 181
    platinum 170, 171
    silver, 68, 69, 90–92, 120, 296, 304, 305
    silver-gold, 235
Nanophotonics, 239, 294, 326
Nanopore sequencing, 212, 219, *222*, 223
Nanoprocessing, 54, 66–68
Nanoribbon, 67, 74
Nanorod, 303, 314, 331
Nanostructure, 329–331, 388
Nanotechnology, 53, 135, 136
Nanowire, 80, 87, 113, 118, 120
Naproxen, 20, *21*
Network, 54, 63, 68, 89, 91, 92, 96
Next-generation sequencing, 299
Nickel
    in coordination polymers, 62
    in guanine quadruplexes, 379–381, 383, 384, 387, 388
    in M-DNA, 66, 87
    in metal-mediated base pairs, 82, 236, 260, 267
    in MOFs, 73
    in nucleobase complexes, *8*, 28, 39, 40, 42
    in peptide complexes, 174, 175
    riboswitch, **406**, 426–428
NIR fluorescence, 294
Nitroxide, 391
NMR spectroscopy, 110, 244, 245, 249, 260, 261, 375, 391, 413, 415, 423
    ^{19}F, 218, 219
NO, 169
Non-covalent interaction, 191, 192, 195, 196, 206, 348, 349
Nucleobases, 232, *233*, *248*; *see also* individual names
    artificial, 214, *259*, 263, 264, *273*
    bifacial, 279, *280*–284
    purine, *53*, *135*
    pyrimidine, *53*, *135*, *215*

OADF, 317, 329
Oncogene, 110, 345, 376

Optically activated delayed fluorescence *see* OADF
Orbital interaction, 347, 352, 360
Organogel, 89, 91, 92
Organometallic nucleobase, 212, 214–219
Osmium, 148–150, 220, 223
Oxalate, 4, 6, 9, 55, 65
Oxaliplatin, 140, 142, 161, 162, 164, 166, 170, 171
Oxido ligand, 44
2-Oxo-imidazole-4-carboxamide, 268
2-Oxo-imidazole-4-carboxylate, 267, 268

p53, 141
PACT, 168, 169
PAGE, 380
Pair-distribution function *see* PDF
Palladium
    catalysis, 179, 180, 182, 183
    complex, 182
    deposition on DNA, 235
    in metal-mediated base pair, 116, 218, 236, 245–249, 260
    nanoparticle, 180
    in nucleobase complex, 126, 127, 233
    in peptide complex, 174
    prodrug, 182
    sensor, 107
Pancreatic cancer, 191
Paramagnetism, 390, 391, 394
Parkinson's disease, 147
Pauli repulsion, 347, 349, 350, 352, 360, 364
PCR, 212
PDEPR spectroscopy, 391–393
PDF, 74
PDT, 168, 169, 171
Peptide, 162, 167, 168, 171–175, 180
1,10-Phenanthroline, 42–45
Phenanthroline diamine, 164
o-Phenylenediamine, 260
Phosphate, 27, 30, 32–38, 40–46
    recognition, 409, 412
Phosphoramidite, 379–381, 393
Phosphorescence, 298, 315
Phosphorothioate, 424
Photoactivated chemotherapy *see* PACT
Photobinding, 169
Photocleavage, 169
Photodynamic therapy *see* PDT
Photoemission, 92, 95
Photoexcitation, 315, 317
Photoluminescence, 234, 238
Photophysical properties, 294–295, 300, 301, 307, 309, 313–315, 318, 320–322, 333–335
Photoreduction, 169, 170

Photosensitizer, 168, 171
Photostability, 294, 295, 329, 333
Photosubstitution, 168
Phototoxicity, 170
π-hole, 122, 128
π-resonance-assisted hydrogen bonding *see* RAHB
π stacking
    of base pairs, 260
    of bipyridine, 44
    in crystal packing, 309
    as fluorescence quencher, 218
    in guanine quadruplexes, 354, 355, 375, 376, 384, 392, 393
    of hemin, 377
    interactions, 2, 15–20, 22, 40, 106, 107, 111, 122, 124, 164, 230, 244–246
    lateral, 353
    in metal-organic frameworks, 2
    of nucleobases, 95
    of purine residues, 128, 311, 414, 415, 420
    of pyrimidine residues, 34, 40, 42, 112, 117, 118, 238, 383
    in riboswitches, 407, 414, 415, 420
    topology, 361
PIPER, 392, 393
Platinum
    complexes, 166, 167
    deposition on DNA, 235
    dinuclear complexes, 191–202
    metallodrug, 139, 140, 141, 142, 151, 152, 160, 206
    nucleobase complexes, 43, 56, 109, 110, 126, 127, 135, 136, 233
    prodrug, 161, 162, 163, 164, 167–172, 180
PMe$_3$, 120, 121
Pollution, 363
Polyacrylamide gel electrophoresis *see* PAGE
Polyacrylonitrile, 142, 143
Polyamine, 197
Polymerase, 265, 266, 269, 272
Polymerase chain reaction *see* PCR
Polymerization, 95
Porosity, 71, 73
Porous material, 2, 14, 21, 22
Porous structure, 36–38
Porphyrin, 377
Potassium
    in cation-π interactions, 123
    dependent folding pathway, 421
    in guanine quadruplex, 345, 384, 385
    in guanine quartets, 120, 137, 151, 152, 259, 353, 355, 356, 358–366, 374
    ion transport, 136
    in riboswitches, 402, **405**–407, 412, 415
    in uracil complex, 63

Index

Prefolding, 403–407, 416
Prequeusine, **405**
Prodrug, 161–168, 170, 178–183
Programmability, 388
Promoter, 376
  region, 344, 363
Propeller twist, 261
9-Propyl-7-deazaadenine, 245, 246
Protein engineering, 386
Proteobacteria, 423
Pterin, 421
Pulsed dipolar electron paramagnetic resonance spectroscopy *see* PDEPR spectroscopy
Pyran, 421
Pyrazole, 191, 192, 194
Pyrene, 175
Pyridine, 236, 259, 260, 264, 265, 380–386, 388, 390–394
  -2,6-dicarboxamide, 116
  -2,6-dicarboxylate, 236, 259, 260
Pyrophosphate, 403–**405**, 410–412
Pyrrolocytosine, 218

QM/MM, 307, 311, 346
Quantum dot, 70, 294, 320, 329, 334
Quantum mechanics/molecular mechanics *see* QM/MM
Quantum yield, 294, 295, 315, 317, 321, 323, 328, 329
Quinolone, 180

RAHB, 350
Rate constant, 193, 194, 274–277
RBS, 418
Reactive oxygen species *see* ROS
Receptor, 30, 31
Recognition, 401, 402, **405**, **406**, 409, 411, 412, 414–417, 419, 421
Redox-based regulation, 285
Regium bond, 106, 107, 121, 122, 128
Relaxation-induced dipolar modulation enhancement *see* RIDME
Reversed Hoogsteen orientation, 262
Rheology, 91
Rhodamine, 170, 180
Rhodium, 9, 141, 169, 233, 235
Riboflavin, 411
Ribosome binding site *see* RBS
Riboswitch
  adenine, 403, **405**, *416*
  adenosylcobalamin (AdoCbl)-specific *btuB*, **404**, 407–409, 418–420
  B$_{12}$, 417–420, 428
  cobalamin, 409, 417–420, 428
  cyclic-di-GMP, 403, 405

flavin mononucleotide (FMN), **404**
fluoride-dependent, 402, 414, 415
glmS, 401, 403, **406**, 412, 427
glutamine, 402, 403, **406**, 413
glycine, 403, **406**, 413
guanidine, 401, **405**, 411
guanine, 405, 415, *416*
Li$^+$, **406**, 422
lysine, 402, **406**, 412, 413
M-box, 407, 422–424
metal-assisted folding, 402–409
Mg^{2+} (*see mgtA* riboswitch and M-box riboswitch)
mgtA, 422–423
Mn^{2+} (*see* yybP-ykoY RNA motif and *mntH* riboswitch)
mntH, **406**, 426
moaA, 421
molybdenum cofactor (Moco), **404**, 420, *421*, 422, 428
Na$^+$, **406**, 422
NiCo, **406**, 426, 427
orphan, 409
ppGpp, **405**, 411, 412
PRPP, **405**, 411, 412
purine, 403, 415, 416
SAM, **404**, 413, 414, 417
THF, 402, 404
thiamine pyrophosphate (TPP), 403, **404**, 410, 411, 417, 427
tungsten cofactor (Wco), **404**, 420–422
yybP-ykoY, **406**, 424, *425*
RIDME, 391
RNA, 112, 344, 353–356, 358, 361, 366, 400–406, 408–411, 413–417, 420–427
  non-coding, 400
  translation, 344
Rod-like structure, 302–304, 310, 314, 317, 319, 333, 334
ROS, 165, 168
Roscovitine, 141
Rotaxane, 171, 172
Rubidium, 151, **355**, 356, 358–361, 363–**365**
Ruthenium, 136, 148, *149*, 150, 164, 165, 169, 172, 179, 180, 182, 233
  prodrug, *165, 172*

SAH, 404, 414
Salphen, 164, 171
SAM, 404, 412–414, 417
SARS-CoV-2, 212
SAXS, 246
SBU, 4, 6–7, 9
Scanned conductance microscopy *see* SCM
Scanning tunneling microscopy *see* STM
SCM, 88, 89

SDSL, 391
Secondary building unit *see* SBU
Secondary structure, 296, 299, 376–381, 384, 386, 387, 393
SELEX, 268
Self-assembly, 61, 80, 82, 86, 87, 89, 95, 98, 99, 151, 152
Self-healing, 56, 73
Self-repair, 91, 92, 95
Semiconductors, *61*, 64, 65, 75
Sensing, 299, 320, 326–329, 335, 407, 414, 416, 422–423, 426
Sensor, 59, 67, 69–70, 73–75
Sequence-structure-property relation, 298, 322, 323, 332
Sequencing, 212, 219, 220, 222, 223
Shine-Dalgarno sequence, 401
Signaling, 402, **405**
Silver; *see also* Argentophilic interaction
 adenine complex, 69
 carbene complex, 141
 cytosine complex, 28, 38, 61, 63, 85–89, 91, 110, 117, 118, 233
 deposition on DNA, 235
 guanine complex, 68, 83, 90
 hydrogels, 152
 inosine complex, 69, 377
 in metal-mediated base pairing, 82, 84, 109, 113, 114, 119, 120, 137–139, 214–218, 234–244, 259–263, 268–272, 277–279, 283, 285
 nanocluster, 92, 93, 99, 293–335
 nanoparticle, 90–92, 120
 purine complex, 56, 126–138
 pyrimidine complexes, *114*
 in regium bonds, 122
 silver/gold nanoparticle, 235
 thioguanine complex, 94–96
Single-chain magnet, 59
Single-molecule measurement, 315, 316, 329
Single-molecule observation, 192, 205
Single-nucleotide polymorphism *see* SNP
Site-directed spin labeling *see* SDSL
Small-angle X-ray scattering *see* SAXS
smFRET, 409, 415
SMOF, 2, 10, 11, **14**, 15, 18, 20, 22
SNP, 212–214, 217–219, 327, 328
Sodium
 bisulfite, 220
 in cation-π interactions, 123
 in C-form DNA, 195
 in guanine quadruplexes, 379, 381
 in guanine quartets, 151, 353–356, 358–361, 363–366, 374
 interaction with nucleic acids, 106, 137, 259
 ion transport, 136

riboswitch, 422
 in riboswitches, **406**, 412, 427
Solid-phase synthesis, 265, 380, 381, 384
Solomonic column, 119
Solvation, 346, 354, 358, 359, 361–363
SPAAC, 218
Spin label, 390–394
Square wave voltammetry, 219
Staphylococcus aureus, 138
Stereochemistry, 402
Stimulus, 269, 272, 273, 283, 377, 380, 390
 -responsive, 54, 56–58, 67–69, 71, 73, 332, 377, 394
STM, 89
Stokes shift, 294, 298, 307, 315, 318–320, 333
Strain energy, 347, 359, 363
Strain-promoted azide-alkyne cycloaddition *see* SPAAC
Strontium, 363–**365**, 407, 424, 407, 424
Succinate, 9
Succinic acid, 145
Sugar edge, *10*, 11, 13
Superatom, 302–304
Supercapacitor, 73
Superexchange, 59, 60
Supramolecular
 assembly, 27, 28, 106, 107, 113, 122, 128
 metal-organic framework (*see* SMOF)
Supramolecule, 279
Surface
 adsorption, 197
 plasmon resonance, 293
Surfactant, 199, 201
Switching, 265, 272–277, 279, 284
Symbiobacterium thermophilum, 409, 419, 420
syn conformation, 262, 263, 375
Synthon, 10, 11, 13–16

T4 phage DNA, 197, 198, 201–203, 205
Tautomer, 3, 5, 11, 107, 108, 136, 137
Telomerase, 327, 376
Telomere, 110, 344, 353, 375, 376
 homeostasis, 344
TEM, *91*, 92, 95, 192, 197, 198, 201, 203, 298
Terbium, 69–71, 107, 409, 421
Terephthalate, 16, *18*, *19*
Terpyridine, 140, 142, 173, 174
Tertiary interaction, 402–**404**, 407, 409, 412, 416, 418
Tetrahymena telomeric DNA (ttel24), 384–386
Tetraloop, 124, 421
Tetrazole, 191, 193, 199, 201–206
TFO, 283, *284*
Thallium, 123
Theobrominate, 16, 17
Thermoanaerobacter tengcongensis, 419

Index

Thiazole, 410
Thioadenine, 142
6-Thiodeoxyguanosine, 62, 98
6-Thioguanine, *53*, 61, 62, 66
Thioguanosine, 94–*96*, 97–99
Thionucleosides, 93, 94, 99
Thioredoxin reductase see TrxR
Thixotropic, 91
Three-way junction, 231, 327, 374, 403, 413–415
Thrombin, 390
Thymine, *3*, 9, 10, *53*, *55*, *109*, *135*, 138, 145–147, *223*, *233*, *240*
Thymine-1-acetate, 55–60, 64, 65, 74
Time-resolved
 emission spectra (see TRES)
 infrared (TRIR) spectroscopy, 305, 333
 single-photon counting (see TRSPC)
Topoisomerase II, 180
Topology, 4, 8, 9, 13, 18, 375, 376, 379, 381, 383–386, 389, 391, 393
Toxicity, 328, 334
TPE, 320
Transcription, 418, 423
Transient absorption spectroscopy, 315, 316
Transition dipole moment, 318
Translation, 401, 418, 423
Transmission electron microscopy see TEM
Transplatin, 259
TRES, 316
1,3,5-Triaza-7-phosphaadamantane, 120
Triple helix, 374, 414
Triplex-forming oligonucleotide see TFO
TRSPC, 315
TrxR, 142
Tungsten, 417, 421, 428
Two-photon excitation see TPE
Tyrosine, 386

Uracil, *3*, 9, *10*, *53*, *55*, *135*
 -1-acetate, 55, 58, 65, 68, 69, 71–73
 -1-propionate, 59–61, 63, 64, 72, 73
Uranyl, 220
5'-UTR, 400, 401
UV crosslinking, 403
UV-vis spectroscopy, 376

van-der-Waals interaction, 419
VDD, 348, 349, 351
Vitamin B$_{12}$, 417
Voronoi deformation density see VDD

Watson-Crick
 base pairs, 56, *111*, 117, 194, 212–214, 218, 224, 237–239, *240*, 241, 250, 258, 261–264, 280, 331, 374, 376, 377, 416
 double helix, 230, 296, 310–313, 330
 edge, *10*, 11, 13, 15, 148
 face, 11, 22, 216, 219, 237, 244, 280, 282, 285
 hydrogen bonds, 110, 233, *240*, 241, 243, 330
 metallo base pairs, 238, *240*, 243, 311, 312
 reverse, 56
Wobble base pair, 56

XANES, 304
Xanthine, **405**, 417
Xeno nucleic acid see XNA
Xerogel, 68
XNA, 334
XPS, 298, 304, 305
X-ray
 absorption near edge structure (see XANES)
 crystallography, 230, 237, 313, 332
 diffraction, *84*, 246, 260, 261, 375, 391, 391
 photoelectron spectroscopy (see XPS)
 spectroscopy, 301, 304, 305
 structure, 238

Yersinia enterocolitica, 423
Young's modulus, 71
yybP-ykoY RNA motif, **406**, 424, *425*

Zinc
 in anion-π interactions, 124, 125
 cofactor, 136
 coordination polymers, 69
 cytosine complex, 32, 33, 113
 DNA interaction, 233
 in guanine quadruplexes, 379
 in M-DNA, 61, 66, 87
 in metal-mediated base pairing, 113, 236, 267, 282
 in metal-mediated base tetrads, 383, 384, 387, 388
 in MOFs, 4–9, 11, 12, 73
 purine complex, 147, *148*
 in supramolecular assemblies, 107
 thymine complex, 247

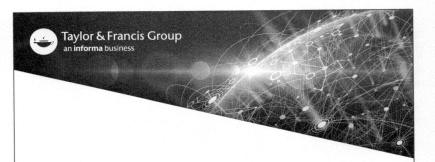